Stuttering
An Integrated Approach to Its Nature and Treatment

Stuttering
An Integrated Approach to Its Nature and Treatment

Barry Guitar, Ph.D.
Professor
Department of Communication Sciences
The University of Vermont
Burlington, Vermont

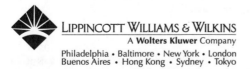

LIPPINCOTT WILLIAMS & WILKINS
A **Wolters Kluwer** Company

Philadelphia • Baltimore • New York • London
Buenos Aires • Hong Kong • Sydney • Tokyo

Acquisitions Editor: Pamela Lappies
Managing Editor: Linda Napora / Kevin C. Dietz
Marketing Manager: Mary Martin
Production Editor: Chrissy Remsberg
Designer: Doug Smock
Compositor: TechBooks
Printer: R.R. Donnelley

Library of Congress Cataloging-in-Publication Data
Guitar, Barry.
  Stuttering: an integrated approach to its nature and treatment/Barry
Guitar. — 3rd ed.
      p. ; cm.
    Includes bibliographical references and index.
    ISBN 0-7817-3920-9 (hardcover)
   1. Stuttering.   2. Stuttering—Treatment.   I. Title.
   [DNLM: 1. Stuttering—diagnosis. 2. Stuttering—etiology.   3. Stuttering
—therapy. WM 475 G968s 2006]
RC424. G827   2006
616.85′54—dc22

                                        2005016239

Contents

Preface

This 3rd edition of *Stuttering: An Integrated Approach to Its Nature and Treatment* contains some major renovations. New research, particularly in brain imaging, genetics, speech motor control, and temperament, has motivated me to expand chapters on the nature of the disorder, particularly Chapter 2 on constitutional factors. I have tried to tame this large body of new information by dividing it into subsections and summarizing each subsection in a table.

The chapters on evaluation and treatment have been reorganized; in part, this has been in response to excellent suggestions by students, colleagues, and reviewers. I have added more data collection procedures and outcome measures and have expanded the chapters on evaluation. The division between fluency shaping and stuttering modification, which was so prominent in the first two editions, has lost its defining edge. Therefore, I have streamlined chapters on each of the developmental and treatment levels. Now, each chapter contains a detailed description of the approach I use, followed by briefer descriptions of other approaches. I have also added a chapter on the nature and treatment of neurogenic and psychogenic stuttering and cluttering.

Further additions, which are still in the works, include video clips to illustrate some of the material in the text and a website with instructional materials and updated evidence supporting therapy approaches.

Acknowledgements

One of the pleasures in writing a book is hearing from readers who have used it. I am deeply grateful to students and colleagues who let me know that the last edition was helpful to them, especially those who suggested what to keep, what to toss, and what to add.

Dick Curlee has again provided masterful editing of my ideas as well as my prose. As in previous editions, he has guided both my writing and my thinking toward greater clarity.

Many at Lippincott Williams & Wilkins have given me generous support during my work on this edition. Foremost among those is Linda Napora, a magnificent managing editor for this and previous editions. I am very appreciative of Kevin Dietz, who has taken over her role and has been a stalwart during the last stages of this project. I also wish to thank Pamela Lappies, Acquisitions Editor, who has been wonderfully encouraging throughout the work on this edition; Caroline Define, Production Editor, who has shepherded this edition through in flawless form; Mary Martin, Marketing Manager, who has helped me get this and the last edition known to many students, teachers, and clinicians; and Susan Katz, Vice President, Publisher Health Professions, for her continuing support.

Although Ted Peters has not directly contributed to this edition, his influence from the first edition (Guitar and Peters, 1991) remains strong. His clinical insights and insistence on a logical structure have been guiding principles for the second and third editions.

Rebecca McCauley and Charles Barasch have been absolute bricks during the writing of this edition. They have read each word of each chapter and commented on the prose, the organization, and the concepts; they have suggested illustrations, developed website material, and listened to the latest theories of stuttering with apparent interest and real patience. They are true friends.

Finally, I wish to thank my wife, Carroll, for the support and nurture she has given both me and this text throughout its three editions. As a judicious editor and masterful reference librarian, she continues to be a major contributor to the book's success.

This edition is dedicated to Cully Gage.

Nature of Stuttering

Chapter 1

Introduction to Stuttering

Perspective

Stuttering is an age-old problem that has its origins in the way the brain has evolved to produce speech and language. The onset of stuttering is influenced by the development of children's communication skills, as well as their emotions and cognitions. Its many variations and manifestations are determined by individual learning patterns, personality, and temperament. Stuttering also provides lessons about human nature; the variety of responses that stuttering provokes in cultures around the world is a reflection of the many ways in which humans deal with individual differences.

This description of stuttering makes it seem like a very complicated problem—one that will take a long time to learn about. You could spend a lifetime and still not know everything there is to know about stuttering. But you don't need to understand everything in order to help people who stutter. If you read this book critically and carefully, you will get a basic understanding of stuttering and a foundation for evaluating and treating people who stutter and for helping their families. Once you start working with people who stutter, your understanding and ability can expand exponentially.

If you continue to work with stuttering, you will soon outgrow this book and begin to make your own discoveries. You will experience the satisfaction of helping adults, adolescents, and children regain their ability to communicate easily. Someday, you may even write about your therapy procedures and your assessment of their effectiveness. Those of us who have spent many years engaged in stuttering research and treatment all began where you are right now, at the threshold of an exciting and rewarding profession.

The Words We Use

In any field, whether it's law, medicine, or speech-language pathology, words may be used in particular ways. Definitions of many of the specialized terms used in our field are defined in the glossary at the back of this book, but some words and phrases deserve to be discussed at the beginning.

People Who Stutter

Until recently, it was common practice to refer to people who stutter as "stutterers." In fact, some of us who stutter refer to ourselves as stutterers and feel some pride in this term. However, many people prefer not to be labeled "a stutterer" and want to be called "people who stutter." They feel, and rightly so, that stuttering is only a small part of who they are.

Adults who stutter often say that changing the way they think of themselves—as people who happen to stutter but with many more important attributes—was one of the most significant things they did to break free of the bonds of stuttering. Such reports remind us that clients are far more than people who stutter. They are people, each with a galaxy of characteristics, one of which happens to be that they stutter. This way of thinking enables us to help not only our clients, but also their families. It helps families listen beyond the sounds of stuttering to the thoughts and feelings their children are communicating. It helps them view disfluencies in perspective, as only a small part of the whole child.

Some authors abbreviate "people who stutter" as "PWS." Personally, I feel that substituting an acronym that highlights stuttering is not really different from using "stutterer," so I won't use that as a euphemism. However, I know that the language in this book would grow stale and cumbersome if I were to use "person who stutters" over and over. So, I often refer to the "adult," "child," or "adolescent you are working with" and may sometimes use "stutterer." That, too, I feel is acceptable when used occasionally. After all, a stutterer may be someone who is proud that he sometimes stutters but doesn't let it get in the way of his life.

Symptom

In the medical literature, the term "symptom" is often used in referring to behavior that is caused by an underlying condition. For example, pain in the lower right abdomen may be a symptom of appendicitis. In the stuttering literature, however, symptom is often used to denote behaviors that are an aspect of the disorder itself, such as multiple part-word repetitions. I use "symptom" and "sign" interchangeably to indicate such behaviors.

Disfluency

In our literature, "disfluency" is used to denote interruptions of speech that may be either normal or abnormal. That is, it can apply to natural pauses, repetitions, and other hesitancies that occur in the speech of persons with normal speech. It can also apply to moments of stuttering and is a handy term to use when describing the speech of young children whose diagnosis is unclear.

I'll use "disfluency" interchangeably with "stutter" to make the writing more varied. When someone's speech hesitancies are unequivocally *not* stuttering, I'll use the term "normal disfluency." I won't use the older term for abnormal hesitations, "dysfluency" with a "y," because it can easily be mistaken for "disfluency" when you see it on the page and because the two are indistinguishable when spoken.

Overview of the Disorder

This section previews the next few chapters on the nature of stuttering and gives me a chance to reveal my own slant on the disorder. It is intended especially for readers who have not had a course in stuttering and who may, therefore, know few details of its nature.

Do All Cultures Have Stuttering?

Stuttering is found in all parts of the world and in all cultures and races. It is indiscriminate of occupation, intelligence, and income; it affects both sexes and people of all ages, from toddlers to the elderly. It is an old curse, and there is evidence that it was present in Chinese, Egyptian, and Mesopotamian cultures more than 40 centuries ago. Moses was said to have stuttered (Garfinkel, 1995) and to have used a trick typical of many of us who stutter, by getting his brother to speak for him. I did something similar when I had to read a prayer aloud in Sunday school.

What Causes People to Stutter?

The cause of stuttering is still something of a mystery. Scientists have yet to discover what causes stuttering, but they have many clues. First, there is strong evidence that stuttering often has a *genetic* basis; that is, something is inherited that makes it more likely a child will stutter. This genetic "something" must be a physical trait, and many researchers believe that it is the way a child's brain is organized for speech and language. For example, the neural connections or pathways for talking may be less well developed or more easily disrupted by an overflow of emotional activity in the brain. Another clue about the nature of stuttering is that most stuttering begins in children between the ages of 2 and

5 years. The onset of stuttering occurs about the same time that many typical stresses of early childhood are occurring. One child may begin to stutter soon after a baby brother or sister is born. Another child's stuttering may first appear when the family moves to a new home. Still another child may start stuttering when a dramatic growth in his vocabulary and syntax is occurring. Many different factors, acting singly or in combination,

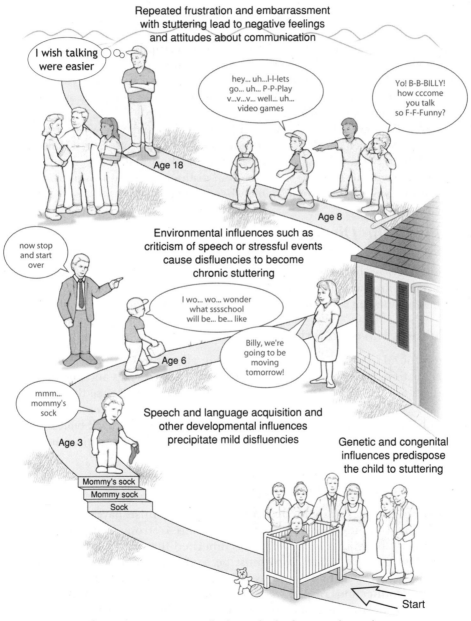

Figure 1–1 *Factors contributing to the development of stuttering.*

may *precipitate* the onset of stuttering in a child who has a neurophysiological *predisposition* for stuttering.

Once stuttering starts, it may disappear within a few months, or it may get gradually worse. When it gets worse, learned reactions may be an important factor in its severity. Playmates at school or thoughtless adults may cause a child to become highly self-conscious about his stuttering. He will quickly learn that an eye blink or an "um" said quickly before trying to say a hard word may short-circuit stuttering temporarily. By the time a child is a teenager, learned reactions influence many of the symptoms. He has learned to anticipate stuttering and may thrash around in a panic when he speaks, trying to escape or avoid it. By adulthood, his fear of stuttering and desire to avoid it can permeate his lifestyle. An adult who stutters often copes with it by limiting his or her work, friends, and fun to those people and situations that put few demands on speech. Figure 1–1 provides an overview of many of the contributing factors in the evolution of stuttering. In this and the subsequent four chapters, I'll describe in detail our current understanding of these influences.

Can Stuttering Be Cured?

Stuttering often cures itself. Some young children who begin to stutter recover without treatment. For others, early intervention may be needed to help the child develop normal fluency and prevent the development of a serious problem. Once stuttering has really become firmly established, however, and the child has developed many learned reactions, a concerted treatment effort is needed. Good treatment of mild and moderate stuttering in preschool and early elementary school children may leave them with little trace of stuttering, except perhaps when they are stressed, fatigued, or ill. Most people who stutter severely for a long time or who are not treated until after puberty make only a partial recovery. They usually learn to speak more slowly or stutter more easily and are less bothered by it. However, some people will not improve, despite our best efforts.

Before I delve deeper into the nature and treatment of stuttering, I will touch briefly on the personal side of the problem. Some of you may never have had a friend who stutters or may never have worked with a stutterer in treatment, so I will present several examples of what stuttering can be like. Even if you are familiar with stuttering, these brief sketches, which portray four individuals who differ widely in age and in their accommodations to stuttering, may expand your sense of what stuttering is like for the person who experiences it.

CASE EXAMPLES

Borderline Stuttering

Ashley was precocious in her language development, speaking in well-formed sentences when she was 18 months old. Her stuttering began when she was 21 months and took the form of multiple part-word repetitions, most often at the beginnings of sentences. Despite the fact that she would sometimes repeat a syllable 10 times before getting the word out, she appeared to be unaware of her stuttering. She continued to develop language rapidly, talk copiously, and socialize easily.

About 6 months after she started stuttering, her parents contacted a speech-language pathologist who evaluated Ashley and counseled them about changes they could make in their interactions with their daughter that might facilitate her fluency. The evaluation indicated that Ashley's language development was advanced for her age, that her phonological development was also advanced, and that she stuttered on 4% of the syllables she spoke. Ashley's parents were relieved to hear that the early onset of her stuttering, her advanced language development, the lack of other family members who stutter, and the fact that she is a girl made it more likely that she will recover from her stuttering naturally. Nonetheless, Ashley's parents wanted to do all they could to make that happen, so the clinician guided the parents in learning to talk more slowly when speaking with Ashley, spending more time with her in child-directed play, and remaining calm and accepting when Ashley stuttered. Ashley's parents also kept a journal of when her stuttering waxed and waned so they could try to determine whether there were factors affecting it that they could change.

For several weeks, the clinician met with Ashley's parents and helped them evaluate their changes and discussed Ashley's fluency with them. Ashley's stuttering began to diminish after 2 weeks of clinician-guided changes; then the clinician began to slowly fade contact with them but kept in telephone and email contact to support their efforts. Within 6 months, Ashley's fluency was close to normal, with occassional increases in stuttering that occurred during periods of excitement, such as when her sister was born and when relatives came to visit over the holidays.

Ashley is now 8 years old, her speech is entirely normal, and she has no recollection of ever having stuttered.

DISCUSSION

Ashley's stuttering may have emerged as the result of advanced language development overtaking the capacity of her speech-motor skills to keep pace. In other words, it may be the classic "old wives tale" of Ashley thinking faster than she could talk. This etiology of stuttering most commonly occurs in girls and sometimes produces stuttering more severe than in this case. As long as Ashley was not frustrated by her stuttering (in fact, she hardly seemed aware of it) and because she was so young, direct therapy was not appropriate.

At this age and with this level of awareness, the child can be treated by indirect therapy. This approach, guided by a clinician, is usually effective in making the child's environment facilitate the development of fluency without making the child unduely focussed on her stuttering. It is possible that Ashley would have recovered without any changes in her environment. However, her parents' level of concern indicated the need for some treatment—preferably an approach that would give them an active role to reduce their anxiety. Continued but gradually fading support by the clinician may be an important component; normal fluency within a few months (or with very young children, within a year) can be expected.

Beginning Stuttering

Katherine developed speech and language normally, speaking her first word at about 1 year old and beginning to combine words at 15 months, with complete fluency. When she was 3 years old, after a particularly hectic Christmas holiday, she began to stutter. Her first disfluencies were easy part- and whole-word repetitions, but she soon appeared to be impatient and began to stop her repetitions by squeezing her larynx or articulators and momentarily blocking the flow of speech until the word "popped out." When she was completely stuck for several seconds, she responded by hitting her parents or crying out in frustration.

Her parents soon brought her to a speech and language clinic, where they received counseling and suggestions for changing the home environment. In addition, Katherine began weekly stuttering therapy, which incorporated both reducing stresses in her home environment and a systemic behavioral treatment provided by Katherine's mother. Her mother also attended a weekly support group with other parents who were using the behavioral approach. At the time of her evaluation, Katherine's stuttering was assessed with the Stuttering Severity Instrument, which rated it as severe. At the beginning of treatment, she was stuttering on 21% of the syllables spoken. (This means that when her speech output was analyzed, and the number of syllables she spoke in a few minutes time was counted, Katherine stuttered on 21% of those syllables, which is a very high percentage for any child.)

After 9 months of treatment, Katherine's therapy was gradually reduced so that she came to the clinic less and less frequently, even though her fluency continued to be monitored via weekly ratings made by her mother. During the year after she stopped coming to the clinic for weekly sessions, Katherine occasionally had bouts of mild stuttering when excited or worried, at which time her mother reinstated speech practice a few minutes each day until her daughter's speech was essentially fluent again. Katherine's mother continues to be in contact with the clinician, but with greater and greater amounts of time between the contacts.

DISCUSSION

Katherine's stuttering was more severe than that of most 3 year olds, but it is not uncommon for preschool-age children to begin to stutter with repetitions and then progress rapidly to tense blocks or even to begin with blocks. Katherine's level of frustration with her stuttering was high, as we could surmise from the way she responded by hitting and crying out when she was "stuck." Katherine's parents were deeply concerned, of course, and this made it crucial for the clinician to provide some immediate actions for the parents to take. The first was to make sure that both her mother and father acknowledged Katherine's stuttering openly and sensitively, especially when she reacted with frustration. The parent-delivered behavioral therapy provided intensive practice in fluency but also relieved the parents' anxiety because it engaged them in so much of the work of therapy. As with any treatment, each aspect of the therapy program had to be adjusted to Katherine's needs and progress toward fluency.

Intermediate Stuttering

David was the second of three children in a family with no history of speech or language disorders. His speech was developing normally until age 4, when he began to show excessive part-word and whole-word repetitions. After several months, when David's stuttering had not decreased, his mother took him to his pediatrician who assured her that it would resolve on its own.

When David was almost 6, his stuttering was growing steadily more severe, and he was avoiding talking in many situations. His mother then decided to consult a speech-language pathologist at a university clinic who evaluated David and determined that treatment was appropriate. In the evaluation, David was stuttering on 8% of his syllables spoken; many stutters were tightly squeezed blocks with evident struggle behavior. Progress was slow the first year of treatment. David resisted the clinician's attempts to talk about stuttering and was reluctant to try to modify his stuttering. In the second year of therapy, a local television station filmed David and the clinician working together. Under this special condition of being "on camera," David was willing to change his hard blocks to looser, controlled stutters. Even better, he was willing to show a video clip from the television production to his second-grade class and share with them his experiences in speech therapy.

Over the next 2 years, David's progress in therapy was slow but steady. To keep him interested in therapy and to counteract the feeling of failure he had about his speech, the clinician created many activities in which David could excel. He was a good athlete and could usually beat the clinician at shooting "hoops" and other games of skill. A major breakthrough came when David was willing to use "slide-outs," which is an easy form of stuttering, in place of his typical, hard stutters. At first, he would only try them when he was given a piece of candy for each real or pretended slideout. Gradually, he began to reinforce himself for slideouts, using a tally sheet when talking to the clinician and to strangers, then cashing in the tally sheet for candies at the end of each session.

Therapy continued intermittantly for several more years, and now, 7 years after he stopped therapy, David speaks with only minor stuttering, which he usually handles with slideouts. He is very open about his remaining stuttering and has been a mentor to several younger children who stutter. Recently, he testified eloquently to the state legislature about the need for more funding for services to school children who stutter.

DISCUSSION

David's therapy history may be typical for some children who are extremely sensitive about their stuttering. His reluctance to work on his stuttering was overcome by the positive attention he received from appearing on television. In addition, the games he won playing the clinician and the tangible rewards he received, in the form of candy, probably gave him a sense of mastery over a situation in which he previously had felt helpless.

Advanced Stuttering

Sergio is a 44-year-old musician who has stuttered since he was 3 years old. Eight of his maternal aunts and uncles stuttered, making stuttering somewhat of a family trait. His stuttering began as multiple repetitions of one-syllable words and parts of words. Much of his speech was fluent, but whenever he was excited or hurried, Sergio's stuttering flared up, sending his parents into a state of alarm and concern for his future. His father tried to fix Sergio's stuttering in early years by hitting him on the head with his knuckles when he blocked. When this failed and Sergio developed physically tense prolongations and blocks that occurred regularly in his speech, his parents took him to various therapists, including a hypnotist and a psychotherapist who prescribed tranquilizers. None of this seemed to have more than a temporary effect, and Sergio's stuttering grew steadily worse. During his elementary and junior high school years, he was frequently ridiculed for his stuttering, even by teachers, and Sergio found himself an outcast among his peers. This changed, however, soon after "Beatlemania" swept through America. Sergio bought a guitar and taught himself to sing, "I Want to Hold Your Hand." As a result, his popularity with schoolmates shot up, even though his stuttering continued to worsen. He had so much difficulty speaking in class and his teachers were so unsympathetic that he finally dropped out of school and pursued a vagabond lifestyle as a singer and songwriter.

As he traveled, working various jobs by day and singing at night, Sergio continued to stutter severely whenever he spoke, with one happy exception. When he was performing with his band, not only did he sing fluenty, but he also spoke to the audience easily, announcing each number and making casual, funny comments between songs. As a result of his constant battle with stuttering, Sergio developed a wide variety of avoidances. He dodged making phone calls, and whenever he received calls, he used elaborate facial grimaces and starter sounds to fight his way though stutters.

At the urging of a friend, Sergio sought out a local support group for adults who stutter and became an active member. In the 8 years since he joined, he has received some informal therapy helping out as a "teaching client" in a graduate class on fluency disorders. As a result of his support group and therapy experiences, Sergio has come to accept himself as someone who stutters, to pride himself on often using "easy stuttering," and to dramatically reduce his avoidances.

DISCUSSION

Sergio's story illustrates the influence that heredity and early life experiences may have on the severity of stuttering. Clearly, with eight aunts and uncles who stuttered, he was at high risk for inheriting stuttering. However, effective treatment during his preschool or school years would probably have improved Sergio's fluency enough to please his father and be accepted by schoolmates and teachers. The fact that he has succeeded as a musician, has many close friends, and has educated dozens of students about stuttering is a tribute to Sergio's creative talents and drive to overcome what was a severe disability during childhood and adolescence.

Definitions

Fluency

By beginning with a definition of fluency, I am pointing out how many elements must be maintained in the flow of speech if a speaker is to be considered fluent. It is an impressive balancing act, and it is little wonder that everyone slips and stumbles from time to time when they talk.

Fluency is hard to define. In fact, most researchers have focused on its opposite, *disfluency*. (I use the term disfluency to appy both to stuttering and to normal hesitations, making it easier to refer to hesitations that could be either normal or abnormal). One of the early fluency researchers, Freida Goldman-Eisler showed that normal speech is filled with hesitations (Goldman-Eisler, 1968). Other researchers have acknowledged this and expanded the study of fluent speech by contrasting it with disfluent speech. Dalton and Hardcastle (1977), for example, distinguished fluent from disfluent speech by differences in the variables listed in Table 1–1. Inclusion of intonation and stress in this list may seem unusual. It could be said that speakers who reduce stuttering by using a monotone are not really fluent. But we would argue that it is not their fluency but the "naturalness" of their speech that is affected. Nonetheless, both will be of interest to the clinician who works to help clients with all aspects of their communication.

Starkweather (1980, 1987) suggested that many of the variables that determine fluency reflect temporal aspects of speech production; such variables as pauses, rhythm, intonation, stress, and rate are controlled by when and how fast we move our speech structures. So, our temporal control of the movements of these structures determines our fluency. Starkweather

---

Table 1–1   Variables Suggested by Dalton and Hardcastle (1977) as Useful in Distinguishing Between Fluent and Disfluent Speech

1. Presence of extra sounds, such as repetitions, prolongations, interjections, and revisions
   - If a speaker says, "I-I-I nnnnneed to have uh my uh, well, I-I-I should get mmmmmy car fixed," he sounds disfluent.
2. Location and frequency of pauses
   - If a speaker says, "Whenever I remember to bring my umbrella (pause), it never rains," he sounds fluent. But if he says, "Whenever (pause) I remember to bring (pause) my (pause) umbrella, it never (pause) rains," he sounds disfluent.
3. Rhythmical patterning in speech
   - English is typically spoken with stressed syllables at relatively equal intervals; in general, stressed syllables are followed by several unstressed syllables. When marked deviations from this pattern occur, as when a speaker with cerebellar disease stresses all syllables equally, the speaker sounds disfluent.
4. Intonation and stress
   - If a speaker does not vary intonation and stress and is, therefore, monotonous, he may be considered disfluent. Abnormal intonation and stress patterns may also be considered disfluent.
5. Overall rate
   - If a speaker has a very slow rate of speech or has bursts of fast rate interspersed with slower rate, he may be considered disfluent.

also noted that the rate of information flow, not just sound flow, is an important aspect of fluency. Thus, a speaker who speaks without hesitations but who has difficulty conveying information in a timely and orderly fashion might not be considered a fluent speaker.

In his description of fluency, Starkweather (1987) also included the effort with which a speaker speaks. By effort, he means both the mental and physical work a speaker exerts when speaking. This is difficult to measure, but it may turn out that listeners can make such judgments reliably. Moreover, it may reflect important componants of what it feels like to be a person who stutters.

In essence, fluency can be thought of simply as the effortless flow of speech. Thus, a speaker who is judged to be "fluent" appears to use little effort when speaking. However, the components of such apparently effortless speech flow are hard to pin down. As researchers analyze fluency more carefully, they may find that the appearance of excess effort may give rise to judgments that a person is stuttering. However, other elements, such as unusual rhythm or slow rate of information flow, may result in judgments that a person is not a fluent speaker, but is not a stutterer either. We will discuss aspects of fluency again in relating components of fluency, such as rate and naturalness, to various therapy approaches.

Stuttering

General Description

Stuttering appears at first to be complex and mysterious, but much of it is based on human nature and can be easily understood if you think about your own experiences. In some ways, it is like a problem you might have with your car.

Imagine you had a car that would suddenly stop when you were driving in traffic. Sometimes it would sputter and jerk when you pulled away from a stop sign. Other times, it would drop into neutral, and the engine would race but the wheels wouldn't turn. Still other times, the brakes would jam on by themselves and wouldn't release until you stomped repeatedly on the pedal.

Compare this with what the "core" of stuttering behavior is: Stuttering is characterized by an abnormally high frequency and/or duration of stoppages in the forward flow of speech. These stoppages usually take the form of (1) repetitions of sounds, syllables, or one-syllable words, (2) prolongations of sounds, or (3) "blocks" of airflow or voicing in speech.

Returning to the car analogy: *After you had had problems with your car repeatedly, you would probably develop some coping strategies to get it going again. You might, for example, turn the engine off and restart it.*

Similarly, a speaker who is stuttering usually reacts to his repetitions, prolongations, or blocks by trying to force words out, or by using extra sounds, words, or movements in his efforts to become "unstuck" or to avoid getting stuck.

If your car's problem persisted for several days or longer, you would probably develop some bad feelings about it. The first time it happened, you would be surprised. Then, as it happened more and more, surprise would give way to frustration. If your car frequently quit in the middle of traffic and other drivers nearly hit you and started honking, you would begin to anticipate problems and feel fear as well.

The child who begins to stutter goes through many of the same feelings of surprise, frustration, embarrassment, and fear. These feelings, in combination with the difficulty he has in speaking, may cause the stutterer to limit himself in school and social situations and at work.

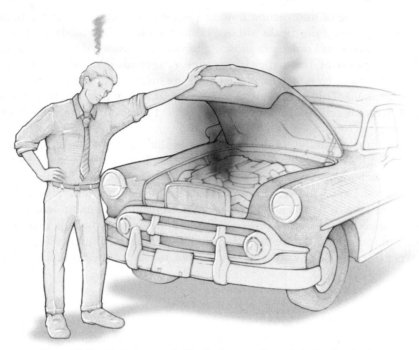

Figure 1–2   *Stuttering can be like having an old car that often breaks down.*

This might be similar to your responses to a troublesome car. After your car quit on you in traffic many times, you'd probably leave it in the garage and walk, or you'd just stay home.

Another aspect of any description of stuttering involves specifying what it is not. For example, an important distinction must be made between the stuttering behaviors just described and normal hesitations. Children whose speech and language are developing normally often display repetitions, revisions, and pauses, which are not stuttering. Neither are the brief repetitions, revisions, and pauses in the speech of most nonstuttering adults when they are in a hurry or uncertain. Chapter 5 describes the differences between normal disfluency and stuttering in more detail to prepare you for the task of differential diagnosis of stuttering in children.

A distinction should also be made between stuttering and certain other fluency disorders. Disfluency resulting from cerebral damage or disease, disfluency resulting from psychological trauma, and cluttering (i.e., rapid, garbled speech) all differ from stuttering that begins in childhood. These disorders may be treated somewhat differently, although some of the techniques that clinicians use with stuttering are also useful with other fluency disorders. These disorders are discussed in Chapter 13.

Core Behaviors

I have adopted the term "core behaviors" from Van Riper (1971, 1982), who used it to describe the basic speech behaviors of stuttering: repetitions, prolongations, and blocks. These behaviors seem involuntary to the person who stutters, as if they are out of his control. They differ from the "secondary behaviors" that a stutterer acquires as learned reactions to the basic core behaviors.

Repetitions are the core behaviors observed most frequently among children who are just beginning to stutter and are simply a sound, syllable, or single-syllable word that is repeated several times. The speaker is apparently "stuck" on that sound and continues repeating it until the following sound can be produced. In children who have not been stuttering for long, single-syllable word repetitions and part-word repetitions are much more common than multisyllable word repetitions. Moreover, children who stutter frequently repeat a word or syllable more than twice per instance, li-li-li-like this (Yairi, 1983; Yairi and Lewis, 1984).

Prolongations of voiced or voiceless sounds also appear in the speech of children beginning to stutter. They usually appear somewhat later than repetitions (Van Riper, 1982), although both Johnson et al (1959) and Yairi (1997a) reported that prolongations, as well as repetitions, may be present at onset. I use the term *prolongation* to denote those stutters in which sound or air flow continues but movement of the articulators is stopped. Prolongations as short as half a second may be perceived as abnormal, but in rare cases, prolongations may last as long as several minutes (Van Riper, 1982). In contrast to my use of the term, older writers include stutters with no sound or airflow, as well as stopped movement of the articulators, in their definitions of prolongations (e.g., Van Riper, 1982; Wingate, 1964).

Repetitions and sound prolongations are usually part of the core behaviors of more advanced stutterers, as well as of children just beginning to stutter. Sheehan (1974) found that repetitive stutters occurred in every speech sample of 20 adults who stuttered. Indeed, 66% of their stutters were repetitions. Although many of their stutters were also prolongations, as defined in the previous paragraph, how many is not clear, because Sheehan's definition of prolongations may differ from mine.

Blocks are typically the last core behavior to appear. However, as with prolongations, some investigators (Johnson et al, 1959; Yairi, 1997a) have observed blocks in children's speech at, or close to, stuttering onset. Blocks occur when a person inappropriately stops the flow of air or voice and often the movement of his articulators as well. Blocks may involve any level of the speech production mechanism—respiratory, laryngeal, or articulatory. There is some evidence and much theorizing that inappropriate muscle activity at the laryngeal level characterizes most blocks (Conture, McCall, and Brewer, 1977; Freeman and Ushijima, 1978; Kenyon, 1942; Schwartz, 1974).

As stuttering persists, blocks often grow longer and more tense, and tremors may become evident. These rapid oscillations, most easily observable in the lips or jaw, occur when someone has blocked on a word. He closes off the airway, increases air pressure behind the closure, and squeezes his muscles particularly hard (Van Riper, 1982). You can duplicate these tremors by trying to say the word "by" while squeezing your lips together hard and building up air pressure behind the block. Imagine this happening to you unexpectedly when you were trying to talk.

People who stutter differ from one another in how frequently they stutter and how long their individual core behaviors last. Research indicates that a person who stutters does so on average on about 10% of the words while reading aloud, although individuals vary greatly (Bloodstein, 1944, 1987). Many people who stutter mildly do so on fewer than 5% of the words they speak or read aloud, and a few people with severe stuttering stutter on more than 50% of the words. The durations of core behaviors vary much less; they average around 1 second and are rarely longer than 5 seconds (Bloodstein, 1944, 1987).

Secondary Behaviors

People who stutter don't enjoy stuttering. They react to their repetitions, prolongations, and blocks by trying to end them quickly if they can't avoid them altogether. Such reactions may begin as a random struggle but soon turn into well-learned patterns. I divide secondary behaviors into two broad classes: escape behaviors and avoidance behaviors. I make this division, rather than follow the traditional approach of dealing with secondary behaviors more specifically as "starters" or "postponements," because my treatment procedures focus on the principles by which secondary behaviors are learned.

The terms "escape" and "avoidance" are borrowed from the behavioral learning literature. Briefly, escape behaviors occur when a speaker is stuttering and attempts to terminate the stutter and finish the word. Common examples of escape behaviors are eye blinks, head nods, and interjections of extra sounds, such as "uh," which are often followed by the termination of a stutter and are, therefore, reinforced. Avoidance behaviors, on the other hand, are learned when a speaker anticipates stuttering and recalls the negative experiences he has had when stuttering. To avoid stuttering and the negative experience that it entails, he often resorts to behaviors he has used previously to escape from moments of stuttering (for example, eye blinks or "uh's"). Or, he may try something different, such as changing the word he was planning to say.

In many cases, especially at first, avoidance behaviors may prevent the stutter from occurring and provide highly rewarding, emotional relief. Soon these avoidance behaviors become strong habits that are resistant to change. The many subcategories of avoidances (e.g., postponements, starters, substitutions, and timing devices such as hand movements timed to saying the word) are described in Chapter 5.

Feelings and Attitudes

A person's feelings can be as much a part of the disorder of stuttering as his speech behaviors. Feelings may precipitate stutters, just as stutters may create feelings. In the beginning, a child's positive feelings of excitement or negative feelings of fear may result in repetitive stutters that he hardly notices. Then, as he stutters more frequently, he may become frustrated or ashamed because he can't say what he wants to say, even his own name, as smoothly and quickly as others. These feelings make speaking harder as frustration and shame increase effort and tension, which hold back speech. Feelings that result from stuttering may include not only frustration and shame, but also fear of stuttering again, guilt about not being able to help himself, and hostility toward listeners as well.

Attitudes are feelings that have become pervasive and part of a person's beliefs. As a person who stutters experiences more and more stuttering, for example, he begins to believe that he is a person who generally has trouble speaking, just as you might believe that your car is a lemon if you continue to have trouble with it. Adolescents and adults who stutter usually have many negative attitudes about themselves that are derived from years of stuttering experiences (Blood et al, 2001; Gildston, 1967; Rahman, 1956; Wallen, 1960). A person who stutters often projects his attitudes on listeners, believing that they think he is stupid or nervous. Sometimes, however, listeners may contribute directly to the person's attitudes. Research has shown that most people, even classroom teachers and speech-language pathologists, stereotype people who stutter as tense, insecure, and fearful (e.g., Turnbaugh, Guitar, and Hoffman, 1979; Woods and Williams, 1976). Such listener stereotypes can affect the way individuals who stutter see themselves, and changing a client's negative attitudes about himself can be a major focus of treatment.

The three components of stuttering—core behaviors, secondary behaviors, and feelings and attitudes—are depicted in Figure 1–3. The core behavior is the individual's block on the N in "New York." The secondary behaviors consist of postponement devices, such as "uh," "well," and "you know," and substitution of "The Big Apple" for "New York."

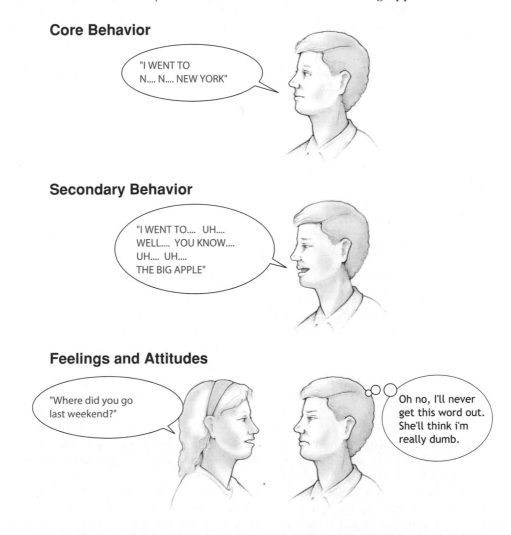

Figure 1–3 *Components of stuttering: core behaviors, secondary behaviors, and feelings and attitudes.*

Feelings and attitudes are depicted as the individual's thoughts that he won't succeed in saying the word fluently and his belief that listeners will think that he is dumb because he stutters.

Disability and Handicap

Some time ago, the World Health Organization (WHO) adopted The International Classification of Impairments, Disabilities, and Handicaps (ICIDH) to describe the consequences of various diseases and disorders (WHO, 1980). A number of authors have applied this framework to stuttering (Curlee, 1993; McClean, 1990; Prins, 1991, 1999; and Yaruss, 1998, 1999). Among these authors, Yaruss (1998) hews most closely to the definitions adopted by the WHO, and I will borrow heavily from his writing as I describe the disablity and handicap that may result from stuttering.

The *disability* of stuttering is the limitation it puts on an individual's ability to communicate. The limitation may come in part from the severity of the stuttering, but it will be heavily influenced by how a stutterer feels about himself and his stuttering, as well as how listeners react to him. You can best understand this rather complicated interaction by comparing two well-known people who stutter. The first is the successful former CEO of General Electric, Jack Welch, who authored *Jack: Straight from the Gut*. His assertive temperament and early acceptance of his stuttering were no doubt important in helping him to succeed in the high pressure world of corporate boardrooms. From an early age, Welch refused to let stuttering stand in the way of his goals (Welch and Byrne, 2001). In contrast, actor James Earl Jones initially reacted to his stuttering in a vastly different way. When he was 6 years old, he was so traumatized by his stuttering, he pretended that he was mute so that he wouldn't have to speak. Only later, with the help of a high school English teacher, did he begin to learn that he could overcome his stuttering by facing difficult situations and practicing reading aloud in front of an audience (Jones and Nevin, 1993). Although stuttering often results in a disability, sometimes it may not, and if it is a disability, its magnitude can be dramatically reduced, even when stuttering remains.

The *handicap* that may result from stuttering is the limitation on a person's life. Handicap is different from disability because it refers to the lack of fulfillment an individual has in his social life, school, job, and community. Disability, on the other hand, refers only to the limitations on communication. It is important to understand that both disability and handicap result more from the way a person and significant listeners respond to his stuttering rather than from the stuttering itself. Prime examples of this are the successful careers of two men who had stuttered severely since childhood but obtained excellent college educations, were highly successful in business, and used their wealth to help others. One is Malcolm Fraser who was a co-founder of the National Auto Parts Association and who created the Stuttering Foundation of America. The other is Walter Annenberg, who established a media empire and later the Annenberg Foundation, a large philanthropic organization.

Many people who stutter limit themselves needlessly because of their difficulty speaking. As a clinician, you may treat your clients' stuttering, but your work can affect their lives by freeing them to communicate effectively and participate fully in the world around them.

Basic Facts About Stuttering and Their Implications for the Nature of Stuttering

This section relates some of the best-known "facts" about stuttering. These are replicated research findings that pertain to the occurrence and variability of stuttering in the population and in individuals. As we discuss these findings, we will note what they suggest about the nature of stuttering. Thus, as you read the rest of this chapter, you will become increasingly aware of my perspective on the nature and treatment of stuttering.

Much has been made of the "heterogeneity" of stuttering; a number of authors have suggested that stuttering is not one disorder, but many. Researchers have proposed various divisions of the disorder, such as Van Riper's (1982) four "tracks" of stuttering development and St. Onge's (1963) triad of speech-phobic, psychogenic, and organic stutterers. My approach is to focus on the majority of people who stutter: those whose stuttering begins during childhood, without an apparent link to psychological or organic trauma. This most common type of stuttering has been called "developmental stuttering," because symptoms usually emerge gradually as a child develops, especially during the period of intense speech and language acquisition. I simply call it "stuttering." In denoting similar fluency problems that are associated with psychological problems, brain damage, cognitive impairment, and cluttering, I refer to their assumed etiology, such as "disfluencies associated with brain damage."

Onset

Information about the onset of stuttering initially came from parents' recollections of events that occurred some time in the hazy past. Thus, these reports were often vague and perhaps unreliable. More recently, researchers have been able to interview parents and record children soon after onset, giving us a much clearer picture of the different ways stuttering manifests itself when it begins (e.g., Yairi, 1997a). Stuttering may start as a gradual increase in the frequency of repetitions and prolongations that are common in children learning to talk. It also may begin suddenly, with disfluencies that are striking in terms of their frequency and duration and the amount of physical tension that the child shows when stuttering.

When it begins, stuttering may be sporadic, appearing for a few days or weeks, then disappearing, then coming back. Or, it may disappear altogether after several months. Sometimes, stuttering just persists consistently from its onset. Researchers generally agree that the onset of stuttering may occur at any time during childhood, from the beginning of multiword utterances, around 18 months, until puberty, around 11 or 12 years of age. Onset is *most likely* to occur between ages 2 and 5 years (Andrews et al, 1983). Because of this characteristic onset, stuttering seems not to be a disorder simply of making sounds, but a problem related to using spoken language to communicate.

Prevalence

The term "prevalence" is used to indicate how widespread a disorder is. Information about the prevalence of stuttering tells us how many people currently stutter. Accurate, up-to-date information on the prevalence of stuttering is difficult to obtain. The research literature contains studies having many methodological differences, which can result in wide differences in estimates of prevalence. For example, the prevalence of stuttering probably varies considerably with age, and not all studies measure stuttering in the same age groups. Moreover, definitions of stuttering may vary from study to study. Some studies may include relatively normally disfluent individuals in their count; others may exclude them.

Beitchman et al (1986) assessed the prevalence of speech and language disorders in kindergarten children, using a representative sample. They retested children who failed the initial screening as well as a random sample of children who passed. The prevalence of stuttering in this sample of kindergarten children was 2.4%. Although this is only one study's finding, the care with which the data were collected increases its credibility.

Bloodstein (1995) reviewed and summarized the results of 37 studies of school-age children in the United States, Europe, Africa, Australia, and the West Indies. These studies showed that the prevalence of stuttering throughout the school years is about 1%. Andrews et al (1983) came to the same conclusion; about 1% of school children worldwide are likely to be stutterers at any given time. If the 2.4% prevalence among kindergartners noted earlier is valid, a considerable number of recoveries must take place between kindergarten and the upper grades.

There appears to be no reliable prevalence data for stuttering in adults. However, both Bloodstein (1995) and Andrews et al (1983) suggest that the prevalence of stuttering is lower after puberty. If so, the prevalence for adults would be less than 1%.

Incidence

The incidence of stuttering is an index of how many people have stuttered at some time in their lives. Like the data on prevalence, incidence figures are not clear-cut because different researchers have used different definitions of stuttering and methods for obtaining their data. Some researchers only report stuttering that lasted 6 months or more, not wanting to include shorter episodes of disfluency. Others report any speech behaviors that informants or parents considered to be stuttering. Estimates of incidence, when reports of informants and parents are considered, are as high as 15%, which is a figure that includes those children who stuttered for only a brief period (Bloodstein, 1995). When only the cases of stuttering that lasted longer than 6 months are included, incidence appears to be about 5% (Andrews et al, 1983). We think the latter estimate may more accurately reflect the chronic disorder we call stuttering, but the former illustrates how close perceptions of normal disfluency and early stuttering may be.

A recent report by Mansson (2000) of all children born on the Danish island of Bornholm supports the suggested incidence of 5%. This population is homogeneous and stable, making a careful, longitudinal study quite possible. Of the 1042 children born on the island in 1990 and 1991, 98% were screened for speech and language problems at age 3. The children were followed for 9 years, and it was then found that 5.19% went through some period of stuttering.

Incidence figures tell us something else about the nature of stuttering. The difference between incidence (5%) and prevalence (1% in school-age children and less in adults) suggests that most people who stutter at some time in their lives recover from it, and we know that prevalence declines after puberty. Thus, unless treatment alone is responsible for such remissions, some aspect of growth or maturation allows many individuals to recover from stuttering.

Recovery Without Treatment

Recovery from stuttering without treatment, also referred to as "spontaneous" or "natural" recovery, has long been a puzzling issue. Putting aside the important question about *why* children recover without treatment, there is debate about what percentage of children who start to stutter recover in this way.

Reviews of early research report findings that range from 20% to 80% natural recovery (Bloodstein, 1995; Andrews et al, 1983). This wide range may be a result of different methodologies used by different studies. Some studies asked large numbers of adults if they ever stuttered when they were children. This method, which is called "retrospective," may be affected by faulty memories, poor definitions of stuttering, and the inclusion of individuals who may have stuttered for only a brief period.

Recent research has proceeded more carefully, by first identifying a group of children close to the onset of their stuttering and then following them for several years without offering treatment and assessing how many recover and how many persist. Those who persist are then referred for therapy. Several studies using this methodology have been published. Yairi and Ambrose (1999) followed a group of 84 children for a minimum of 4 years after the onset of their stuttering and determined that, over this span of time, 74% had recovered without treatment. Kloth et al (1999) followed 23 children for 6 years and discovered that 70% had recovered. Mansson (2000) identified 51 children between the ages of 3 and 5 years who started to stutter and found that 71% recovered within 2 years. When follow-up continued for another couple of years, until the children were 8 or 9 years old, recoveries were up to 85%. However, this figure may be affected by speech therapy given to some after the 2-year follow-up.

Several studies have compared children who recover and those who persist to determine what might characterize children who recover. In a study of 32 preschool children, Yairi et al (1996) found that the 12 children who recovered could be differentiated from those who persisted. Those who recovered: (1) had no relatives who ever stuttered or, if the child had relatives who stuttered, all had recovered; (2) showed an earlier age of onset; (3) demonstrated stronger phonological and other language skills; (4) scored higher on tests of nonverbal intelligence; and (5) were more likely to be girls. In a later study of the extended families of 66 children, including those 32 children just mentioned, Ambrose, Cox, and Yairi (1997) confirmed the importance for recovery of being a girl and coming from a family in which any relatives who did stutter had recovered. Later, Yairi and Ambrose (1999) expanded the group to 84 children and again found that being a girl was important in recovery, as were good phonological skills. Unlike the results of Yairi et al (1996), no differences in other language skills beside phonology were found to be related to recovery.

Two other studies examined factors associated with recovery. A longitudinal study by Brosch et al (1999) followed a group of 79 stuttering children for several years. The group that persisted in stuttering had a significantly larger proportion of left-handed children. Because this is a preliminary report from an ongoing study, caution should be exercised in considering this factor as critical to recovery. Nonetheless, the factor of laterality may be one of the additional genetic factors that influence recovery; replication of this work is critical.

In the study by Kloth et al (1999) described earlier, results indicated that children who recovered had a more mature (less variable) speech motor system, a slower speaking rate, and a mother whose interaction style was non-directive and whose language was less complex. Rommel et al (2000) followed 71 children who were identified as stuttering soon after onset and followed them for 3 years. The mothers of those children who recovered naturally had less complex syntax and used a smaller number of different words when talking to their child compared with the mothers of children who persisted.

In summary, I can say that early studies of recovery reported wide variations in results. Their findings depend on many factors, such as the accuracy with which stuttering is differentiated from normal disfluency, whether the study is retrospective or longitudinal, the size of the group studied, and other factors. The most careful studies are longitidinal assessments of children who are identified soon after the onset of stuttering and who are followed for several years. In these studies, about 75% of the children who begin to stutter recover without formal treatment. Many factors have been suggested as associated with recovery. These include speaking more slowly, having a more stable speech-motor system, having a mother who has a non-directive interaction style and uses less complex language when speaking to the child, being right-handed, having less severe stuttering (although some studies dispute this), having relatives who recovered from stuttering or no relatives who stuttered, having good phonological, language, and nonverbal skills, and being female. The most robust (i.e., repeatedly found) factors are good phonological skills and being female. We will now consider the latter variable, the sex factor, in more detail.

Sex Ratio

Studies of the sex ratio in stuttering were first published in the 1890s and have been published every decade since. With this steady stream of information, we ought to have reliable data on this phenomenon. In fact, we do. The results from studies of people who stutter at many ages and in many cultures put the ratio at about three male stutterers to every one female stutterer. There is strong evidence, however, that the ratio may increase as children get older. For example, Yairi (1983) reported that, of 22 children who were 2 and 3 years of age and whose parents believed they were stuttering, 11 were boys and 11 were girls. In a larger study of 87 children between 20 and 69 months, Yairi and Ambrose (1992b) found a male to female ratio of 2.1:1 overall, although the 20 youngest subjects, those under 27 months, showed a 1.2:1 ratio.

Bloodstein's (1995) review indicated that the male to female sex ratio is about 3:1 in the first grade and 5:1 in the fifth grade, confirming the hypothesis that the sex ratio increases as children get older. Evidence of the increasing male to female ratio was provided by two recent studies. Kloth et al (1999) found a male to female ratio of 1.1:1 near onset, which rose to 2.5:1 six years later. Mansson (2000) found a male to female ratio of 1.65:1 at the initial screening (age, 3 years), which rose to a ratio of 2.8:1 two years later. The nearly even sex ratio among very young children who stutter and the gradually increasing proportion of boys who stutter may be a consequence of several factors. West (1931) presented data indicating that the change in sex ratio was the result of an increasing proportion of boys beginning to stutter in the late preschool and early school age years. However, recent data indicate that girls begin to stutter a little earlier (Yairi, 1983; Yairi and Ambrose, 1992b) and recover earlier and more frequently (Andrews et al, 1983; Yairi and Ambrose, 1992b; Yairi, Ambrose, and Cox, 1996; Yairi and Ambrose, 1999).

Females who stutter and don't recover by adulthood may be an interesting subpopulation to study. They may have inherited a stronger predisposition to stutter or have been subjected to strong environmental pressures on their speech, or both (Andrews et al, 1983). Alternately, they may lack the "recovery factor" that most young female stutterers appear to have or may have inherited additional factors that interact with stuttering to inhibit recovery.

Variability and Predictability of Stuttering

Another important piece of background information about stuttering is how it varies, and yet, it is surprisingly predictable in its occurrence, despite the fact that it seems so inconsistent and so idiosyncratic. This predictability is an important clue to its nature. As we trace the research on stuttering's variability, we will see how this information reflects changing theoretical perspectives on the disorder.

Before the 1930s, stuttering had been commonly regarded as a medical disorder. Lee Edward Travis, the first person trained as a Ph.D. to work with speech and hearing disorders, set up a laboratory at the University of Iowa in 1924 to study stuttering from a neurophysiological perspective. He hypothesized that stuttering was the result of an anomalous or inefficient organization of the brain's two cerebral hemispheres. To Travis and his fellow researchers, the variability of stuttering behaviors was seen as part of an organic disorder, and an unimportant part at that. Far more relevant to their research were stutterers' brain waves, heart rate, and breathing pattern. But in the 1930s, psychologists at Iowa and elsewhere began taking a keen interest in behavioral approaches to the study of human disorders, which spilled over into research on stuttering. Scientists who had been trying to understand the neurophysiology of stuttering gradually began trying to examine the social, psychological, and linguistic factors that govern its occurrence and variability (Bloodstein, 1995).

Anticipation, Consistency, and Adaptation

Much of the early research into behavioral aspects of stuttering focused on how stuttering varies in predictable ways. Researchers found, for example, that when stutterers were asked to read a passage aloud, many of them could forecast with surprising accuracy which words they would stutter on (Johnson and Solomon, 1937; Knott, Johnson, and Webster, 1937; Milisen, 1938; Van Riper, 1936).

Researchers also discovered that, when stutterers read a passage aloud several times, they tended to stutter on many of the same words each time (Johnson and Inness, 1939; Johnson and Knott, 1937). They also found that, when people who stutter read a passage repeatedly, their stuttering usually occurred less and less often through about six readings (Johnson and Knott, 1937; Van Riper and Hull, 1955). These studies were usually carried out by giving the stutterer a passage and asking him to read it aloud. If the experimenter were studying consistency, for example, he would have his own copy of the passage on which he would mark every word the stutterer stuttered on. Then he would ask the stutterer to read it again, and the experimenter would again mark the words stuttered in the second reading. From this, he could calculate the percentage of words stuttered in two (or more) readings. These findings, called anticipation, consistency, and adaptation, changed some assumptions about the disorder. Stuttering, it seemed, was not simply a neurophysiological disorder. It showed characteristics of learned behavior as well.

These studies not only changed existing views of stuttering, they also opened the door to new treatment possibilities. If much of stuttering is learned, it may be unlearned. The challenge was to determine how much is learned and how to help people who stutter develop new responses. Many of the treatment approaches we discuss later in the book were developed using this orientation.

Language Factors

One of the Iowa researchers, Spencer Brown, pushed investigations of the predictability of stuttering into the realm of language. In seven studies completed over a stretch of 10 years, Brown found correlations between stuttering and seven grammatical factors during reading aloud. These findings were reported in a remarkable series of papers Brown published from 1935 to 1945 (Brown, 1937, 1938a, 1938b, 1938c, 1943, 1945; Brown and Moren, 1942; Johnson and Brown, 1935). Brown showed that most adults who stutter do so more frequently (1) on consonants, (2) on sounds in word-initial position, (3) in contextual speech (versus isolated words), (4) on nouns, verbs, adjectives, and adverbs (versus articles, prepositions, pronouns, and conjunctions), (5) on longer words, (6) on words at the beginnings of sentences, and (7) on stressed syllables. Evidently, stuttering is highly influenced by these linguistic factors.

Later investigators applied Brown's hypotheses to the speech of children who stutter. An advantage in studying language factors in children's stuttering is that the loci (places where it occurs in speech) and frequency of stuttering might be less influenced by responses learned from years of stuttering and more by innate language processing difficulties. Indeed, researchers discovered that, although stuttering in elementary school children follows the same linguistic patterns as adult stuttering, the loci and frequency of stuttering in preschool children are different. Stuttering in these very young children occurs most frequently on pronouns and conjunctions, not on nouns, verbs, adjectives, and adverbs. It occurs *not* as repetitions, prolongations, or blocks of sounds in word-initial positions, but as repetitions of parts of words and single syllable words in sentence-initial positions (Bloodstein, 1995; Bloodstein and Gantwerk, 1967). This led researchers to hypothesize that, in its incipient stage, stuttering is located at the beginning of syntactic units (sentences, clauses, and phrases), as if the task of linguistic planning and preparation was a key ingredient in the recipe for disfluency (Bernstein Ratner, 1997; Bloodstein, 2001, 2002).

Conture (2001) and others have focused particular attention on the phoneme or sound selection component of linguistic planning in individuals who stutter. Findings that recovery from stuttering may be associated with good phonological skills, a slower speech

production rate, and a stable speech-motor system suggest that some individuals who stutter may overcome a linguistic planning delay by relying on strengths in related language areas or by slowing their rate of speech production to compensate for such a deficit.

Fluency-Inducing Conditions

One of the researchers at the University of Iowa, Oliver Bloodstein, wrote his Ph.D. dissertation on "Conditions Under Which Stuttering Is Reduced or Absent" (Bloodstein, 1948, 1950). In studying the speech of stutterers in 115 conditions, Bloodstein found that stuttering is markedly decreased in many of these conditions. Some of these conditions are speaking when alone, when relaxed, in unison with another speaker, to an animal or an infant, in time to a rhythmic stimulus or when singing, in a different dialect, while simultaneously writing, and when swearing. In later studies, reviewed in Andrews et al (1982), additional conditions were found to reduce stuttering. These conditions included speaking in a slow prolonged manner, speaking under loud masking noise, speaking while listening to delayed auditory feedback, shadowing another speaker (repeating what they say immediately afterwards), and speaking when reinforced for fluent speech.

Various explanations have been proposed to account for the impact of these conditions. Most are compatible with the idea that stuttering has a substantial learned component and is affected by such external stimuli as communicative pressure. Recently, however, new explanations have appeared, reflecting new trends of thought about stuttering. It has been suggested that "reduced stuttering is associated with conditions in which the neurophysiological demands of speech motor control and language formulation are reduced" (Andrews et al, 1982). For example, conditions such as speaking in time to a rhythmic stimulus reduce the demands on both linguistic and motor systems to generate the prosody for speech; whereas speaking slowly reduces the demands on language formulation and motor coordination functions. Some studies suggest that reduced demands may be needed because the brain organization of adults who stutter may not favor the rapid processing of motor speech and language functions.

An Integration

Modern research on stuttering has taken a long and complex journey from Travis's laboratory in Iowa in 1924. Yet, in many ways, its origins have not been forgotten. Travis's theory of stuttering as a problem of coordinating the two sides of the brain for speech has re-emerged as a view of stuttering as a problem of coordinating multiple brain networks for speech with those for language, cognition, and emotion. This juggling act breaks down in all speakers when the resources needed to process language, cognition, or emotion momentarily drain available central nervous system capacities, leaving too little attention for the intricacies of rapid, smooth speech production. The result is normal disfluency. Those individuals who stutter appear to have trouble allocating resources to speech production under conditions of high demand. They have inherited or acquired a more vulnerable speech production system, one that is less able to deal with the norm of rapid, smooth speech under a wide variety of conditions.

This vulnerable speech production system may soon heal itself and become more resistant to disruption in children who recover naturally from stuttering. Some of these children who recover may simply catch up to their peers when their speech production systems mature and become robust enough to function smoothly in spite of stress. Others may recover because they learn to compensate by speaking more slowly or finding other ways to marshall their resources to resist disruption. The children who don't recover appear to fall into a cycle of reacting to their disfluencies by tensing muscles, struggling to escape, and even avoiding difficult words and situations. These highly learned reactions, which are influenced by an individual's personality and the people around him, become part of an individual's stuttering patterns and influence the way he thinks and feels about speaking.

This updated view is essentially the model of stuttering presented in this book. To state it more formally, stuttering is an inherited or congenital disorder that first appears when a child is learning the complex and rapid coordinations of speech and language production. Children who do not recover but persist in stuttering are those who learn maladaptive responses to their disfluencies. This learning is influenced by their biological temperament, developing social and cognitive awareness, and the response of the environment to their speech.

The next few chapters expand on this theme and prepare you to use this information in diagnosis and treatment.

Summary

- Stuttering appears in all cultures and has been a problem for humankind for at least 40 centuries.

- It is characterized by a high frequency or severity of disruptions that impede the forward flow of speech.

- It begins in childhood and usually becomes more severe as the child grows to adulthood, unless he recovers with or without formal treatment.

- Core behaviors of stuttering are repetitions, prolongations, and blocks. Secondary behaviors are the result of attempts to escape or avoid core behaviors, which include physical concomitants of stuttering, such as eye blinks, or verbal concomitants, such as word substitutions. Feelings and attitudes can also be important components of stuttering that reflect the stutterer's emotional reactions to the experience of being unable to speak fluently and to listener responses to his stuttering. Feelings are immediate emotional reactions and include fear, shame, and embarrassment. Attitudes crystallize more slowly from repeated negative experiences associated with stuttering. An example is a stutterer's belief that listeners think he is stupid when they hear him stuttering.

- Stuttering begins between 18 months of age and puberty, but most often between ages 2 and 5 years. Its first appearance may be either a gradual increase in easy repetitions of words and sounds or, less likely, a sudden onset of multiple, tense repetitions, prolongations, or blocks.

■ Prevalence of stuttering is about 1%. Incidence is about 5%. Recovery rate without professional treatment is about 75% of children who ever stuttered. The male to female ratio in school children and adults is about 3:1 but may be lower, close to 1:1, in very young children who start to stutter. More girls recover during early childhood, increasing the proportion of males with the disorder after the preschool years.

■ Many persons who stutter are able to predict the words in a reading passage they will stutter on before reading it aloud (anticipation), and most tend to stutter on many of the same words each time in repeated readings of a passage (consistency). Stuttering frequency decreases for most stutterers when they read a passage over many times (adaptation).

■ Stuttering occurs more frequently in certain grammatical contexts. The nature of these grammatical contexts differs somewhat for adults and children.

■ A variety of conditions reduces the frequency of stuttering. Their effects may be attributable to changes in speech pattern, reductions in communicative pressure, or both. Research on these fluency-inducing conditions suggests that stuttering may be decreased by conditions that reduce the demands on speech motor control and language formulation functions.

Study Questions

1. What makes some children's core behaviors change from repetitions to prolongations to blocks?

2. What are the differences between core and secondary behaviors in stuttering?

3. When stuttering is defined, what other kinds of hesitation must it be distinguished from?

4. What are some feelings and attitudes persons who stutter might have, and what is their origin? Do nonstutterers ever have these feelings?

5. What is the age range for the onset of stuttering (the youngest and oldest ages at which onset is commonly reported)? Why might it occur at that time?

6. What is the difference between "incidence" and "prevalence"?

7. What problems do researchers encounter when they try to determine how many stutterers recover without treatment?

8. Why might the ratio of male to female stutterers change with age?

9. In what ways is stuttering predictable? In what ways does it vary?

10. Why is it difficult to answer the question what is THE cause of stuttering?

11. Will a person whose stuttering results in a significant *disability* necessarily have a significant *handicap* because of it?

12. Can you think of a situation in which someone who stutters has little *disability* from it but a significant *handicap*? Why might this happen? How could treatment help?

13. How would you describe the etiology of stuttering to a parent who has had limited education and is not used to discussing abstract concepts?

SUGGESTED PROJECTS

(1) Enlist the help of an adult who stutters and have him teach you to stutter. Then ask him to go with you while you use some voluntary stuttering in public. Write a brief report of what feelings you experienced and how people reacted to you.

(2) Use an internet search engine (for example, www.google.com) to find an on-line discussion group of people who stutter and clinicians. Join the group and observe what issues they discuss.

(3) Attend a support group for people who stutter.

(4) Listen to a group of preschool children playing and note their normal disfluencies. Then listen to elementary school children playing and talking and compare their disfluencies to those of the preschool children.

(5) If you are a fluent speaker, record your own speech and observe the types of disfluencies you hear. Do they differ from stuttering? In what ways?

(6) Conduct a search on the internet for resources that guide you to critically evaluate websites (for example, http://www.library.ucla.edu/libraries/college/help/critical). Using that format, critically evaluate a website you find when searching for "stuttering" sites with your search engine.

Suggested Readings

Bloodstein, O. (1993). *Stuttering: The Search for a Cause and Cure.* **Boston: Allyn & Bacon.**
This book is part history and part analysis and written with charm and clarity. Bloodstein covers early treatments for stuttering, the burgeoning of research in the 1930s, 1940s, and 1950s, and more recent findings in the realm of neurophysiology. His own orientation on the learning-environmental bases of stuttering comes through, but he gives good coverage of other possible factors as well. Bloodstein is particularly good at conveying the excitement that accompanies research.

Bobrick, B. (1995). *Knotted Tongues—Stuttering in History and the Quest for a Cure.* **New York: Simon & Schuster.**
A highly readable account of various treatments for stuttering throughout the ages and of famous people who stutter.

Carlisle, J. (1985). *Tangled Tongue: Living With a Stutter.* **Toronto: University of Toronto Press.**
An eloquent autobiography by a man with a severe stutter and a great sense of humor.

Helliesen, G. (2002). *Forty Years After Therapy: One Man's Story.* **Newport News, VA: Apolo Press.**
An autobiography of someone who stuttered severely and was treated by Charles Van Riper, the world-renowned stuttering clinician. This book presents a unique view of stuttering therapy from the client's perspective.

Jezer, M. (1997). *Stuttering: A Life Bound Up in Words.* **New York: Basic Books.**
A compelling, sensitive book about the frustrating and sometimes funny things that happen to someone growing up with a severe stuttering problem and learning to cope with it.

Johnson, W., and Leutenegger, R. (1955). *Stuttering in Children and Adults.* **Minneapolis: University of Minnesota Press.**

These authors compiled the research papers from one of the most productive research efforts ever applied to stuttering. These studies, conducted between 1930 and 1950 at the University of Iowa, uncovered many of the basic facts we have about the variability and predictability of stuttering. The first chapter, "The Time, the Place, and the Problem," gives a historical perspective on this research.

Murray, F.P. (undated). *A Stutterer's Story.* **Memphis: Stuttering Foundation of America (www.stut teringhelp.org).**

An autobiography depicting the long struggle of someone who stuttered severely and spent his life searching for answers. The author describes his acquaintance with many of the pioneers of stuttering therapy.

St. Louis, K. (Ed) (2001). *Living With Stuttering—Stories, Basics, Resources, and Hope.* **Morgantown, WV: Populore Publishing Company.**

Twenty-five life stories by people who stutter about how they have coped with their stuttering.

Shields, D. (1989). *Dead Languages.* **New York: Knopf.**

This is a novel about a young boy who stutters. It conveys the feelings associated with being a stutterer in a world that prizes spoken language. It is recommended for students who would like to understand a child who stutters.

Wingate, M. (1988). *The Structure of Stuttering: A Psycholinguistic Approach.* **New York: Springer-Verlag.**

Wingate builds a logical case for the explanation of stuttering as a neurological disorder, which has overt symptoms that are the result of a dyssynchrony in utterance planning and assembly. It reflects current thinking that stuttering has an important language component.

Chapter 2

Constitutional Factors in Stuttering

Biological Background

Hereditary Factors

A well-known fact about stuttering is that it often runs in families. For many years, researchers debated about what this meant. Some suggested that the appearance of stuttering in several generations of a family must mean that it is caused by an inherited physiological difference or "anomaly" that is inherited. Others disagreed, noting that political beliefs often run in families too, but they aren't inherited. These researchers argued that stuttering develops in response to a critical attitude toward normal disfluency that has been handed down from one generation to the next (Johnson et al, 1959). A child whose parents were critical of her normal disfluencies would grow afraid and would "hesitate to hesitate." This would start a spiral of more hesitations leading to greater fear, and so on.

For many years, researchers aligned themselves with one side of this argument or the other. Currently, however, there is broad agreement that stuttering can be inherited (Curlee, 2004). In other words, for many people who stutter, one or both of their parents had some predisposition for stuttering in their genes that they passed along. In part, the current thinking may be due to strong new evidence about heredity in stuttering, but it is probably also due to a less deterministic view of heredity. Research has shown, for a number of inherited disorders, that genes do not work alone. Stuttering, asthma, migraine headaches, and certain other disorders are seen as the result of heredity *and* environment acting together, with elements of chance thrown in (Kidd, 1984).

In this chapter, I will review three approaches to the study of heredity and stuttering: family studies, twin studies, and adoption studies. These different ways of gathering evidence all suggest that, for many individuals, stuttering is partly attributable to heredity. The insights we gain from these studies are vital to us in counseling individuals and families about the nature of stuttering.

Family Studies

In family studies, researchers gather evidence of the inheritance of stuttering by studying family trees. They begin with a group of individuals who stutter—for example, a group of 100. They then make up a group of 100 individuals who don't stutter, matched with the first group by age and gender. The researchers interview all the relatives in each group member's family to determine the average number of stuttering relatives each stutterer has. They then compare the findings in each group to answer the question: Do individuals who stutter have more relatives who stutter than individuals who don't stutter?

As scientists study family trees of stutterers, they also search for patterns of occurrence of stuttering. Geneticists know that certain inherited traits occur in specific patterns in families. For example, some traits appear only if both the mother and father have the trait; other traits are more common in children when the mother has the trait than if the father has the trait. Therefore, when scientists find these patterns of family occurence in a disorder like stuttering, it provides more evidence to support the idea that the disorder is likely to be inherited rather than simply the result of imitation or critical family attitudes about disfluency.

The first "modern" reports on the genetics of stuttering were published by a group of researchers in Newcastle, England (Andrews and Harris, 1964; Kay, 1964). They investigated the family histories of 80 stuttering children and compared them with nonstuttering children. They found that (1) children who stuttered had far more stuttering relatives than children who didn't stutter, (2) male children were at higher risk for developing stuttering than female children, and (3) female children who stuttered were more likely to have stuttering relatives than male children who stuttered. Thus, a pattern of family occurrence was seen, supporting a genetic explanation. These results supported a model in which stuttering was transmitted by either a single gene or a combination of several genes contributing different factors. This early insight into the possibility of multiple genes is supported by more recent work. My own working hypothesis is that chronic or persistent stuttering is the result of genes affecting not only speech motor control but also language and temperament.

Ten years later, researchers at Yale University conducted further family studies of stuttering (Kidd, 1977; Kidd, Kidd, and Records, 1978; Kidd, Reich, and Kessler, 1973). Using the data from England (Kay, 1964), combined with new data they gathered themselves in the United States, the researchers were able to develop statistical models that predicted patterns of inheritance. They found, as in Kay's earlier study, that males were more likely to stutter than females and that females who stuttered were more likely to have relatives who stuttered. Kidd (1984) concluded that these patterns were best explained by an interaction between the environment and a combination of several genes.

The Newcastle and Yale family studies focused on children and adults, most of whom had been stuttering for several years. A different approach was used by researchers at the University of Illinois. Ambrose, Yairi, and Cox (1993) studied the family histories of children who had just been diagnosed with stuttering, which made the population they studied decidedly younger and closer to onset than that of the Newcastle and Yale studies. Looking at the families of 69 very young children, they found that two-thirds of these children had relatives who stuttered and that, as in earlier studies, more male relatives than female relatives stuttered. Unlike past studies, however, these researchers found that male and female children who stutter had similar chances of having relatives who stuttered. This difference is likely to have come from the fact that females in the Kay and Kidd studies were older with persistent rather than transient cases of the disorder. So they may have carried higher "genetic loadings" (i.e., more genetic predisposition) for stuttering, which means their relatives were also more likely to have received or passed on more of such genetic material. On the other hand, Ambrose et al's (1993) very young female subjects often recovered quickly from stuttering and thus may have had lower genetic loadings and fewer relatives who stuttered.

Kay's (1964) and Kidd's (1984) hypotheses that stuttering may be transmitted by several genes rather than a single gene received support from a study that investigated differences between those young children who recover from stuttering without treatment and those who persist. Ambrose, Cox, and Yairi (1997) analyzed the family trees of 66 children who were identified soon after the onset of stuttering. The children were followed for several years and eventually grouped into those who persisted in stuttering and those who recovered. The researchers found that the sex ratios of the two groups were quite different. The male to female ratio was 7:1 in the persistent group but about 2:1 in the recovered group, indicating a much higher percentage of boys in the persistent group. This provides more evidence that girls are more likely to recover than boys. A second finding was that persistence runs in families. In other words, children who did not outgrow their stuttering were likely to come from families in which relatives who stuttered also persisted in their stuttering. Conversely, children who recovered were likely to come from families in which relatives who stuttered also became fluent speakers. Further analysis of their data led the authors to propose that persistent and recovered stuttering are transmitted by the same major gene or genes but that those individuals whose stuttering persists have additional genetic factors that hamper recovery. It is also possible that those who recovered have additional genetic factors that facilitate recovery.

The researchers in Illinois have examined a number of genetic and nongenetic factors that might predict recovery or persistence and thereby might be useful in deciding which children are in immediate need for treatment. Yairi et al (1996) found that predictors of recovery include (1) good scores on tests of phonology, language, and nonverbal skills, (2) family members who had recovered from stuttering, and (3) early age of onset of stuttering. Some of the factors that impede recovery, such as problems in phonology or language, might be determined by the other genes that may accompany a gene that is related to the initial onset of stuttering.

Before we leave the topic of family studies, it is worth mentioning several criticisms that have been made about genetic studies in reviews by Felsenfeld (1997) and Yairi, Ambrose, and Cox (1996). Many of the genetic studies used no matched control group, but instead, they relied on incidence figures from other studies. Other problems in past studies include the inadequacy of a definition of stuttering when searching for stuttering among relatives of children or adults who stutter and relying on testimony of others, rather than direct assessment, to determine whether or not a relative stutters. These researchers suggest that future studies (1) look for subgroups of stutterers that may have different genetic etiologies, (2) examine family members who do not stutter to find factors that may resist stuttering, and (3) search for environmental factors that may interact with genetic factors to precipitate or maintain stuttering.

In summary, despite the small number of studies and their limitations, family studies have provided strong evidence for a genetic predisposition in many individuals who stutter. Some evidence also suggests that there may be two genetic mechanisms involved in chronic stuttering: one or more genes that carry the predisposition for the speech breakdown evident in children who begin to stutter and an additional genetic predisposition that prevents natural recovery from stuttering.

Twin Studies

The genetic transmission of stuttering can also be investigated by comparing the incidence of stuttering in fraternal and identical twins. Identical twins (also called monozygotic twins) have completely identical genes. In fraternal twins (dizygotic), only 25% of their genes are identical, like any other two siblings. Greater similarities in the traits of identical twins compared with those of fraternal twins are generally attributed to inheritance. Twin studies of stuttering have shown that stuttering occurs much more often in both members of identical twin pairs than in both members of fraternal, same-sex twin pairs (Andrews et al, 1990; Felsenfeld et al, 2000; Howie, 1981; Luchsinger, 1944; Seeman, 1937). To use the vocabulary of genetics, there is higher "concordance" of stuttering in identical compared with fraternal twins. This supports the hypothesis that stuttering is inherited, but it does not reveal what is inherited. How does a gene (or several genes) affect a child's speech so that stuttering results? No one is sure. In addition to providing evidence of genetic factors in stuttering, twin studies demonstrate that heredity does not work alone. In one of the twin studies previously cited, although there was higher concordance for stuttering among identical twins, some pairs were discordant (Howie, 1981). Specifically, Howie found that in six of the 16 identical twin pairs, one twin stuttered, but the other did not. This means that, even though both members of the twin pair had the same genetic inheritance, only one of them stuttered, indicating that genes alone do not explain stuttering. However, this may not be surprising because genes must interact with the environment to produce their effects (LeDoux, 2002). A gene might not express itself in stuttering unless, for example, there is some kind of prenatal stress on the child, unless the family environment creates a certain level of communicative pressure, or unless the child's language development proceeds at too fast or too slow a pace. In the case of stuttering, where there appears to be several genes working together to produce a chronic disorder, the situation is even more complex because several genetic tendencies may need to interact with different aspects of the child's internal and external environment to create stuttering. No wonder there were six discordant pairs in the Howie study.

An estimate of the relative proportions of genetic and environmental influences was suggested in a later study involving 3810 unselected twin pairs (Andrews et al, 1990). They were deemed "unselected" because they were all part of the Australian Twin Registry rather than a population selected because of stuttering, making the sample less likely to be influenced by "ascertainment bias." This kind of bias might occur, for example, if subjects were found through newspaper ads; only individuals who read the ads in newspapers and were motivated to be in the study would participate in the study. Analyses of these data estimated that 71% of the variance (the probability of whether or not one would stutter) is accounted for by genetic factors, and 29% is accounted for by the individual's environment (including factors influencing the fetus, as well as factors after birth). Felsenfeld et al (2000) recently followed up this study by contacting a group of twins in the Australian Twin Registry that was different from the group studied by Andrews et al (1990). Felsenfeld et al (2000) screened 1567 pairs of twins and 634 individuals using questionnaires and telephone interviews. They found 17 monozygotic and eight dizygotic twins who were concordant for stuttering (both twins stuttered at some time in their lives) and 21 monozygotic and 45 dizygotic twins who were discordant for stuttering (only one of the twins ever stuttered). Statistical analyses estimated that "additive genetic effects" (the effects of different genes working together) accounted for 70% of the variance and that an individual's unique environment (influences on one of the twins but not the other, such as illness) accounted for 30% of the variance. These proportions are essentially the same as those found by Andrews et al (1990) and support current thinking that genes and environment interact to set the stage for stuttering. Unfortunately, there were no data on the chronicity of stuttering in any of the twin groups. Such information might help us understand more about the factors influencing persistence and recovery.

Adoption Studies

One of the most powerful ways to examine the relative contributions of genes and the environment to stuttering is to look at the families of stutterers who were adopted soon after birth. A higher incidence of stuttering among the biological relatives of adopted stutterers would support a greater role of genetics in causing stuttering, whereas a higher incidence among adoptive relatives would support a greater role of the environment.

Because the birth records of adopted children are difficult to obtain, studies of adopted stutterers are rare. Bloodstein (1995) presented information obtained from 13 adopted stutterers who he interviewed about stuttering in their adoptive families (information on their biological families was not available). Four of the 13 stutterers reported having relatives who stuttered in their adoptive families, which is higher than would be expected by chance. This small sample, without data from biological families, supports the possibility that environmental factors may have an effect. If the relatives in the adoptive family were key figures, such as a parent or older sibling who was close to the child, this would be stronger evidence for the influence of the environment. Unfortunately, this information is not available.

Felsenfeld (1997) reported some preliminary data on a small sample of adopted children who had speech disorders (primarily stuttering) and for whom data were available from *both* adoptive and biological families. These data indicated that a history of stuttering in the biological families was slightly more predictive of disorders in these children than was stuttering in the adoptive family.

In short, the evidence suggests that both genetic and environmental factors influence whether or not a child will stutter and that genetic inheritance appears to contribute more strongly.

Genes

A number of researchers are currently looking for the gene (or genes) that predisposes children to stutter. Dennis Drayna (1997) at the National Institutes of Health has begun genetic linkage studies using large numbers of families to try to isolate the gene for stuttering. Linkage analysis compares the chromosomes of family members who have a trait (the appearance of a trait in a person is called a "phenotype") with those of family members who do not. In this way, the chromosomal location of the stuttering gene or genes can be identified. He is currently seeking families in which there is more than one individual who stutters. His work has recently brought him into contact with a family in Cameroon, Africa, in which 42 of 100 family members stutter. Preliminary results suggest genes on chromosome 18 may be related to stuttering, a set of genes that control intercellular communication (Shugart et al, 2004). Susan Felsenfeld is collaborating with other researchers in studies of the citizens of Iceland (a largely homogeneous population) to look at patterns of inheritance and examine genetic material that may provide details about how and what is inherited in stuttering (Willig and Moss, 2000). Cox and Yairi (2000) have been studying individuals who stutter in a North Dakota community of Hutterites. This group is of interest because they do not marry outside the community, resulting in a homogeneous gene pool. These researchers have identified three chromosomes (numbers 1, 13, and 16) that may include the genes involved in stuttering. Workers in Britain studying a family with many members who have developmental verbal dyspraxia (difficulty producing sequences of sounds) have located a gene (FOXP2) that they suggest "is involved in the developmental process that culminates in speech and language" (Lai et al, 2001). Perhaps this discovery and other studies by the Human Genome Project will lead to a better understanding of how stuttering may be related to the development of speech and language and to other disorders.

I suspect that there are several genetic pathways that lead to stuttering. Difficulties with speech motor control, language and learning ability, or sensory processing (and the interactions of difficulties in these areas), as well as a vulnerable temperament, may be among those factors with genetic bases which can, in combination with environmental factors, result in stuttering. Studies yet to be done include those that can identify characteristics other than stuttering (such as language and learning difficulty) which, in other family members and in the child, put the child at risk for stuttering and may predict severity or recovery. Studies may eventually show that those stutterers who have no family history of stuttering do have family members with other speech, language, or learning difficulties that the child also has and that predispose her to stuttering. It is hoped that these studies will also look at the inheritance patterns of those who persist in stuttering compared with those who recover early.

Table 2–1 summarizes the important hereditary factors in stuttering that I have described in this section. Some of the major clinical implications of these factors are also given.

Congenital and Early Childhood Factors

It has been estimated that 30% to 60% of individuals who stutter have a family history of stuttering (Yairi et al, 1996). Therefore, 40% to 70% of individuals who stutter have *no* family history and may have developed the disorder by mechanisms other than inheritance of a predisposition that has caused stuttering in relatives. However, we do not know how many of these individuals inherited a factor or several factors that predisposed them to stuttering but did not produce stuttering in other family members. On the other hand, some individuals who stutter may not have inherited any factor that predisposed them to stutter. Instead, they may have experienced a physical or psychological trauma that predisposed them to stuttering or even precipitated its onset. Such traumas may have occurred at or near birth and would be viewed as "congenital" factors. Some events or factors may also have occurred during early childhood, but for simplicity's sake, I will refer to them all in the remainder of this section as congenital.

There is relatively little research on congenital factors related to stuttering. West, Nelson, and Berry (1939) carefully examined the family histories of a sample of 204 people who stuttered and found that 100 of them had no family history of stuttering. Eighty-five of these 100 people reported congenital factors that may have been related to the onset of stuttering. These factors included infectious diseases, diseases of the nervous system, and injuries, which were all reported to have occurred just prior to stuttering onset, although the exact proximity to onset was not reported. Boehme (1968) investigated a sample of 313 individuals who had sustained brain damage at birth or in early childhood and reported that 24% developed stuttering (compared to 5% in the general population). In a more recent study, Poulos and Webster (1991) found that 57 of the clients in a clinic sample of 169 adults and adolescents who stuttered reported no family history of

Table 2–1	Summary of Hereditary Factors in Stuttering	
Area of Interest	**Important Findings**	**Major Clinical Implications**
Family Studies	Stuttering appears to be inherited in many cases. May be single gene for transitory stuttering and that gene combined with others for persistent stuttering.	Parents should be told that stuttering is often inherited rather than the result of their parenting.
	Sex ratio at onset is fairly equal: less than 2:1, males to females. Females more likely to recover within 2 years, making the ratio 3:1 in early school years.	
	Factors that predict recovery include: (1) being female, (2) no family members who stuttered or only transitory stuttering, (3) early onset of stuttering (prior to age 3), and (4) good language, phonological, and non-verbal abilities.	Prognosis improves as more of the four recovery factors are true for child.
Twin Studies	Greater concordance among identical compared to fraternal twins.	
	Two-thirds of the influence on the occurrence of stuttering appears to be related to genes, one-third to environmental factors.	Both genetic and environmental factors are important, so that the child's home environment might be an influence in occurrence of stuttering and recovery.
Adoption Studies	More than chance occurrence of bio-logical and adopted relatives who stuttered among adopted children. These studies provide evidence for the importance of both genetic and environmental factors.	Presence of relatives who stutter does not make it certain that child will stutter.
Genes	One study found evidence for trans-mission of stuttering transmission via chromosome 18; another study found evidence via chromosomes 1, 13, and 16.	Research underway to identify genes associated with stuttering; may lead to earlier identification and preventive treatment.

stuttering. Of these clients, 37% reported congenital factors that may have been associated with the onset of stuttering, whereas only 2.4% of the clients having a positive family history of stuttering reported such factors. The factors reported included anoxia at birth, premature birth, childhood surgery, head injury, mild cerebral palsy, mild retardation, and experiencing intense fear.

The fact that physical and psychological traumas may be associated with childhood stuttering in those without a family history of stuttering is not surprising. Adult onset of stuttering may also be associated with head injury, neurological disease, or intense fear, as I will describe in Chapter 13. Thus, mechanisms similar to those precipitating adult onset may be involved in childhood stuttering in the absence of family history of stuttering, but this possibility raises as many questions as answers. Why would some children (and adults), but not others, begin to stutter as a result of intense fear? Which brain structures and functions affected by head injury and neurological disease result in stuttering? How are they similar to and how do they differ from the effects of inheriting a predisposition to stutter?

The important findings and clinical implications regarding congenital and early childhood constitutional influences on stuttering are summarized in Table 2–2.

Brain Structure and Function

Whether an individual's stuttering results from an inherited predisposition or from an early brain injury, structures or functions in the central nervous system would be affected. The search for how these brain structures or functions are different in people who stutter has been under way at least since the experiments of Travis at the University of Iowa in the 1930s, which were described in Chapter 1. In the following sections, I will briefly review the older studies and then focus on recent brain imaging research that has produced many promising leads. Figure 2–1 shows areas thought to be involved in speech and language production, in both stutterers and nonstutterers.

Electroencephalographic (EEG) Studies

Motivated by a theory that stuttering was caused by a lack of dominance of one cerebral hemisphere over the other (Travis, 1931), Travis and his students used EEG to measure brain waves in stuttering and nonstuttering subjects. Their hope was to find proof that the brains of stutterers didn't show the normal left-hemisphere dominance during speech. EEG studies are carried out by pasting electrodes on the surface of the scalp to measure the electrical activity of brain. This procedure, like any assessment of the brain,

Table 2–2 Summary of Congenital and Early Childhood Factors

Area of Interest	Important Findings	Major Clinical Implications
Congenital and Early Childhood Factors	40% to 70% of stutterers have no family history of stuttering.	Heredity shouldn't be assumed to be the only cause of stuttering; clinician should ask family about with child's experiences and events near the time of stuttering onset.
	Onset of stuttering, especially in cases without family history, has been associated with such factors as brain injury before or soon after birth, premature birth, surgery, head injury, retardation, and intense fear.	Clinician should be mindful that a purpose of exploring etiology is to relieve guilt of parents; statements about cause should be made tentatively and without blaming family.

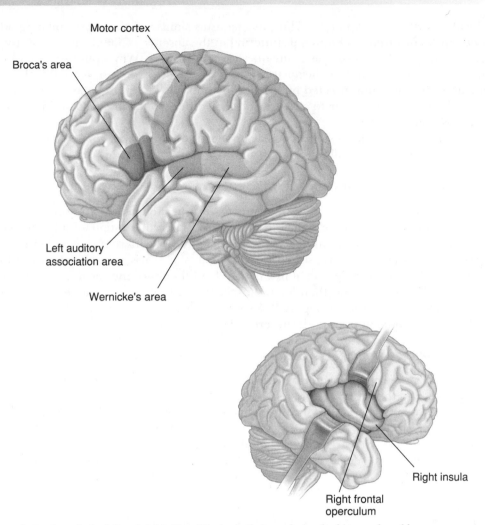

Figure 2–1 *Areas in the left and right sides of the brain that may be involved in speech and language processing in stutterers and nonstutterers.*

was fraught with methodological quandaries (Bloodstein, 1995). How faithfully would electrical activity on the scalp plumb the activity of brain cells several centimeters below? How do you know that the electrical activity recorded isn't created by muscle contractions during speech or even the result of the subject blinking her eyes or wiggling her nose? How do you know which part of the brain is active when you see the squiggles on the chart paper that represent electrical impulses? These uncertainties make it likely that the EEG studies by different scientists in different laboratories will produce widely different findings due to different methodologies and different interpretations of the data.

Despite these problems, many EEG studies of stutterers and nonstutterers have been conducted, and some interesting findings have turned up. As with other experimental results, one should be cautious about accepting the results as final proof. Several EEG studies supported the notion that stutterers' brains were somehow wired differently, although other studies did not. Studies by Travis and Knott (1937), Douglass (1943), Zimmerman and Knott (1974), Ponsford, Brown Marsh, and Travis (1975), Moore et al (Moore and Haynes, 1980; and many more), and Boberg et al (1983) showed in different ways that individuals who stutter tend to have more activity on the right side of the brain during speech and especially during stuttering than nonstutterers. This activity seemed to involve structures in the right hemisphere in the same locations as those in the left hemisphere that control speech and language. Although this was not exactly what Orton and Travis had predicted, it was close. Whereas the Orton-Travis theory hypothesized that stutterers lacked hemispheric dominance, findings from these EEG studies suggested that rather than lacking dominance, stutterers may have a *right* hemisphere dominance for language (whereas nonstutterers have left hemisphere dominance). Interestingly, two EEG studies have also shown that therapy can affect which hemisphere is most active during speech. MacFarland and Moore (1982) and Boberg et al (1983) found evidence of high levels of brain activity in the right hemisphere during speech prior to stuttering treatment and proportionally greater activity in the left hemisphere after treatment. This apparent switch could also be caused by a reduction in negative, right hemisphere emotions after treatment, which would appear to lessen the proportion of right hemisphere activity in relation to the amount of activity in the left hemisphere.

Cerebral Blood Flow (CBF) Studies

In the 1970s and 1980s, researchers developed new technology that was more precise in detecting where brain activity was occurring by measuring the amount of blood flowing to those areas. CBF is usually detected by injecting a radioactive tracer into the blood stream and taking the equivalent of x-ray pictures of the amount of radioactivity given off. The greater the amount of neural activity in an area, the greater the blood flow in that area and the greater the amount of radioactivity given off.

Interpretation of CBF and other brain imaging studies must take into account many different variables that can influence the results (Ingham, 2001). Two such variables are the spatial and temporal resolution of each technology. In other words, how accurately can CBF determine exactly *where* the activity is occurring and *when* it's occurring? Early studies could only observe areas of the brain in a relatively general way, but improved technologies have allowed later studies to differentiate the activity of different areas in more detail and reveal interactions among brain areas. Besides the problem of how good the resolution is, other variables that can influence outcomes of brain imaging studies are the gender of the participants, the severity of their stuttering, whether or not they've had therapy, what tasks the participants perform in the study, and techniques used to analyze the data (Lauter, 1995, 1997). Keep these in mind as you read about the research in this area.

The first study of CBF in stuttering was published by Wood et al (1980) but used only two participants. They found greater right than left hemisphere activity in Broca's area during stuttering before treatment with the drug Haloperidol. After 2 weeks of therapy with the drug, both participants showed that the greatest activity had shifted from right to left hemisphere speech areas. The second CBF study of stuttering was not published until 11 years later. Pool et al (1991) studied the brains of 20 adult stutterers using single emission computed tomography (SPECT), an improved technology that enabled scientists to view the brain from multiple angles and obtain better images of what was going on. The principal finding from this study, in addition to lower absolute levels of CBF overall, was that the stuttering group showed less left hemispheric dominance in areas that are believed to be related to motor initiation, speech motor control, and language processing.

Positron Emission Tomography (PET) Studies and Beyond

Four years later, another CBF study took advantage of a new brain imaging tool, positron emission tomography (PET), which allowed researchers to make more accurate inferences about where increased blood flow was occurring in the brain. A large team of researchers, Wu et al (1995), studied the brains of four adults who stuttered and a matched group of control participants in two conditions: reading aloud and reading in unison with someone else (called "choral reading"). As you may remember from Chapter 1, when individuals who stutter read aloud along with someone else, they become fluent. These researchers' findings suggested that two important speech and language areas of the brain, Broca's area and Wernicke's area, both in the left hemisphere (see Fig. 2–1), showed decreased activity (compared with their normal-speaking controls) when participants were stuttering compared with when they were fluent during choral reading. Broca's area is thought to be the major cortical area responsible for organizing and executing speech motor output. Wernicke's area, on the other hand, is vital for speech and language comprehension but may also be involved in speech output because it appears to be the storehouse for the sounds that form words—the phonological representations that are called upon before the motor commands are given.

In November 1995, four different research groups presented their findings at the annual convention of the American Speech-Language-Hearing Association in Orlando, Florida (De Nil et al, 1995). As the presentations were given, the excitement in the room was palpable because so many of their findings were similar, although the groups were working entirely independently. Here at last was clear evidence that the brains of people who stutter worked differently than those of nonstutterers. Years of previous speculation and studies suggesting anomalous cerebral dominance, inadequate laterality, auditory processing problems, and language dysfunction in stuttering seemed to be confirmed. These findings and others are reviewed in the following sections.

Right Hemisphere Over-Activation During Stuttering

A common finding by several of the brain research teams in 1995 and afterwards is that individuals who stutter demonstrate high levels of activity in the right hemisphere when they are speaking, especially when stuttering, as illustrated in Figure 2–2. The focus of this activity is greatest in right hemisphere structures that are homologous to those in the left hemisphere used by normal speakers (Fox et al, 1996; Fox et al, 2000; Braun et al, 1997; De Nil et al, 2000). One of those areas is called the *right frontal operculum* (see Fig. 2.1) and is in the same location in the right hemisphere that Broca's area is located in the left hemisphere (Fox, 2003). Broca's area is thought to be active in planning the phonetic structure of an utterance to be spoken (Kent, 1997). Another area in the right hemisphere commonly found to be active during stuttering is the right *insula* (Fox, 2003). In the left hemisphere, the insula may function as a connection

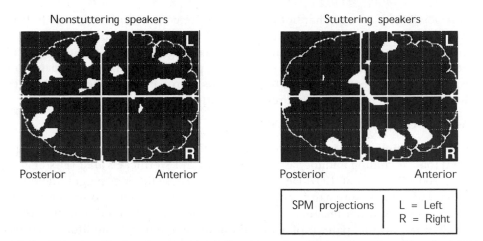

Figure 2–2   *PET scans of brains of nonstuttering (left) and stuttering (right) adults while reading aloud. SPM, statistical parametric mapping. (From De Nil, L., Kroll, R., Kapur, S., and Houle, S. (1995). Silent and oral reading in stuttering and nonstuttering adults: A positron emission tomography study. Paper presented at the Annual Convention of the American Speech-Language-Hearing Association, Orlando, FL, December.)*

between Wernicke's area (which may be important for phonological representations of words and auditory monitoring of one's own speech) and Broca's area (Ingham et al, 2003).

Researchers have considered two possible explanations for the over-activation of these right hemisphere structures during stuttering. One explanation is that during embryonic development the right side of the brain becomes "wired" to be the primary speech and language area (e.g., Geshwind and Galaburda, 1985). This may result in some difficulty speaking because right hemisphere structures are not generally suited for the rapid processing of signals required for speech (such as the quick transitions in many consonant-vowel transitions). When a child with this right hemisphere "wiring" for speech develops language beyond the single word stage, stuttering may emerge as she tries to produce multi-word utterances at the typically fast speech rates used for longer sentences (Kent, 1984). A second hypothesis is that the child who stutters initially tried to use left hemisphere regions for speech and language, but the neural networks for speech and language failed to function adequately and resulted in stuttering. Only then did the child's brain begin to use right hemisphere structures in a compensatory way, to try to achieve more normal speech, similarly to the way in which some individuals with aphasia use right hemisphere structures to compensate for damaged areas in the left hemisphere (e.g., Sommer et al, 2002; Weiller et al, 1995).

Several researchers have provided evidence in favor of the second (compensation) hypothesis. Braun et al (1997) found that activations of right hemisphere sensory areas were negatively correlated with stuttering; that is, these regions became more active as speech became more fluent. Moreover, researchers in Germany (Neumann et al, 2003) found that right hemisphere activations were greater in participants who stuttered moderately compared with those who stuttered severely, suggesting that right hemisphere activity may indeed be a way in which individuals could partially overcome dysfunctions in the left hemisphere areas. In other words, the moderate stutterers used more compensatory right hemisphere activity to reduce the severity of their stuttering.

It is possible, of course, that both hypotheses are correct and that some individuals develop right hemisphere processing for speech and language before they begin to stutter and others develop right hemisphere processing after they begin to stutter, as a compensatory response. Still others, in fact, may process speech and language in both hemispheres simultaneously. Each of these options is probably inefficient and may create the dyssynchrony in processing that results in stuttering.

Left Auditory Cortex Inactivity During Stuttering

Many brain imaging studies of stuttering have shown a lack of activity in the left superior temporal lobe, including auditory association areas and Wernicke's area (Fox et al, 1996; Fox et al, 2000; Braun et al, 1997; De Nil et al, 2003). These findings suggest the possibility that when individuals stutter they are not using auditory feedback to monitor and control their speech. Another imaging study (Salmelin et al, 1998) found that stutterers have a reversal of the normal pattern of activation of the left and right auditory cortices during stuttering. Evidence of auditory dysfunction during stuttering is especially pertinent in light of the many studies that have shown that stutterers may have difficulty performing auditory processing tasks (e.g., Barasch et al, 2000; Molt, 1997) and that fluency can be induced by changing the way stutterers hear their own speech (e.g., Brayton and Conture, 1978; Howell, El-Yaniv, and Powell, 1987).

How does auditory self-monitoring affect fluency? It may provide a stimulus to time or integrate the sequence of activities that run in parallel when a speaker decides what she will say, selects the linguistic elements for it, and executes the utterance. Thus, the dyssynchrony or timing disturbance that many researchers see as the basis of stuttering (e.g., Perkins, Kent, and Curlee, 1991; Van Riper, 1982) may be caused by a paucity of signals that synchronize the sequence for speech output. Therapies (e.g., Van Riper, 1973) that emphasize proprioception may be giving the client another feedback modality to use for timing; therapies that focus on the use of slow speech, gentle onsets, and light articulatory contacts may develop the client's auditory as well as proprioceptive monitoring of speech.

Other functions besides monitoring one's own speech may also reside in the deactivated regions of the superior temporal lobe. For example, Wernicke's area may be important for storing the phonological representations of words (Caplan, 1987; Paulesu, Frith, and Frackowiak, 1993). Therefore, activation of this region of the brain may be a key stage in phonological planning for speech production. Lack of activation during stuttering may reflect a deficit in the sequence of phonological selection, phonetic planning, and motor execution.

Neuroanatomical Differences in Individuals Who Stutter

Most of the studies of stuttering just reviewed have examined brain activity patterns that describe the *functions* of stutterers' brains, rather than their *structures*. In contrast, three studies have examined the brain anatomy of individuals who stutter by measuring the shape and size of speech and language areas. In the first study, researchers at Tulane University in New Orleans (Foundas et al, 2001) used magnetic resonance imaging (MRI) to assess the size of the *planum temporale (PT)*, a part of Wernicke's area thought to be associated with higher level auditory processing. Their results found that the PT in nonstutterers was larger in the left hemisphere than the right, but in stutterers, it was symmetrical in size in the two hemispheres or, in some cases, larger on the right. The researchers pointed out that a similar lack of asymmetry on the left has been found in individuals with dyslexia and specific language impairment. An additional anomaly found in participants who stuttered were differences in various *gyri* (folds) in the speech and language areas of the brain. The authors of the study speculated that these differences in the brains of those who stutter may reflect deficits that interfere with information flow between Wernicke's area (auditory cortex) and Broca's area (speech motor).

A follow-up study by Foundas et al (2004) was launched to find evidence of abnormal function associated with the abnormal structure shown in the earlier study. These researchers found that matched groups of stutterers and controls had approximately the same PT asymmetry (64% had leftward asymmetry and 36% had rightward asymmetry in each group). However, the subgroup of stuttering participants who had rightward asymmetry were more severe stutterers and, interestingly, had a significantly greater response to the fluency-inducing condition of delayed auditory feedback. The authors attributed this finding to the fact that the PT is thought to be important in auditory processing of language and perhaps in coordinating auditory feedback of speech with ongoing speech output. Delayed auditory feedback may have corrected an auditory feedback processing deficit, causing stuttering in those with rightward PT asymmetry.

The third neuroanatomical study was conducted in Germany by Sommer et al (2002). Using a process called diffusion tensor imaging, these investigators examined the density of white matter fiber tracts in the area of the left Rolandic operculum, fibers which are thought to connect sensory, planning, and motor areas of the brain (Fig. 2–3). They chose this area of the brain to study because, 2 years earlier, other researchers studying activity in the left operculum found dyssynchrony in the sequencing stages of speech processing in stutterers (Salmelin et al, 2000). Sommer et al (2002) indeed found what they suspected; fibers in the left operculum in stuttering participants were less dense than those in fluent participants. These results suggested to them that this structural difference in stutterers' brains could be the basis for the dyssynchrony in processing found by Salmelin et al (2000). These results complement the findings of Foundas et al (2001; 2004) who also reported anomalies in this region of the brain.

The findings just described indicate that stutterers' left hemisphere structures for speech and language have anomalies or differences from those in normal speakers. These differences appear to reflect the lack of activation or the unusual sequencing of activation and may account for compensatory activity seen in homologous right hemisphere structures.

Changes in Brain Activity with Increases in Fluency

There is a consensus among researchers that when stutterers become fluent, either through a temporary procedure like choral reading or through a treatment program, their right hemisphere over-activations are reduced and cortical activity is more lateralized to the left hemisphere (including the auditory cortex) (De Nil et al, 2003; Ingham, 2003; Stager, Jeffries, and Braun, 2003; Neumann et al, 2003).

Figure 2–4 depicts the differences in brain activity between stutterers and nonstutterers before and after treatment. It is evident, particularly in the coronal sections in Figure 2–4 before treatment and immediately after treatment, that activity levels shift from greater in the right hemisphere to greater in the left hemisphere.

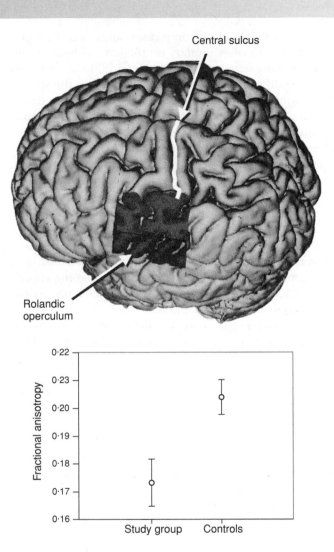

Central sulcus

Rolandic
operculum

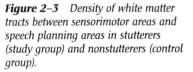

Figure 2–3 *Density of white matter tracts between sensorimotor areas and speech planning areas in stutterers (study group) and nonstutterers (control group).*

Brain imaging studies suggest that temporary fluency, induced by choral reading or singing, appears to activate not only the speech motor areas of the left hemisphere, but also the primary auditory cortex and auditory association cortex, which are areas that are typically active when nonstuttering speakers monitor their own speech and voice. The fluency thus produced in stutterers may be a result of "more effective coupling of auditory and motor systems" to control speech (Stager et al, 2003, p. 333).

Brain imaging studies of stutterers before and after behavioral treatment have found changes in cerebral activity similar to those created by temporary fluency (De Nil et al, 2003). There was, for example, greater activity in left hemisphere "auditory and frontal speech motor planning and execution areas" (Neumann et al, 2003, p. 404). The results of one study (Neumann et al, 2005) indicate that regions of the brain that became newly active after therapy (left insula and left Rolandic operculum) were remarkably close to the very regions where deficits in white matter tracts were reported earlier by Sommer et al (2002). This finding may indicate that the immediate effect of treatment is

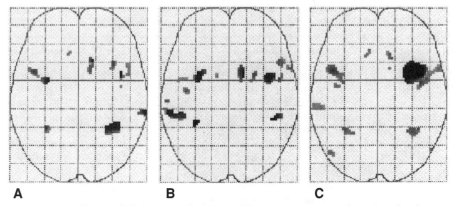

Figure 2–4   *Overt reading: statistical parametrical maps of between-group comparisons (people who stutter versus people who do not stutter) (A) before therapy, (B) immediately after therapy, (C) 2 years after therapy (Neumann et al, 2003).*

to re-establish functions in the cerebral neighborhood where they "belong," that is, in a part of the brain that was originally designed for the rapid transfer of information in the service of speech and language.

Brain Imaging Studies of Long-Term Outcome

As reported in the preceding section, stutterers show a decrease in right hemisphere over-activity and an increase in left hemisphere activity immediately after treatment. However, a year or two after treatment, some right hemisphere over-activity reappears, as depicted in Figure 2.4C and described in De Nil et al (2003) and Neumann et al (2003). Both of these studies found that increases in right hemisphere activity in the groups at 1 and 2 years of follow-up were accompanied by slight increases in stuttering. Thus, the reappearance of right hemisphere activity may be causally related to increased stuttering. Studies of groups who had successful long-term outcome versus groups who did not would shed more light on this question.

The results of long-term outcome also show a general decrease in level of brain activity in both hemispheres compared with pre-treatment and immediately post-treatment levels (De Nil et al, 2003; Neumann et al, 2003). This decrease is unlikely to be the result of simply less stuttering because participants are usually fluent during brain imaging tasks, even pre-treatment. De Nil et al (2003) suggests that treatment and maintenance programs may be responsible for making fluent speech a more automatized skill, requiring less brain activity.

The major findings related to brain structure and function in stuttering are presented in Table 2–3, along with clinical implications.

Performance

In the preceding section, you learned that certain brain structures and functions related to speech and language in individuals who stutter are different from those in individuals who don't stutter. These findings about the brain are supported by research on how individuals who stutter perform on sensory and motor tasks. This section on performance

Table 2–3 Summary of Brain Structure and Function in Stuttering		
Area of Interest	**Important Findings**	**Major Clinical Implications**
EEG Studies	Stutterers differ from nonstutterers in showing more activity on right side of brain in structures similar to those on left side active in nonstutterers. Stutterers show more left hemisphere activity during speech after treatment	Evidence that treatment is associated with greater activity in left hemisphere during speaking; may have implications about the neurological changes that accompany improvement in fluency.
Brain Imaging Studies Using MRI, PET, and Modern Techniques	Stutterers show the following differences from nonstutterers: over-activation of many areas of right hemisphere during speaking, especially when stuttering; activity greatest in right frontal operculum and right insula; deactivation of left auditory cortex during stuttering; anomalous symmetry in planum temporale (part of Wernicke's area) in stutterers; less dense fibers in white matter tracts of left operculum, which are thought to connect sensory, planning, and motor areas. After either transitory or long–term fluency is induced, right hemisphere over–activations are reduced and left hemisphere speech, language, and auditory areas are activated.	As above, evidence that improvement in fluency is associated with increase in left hemisphere activity and decrease in right hemisphere activity; potential to refine treatments by increasing activities that involve left hemisphere speech, language, and auditory areas.

will summarize this research and highlight how the findings may be related to brain structure and function.

Some Caveats About Finding the Causes of Stuttering

As researchers have searched for the causes of stuttering, they have been hampered by the difficulty in demonstrating cause and effect relationships. In particular, the brain differences described in the preceding section could be the cause of the disorder or the result of how the brain has responded to years of stuttering. Moreover, brain activity during stuttering may also be indirectly related to the behavior of stuttering; for example, some right hemisphere activity may be a manifestation of stutterers' fears and anxiety about stuttering. These fears might not cause the disorder in the first place, but they may make it worse.

In some speech disorders that have a more clear-cut physical basis, cause and effect can be directly investigated. There may even be animal models of the disorder to work from. In a disorder that can occur in animals, factors thought to cause the disorder can be manipulated, and their effects can be measured. For example, interfering with the genes or the embryonic development of dogs or cats or rabbits can produce the clefting or spasticity similar to cleft palate or cerebral palsy seen in humans. Thus, scientists can infer how inheritance, embryonic development, or brain trauma can cause these disorders. However, communication through spoken language does not occur in animals, which eliminates their use in looking for the cause of disorders like stuttering that occur only in spoken communication. And obviously, selective breeding or surgery to create stuttering is not an option in humans. Therefore, researchers have turned to indirect approaches, or **descriptive** rather than experimental approaches. They compare groups of stutterers and nonstutterers on tasks they believe are related to speech fluency. If they find, again and again, that the two groups perform differently in certain tasks, they may have a clue about the disorder.

Such indirect research is complicated because the differences that are found might be a *result* of stuttering and not a cause of it. For example, reaction time studies of how quickly subjects can say a word that is flashed on a screen might show that subjects who stutter are slower than subjects who don't. This difference, however, might be the result of subjects who stutter saying words more slowly to keep from stuttering. Even if a difference were not the result of trying not to stutter, it is more likely to be only a correlated factor that has no **causal** relationship to stuttering. Even if groups of stutterers do respond more slowly, slower reaction times alone probably do not cause stuttering. If they did, people would start stuttering as they grew older or after they imbibed a few beers. Finding something that co-occurs with something else but doesn't cause it is like finding that most basketball players have larger shoe sizes than most gymnasts. Shoe size itself doesn't determine who is better suited for each of these sports, but height may be a determining factor. Both shoe size and height are related to one's genetically determined bone size, so they end up being different in gymnasts and basketball players, but shoe size itself doesn't make one a better basketball player or gymnast.

Another problem with descriptive studies rather than experimental approaches to studying the nature of stuttering is that when comparing groups of people who do and do not stutter there is often a great deal of overlap in the two groups' performances even though their averages might be statistically different. For example, some of the people who stutter usually will show coordination as good as the average person in the group of nonstutterers on a typical test of motor coordination, and some of the people who don't stutter will demonstrate the same level of coordination as an average person in the stuttering group. These overlaps remind us that we are usually not studying factors that are necessary or sufficient by themselves to cause stuttering in persons. However, such underlying differences between people who stutter and people who don't may provide us with clues. And, with those clues in hand, we may look more closely at certain abilities, brain functions, and neuroanatomical sites to see whether there truly are things that distinguish all stutterers from all nonstutterers. Failing to find that, we see whether there may be subgroups of stutterers, some of whom differ from nonstutterers in one way, and others who differ in another way. This may help us discover other paths leading to a better under-standing of stuttering.

In the next section, I will review some of the literature on stutterer/nonstutterer per-formance differences. As you will see, when scientists try to repeat others' experiments to verify their results, inconsistent research findings are common. One study finds a differ-ence; another study reports it isn't there. Differences in the findings of two studies may occur because different subjects were involved or because there were small differences in the way that the studies were done. For example, one study may use a 1000-Hz tone as a stimulus, and another study may use a recording of the word "go." Despite the inconsis-tencies in many results, there are areas of agreement or trends that many studies find. As you read, try to determine for yourself which areas give us solid leads. In my summaries, I will share my own interpretation of these areas of overlap.

Sensory Processing

You might wonder why research has been conducted on the ability of individuals who stutter to process such sensory information as auditory, visual, and tactile signals. Stut-tering, after all, appears to be a motor rather than a sensory problem. The answer is two-fold. First, as patients with various injuries and diseases have taught us, normal speech depends on intact auditory as well as tactile feedback, and researchers have been curious to see if stutterers' abnormal speech might be the result of some disturbance of feedback. Second, experiments that have altered sensory processing, such as delayed auditory feed-back (Black, 1951; Lee, 1951), have created repetitions, prolongations, and blocks in nor-mal speakers, prompting scientists to ask whether this might be the cause of stuttering.

The findings that I'm about to review may be related to the results of the brain imag-ing studies discussed earlier. Remember that many studies found that areas of the audi-tory cortex, particularly the superior temporal lobe regions, are under-activated during stuttering. It would not be surprising, then, if anomalies in this area affect both the flu-ency of speech production and the accuracy of speech perception. For example, the superior temporal gyrus has been shown to contain systems that are important in the phonemic planning of utterances and the understanding of speech (Hickok, 2001). Moreover, efficient functioning of the auditory cortex is likely to be critical for fluent speech production because of the crucial role of auditory feedback in normal speaking and the deleterious effects on fluency of delaying auditory feedback.

Central Auditory Processing

Research has assessed how well individuals who stutter can process auditory signals in various parts of the brain. A number of studies have used the Synthetic Sentence Iden-tification/Ipsilateral Competing Message test (SSI-ICM) to compare stutterers and nonstutterers. This test requires participants to identify words in a nonsense phrase (such as "small boat with a picture has become") when competing noise is presented in the same ear. Three studies using this test found that stutterers performed worse than normal participants (Hall and Jerger, 1978; Molt and Guilford, 1979; Toscher and Rupp, 1978). The same test was given to two groups of normal speakers: those who were judged to be more fluent and those who were judged to be less fluent. The more fluent normal speakers performed significantly better than the less fluent normal speakers (Wynne and Boehmler, 1982). This finding suggests that stuttering and normal disfluencies are not entirely different phenomena; both may be associated with some difficulty in central auditory processing. This difficulty may give rise to disfluencies in many children, only some of whom develop chronic stuttering. Some other factor in addition to an auditory processing difficulty may be necessary for high levels of normal disfluency to become stuttering.

In contrast to these studies, Hannley and Dorman (1982) found no differences between stutterers and nonstutterers on the SSI-ICM, but the stutterers in their study had all recently completed a treatment program. This finding is intriguing in light of evidence from brain imaging studies that individuals who stutter who had demonstrated an absence of activity before treatment in the left auditory cortex showed normal levels of activity immediately after treatment (De Nil et al, 2003; Ingham, 2003; Stager et al, 2003; Neumann et al, 2003).

Another tool for assessing central auditory processing is the Masking Level Difference (MLD) test, which requires listeners to detect the onset and offset of a tone in the presence of a masking noise. When masking noise is played in the same ear as the tone, there are fewer cues for listeners to use in "filtering" the tone from the masking noise. Listeners must use very subtle temporal cues to detect the tone; under these conditions, persons who stutter perform more poorly than groups of nonstutterers (Liebetrau and Daly, 1981; Kramer, Green, and Guitar, 1987). These results may be interpreted to support the outcome of the SSI studies because both tests require the participants to use temporal information—in one case (SSI), rapidly changing formant frequencies in identifying words, and in the other case (MLD), detection of the onset and offset of a tone in masking.

Two other studies of central auditory processing tested the hypothesis that people who stutter have difficulty resolving temporal differences. Herndon (1966) found that stutterers were poorer than nonstutterers at distinguishing which of two brief tones was longer. Barasch et al (2000) administered the Duration Pattern Sequence (DPS) test, which involves judging the relative lengths of three tones, and another measure in which subjects estimated the durations of tones and silent intervals. These tests failed to distinguish between the stuttering and nonstuttering participants as groups, but they showed that less-fluent participants in each group scored worse on the DPS than more fluent participants. In addition, more disfluent subjects in both groups judged temporal intervals to be longer than less disfluent subjects. This finding is evidence that there may be a connection between normal disfluency and stuttering. The authors speculated that one of the possible connections between increased disfluency and longer protensity estimates is the effect of fear and anxiety on speaking. It has been suggested that fear and anxiety affect temporal processing (Fraisse, 1963) and that anomalies in temporal processing may be an underlying cause of both stuttering (Kent, 1984) and high levels of normal disfluency (Wynne and Boehmler, 1982). Given the evidence that stutterers are no more anxious than nonstutterers (Guitar, 1998), one might ask the following question: why should stutterers' temporal processing for speech be any more susceptible to negative emotions than temporal processing in nonstutterers? The answer may be found in evidence that negative emotions, such as fear and anxiety, appear to be regulated by the right hemisphere, along with evidence that stutterers process speech in widely distributed areas of the right hemisphere. Thus, the close proximity of areas regulating negative emotions and speech production may allow cross-talk between these areas to interfere with speech, producing disfluency. It remains to be seen whether highly normally disfluent speakers also use right hemisphere structures for speech production.

Brain Electrical Potentials Reflecting Auditory Processing

Studies of electrical brain activity in response to auditory stimuli have provided further evidence that auditory processing is abnormal in individuals who stutter. Studies by Hood (1987) and Dietrich, Barry, and Parker (1995) reflecting both subcortical and cortical activity have found group differences between stutterers and nonstutterers. However, the first study found stutterers' responses to be slower than nonstutterers' responses, and the second study found them to be faster than nonstutterers' responses. A study by Molt (1997) is more relevant to the question raised by brain imaging studies of whether persons who stutter have a deficit in the left auditory cortex. Molt found that stutterers (compared with nonstutterers) had longer latencies and lower amplitudes of brain waves in the cortex when they were asked to make decisions about semantic incongruencies in sentences they listened to.

Dichotic Listening Tests

More support for the notion that stutterers have abnormal auditory processing comes from speech perception studies. In the early 1960s, a procedure was developed to assess hemispheric dominance for speech and language by testing which ear was more accurate at hearing speech sounds. Kimura (1961), a Canadian psychologist, invented the dichotic listening test, which simultaneously presented two different syllables (like "ba" and "da") dichotically (a different one to each ear). Listeners reported which syllable they heard. Auditory nerves connecting the ears to the cerebral hemispheres carry more information to the hemisphere on the opposite side than to the hemisphere on the same side. Results with normal speakers indicated that syllables presented to the right ear (opposite the left hemisphere, which is dominant for speech and language) were most frequently reported as heard, which was called a right-ear advantage for speech. This procedure has been used to assess laterality differences between stuttering and nonstuttering groups. A number of experiments found that many persons who stutter do not show the typical right ear advantage that nonstutterers do, which is evidence that people who stutter do not have left hemisphere dominance for language (Blood, 1985; Curry and Gregory, 1969; Davenport, 1977; Liebetrau and Daly, 1981; Sommers, Brady, and Moore, 1975). Some dichotic studies, however, found no differences between stutterers and nonstutterers (Dorman and Porter, 1975; Pinksy and McAdams, 1980; Slorach and Noer, 1973). Other studies found no significant group differences but found that fewer stutterers than nonstutterers showed the expected right-ear advantage (Brady and Berson, 1975; Quinn, 1972; Rosenfield and Goodglass, 1980; Strong, 1977). Like much research in this area, dichotic testing of stutterers suggested there might be group differences or at least subgroups of stutterers who differ from nonstutterers on a critical dimension. Examples of such subgroups might be those with more severe stuttering (Davenport, 1977) or those who show several positive signs on a neuropsychological test battery, suggesting an "organic" origin of their stuttering, or those showing only a few positive signs, suggesting a "functional" origin (Liebetrau and Daly, 1981). An additional finding was that the more linguistically complex the stimulus (for example, words vs. syllables), the more likely that differences between stutterers and nonstutterers would be found.

These findings point to the likelihood that any auditory processing anomaly related to stuttering is likely to be on a continuum, rather than simply present or absent. Moreover, more severe or more neurologically involved stutterers may have more abnormal auditory processing.

Auditory Feedback

Ever since the ancient Greek stutterer Demonsthenes improved his speech by orating above the roar of the Mediterranean Sea, it has been observed that changes in auditory feedback can affect fluency. Masking noise, delayed auditory feedback, frequency shifts, and other alterations in the properties of the auditory signal can create temporary fluency in persons who stutter (see Van Riper, 1982, for a review). On the other hand, delayed auditory feedback can create an artificial stutter in normal speakers (Black, 1951; Lee, 1951). A variety of explanations for the effects of altered feedback have been offered, including that it (1) is a distraction, (2) causes stutterers to change how they talk (becoming louder, for example), and (3) compensates for a defect in stutterers' auditory monitoring of their speech (Bloodstein, 1995; Garber and Martin, 1977).

One interesting hypothesis about how impaired auditory feedback affects speech was proposed by Stromsta (1957, 1972, 1986). His research on auditory feedback led him to suggest that stutterers' abnormal brain rhythms impair the integration of auditory feedback and speech output. The result, he suggested, is interruptions of phonation and improper coarticulation of sounds (Stromsta, 1986). This proposal foreshadows the results of recent brain imaging studies reviewed earlier. Stager et al (2003) suggested that their brain scans during fluency-inducing conditions indicated increased activity in stutterers' auditory areas, reflecting "more effective coupling of auditory and motor systems" (p. 334) so that auditory feedback could help to integrate the sequencing of speech motor output.

Other Sensory Feedback

The findings reviewed in the last few sections are related to the auditory system, but other sensory systems are important for the control of speech, specifically touch and movement. The few studies that have been conducted on these systems also show some deficits, but the results are mixed. Baker (1967) found that people who stutter performed more poorly than nonstutterers on tests of oral sensation. However, this finding was not replicated by Jensen et al (1975). On a test that required subjects to match spatially ordered visual patterns with temporally ordered auditory patterns, Cohen and Hansen (1975) found that individuals who stutter performed more poorly than those who do not stutter. Chuang et al (1980) evaluated stutterers' ability to make the smallest movements possible with their jaws and tongues. The stuttering group had significantly larger "difference limens," with or without the assistance of visual feedback, for such movements. This means that they did not have the degree of fine sensory-motor control of the jaw and tongue that the nonstuttering group did. De Nil and Abbs (1991) followed up on this study and demonstrated that stutterers had less sensorimotor control for minimal movements with their jaw, lip, and tongue (but not finger movements) compared with nonstutterers when using only kinesthetic feedback. There were no differences between the groups when using visual feedback. These studies, together with the findings about the auditory system, may indicate that, as a group, individuals who stutter have some difficulty using auditory, touch, and movement information to control speech. Indeed, it has been suggested that, because left hemisphere sensory areas are deficient in stutterers, they try to use a homologous right hemisphere system that "integrates auditory and oralingual-laryngeal somaesthetic information" to regulate speech and thereby increase fluency (Braun et al, 1997, p. 779). The topic of sensory-motor control of speech will be taken up in the next section.

Some of the most important findings regarding sensory processing and stuttering are summarized in Table 2–4, along with the clinical implication of these findings.

Sensory-Motor Control

On the surface, stuttering appears to be a disorder of speech motor control. Fluent speech depends on the muscles that move speech structures to produce airflow, voicing, and articulation in a coordinated fashion so that speech sounds are produced smoothly in a specified sequence and at a reasonable rate. Stuttered speech, then, must be the result of some disturbance in the smooth, sequenced muscle contraction for structural movements. Van Riper described this as "a temporal disruption of the simultaneous and successive programming of muscular movements" (Van Riper, 1971, p. 404; 1982, p. 415).

The control of the smooth movements of speech depends, in part, on sensory input as well as motor output. In fact, part of the control of any complex movement uses sensory

Table 2–4 Summary of Sensory Processing and Stuttering

Area of Interest	Important Findings	Major Clinical Implications
Sensory Processing	Stutterers show the following differences from nonstutterers: poorer central auditory processing, especially with regard to temporal information; auditory evoked potentials of stutterers may have longer latencies and lower amplitudes when listening to linguistically complex stimuli; some dichotic listening studies have found that stutterers have less right ear/left hemisphere advantage (more evident in more severe stutterers; more likely when stimuli are linguistically complex); a small number of studies suggest stutterers may be poorer at processing tactile and visual information	Dysfunction of auditory system implicated in stuttering. Use of other sensory feedback for speech, such as proprioception, may be helpful as a therapeutic strategy.
	Masking and other changes in the way that stutterers hear themselves speaking can decrease the frequency and severity of stuttering.	Temporary fluency can be obtained by masking or distorting auditory feedback.

information about where the structure is now and where it's going to produce just the right amount of contraction of all the muscles involved. When the brain plans the movements needed to produce sounds, it uses stored memories of past movements and their consequences in planning what must be moved, as well as when and how to produce the desired acoustic and perceptual result (the sounds of speech). This section reviews several areas of research that have looked at stutterers' speech and nonspeech motor control. It is important to remember that, even if it is not explicitly stated by researchers, investigations of motor skills are, in fact, investigations of sensorimotor skills.

Reaction Time

Figure 2–5 depicts an example of a reaction time experiment. The participant is told to watch the computer screen for a picture of an object and to say the name of the object

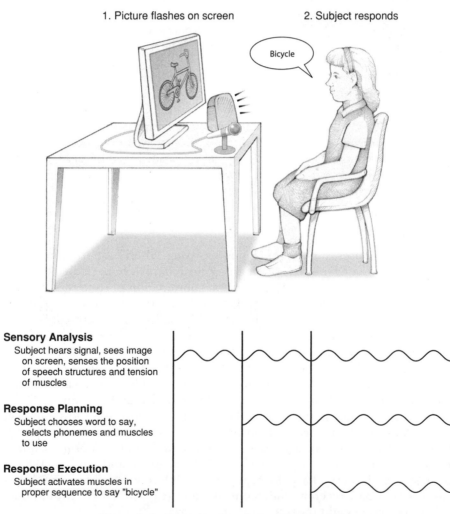

1. Picture flashes on screen   2. Subject responds

Bicycle

Sensory Analysis
Subject hears signal, sees image on screen, senses the position of speech structures and tension of muscles

Response Planning
Subject chooses word to say, selects phonemes and muscles to use

Response Execution
Subject activates muscles in proper sequence to say "bicycle"

Figure 2–5   *Processing stages in a reaction time task.*

the instant it appears. The time between the appearance of the object on the screen and the first sound or movement made by the participant is her reaction time. As indicated, reaction time involves sensory analysis, response planning, and response execution. Therefore, reaction time is a potentially useful measure in stuttering research if it is thought that the core deficit is a delay in some aspect of sensory processing, planning, or motor execution.

The first experiments on people who stutter found that they were slower than non-stutterers in initiating and terminating a vowel in response to a buzzer (Adams and Hayden, 1976; Starkweather, Hirschman, and Tannenbaum, 1976). Later experiments showed that stutterers were slower than nonstutterers in reacting with respiratory (exhalation) and articulatory movements (lip closing) (McFarlane and Prins, 1978; Watson and Alfonso, 1987) and were also slower whether they were responding to auditory or visual signals (Cross and Cooke, 1979). Children who stutter were also found to have slower reaction times in similar studies (Cross and Luper, 1979, 1983; Cullinan and Springer, 1980; Maske-Cash and Curlee, 1995; Till et al, 1983).

Although not all studies showed group differences, De Nil (1995) pointed out that about 75% of the 44 voice reaction time studies that he reviewed found that people who stutter were significantly slower than people who do not stutter and that most of the other studies showed trends in that direction. He further noted that, when investigators used linguistically meaningful stimuli to test reaction time (words or sentences, rather than isolated sounds), 80% of the studies found significant differences between stutterers and nonstutterers. These findings are likely to be related to the evidence from brain imaging studies indicating that individuals who stutter have anomalies in areas used for sensorimotor processing of speech and language. Not surprisingly, these anomalies may affect sensorimotor reaction times on nonspeech tasks but are most evident in tasks requiring linguistic processing.

Fluent Speech

Reaction time responses, such as lip closing or saying "ahhh," are indirect measures of speech processing under normal conditions. Researchers have been able to make more direct assessments by examining the speed and coordination of stutterers' speech movements when they are talking fluently and by analyzing the sound waves of their fluent speech. Acoustic studies have demonstrated that stutterers, on average, have longer vowel durations, slower transitions between consonants and vowels, and delayed onsets of voicing after voiceless consonants (Colcord and Adams, 1979; DiSimoni, 1974; Hillman and Gilbert, 1977; Starkweather and Myers, 1979). The findings of these acoustic studies have been supported by "kinematic" research, which has measured the movements of speakers' speech structures (e.g., Alfonso, Story, and Watson, 1987; Zimmerman, 1980). As a group, stutterers have been found to move their lips and jaws more slowly, even during fluent speech, than nonstutterers (e.g., Zimmerman, 1980). Kinematic research has also shown that some stutterers demonstrate abnormal sequencing of articulator movement onsets and velocities (Caruso, Abbs, and Gracco, 1988). Other kinematic studies, however, have not found group differences or have found them only in stutterers who had recently undergone therapy (e.g., McClean, Kroll, and Loftus, 1990) that may have taught them to speak more slowly.

So what does this mean? Why might many stutterers speak more slowly or use different sequences of articulatory movements than nonstuttering speakers even when they are fluent? Some researchers think that these findings reflect delays or other dysfunctions in processing incoming and outgoing signals. Stutterers may be unable to process neural signals fast enough to make the rapid, precise movements of normal conversational speech, especially when they are under the stress of planning a complex sentence or competing with other talkers. Their delays in voicing onset, slower transitions, and abnormal sequencing during fluent speech may just reflect a slower mechanism working at its normal rate. A different view, suggested by more skeptical researchers, is that such differences simply reflect the way stutterers have learned to talk to avoid stuttering, either on their own or as a result of therapy, and this way of speaking keeps them fluent even with an inefficient speech motor system.

Another interpretation of these slower movements is that they are the result of heightened tension in muscles having antagonistic functions for speech production (Starkweather, 1987). For example, increased tension in muscles that move a structure forward (agonists), as well as muscles that hold it back (antagonists), would make movement of that structure considerably slower. Imagine two people pulling a rope in opposite directions. Even if one were stronger, she would make slow progress in her direction because the other, weaker person would create a drag. The slowed movements of stutterers' speech structures would account for not only slower reaction times, but also the longer movement durations in their fluent speech. Findings from a number of studies support this view. They have reported that stutterers co-contract agonist and antagonist muscles of both the laryngeal (Freeman and Ushijima, 1975; Shapiro, 1980) and articulatory (Guitar et al, 1988) muscle groups during stuttering. These studies, like Starkweather's (1987) review, have noted that such co-contraction of agonist and antagonist muscles appears even in some of the apparently fluent speech of stutterers. This finding has led many researchers to posit that stuttering is not an all or nothing event (Adams and Runyan, 1981; Bloodstein, 1987). Sometimes, stutterers may speak freely, without a trace of excess tension. Sometimes, they may have excess tension that isn't heard by listeners as stuttering. And sometimes, muscle tension may be so great that both the listeners and the person who stutters are acutely aware of the stuttering. This continuum of fluency reflects the subjective impression of many stutterers, including this author.

Nonspeech Motor Control

Following in the wake of studies that showed that individuals who stutter often have slower than normal reaction times and slower segments in their fluent speech, researchers began to examine complex motor coordinations of nonspeech muscles and structures. One advantage of this approach is that it eliminates the effect of learned coping responses that may be contaminating measures of speech movements. Second, complex motor coordinations, such as sequential finger movements, appear to be planned and organized by areas of the brain, such as the supplementary motor area (SMA), which also appear to be involved in the sequential articulatory movements of speech (Goldberg, 1985). Interestingly, neurophysiological evidence that sequential finger movements are regulated by the same brain regions that control speech has been supported by arguments that spoken language in humans evolved from right-hand/left-hemisphere specialization for manipulating objects and hand gesturing in earlier hominids (Kent, 1997; MacNeilage, 1987).

In a study of both sequential finger movements and sequential counting aloud fluently, Borden (1983) found that severe stutterers, but not mild stutterers, were slower than nonstutterers in executing both finger movement and speech tasks. Thus, severe stutterers may have substantial deficits in certain sensory-motor tasks, but mild stutterers may have only slight deficits, and these deficits may require special task conditions to be revealed.

Ten years later, Webster (1993) developed a finger movement task in which participants tapped four numbered keys in a predetermined sequence. To make the task somewhat like speech, participants were assigned a novel sequence of keys at the beginning of each trial (3-2-4-1 or 4-1-2-3, etc). In both timed and untimed tests, stutterers made more errors sequencing and were slower initiating the task but were comparable to nonstutterers in execution time. Unlike Borden's study, no effort was made to analyze the results by subjects' stuttering severity. Webster thought that these results suggested that stutterers may have difficulty in "response planning, organization, and initiation" (Webster, 1993, p. 84) of novel sequences of movements.

To answer the question of why this difficulty may be present only intermittently in individuals who stutter (after all, they have a great deal of fluent speech), Webster (1993) postulated what others (Cross, Sweet, and Bates, 1985; Curlee, personal communication, 1990; Peters and Guitar, 1991) have also considered, that at times, such as under stress, there is cross-talk or interference between the hemispheres. Specifically, activity in the right hemisphere interferes with sequential movement control in the left hemisphere.

To test this, Webster used a task in which participants performed sequential finger tapping with the right hand while turning a knob with the left hand, in response to an auditory signal. If his hypothesis were true, the stuttering group's left hemisphere–controlled finger tapping would be vulnerable to interference by the right hemisphere–controlled knob turning. Indeed, the stuttering group's performance was significantly poorer than that of the nonstuttering group on both tasks.

Webster (1997) then wondered if interference of left-hemisphere sequential movement control mechanisms might be the result of stutterers' inability to focus attention on the left-hemisphere task and ignore interference from a competing source, whether from the right or left hemisphere. To test this, Webster used a procedure developed to investigate attention focus in right- and left-handed people. Participants were required to tap twice with one hand for every tap they made with the other hand. They were tested with the right hand double tapping and the left hand single tapping, and vice versa. The nonstutterers were able to perform the task significantly better when they tapped twice with the right hand and once with the left; however, stutterers and nonstuttering left-handed subjects performed the task equally well with either hand doing the double tapping. Webster interpreted this outcome as suggesting that stutterers and left-handed nonstutterers did not have the ability to focus predominantly on the left hemisphere but had equal focus on both, making their left hemispheres vulnerable to interference from other activities. Webster's model of stuttering, derived from these experiments, postulates that individuals who stutter are unable to protect the integrity of speech production centers from interference or cross-talk from emotions or other on-going processes. It is not clear why, then, all left-handed people do not stutter. I would presume that this model proposes that stutterers have both a deficit in the sequencing of processing underlying speech production as well as an inability to focus on the left hemisphere.

The last studies of nonspeech motor control I will review concern the use of auditory input to control motor output. A common paradigm in these studies is to have participants track or follow the changing frequency (pitch) of a target sound with a second sound, called a cursor. A computer controls the pitch changes in the target's sound, and participants follow these changes by using their hand or their jaw to move a lever that changes the pitch of the cursor. Using this paradigm, Sussman and MacNeilage (1975) found that normal speakers made fewer errors tracking the target sound when the cursor tone was presented to the right ear and the target tone was presented to the left ear. Persons who stuttered, on the other hand, made equal numbers of errors whether the cursor tone was in the right ear and the target tone was in the left ear or vice versa, suggesting that they did not have a left hemisphere advantage for integrating auditory information with motor output, as the nonstutterers did.

Researchers in Australia replicated and extended this work on tracking (Neilson, 1980; Neilson and Neilson, 1987, 1988), using both visual and auditory targets and cursors. They demonstrated that participants who stuttered were significantly poorer using auditory targets and cursors than when using visual ones. They also showed that, when both stuttering and nonstuttering participants practiced the tasks beforehand, the differences between the groups was even larger than when they had not practiced. The Neilsons proposed that stutterers were slow in developing a mental auditory-motor model of the relationship between their movement of the cursor control and the resulting sound change. They further hypothesized that the basic deficit in stuttering is difficulty in forming or accessing auditory-motor models of what speech movements are needed to produce the sounds they want to make. I suspect that the Neilsons would agree that stutterers can use their auditory-motor models better in situations where the demands on their neural resources are low but that they have more trouble when the demands are high.

As the Neilsons were working on their experiments in Australia, researchers at Baylor College of Medicine in Texas were also studying the auditory-motor tracking abilities of persons who stutter. In a series of publications (Nudelman et al, 1987; 1989; 1992), the researchers described experiments that required participants to hum along with a tone that suddenly changed pitch. The pitch of the target tones was sometimes changed rapidly and sometimes changed slowly, while researchers measured how quickly participants could change their humming to match the changing pitch of the auditory target tone. The researchers found that stutterers were significantly slower than nonstutterers in detecting changes in the target's frequency, suggesting that stutterers need more time to process auditory signals. Once again, we find that research has produced evidence that, as a group, people who stutter have difficulty performing auditory processing tasks.

The major findings regarding stutterers' abilities in speech and nonspeech sensory-motor control and the clinical implications are given in Table 2–5.

Table 2–5   Summary of Sensory-Motor Control and Stuttering

Area of Interest	Important Findings	Major Clinical Implications
Sensory-Motor Control	Compared with nonstutterers, individuals who stutter appear to have these differences: stutterers' reaction times are slower, especially when linguistically meaningful stimuli are used; stutterers' fluent speech is slower (longer vowels, slower transitions, delayed onset of voicing); stutterers are slower and make more errors on nonspeech tasks of sequencing (may be more true for more severe stutterers); hand tapping task suggested that stutterers are not as able to focus on left hemisphere motor control (may be vulnerable to interference from right hemisphere or other areas of left hemisphere); stutterers are poorer at auditory-motor tracking (may not have left hemisphere advantage for auditory-motor tracking; may be slower at developing a mental model of auditory-motor relationships).	Possibility that training in auditory-speech motor control could improve fluency. Evidence that stutterers are slower at a variety of tasks suggests that slower speech rate may facilitate fluency.

Language

In chapter 1, I described research findings indicating that stuttering is influenced by language. First, there is evidence that the onset of stuttering generally occurs at ages when language growth is greatest (Bloodstein, 1995). Second, studies have shown that disfluencies increase when speakers produce longer, more linguistically complex sentences (Bernstein Ratner, 1997). And finally, when and where stuttering is likely to occur in spoken language is influenced by such linguistic factors as the lexical class of a word, its length, and its location in a sentence (Wingate, 1988).

Although stuttering may be precipitated or exacerbated by language factors, a recent brain imaging study provided evidence that language difficulty may not be the primary cause of stuttering. De Nil, Kroll, and Houle (submitted) compared brain scans of stutterers and nonstutterers while they performed two tasks: reading single words aloud and generating verbs. Although both tasks involved saying single words aloud, the verb generation task engaged more language processing, specifically, semantic and phonological searching and encoding. To assess whether the two groups differed on the two tasks, the experimenters "subtracted" the scans of reading the words aloud from the scans of generating verbs. In other words, they wanted to see if just the extra demand of generating verbs showed a big difference between the two groups, so they took out all activity in the verb generation task that was also present just in reading words aloud. The subtraction indicated that there were minimal differences between the groups in the more linguistically involved task of generating verbs, although there were large differences between the groups in reading words aloud. This suggested that the added linguistic burden of having to think of verbs was not particularly more demanding on the stutterers than on the nonstutterers.

Studies of stutterer–nonstutterer differences on performance tasks, reviewed earlier in this chapter, however, support the notion that language factors are important in stuttering, affecting both speech and nonspeech tasks. For example, the results of dichotic listening studies and reaction time experiments indicate that there are greater stutterer–nonstutterer differences when the stimuli used are more linguistically complex and more meaningful (e.g, Curry and Gregory, 1969; De Nil, 1995). Moreover, Kleinow and Smith (2000) found that linguistic complexity affected the stability of speech motor control in stutterers. Using a measure called the spatiotemporal index, which reflects the amount of variability in articulator movement when a sentence is said over and over, Kleinow and Smith demonstrated that longer and more syntactically complex sentences produced significantly more instability in stutterers' speech production than simpler and shorter sentences. The same was not true for nonstutterers. Kleinow and Smith (2000) interpreted these findings as suggesting that stutterers' speech production systems are more vulnerable to breakdown when language demands are high.

How does one reconcile these different views? On one hand, there is evidence from a brain imaging study that the basic problem of stuttering may be in "sensorimotor processes involved in speech production" rather than in the "cognitive language formulation processes" involved in speech production (De Nil, 2004, p. 123). On the other hand, there is strong evidence that when linguistic complexity is greater, stutterers show poorer performance on both perception and production tasks. These two views may be reconciled if one assumes that the basic defect is in sensorimotor control of speech but that individuals who stutter achieve fluency by compensating for that sensorimotor defect by using additonal neuronal resources, additional attention, or simplifying their task by slowing their speech rate. When language becomes more complex and/or sentences become longer, speech rate increases (Starkweather, 1981), and it would seem, from evidence that there is more distributed brain activity when language is more complex, that more neuronal resources and attention are devoted to the greater language demands. Thus, fewer extra resources are available to compensate for the sensorimotor defect and more stuttering results. The notion that stutterers have a limitation on their neural resources during speech and language production is supported by De Nil and Bosshardt (2001), who showed that stutterers perform more poorly than nonstutterers on phonological and semantic tasks when engaged in two tasks simultaneously. The major findings and clinical implications regarding language and stuttering are presented in Table 2–6.

Table 2–6   Summary of Language Factors in Stuttering

Area of Interest	Important Findings	Major Clinical Implications
Language	Stuttering onset is often associated with language development. More stuttering occurs in longer, more complex sentences; stuttering influenced by linguistic factors such as lexical class of word, length, and location in sentence. More linguistically complex stimuli result in poorer performances by stuttering on many performance tasks.	Decreasing linguistic load on children who are beginning to stutter may reduce their stuttering.

Emotion

Because people who stutter are a heterogeneous group, the relationship between emotion and stuttering, like the relationship between language and stuttering, will vary among individuals. For some, emotion may be an important etiological factor that triggers the onset of stuttering and makes recovery difficult. For others, although emotion in strong doses may cause stuttering to change (sometimes for the worse and sometimes for the better), it may not be a major factor in its cause. Conversely, the experience of stuttering generates emotions, such as frustration, fear, and anger, in everyone who stutters.

We will begin a discussion of emotion and stuttering with a review of the research that has studied the link between stuttering and anxiety and then examine the evidence suggesting that many people who stutter have more sensitive temperaments than fluent speakers.

Anxiety and Autonomic Arousal

The average listener may think that people stutter because they are nervous. Scientists, following up on this impression, have used such terms as "anxiety," "autonomic arousal," and "negative emotion" to specify the emotional states that may cause or accompany stuttering. In one of the more interesting early studies, Hill (1954) demonstrated that nonstutterers showed stuttering-like repetitions and prolongations when a red light that was associated with electric shock flashed on when they were speaking. The expectation of shock, Hill reasoned, created a momentary sensation of anxiety that resulted in the disfluencies.

In an early study of anxiety and stuttering, Horovitz et al (1978) looked at a phenomenon called the stapedial reflex, which had been previously shown to increase during anxiety in normal speakers. The stapedial reflex is a muscle contraction in the middle ear, triggered by activation of the laryngeal nerve just prior to speaking, that decreases the loudness with which a speaker hears his or her own voice. Horovitz et al found that stutterers demonstrated an increased stapedial reflex when they became more anxious (as measured by a physiological assessment of anxiety) compared with a no-anxiety condition. A group of matched nonstutterers showed no increase in stapedial reflex. Participants in both groups increased their anxiety by imagining themselves in a stressful speaking situation. Although the results of this study are hard to interpret, it appears to show that an increase in anxiety in stutterers may result in changes in speech-related physiology when only imagining some difficulty speaking. It may be relevant that the increase in stapedial reflex may have been brought about by an increase in laryngeal nerve activity. This connection between autonomic arousal and heightened laryngeal muscle activity may reflect a conditioned response that becomes part of the learning, which maintains stuttering in some individuals.

More recently, researchers have asked whether people who stutter are more anxious than people who do not stutter. To answer their questions, they have used various measures of physiological arousal, such as heart rate, skin conductance, and level of cortisol (a chemical secreted by the brain under conditions of stress) in saliva secretion.

Four studies (Caruso et al, 1994; Miller, 1993; Peters and Hulstijn, 1984; Weber and Smith, 1990) found that both stutterers and nonstutterers show high levels of autonomic arousal when they have to speak or read aloud, indicating that people who stutter are not more anxious or more nervous than people who do not stutter. However, several studies of autonomic arousal have reported that higher levels of arousal are associated with more disfluency in stutterers (Caruso et al, 1994; Miller, 1993; Weber and Smith, 1990). Although most speakers may show increased arousal when they have to speak, it may be that only the speech of those who stutter is vulnerable to breakdown (unless arousal is unusually high, as in the Hill, 1954, experiment). If so, this appears to be analogous to the findings of Kleinow and Smith (2000), which were cited in the previous section, that indicated that the speech production systems of stutterers, but not nonstutterers, become more unstable in response to high language load. We may be seeing, in both cases, the effect on speech production of any other task requiring attention or using a sizable amount of neural resources.

Temperament

Many of us who work with children who stutter have often heard parents describe their child as particularly sensitive. Upon questioning, these parents frequently say that, even before stuttering began, the child was more easily upset by changes in routine or was shyer with strangers than his or her siblings. These emotional and behavioral characteristics may be a part of the child's inherited physiology. Some children seem to be born with a sensitive or inhibited temperament and are more likely to react to new people and novel situations with increased muscle tension and physiological signs of stress (Kagan, Reznick, and Snidman, 1987).

A number of authors have speculated about the possible importance of considering temperament in gaining a better understanding of the nature of stuttering (e.g, Bloodstein, 1987, 1995; Conture, 1991; Guitar, 1997, 1998, 1999, 2000; Peters and Guitar, 1991). A reactive temperament, for example, might trigger increased physical tension in a child when he or she is disfluent and thus create a learned cycle of disfluency begetting more severe disfluencies, leading to chronic stuttering. On the other hand, a placid temperament in an equally disfluent child might allow the child to stay relaxed, ignore the disfluencies, and thereby outgrow early stuttering.

Data on the sensitivity of people who stutter are meager. In a questionnaire study, Oyler (1992) found that adults who stutter were more emotionally sensitive than adults who do not stutter; however, this hypersensitivity could be the result of many years of stuttering. Greater sensitivity in children who stutter has been reported by several studies. Fowlie and Cooper (1978) reported that mothers of children who stutter viewed them as more sensitive than mothers describing children who do not stutter. Oyler and Ramig (1995) found that parents of children who stutter rated them as more sensitive than control parents who rated their nonstuttering children. Using the concept of "difficult" temperament, which includes some aspects of sensitivity as well as restlessness and impulsiveness, both Wakaba (1998) and Embrechts and Ebben (1999) found that parents of stuttering children rated their children as having this type of temperament to a greater degree than parents of nonstuttering children. LaSalle (1999) presented a paper indicating that, in contrast to parents of young children who don't stutter, parents of young children who do stutter rated them as having high frustration reactions and lack of persistence. Both of these traits have been associated with sensitive temperament (Thomas and Chess, 1977). Anderson et al (2003) found that parents of children who stutter rate their children as more sensitive, compared with parents of nonstuttering children, on the Behavioral Style Questionnaire (McDevitt and Carey, 1978).

Using a physiological measure of sensitivity, Guitar (2003) found that the acoustic startle responses of adults who stutter were significantly greater than those of adults who do not stutter. The startle paradigm, which measures the magnitude of the eyeblink in response to a burst of white noise, is believed to differentiate individuals whose nervous systems have a low threshold of arousal from those whose nervous systems require a larger stimulus to react (Vrana, Spence, and Lang, 1988). Moreover, it has demonstrated differences in children who have been categorized as temperamentally inhibited and temperamentally uninhibited (Snidman and Kagan, 1994). Guitar (2003) also found substantial correlations between startle responses and scores on the Nervous subscale of the Taylor-Johnson Temperament Analysis (Taylor and Morrison, 1996).

With evidence in hand that at least some individuals who stutter have more sensitive temperaments, we need to ask how this may shed light on the disruption of fluency by emotion. Psychologists who study temperament have looked carefully at the regulation and expression of emotion in persons with sensitive temperaments. There is good evidence from studies of both normal and brain-damaged patients that the regulation of emotion is a lateralized function (Kinsbourne, 1989; Kinsbourne and Bemporad, 1984). Emotions regulated by the left hemisphere appear to motivate such behaviors as approach, exploration, and action, whereas emotions regulated by the right hemisphere motivate behaviors such as avoidance, withdrawal, and the arrest of action. Studies of electrical activity in the brain indicate that individuals with sensitive temperaments are right hemisphere dominant for emotionally based behaviors (Ahern and Schwartz, 1985; Calkins and Fox, 1994). This means that, if stutterers are temperamentally reactive as a group, they may have an inborn proclivity toward behaviors motivated by right hemisphere emotions, such as avoidance, withdrawal, and the arrest of action.

How this may affect speech is not yet clear, but Webster (1993) speculates that when individuals who stutter are emotionally aroused, right hemisphere proclivities, such as avoidance and withdrawal, could affect their left hemisphere supplementary motor area, interfering with its planning and initiation of speech. My own speculation about the relationship between emotion and stuttering is that one important aspect of right hemisphere–dominant, emotionally based behaviors is the arrest of ongoing behavior. This phenomenon is especially well described by Jeffrey Gray (1987), a psychologist who has studied the central nervous system's response to stress. He proposes that, when an individual experiences fear or frustration, a behavioral inhibition system in the brain increases three distinct forms of behavior: (1) freezing, which involves widespread muscular contractions that produce tense and silent immobility, (2) flight, and (3) avoidance. It is possible that such behaviors may be manifested in speech by both core behaviors (repetitions, prolongations, and blocks) and secondary behaviors (escape and avoidance).

Indirect support for this possiblity may be the findings by Kagan, Reznick, and Snidman (1987) that more sensitive children manifest their reactivity by generating higher levels of physical tension, particularly in laryngeal muscles, when they are speaking in unfamiliar or threatening situations. I suspect that some children who are both sensitive and have a vulnerable motor speech system may respond to early repetitive disfluencies with increased tension, especially in the laryngeal region. This tightening may further interfere with speech, producing the abruptly terminated repetitions, prolongations, and blocks that develop in many children when stuttering persists. Other children who are highly sensitive and predisposed to have motor speech breakdowns may begin their disfluencies with tense prolongations and blocks in response to emotionally difficult situations. The heterogeneity of individuals who stutter and their unique patterns of stuttering will be discussed further in upcoming chapter sections on developmental factors and learning.

Brain imaging studies have shown extensive activity during stuttering in the right insula (Fox, 2003) and the anterior cingulate cortex (Braun et al, 1997; De Nil et al, 2000). Both of these areas have strong connections with the amygdala (Allman et al, 2001; Habib et al, 1995), which is a major structure in fear conditioning (Le Doux, 2002). It is possible that some of the right hemisphere activity heightened during stuttering and reduced during induced fluency may reflect negative emotional arousal. My reasoning is that, first, many of the studies reviewed in this chapter suggest that, in stutterers, speech planning and production are localized in right hemisphere regions homologous to Broca's, Wernicke's, and interconnecting areas. Second, emotions lateralized to the right hemisphere in the human brain are those associated with fear, such as avoidance, escape, and arrest of ongoing behavior (Kinsbourne, 1989). Third, because strong emotions tend to dominate the neural processes in surrounding areas (Le Doux, 2002), these emotions may disrupt ongoing speech processing in ways analagous to how they affect all behavior (avoidance behaviors, escape behaviors, and blocks).

Major findings and clinical implications regarding emotional factors in stuttering are summarized in Table 2–7.

In this chapter, I have reviewed the evidence for a constitutional basis for stuttering. In the next chapter, I will discuss developmental and environmental factors that may

Table 2–7 Summary of Emotional Factors in Stuttering

Area of Interest	Important Findings	Major Clinical Implications
Emotion	Stutterers do not appear to be more anxious than nonstutterers, but anxiety or autonomic arousal in stutterers is associated with stuttering. Some evidence suggests that stutterers tend to have a more sensitive or inhibited temperament.	For many persistent stutterers, treatment programs may benefit from components that facilitate the unlearning of fear-based stuttering behaviors.

interact with constitutional factors to produce the disorder. In the subsequent chapter, I will integrate these findings to provide a comprehensive view of how all of the factors may combine to precipitate stuttering in an individual.

Summary

- Stuttering appears to have a genetic basis in many individuals. However, studies of twins and adoption studies confirm that genes must interact with environmental factors for stuttering to appear.

- Stuttering may have its etiology in congenital factors for some stutterers. These factors may include physical trauma at birth, cerebral palsy, retardation, and emotionally stressful situations.

- Slightly more boys begin to stutter than girls, but girls are more likely to recover, so that by school age and beyond, there are many more boys who stutter than girls.

- Early childhood stuttering may be either *transitory,* in which the child recovers naturally within 18 months with no or minimal treatment, or *persistent,* in which the child, if not treated, stutters for 3 years or more.

- Persistent and transitory stuttering appears to be the result of a common genetic factor (either a single gene or several), but the persistent form of stuttering probably has additional genetic factors that impede recovery.

- Natural recovery from stuttering appears to be associated with the following factors: (1) good scores on tests of phonology, language, and nonverbal skills, (2) either no family history of stuttering or family members who had natural recovery from stuttering, (3) early age of onset of stuttering, and (4) being a girl.

- Brain imaging studies of adults who stutter have shown various anomalies during speaking and especially during stuttering. One anomaly is over-activation in right brain areas homologous to left hemisphere speech and language structures typically used by nonstutterers. Another anomaly is deactivation in the left auditory cortex.

- Neuroanatomical differences seen via brain imaging include (1) anomalies in the planum temporale and in gyri in speech and language areas and (2) less dense fiber tracts connecting speech perception, planning, and execution areas.

- Inducement of short-term or long-term fluency in stutterers is accompanied by decreases in right hemisphere activations and increases in activation of left hemisphere speech, language, and auditory areas.

- On tasks of sensory processing, stutters have less accurate and slower processing, particularly of auditory stimuli, and lack of left hemisphere dominance for processing. Greatest performance deficits occur when linguistically complex stimuli are used. Masking and other changes in auditory feedback creates temporary fluency, suggesting that distortions, deficits, or delays in auditory feedback may be associated with stuttering.

- On tasks of sensory-motor control, stutterers demonstrate slower reaction times, especially when stimuli are linguistically more complex. Stutterers are slower, less accurate, and less left hemisphere dominant when performing sequential motor tasks and auditory-motor tasks.

- When there is a greater linguistic load, stutterers' speech motor systems are more variable; greater linguistic load is also associated with more stuttering.

- Stutterers do not appear to be more anxious than nonstutterers, but there is evidence that when their autonomic arousal levels are high, more stuttering is likely to occur.

- As a group, stuttering children and adults have a more sensitive temperament; this sensitivity may be associated with more physical tension in laryngeal muscles.

Study Questions

1. How do each of the areas of family studies, twin studies, and adoption studies provide evidence that stuttering is inherited?

2. A couple comes to you for advice. They tell you they are thinking of having children but are worried because each has a relative who stutters. What more information would you like to get from them? What would you tell them about the likelihood that they would have a child who stutters and whether they should be concerned?

3. Are there studies that provide evidence that stuttering is a product of both heredity and environment?

4. How would you summarize the brain imaging studies to someone who is not a professional in our field?

5. Why do almost all the brain imaging studies use right-handed males as participants?

6. Researchers have found many differences between groups of stutterers and nonstutterers. Why can't we say that these differences *cause* stuttering?

7. Explain how the deficits in sensory processing in people who stutter could be related to the actual behaviors of stuttering?

8. What are the differences between sensory processing and sensory-motor control?

9. Do you think difficulty with language processing may be a cause of stuttering for some individuals? Why or why not?

10. Describe the relationships between emotion and stuttering.

11. What research finding in this chapter do you think has the most relevance for the treatment of stuttering. Defend your answer.

SUGGESTED PROJECTS

(1) Talk to someone who stutters and plot out his or her family tree for relatives who stutter and relatives who have other speech, language, or learning problems.

(2) Make a family tree of your own relatives indicating which, if any, currently have or have had in the past a speech, language, hearing, or learning disability. Describe how you got the information and what the disabilities are.

(3) On which side of the brain do you process speech and language? Find out how you could ascertain this information by asking speech–language pathology researchers or audiologists you know if they have tests you could take to find out. If this doesn't lead to a test for this kind of laterality, search the Internet for self-administered tests, which tell you whether you are more "left-brained" or more "right-brained."

(4) Use a digital stopwatch (how fast can you turn it on and off?) or similar instrument to determine your reaction time. Try this under many different conditions, such as at several times during the day or when sick or tired versus when feeling alert. Determine what variables affect your reaction times, and see whether these variables affect other people as well. Using this information, suggest why different studies of reaction times in stutterers get different outcomes.

(5) Find a temperament test, such as those available on-line, and administer it to both a group of people with a speech, language, hearing, or learning disorder besides stuttering and to a matched group of people with typical functioning and see whether there are differences in temperament.

Suggested Readings

Yairi, E., and Ambrose, N.G. (2005). *Early Childhood Stuttering: For Clinicians by Clinicians.* **Austin, TX: Pro-Ed.**

The authors describe in depth the results of 14 years of research on the development of stuttering conducted at the University of Illinois. Chapters are devoted to the onset and development of stuttering; characteristics of children's disfluency; genetics; and cognitive, psychosocial, and motor factors in stuttering. Elaine Paden and Ruth Watkins contributed chapters on phonological and language abilities, respectively, of children who stutter. Like Wendell Johnson's magnum opus *The Onset of Stuttering*, this book pulls together a monumental effort focused on childhood stuttering.

Maassen, B., Kent, R., Peters, H., van Lieshout, P., Hulstijn, W. (Eds.) (2004). *Speech Motor Control in Normal and Disordered Speech.* **Oxford: Oxford University Press.**
   This book contains updated chapters by many scientists who presented their findings at a conference on speech motor control in 2001. Although not all of the contents are directly related to stuttering, there is much of great interest to clinicians and researchers interested in the neurophysiological bases of speech and stuttering.

Van Riper, C. (1982). *The Nature of Stuttering* **(ed 2). Englewood Cliffs, NJ: Prentice-Hall.**
   Although now dated, this book reviews an impressive amount of world literature on stuttering, from as long ago as the 20th century B.C. In his attempted synthesis, Van Riper presents his venerable hypothesis that stuttering is a disorder of timing.

Curlee, R., and Siegel, G. (Eds.) (1997). *Nature and Treatment of Stuttering: New Directions* **(ed 2). Boston: Allyn & Bacon.**
   This edited text brings together chapters by leading clinicians and researchers in stuttering. The editors elicit considerable homogeneity among the authors' styles so that it is not difficult to read. A new edition should be available in 2006.

Chapter 3

Developmental, Environmental, and Learning Factors

Many factors, both in a child and in his or her environment, create the conditions under which stuttering first emerges and then grows progressively worse, stabilizes, or disappears. Some of these factors are part of the child's normal development, such as the explosive growth of speech and language skills during preschool years. Other factors may be common situations that most children take in stride as they grow up, such as competing with siblings for attention and speaking time in a busy home. These developmental and environmental influences do not seem to be the cause of stuttering by themselves but may interact with constitutional factors, such as those discussed in Chapter 2, to precipitate stuttering from the time a child begins to speak in phrases and sentences until puberty. Figure 3–1 depicts the interaction of constitutional factors that predispose a child to stutter with those developmental and environmental factors that contribute to the emergence of stuttering during the busy and sometimes stressful years of childhood.

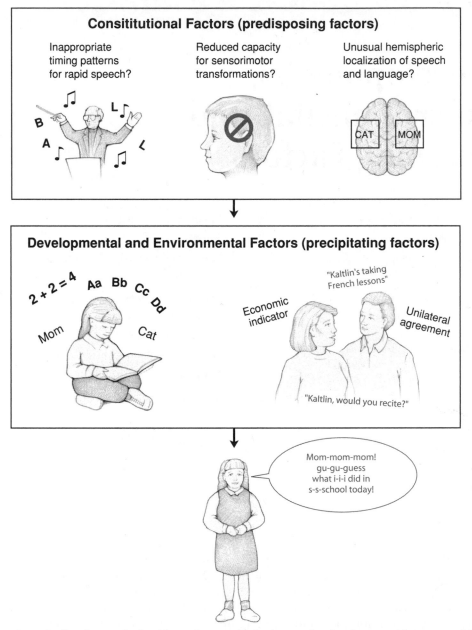

Figure 3–1   *Predisposing constitutional factors interact with developmental and environmental factors to precipitate or worsen stuttering.*

In addition to developmental and environmental factors that may precipitate stuttering, there are also factors that perpetuate it or may even cause it to grow worse. These are various types of learning: classical, operant, and avoidance conditioning. Learning, of course, affects all of our behaviors throughout our lifetime. Learning may cause a child who initially stuttered only when she was excited, tired, or stressed to eventually stutter in ordinary circumstances, day after day. Learning can escalate mild, repetitive stuttering to severe blocking with a complex pattern of extra sounds, substituted words, and avoidance of speaking situations. Understanding the principles of learning will help you understand what may have created the individual stuttering patterns of clients. More importantly, this knowledge will guide treatment procedures as you help your clients acquire more effective communication behaviors and skills.

The interaction of constitutional factors with developmental and environmental factors to precipitate stuttering is ongoing, day by day. Such factors have a gradual, cumulative effect, just like the forces of weather have on the surface of the earth. For most children, there is not a sudden landslide of stuttering but a more gradual erosion of their fluency. Conditions at the onset of stuttering are typically not dramatic; the child is usually not under great stress, nor has the child just experienced a traumatic event. The ordinariness of situations when stuttering first appears is reflected in this observation by Van Riper (1973, p. 81):

> In the great majority of children we have carefully studied soon after onset, we were unable to state with any certainty . . . what precipitated the stuttering. In most instances there simply were no apparent conflicts, no illnesses, no opportunity to imitate, no shocks or frightening experiences. Stuttering seemed to begin under quite normal conditions of living and communicating.

Because children's lives are often so normal when stuttering first emerges, research to determine critical developmental and environmental factors affecting its onset and progression has not produced notable results. This is a domain of educated guesses and tentative conclusions. Evidence for developmental factors is inferred from the fact that almost all onsets of stuttering occur when children are developing most rapidly during their preschool years (Andrews et al, 1983; Wingate, 1983). Evidence of environmental influences comes in part from clinical reports of particular stresses sometimes associated with the onset of stuttering and its remission when these stresses are lessened (e.g., Van Riper, 1973, 1982). Environmental factors are also implicated by higher incidences of stuttering in those cultures that are more achievement- and conformity-oriented (Bloodstein, 1995). Finally, some sources of evidence for genetic factors in stuttering are also evidence for environmental factors. Studies by Andrews et al (1991), Howie (1981), Kidd, Kidd, and Records (1978), and Yairi et al (1996), for example, indicate that both genetic and environmental influences contribute to stuttering onsets. Andrews et al indicated that, for his subject pool of 3810 twin pairs, the best fit statistical models assigned 71% of the etiology in stuttering to genetic factors and 29% to the individual's unique environment. However, this finding does not suggest which environmental factors might be involved. Because of the paucity of objective data on specific developmental and environmental factors, this chapter is more speculative than the last. Wherever I can, however, I try to tie speculations to facts.

In this chaper, I have divided developmental, environmental, and learning factors into separate sections, although they do not operate alone; their actions are influenced by each other and by constitutional factors, such as those described in Chapter 2. A developmental variable, such as cognitive level, may determine at what age avoidance conditioning may occur. An environmental variable, such as the stress of moving to a new neighborhood, may have different effects on different children, depending on such factors as a child's sensitivity, physical development of speech production, and language maturation. It is also critical to keep in mind, when evaluating and treating clients, that every client is an individual whose stuttering has evolved from unique contributions of developmental, environmental, learning, and constitutional factors.

Developmental Factors

My view of how developmental factors affect children's fluency assumes that the brain must share its resources in coping with many demands. Like a computer, the brain can work on several things at once, but like a computer, the more tasks it performs simultaneously, the slower and less efficiently it does each one. Unlike a computer, if the tasks are dissimilar, such as driving a car and talking about the weather, there is less interference between them. But if the tasks are similar, such as rubbing your stomach while patting your head, there is more interference between them (Kinsbourne and Hicks, 1978). The problem of shared resources is more acute in children because their immature nervous systems have less processing capacity to share (Hiscock and Kinsbourne, 1977, 1980). Some children are especially at risk for straining their developing resources. Their development of speech and language skills may be delayed, yet they have to compete in a highly verbal environment. Or, their language development may surge ahead of their speech motor control skills, giving them much to say but limited capacity to say it. Such children may become excessively disfluent as other developmental demands outpace their ability to coordinate the complex movements of rapid, articulate speech.

Here is an example of this competition between burgeoning language and slower motor abilities. Several years ago, I evaluated a 4-year-old girl whose uncle and grandmother stuttered. Her parents were concerned because she had been repeating words and sounds excessively, sometimes up to 20 times per instance, for a year and a half. However, her language development was well above average; she began to talk with single words at 9 months and to produce sentences intelligibly at 12 months. In contrast, her motor development was somewhat slower; she had not walked until 18 months. I think it is possible that her disfluencies emerged as a result of a high proportion of her cerebral resources being used to formulate and express language with less mature capacities for motor activities, including fluent speech. In other words, a disparity between language facility and motor speech ability may have been an important contributor to the emergence of stuttering.

To appreciate how many skills and abilities the child is developing at the same time, look carefully at Figure 3–2. This chart covers only social, motor, and language domains, but it is clear that children have to master many different abilities simultaneously. If a child's development is slower in one or more areas, her road to maturity may be steep and difficult at times. So, let us look at some of the domains of development and how they might contribute to the onset of stuttering.

Physical Development

Between the ages of 1 and 6 years, children grow by leaps and bounds. Their bodies get bigger. Their nervous systems form new pathways and new connections. Their perceptual and motor skills improve with maturation and practice. This intensive period of growth is a two-edged sword for children predisposed to stuttering. Neurological maturation may provide more "functional cerebral space" that supports fluency, but it also spurs development of other motor behaviors that may compete with fluency for available neuronal resources. An example of such competition is the common observation that children learn to walk first or talk first, but not both at the same time. For example, Netsell (1981, p. 25) said of this trade-off, "The practice of walking *or* talking seems sufficient to 'tie up' all the available sensorimotor circuitry because the Toddler seldom, if ever, undertakes both activities at once." Likewise, Berk (1991, p. 194) suggested that "when infants forge ahead in spoken language, they seem to temporarily postpone mastery of new motor skills or vice versa." Studies are needed to explore the specific effects on speech and language of mastering other skills.

The momentary lags and spurts of motor skill and language development may explain normal disfluency as well as stuttering. If a child is learning new language constructions, which temporarily postpones mastery of *speech* motor skills, her expression of more complex language forms may be impaired until speech motor skills catch up. For reasons we don't yet understand, this may account for reduced speech intelligibility in some children, disfluency in others, and both problems in still other children.

I suspect that a significant delay in development of fine motor speech skills in a child with a strong urge to communicate and rapidly developing language abilities may set the stage for more serious disfluency. There is some evidence that children who stutter are slower developing fine motor coordination, but many conflicting results suggest that this is not a simple issue. A review of studies on motor coordination in people who stutter can be found in Bloodstein (1995).

Another challenge of normal physical development are rapid changes in the size and shape of the vocal tract. Between ages 2 and 5 years, structures in the child's head, neck, and torso undergo their most rapid growth; moreover, different structures grow at different rates (Kent and Vorperian, 1995). Thus, the child must learn to produce vowels and consonants that consistently sound the same, even though the shape, size, and biomechanical properties of her muscles and bones are changing from day to day, and the changes in some areas of the vocal tract are more rapid than in others. Callen et al (2000) propose that a child maintains a stable speech output by using the auditory feedback from speech production to continuously update the commands she sends to her muscles to produce specific sounds, despite almost daily changes in her speech structures. Thus, what her muscles were told to do yesterday must be adapted to the new size, shape, and biomechanical properties of the vocal tract today. The theory behind this proposal may be important for understanding parts of the next chapter, so we will spend a little extra time explaining it. A key assumption about learning to speak is that the newborn is learning the relationship between what she does with her muscles (motor commands) and what sounds come out of her mouth beginning with her very earliest cries and babbles. As she begins to attend to the speech around her, she develops an auditory memory of those sounds and then automatically develops the motor commands needed

Age	SOCIAL	SELF-HELP	GROSS MOTOR	FINE MOTOR	LANGUAGE
5-0 yr.	Shows leadership among children	Goes to the toilet without help	Swings on swing, pumping by self	Prints first name (four letters)	Tells meaning of familiar words
4-6	Follows simple rules in board games or card games	Usually looks both ways before crossing street	Skips or makes running "broad jumps"	Draws a person showing at least three parts—head, eyes, nose, mouth, etc.	Reads a few letters (five+)
4-0 yr.	Protective toward younger children	Buttons one or more buttons	Hops around on one foot without support	Draws recognizable pictures	Follows a series of three simple instructions
		Dresses and undresses without help, except for tying shoelaces			Understands concepts —size, number, shape
3-6	Plays cooperatively, with minimum conflict and supervision	Washes face without help	Hops on one foot without support	Cuts across paper with small scissors	Counts five or more objects when asked "how many?"
				Draws or copies a complete circle	Identifies four colors correctly
3-0 yr.	Gives directions to other children	Toilet trained	Rides around on a tricycle, using pedals		Combines sentences with the words "and," "or," or "but"
3-0 yr.	Plays a role in "pretend" games—mom-dad, teacher, space pilot	Dresses self with help	Walks up and down stairs—one foot per step	Cuts with small scissors	Understands four prepositions—in, on, under, beside
2-6	Plays with other children—cars, dolls, building	Washes and dries hands	Stands on one foot without support	Draws or copies vertical lines	Talks clearly, is understandable most of the time
2-6	"Helps" with simple household tasks	Opens door by turning knob	Climbs on play equipment—ladders, slides	Scribbles with circular motion	Talks in two- to three-word phrases or sentences

Figure 3-2 Child development in the first 5 years. (Courtesy of Harold Ireton, Ph.D.)

Age	Social	Self-Help	Gross Motor	Fine Motor	Language
Birth	Social smile	Reacts to sight of bottle or breast	Lifts head and chest when lying on stomach	Looks at and reaches for faces and toys	Reacts to voices; Vocalizes, coos, chuckles
6 mo.	Distinguishes mother from others	Comforts self with thumb or pacifier	Turns around when lying on stomach	Picks up toy with one hand	Vocalizes spontaneously, social
			Rolls over from back to stomach		Responds to name—turns and looks
9 mo.	Reaches for familiar persons	Feeds self cracker	Sits alone, steady, without support	Transfers toy from one hand to the other	Wide range of vocalizations (vowel sounds, consonant-vowel combinations)
	Pushes things away he/she doesn't want		Crawls around on hands and knees	Picks up object with thumb and finger grasp	Word sounds—says "ma-ma" or "da-da"
12 mo.	Plays social games, peek-a-boo, bye-bye; Plays patty-cake	Picks up a spoon by the handle	Walks around furniture or crib while holding on	Picks up small objects—precise thumb and finger grasp	Understands words like "no," "stop," or "all gone"
	Wants stuffed animal, doll, or blanket in bed	Lifts cup to mouth and drinks	Stands without support	Stacks two or more blocks	Uses one or two words as names of things or actions
18 mo.	Gives kisses or hugs; Greets people with "hi" or similar	Feeds self with spoon; Insists on doing things by self, such as feeding	Walks without help; Runs	Picks up two small toys in one hand; Scribbles with crayon	Talks in single words; Asks for food or drink with words
	Sometimes says "no" when interfered with		Kicks a ball forward	Builds towers of four or more blocks	Follows simple instructions
2-0 yr.	Shows sympathy to other children, tries to comfort them; Usually responds to correction—stops	Eats with fork; Eats with spoon, spilling little; Takes off open coat or shirt without help	Runs well, seldom falls; Walks up and down stairs alone	Turns pages of picture books, one at a time	Uses at least ten words; Follows two-part instructions

77

to produce them. She maintains and updates the relationships between motor commands and acoustic output from the information provided by the auditory feedback of her own speech and feeling the touch and movement her articulators made to produce it. If auditory information is as critical as it seems to be, it is important to remember that a common finding of the brain imaging studies reviewed in the previous chapter was that at least some adults who stutter do not process auditory information like nonstuttering speakers do and may not integrate it with other sensory information in planning and producing speech. Much additional research remains to be done on whether anomalous auditory processing is a cause of stuttering and, perhaps, of normal disfluencies as well.

Cognitive Development

Cognitive Development and the Onset of Stuttering

We use the phrase "cognitive development" to refer to the development of the processes of perception, attention, working memory, and executive functions that play a role in spoken language but are separate from it. This is a complex area, with more questions than answers. We don't know, for example, where to draw the line between language and cognition, or even if such a division makes sense.

The relationship between cognition and fluency is also complex. Persons with cognitive deficits, especially when deficits are relatively severe, have a high incidence of stuttering (Van Riper, 1982). This may occur for more than one reason. In the first place, typically rapid and complex speech and language production depend on fully functioning perception, attention, working memory, and executive functions. When these processes are compromised, breakdowns in spoken language are likely to result. As an example, consider the effect of a faulty working memory on rapid retrieval of vocabulary or syntax. If some components of language are mistimed in relation to others, repetitions of words or syllables may result, just as an engine without a steady fuel supply will stop and start stutteringly. Another way in which cognitive retardation may affect fluency has been suggested by Starkweather (1987). He notes that developmentally delayed individuals are slower in their overall acquisition of speech and language. Their extended period of acquisition may make them more vulnerable to speech breakdown because competition for limited neurological resources occurs over a relatively long period of time.

Findings from a study by Yairi et al (1996) provide some evidence that poorer cognitive skills, even in nonretarded individuals, are associated with lack of ability to recover from stuttering. Of the 32 children in their study who began to stutter, 12 continued to stutter for 36 months or more. The two groups of stutterers, those who recovered and those who did not, were compared with a control group of nonstuttering children on an intelligence test, the Arthur Adaptation of the Leiter International Performance Test (Arthur, 1952). The group of children who continued to stutter scored significantly lower than the nonstuttering control group, although their mean score was not below the norm for the test. However, the children in the recovered group did not score significantly lower than the controls. Thus, some abilities associated with cognition may be related to a neural resilience allowing recovery from stuttering. In other words, children with slightly higher cognitive functioning may have the extra resources needed to reorganize their speech and language processing, allowing them to develop a workaround (as computer programmers say) for the problem causing them to stutter.

Let us now consider the sorts of demands that concurrent development of cognitive processes may exert on the development of spoken language. To the extent that cognition and language are separate processes, some aspects of cognitive development may compete with spoken language development for the same neuronal resources, thereby jeopardizing fluency. Consider a key stage of cognitive development described by the Swiss psychologist, Jean Piaget. He believed that children progress through a Preoperational Period from 2 to 6 years, in which they come to understand numbers, to classify, and to reason at a very basic level. During this period, it seems to me, children's focus on developing higher level cognitive abilities occurs at the expense of such sensorimotor processes as expressing language using newly emerging motor speech skills.

Lindsay (1989) pointed out that, during this period of cognitive development, a child goes through a series of transitions in which new cognitive learning must be assimilated and consolidated with current knowledge. These transitions are times when a child's linguistic and cognitive systems are temporarily unstable, before new concepts are mastered. As a consequence, children's speech and language production during this period of adjustment may be vulnerable to disfluencies.

Cognitive Development and Reactions to Stuttering

In the preceding section, I have suggested that children's cognitive development may influence the onset of stuttering through competition for resources in the child's brain. Now, I would like to argue that the role of cognitive development is also important in explaining how and when a child begins to form negative attitudes and beliefs about herself and her speech.

Between the ages of 3 and 4 years, children's cognitions mature enough so that they internalize the standards of behavior of those around them, including peers. It is only at this point, according to Lewis (2000), that children can evaluate how they are performing in comparison to others and will experience the "self-conscious" emotions of embarrassment, pride, shame, and guilt. These emotions may play an important role in stuttering and its persistence. It appears that children who don't naturally recover from stuttering develop maladaptive responses, which are influenced by social, cognitive, and emotional factors. The embarrassment and shame some children feel about their stuttering are probably the most important cognitive-emotional factors that give rise to increases in tension, escape, and avoidance responses that make stuttering a self-sustaining disorder and increasingly difficult to recover from.

Social and Emotional Development

Interference with Speech by Emotion

In early childhood, a child's immature nervous system may permit "cross-talk" or interference between limbic system structures and pathways involved in the regulation and expression of emotion and the structures and pathways used for speech and language. Such interference may be even more likely among children predisposed to stutter, whose slower maturing speech and language functions may not be optimally localized or adequately buffered from interference and are closer to centers of emotion in the right hemisphere, a hypothesis I discussed in Chapter 2. Thus, when such children are emotionally aroused, fluency may suffer because neural signals for properly timed and sequenced muscle contractions may be interrupted in some way. I see evidence of this when I ask parents when their child first began to stutter. They frequently tell me that they noticed stuttering for the first time when their child was highly excited about something.

Excitement is commonly mentioned in the literature as a stimulus that elicits disfluency. Starkweather (1987) noted that "all children speak more disfluently during periods of excitement." Dorothy Davis (1940), who conducted one of the first studies of normal disfluency, reported that, of the 10 situations in which children showed repetitions in their speech, "excitement over own activity" was when they most frequently repeated sounds and words. Johnson et al (1959) asked parents of children identified as stutterers to describe the situation in which they first observed their child's stuttering. They most often reported that the first appearance of stuttering occurred when the child was in a hurry to tell something or was in an excited state. Thus, both stuttering and normal disfluency seem to occur most often or noticeably during states of transitory emotional arousal.

Stages of Social and Emotional Development

Some stages of development may provide more social and emotional stress than others. For example, the processes of separation and individuation are known to be periods of stress. After a child passes his second birthday, he strives harder for autonomy, creating the conflicts of the "terrible twos." Most parents gradually relinquish control, while at the same time helping their child learn the limits of his freedom. In some cases, however, the transition from a dependent infant to an independent preschooler may occur too rapidly for a parent or a child. If the child is pushed toward independence faster than he wants, he may feel frustrated and insecure because his mother seems less nurturing. A mother may become alarmed if she isn't ready for her child's quest for independence and may try to restrain her. A child may conform to these restraints but feel angry and frustrated. Yet, she cannot easily express these feelings to someone she depends on so much, and disfluency may result in those interactions in which such emotional ambivalence and conflict affect motor control of speech (Lidz, 1968).

Security

As a young child grows older, other members of the family besides the mother play a role in social and emotional changes. Although a child's father and brothers and sisters comprise a wider support system, a child's resentment at having to share his mother's attention may elicit feelings of anger, aggression, and guilt. It seems possible that if such feelings are punished or ignored, transient disfluency or more severe stuttering may result in some childen.

One of the more common provocations for feeling resentment is the birth of a sibling. We discuss the effect of a sibling's birth on fluency later in the section on environmental factors, but it warrants mentioning here, too, because a child's strong feelings may often reflect his developmental level as well as the environmental event. Theodore Lidz (1968, p. 246), a developmental psychiatrist with interests in speech and language, provided this example:

Psychoanalytically oriented play therapy with children also indicates that many of their forbidden wishes and ideas have relatively simple access to consciousness. A six-year-old boy who started to stammer severely after a baby sister was born was watched playing with a family of dolls. He placed a baby doll in a crib next to the parent dolls' bed and then had a boy doll come and throw the baby to the floor, beat it, and throw it into a corner. He then put the boy doll into the crib. In a subsequent session, he had the father doll pummel the mother doll's abdomen, saying, "No, no!" At this point of childhood, even though certain unacceptable ideas cannot be talked about, they are still not definitely repressed.

Although we feel, as does Lidz, that stuttering may be triggered by the birth of a sibling, our belief about the underlying cause is not so Freudian. Many threats to feelings of security can create emotional stress that may disrupt the speech of children who are predisposed to stutter. As will be seen in the section on treatment, we have found that therapy strategies that increase a child's sense of security and help him learn to speak more fluently will suffice for many children who begin stuttering.

Self-Consciousness and Sensitivity

As we noted earlier in the section on cognitive development, the emergence of self-consciousness, which begins during the child's second year, may be another source of social and emotional stress. This reflects the child's growing awareness of how he is performing relative to adult expectations. Although this process is not thoroughly understood, Jerome Kagan presents an interesting description of it in his book, *The Second Year: The Emergence of Self-Awareness* (1981). In a relevant example, Kagan proposes that the self-corrections a child makes in his speech are evidence of this self-awareness. Taking this further, we can surmise that increasing self-awareness in a child who is excessively disfluent might lead to self-corrections that only worsen the problem.

In Chapter 2, we briefly discussed clinical reports and a few studies suggesting that persons who stutter, as a group, may have unusually sensitive temperaments. Research on temperament in nonstuttering children, especially the longitudinal studies of Calkins and Fox (1994) and Kagan and Snidman (1991), indicates that the social-emotional traits of fearfulness and withdrawal that accompany more sensitive temperaments can change over the course of a child's preschool years. Some children become better able to modulate their temperamental tendencies, but others remain hostages to their temperaments. Such individual adaptations may be crucial in determining which children who begin to stutter will continue to do so and which will stop.

Before ending this section, I want to comment on stutterers' psychological adjustment in general. Many people who have little exposure to stuttering believe that stutterers are essentially nervous people or that stuttering is a sign of neurosis. If this were true, we should have found evidence of psychological maladjustment or excessive anxiety in people who stutter, particularly when stuttering first begins in childhood. However, research on the personality and adjustment of people who stutter has found no convincing evidence that they differ from nonstutterers in these ways (Bloch and Goodstein, 1971; Bloodstein, 1995; Van Riper, 1982). A few findings suggest that adults who stutter may not be as well adjusted socially as those who do not, but this may reflect the influence of stuttering on social experiences (Bloodstein, 1987).

Summarizing the effect of social and emotional development on fluency, I have suggested that many of the normal social and emotional stresses that children experience may result in disfluent speech, although the evidence is mostly anecdotal. Moreover, we suspect that children who are neurophysiologically vulnerable to stuttering may be especially prone to difficulty when social conflicts and emotions create extra "noise" in their neural circuitry for speech. Children who stutter appear to be as psychologically well adjusted as those who do not stutter, despite the extreme emotional stress that stuttering itself can impose.

Speech and Language Development

The Onset of Stuttering

Most stuttering begins between ages 2 and 6, when speech and language are developing most rapidly (Bloodstein, 1995; Peters and Starkweather, 1990; Van Riper, 1982). As with other developmental factors, we don't believe that the demands of speech and language development *cause* stuttering but that, for many children, these demands may be a precipitating factor.

Many writers have commented eloquently on the connection between the onset of stuttering and language acquisition. Peggy Dalton and W. J. Hardcastle (1977), for example, commented that "it is tempting to see the ever-increasing demands on linguistic competence and articulatory proficiency as major factors in the onset of some disfluency." Joseph Sheehan (1975, p. 142) said, "The age of onset of stuttering is consistently related to certain stages in the developmental sequence. Most notably, the 'period of resonance,' or high readiness in language learning, noted by Lenneberg . . . is also the period during which stuttering develops and flourishes." Andrews et al (1983, p. 239) pointed to the demands placed on speech by rapidly developing language in noting that, "stuttering [has] a maximal frequency of onset at a time when an explosive growth in language ability outstrips a still-immature speech-motor apparatus."

Many studies have found that increased complexity of language is associated with more stuttering. Research on natural conversational speech of children who stutter has shown that more complex utterances contain more stuttering (Gaines, Runyan, and Meyers, 1991; Logan and Conture, 1995; Brundage and Bernstein Ratner, 1989; Yaruss, 1999). Some research suggests that utterance length may have a greater effect on stuttering than does complexity (Logan and Conture, 1997; Wilkenfeld and Curlee, 1997; Yaruss, 1999). Experimental studies, in which children were asked to produce both more and less complex utterances, show that both stutterers (Bernstein Ratner and Sih, 1987; Stocker and Usprich, 1976) and nonstutterers (Gordon, Luper, and Peterson, 1986; Haynes and Hood, 1978; Pearl and Bernthal, 1980; Yaruss, Newman, and Flora, 1999) increase their disfluencies as language complexity is increased. Unfortunately, there is little longitudinal research that directly bears on the question of how and when emerging language is associated with normal disfluency or stuttering.

One of the few descriptive studies was Norma Colburn's analysis of the disfluencies of four nonstuttering children using data originally gathered by Lois Bloom for her work on normal language development. Published reports of her analysis (Colburn and Mysak, 1982a,b) suggested that these children's normal disfluencies did not emerge when they first learned a new language construction but as they began to master it and started using it regularly. Explanations suggested for this result include the possibility that a child who has not completely automatized the use of a new construction allocates fewer resources than are necessary for its production (Kent and Perkins, 1984) or that when a child masters the new construction she produces it at an increased rate, thereby straining capacity (Starkweather, 1987).

A single-case study was used to explore the relationship between syntax acquisition and normal disfluencies by Frank Wijnen (1990). Weekly speech samples were obtained from a boy from age 2 years 4 months to 2 years 11 months. The number of repetitions, revisions, and incomplete phrases were assessed in relation to the length and complexity of utterances. It was reported that disfluencies were randomly distributed initially but eventually clustered on function words and sentence-initial words, and then declined. Although speech rate was not measured and increased rate might have accounted for some of the increase in the child's disfluencies, the number of disfluencies was not highly correlated with length of utterance. Instead, Wijnen concluded that the decline in the child's disfluencies was associated with his development of a routine type of sentence (pronoun + verb + some other word) and that learning this routine involved so much of his processing capacity that speech production was short-changed. This preliminary study needs to be followed up with many more cases to test the hypothesis that learning to make sentence productions more automatic through routinization of several sentence types is related to increased normal disfluency. With a larger sample size, multiple regression analyses could be used to determine which of many possible factors best predict instances of or increases in disfluency.

Having looked at the evidence of an association between increasing sentence complexity and/or sentence length and the frequency of stuttering in children, let's consider what, specifically, may be interfering with fluency as the child acquires language. I'll begin by recounting what the child acquires during this period of time. Between ages 2 and 3 years, a child's vocabulary jumps from 50 to well over 500 words; in fact, toward the end of this year, five to seven new words may be learned each day (Studdert-Kennedy, 1987). At the same time, the child's single word utterances develop into successive single-word pairs with sentence-like intonations and durations and then to multiword sentences (Branigan, 1979). Thus, the child's speech graduates from a simple "syllable-timed" prosody for single words to complex prosodic rhythms that span multiple words (Allen and Hawkins, 1980). As the child expands sentences, she also overhauls her language storage system. At first, her shelves are stocked with whole words in the form of articulatory routines or gestural patterns; then, she must change strategies and stock, not whole words, but segments that can be combined in various ways to form a multitude of words (Kent, 1985; Nittrouer, Studdert-Kennedy, and McGowan, 1989; Stemberger, 1982). During these same early preschool years, the child also progressively learns active, negative, and passive constructions as well as present, future, and past tenses. At the same time, she increases the length and linguistic complexity of her sentences together with the rate of her utterances as she increasingly tries to synchronize the rates and rhythms of her speech with those of her family, with whom she has a growing urge to communicate.

This huge array of language and speech production tasks is a challenge even to the fluency of nonstuttering children. Normal disfluencies of children also increase from ages 2 to 4 years, peaking when they tackle the task of producing long, complex sentences (Ito, 1986). It is not surprising, then, that children who are predisposed to stutter because of genetic or congenital factors tend to begin stuttering during this same period.

We now move from *what* may interfere with a child's fluency to consider *how* it may occur. Imagine that a child's brain has a limited amount of space that is chock-full of highly interconnected networks of neurons (Kinsbourne and Hicks, 1978). Because the child's brain is immature but tightly packed, neural networks may not be well insulated from one another. The insulation of axons is provided by myelin sheaths, fatty protective coatings that develop slowly throughout childhood. Thus, in a younger child, myelinization is incomplete, allowing cross-talk among axons of different neural networks, creating interference in the transmission of information.

Another challenge to the child developing language may be introduced by different neuronal groups maturing at different rates. Neuronal groups working on vocabulary may be more efficient than those working on syntax, or vice versa. In addition, structures, such as the corpus callosum, that link prosodic functions of the right hemisphere with syntactic functions in the left may be slower to develop than other structures involved in speech-language production. All these differences may account for why a young child may have trouble synchronizing the tasks required for speech, some of which are simultaneous, while others are sequential. As a child grows, however, her brain gains more functional space with expanded neural networks that can function more independently from one another. As different groups of neurons mature and become more efficient, they can synchronize their actions more easily. Thus, when the child becomes a teenager, she can rub her tummy and pat her head with less disruption of either task.

Returning now to the realm of speech and language production, when a young child is at the one-word stage of language development, the amount of simultaneous activity in different neural networks may be relatively small. The child's task is to select a word from a small shelf of whole words and then produce it with simple prosody. But when the child moves to the two-word stage and beyond, she must select several words to make each sentence, and her chosen words must be assembled from a large storehouse of smaller segments rather than a storehouse of whole words. She must also work out a grammatical plan for the sentence and align it with a complex rhythm that spans the entire sentence. Some of the planning for the later parts of the sentence is going on at the very time she is beginning to produce the first words of the sentence, putting greater stress on developing cognitive factors such as memory. Clearly, these simultaneous but different tasks involving interconnecting neural networks that are not fully mature will sometimes interfere with each other. Think of the errors we all make when we try to do too many different things at the same time. The hesitations, pauses, and repetitions in the speech of normal children who are learning to talk in sentences may be the equivalent of the stops and starts and confusion that children show when simultaneously performing tasks that interfere with each other.

Now let's consider what may be happening to create an *excess* of disfluencies in the speech of children who begin stuttering during the period of rapid speech and language development. You will remember from Chapter 2 that brain imaging studies of adults who stutter have shown some unexpected patterns of activity during speech. For example, there are abnormally high levels of activity in some regions of the right hemisphere and abnormally low levels in some areas of the left hemisphere. It is possible, then, that some aspects of the brain are different in children who will develop stuttering. Planning and production of speech and language may use atypical neural pathways that may be slow or inefficient. But the demands grow ever greater as a child produces longer, faster, and more complex sentences. Tasks using different neural networks for segment selection, grammatical formulation, and prosodic planning must be orchestrated precisely so that each element is in place at the proper time as utterances are produced. If some components are ready but others are delayed, initial sounds or syllables may be repeated or prolonged or even blocked, while waiting for the whole sentence to be compiled. A child's reaction to this speech traffic jam may determine whether maladaptive learning occurs or whether such jams happen only temporarily, until compensatory strategies help the child develop normal speech.

Delayed and Deviant Speech and Language Development

If stuttering arises from constitutional differences (for example, inheritance or congenital injury) in some children, it is natural to wonder if other speech and language abilities besides fluency are affected. It is also important to understand how delays in speech and language development might be related to the appearance of stuttering or disfluency. In general, research has found that speech and language delays or difficulties are more common among children who stutter than those who don't, but the findings are neither simple nor clear-cut, and their implications are unclear.

When assessed on such measures as the ages when children said their first word and first sentence, size of receptive vocabulary, mean length of utterance, and expressive and receptive syntax, children who stutter often score lower than their nonstuttering peers (Andrews and Harris, 1964; Arndt and Healey, 2001; Berry, 1938; Darley, 1955; Kline and Starkweather, 1979; Murray and Reed, 1977; Okasha et al, 1974; Wall, 1980; Westby, 1979; Williams, Melrose, and Woods, 1969). However, other studies have not found language differences (e.g., Johnson, 1955; Miles and Ratner, 2001; Peters, 1968; Seider, Gladstien, and Kidd, 1982; Watkins, Yairi, and Ambrose, 1999).

Young children who stutter have also been shown to have difficulty achieving age-appropriate speech. In the clinic, we often observe children in the early stages of stuttering who have multiple articulation or phonological errors and speech that can be difficult to understand. Research has repeatedly confirmed the finding that stutterers have roughly two and a half times the incidence of articulation disorders as that found in same-age nonstutterers (Andrews and Harris, 1964; Berry, 1938; Bloodstein, 1958; Kent and Williams, 1963; Williams, Silverman, and Kools, 1968). Nevertheless, several studies have found no differences in the articulation abilities of children who do and do not stutter (Ryan, 1992; Seider, Gladstien, and Kidd, 1982).

Two excellent, critical reviews of the research on language, phonology, and stuttering have been published. Nippold (1990) suggested, for example, that research does not clearly support the hypothesis that children who stutter are also likely to have language or articulation difficulties. Rather, she proposed that there may be subgroups of children who stutter who have language or articulation problems related to their stuttering. Bernstein Ratner (1997) concurred and noted that the differences found between groups of children who stutter and children who do not stutter have been very subtle. She suggested that future research should use more sophisticated tests of language and phonology and look for subgroupings, not only in children but also in adults who stutter.

Findings of deficits in articulation and language performance, at least in some children who stutter, can be interpreted in several ways. Some authors have suggested that children who have articulation or language difficulties will start to believe that speaking is difficult. Their anticipation of such difficulty is hypothesized to lead to hesitation and struggle and then to stuttering (Bloodstein, 1995, 1997). An alternative view is that stuttering, language disorders, and articulation errors all result from a common deficit, which might be passed on genetically. Because specific regions and pathways of the brain are responsible for speech and language-related functions, delayed development of (or damage to) these areas may result in language, articulation, or fluency problems in any combination. Small differences in how the brain processes such functions could tip the balance toward any of these disorders.

The literature on disfluencies of language-impaired children who are not considered stutterers provides support for a slightly different hypothesis about the relationship between language deficits or delays and stuttering. Several studies of language-impaired children have found that they, or a subgroup of them, evidence high frequencies of the types of disfluencies that are seen more often in children who stutter than in normal children, even though they wouldn't be considered stutterers (Boscolo, Ratner, and Rescorla, 2002; Hall, Yamashita, and Aram, 1993; Hodge, Rescorla, and Ratner, 1999). These authors speculate that the excess disfluencies result from difficulties in formulating and executing utterances just beyond the limits of their language abilities. Thus, when language resources are strained, fluency must be sacrificed in order to meet the demands of language production. Perhaps these children need extra time to meet these demands, and part- and whole-word repetitions provide the needed time, or this may be what results when a speech production system is spinning its wheels, waiting for elements of the language plan to be ready for execution. These findings suggest that the association between stuttering and language delay or deficit may emerge from the demands of normal development on weak language formulation/production systems and result in high frequencies of stuttering-like disfluencies. Other factors, such as a vulnerable temperament, environmental pressures, or a traumatic life event, may turn these disfluencies into real stuttering.

In addition to the evidence that children who stutter have a higher incidence of language or articulation problems, researchers are finding evidence that articulation or language delays and disorders may be related to whether or not a child recovers from stuttering. This is reflected in the research of Conture, Louko, and Edwards (1993), St. Louis (1991), and Yairi et al (1996), whose findings suggest that children who stutter and also have phonological or language differences are more likely to persist in stuttering or take longer in treatment. As part of a large ongoing study of children identified and assessed close to the onset of stuttering, Yairi et al (1996) found that children who later recovered from stuttering without treatment had higher scores on the Preschool Language Scale (Zimmerman, Steiner, and Pond, 1979) than the children who did not recover. It is noteworthy, however, that the children who later recovered as well as those whose stuttering persisted scored above the norms on this test. A more recent study of an extended cohort of these same children (Watkins, Yairi, and Ambrose, 1999) did not replicate the study's initial finding. Specifically, lexical, morphological, and syntactic analyses of the cohort's spontaneous language showed no differences between recovered and persistent groups of children. However, in looking at the phonological development of both groups near onset of stuttering, Paden, Yairi, and Ambrose (1999) found that the children who recovered from stuttering scored significantly higher on the Assessment of Phonological Processes—Revised (Hodson, 1986) than the children who did not recover. Thus, it appears that a child's phonological status, but not expressive language status, near the onset of stuttering may predict recovery. Children with delayed phonology are at risk for stuttering to persist.

Environmental Factors

Some children may show initial signs of stuttering in response to developmental pressures alone, but most who become stutterers are probably affected by environmental pressures as well. Such pressures typically result from attitudes, behaviors, or events that occur in their homes. One example is a family's anxiety about the child's speech, which is readily apparent in the facial expressions of parents and siblings when the child is disfluent. Another may be the conversational style in the child's home that is distinguished by lots of interruptions and rapid, complex speech.

When I described the effects of developmental factors on a child's speech, I used the analogy of a computer that is overloaded by too many simultaneous tasks. The computer analogy is also appropriate to depict environmental factors, but now you need to imagine that a computer is being used for programs that exceed its processing or memory capacities, is subjected to periodic power surges, or is given commands its programs cannot process. It is easy to imagine that such circumstances would likely create fluency breakdowns in a vulnerable child. These kinds of environmental pressures can also worsen the symptoms of stuttering, as I describe in Chapter 5. I will begin this discussion of environmental factors by reviewing research on the most important factor in family environments, the parents.

Parents

In the 1930s and 1940s at the University of Iowa, Wendell Johnson developed the "diagnosogenic" theory of stuttering. This theory, which is described more fully in a later section, proposes that a child's parents misdiagnose normal disfluencies as stuttering. Their reaction then causes the child to try to avoid these normal interruptions of speech and struggle in a way that becomes real stuttering. Johnson's diagnosogenic theory generated a great deal of research on parents of stutterers. Were they different from the parents of nonstutterers? Were they unusually critical? Did they have unreasonably high standards of speech?

One of the first studies of parents of stuttering children was conducted by John Moncur (1952). He interviewed the mothers of both stuttering and nonstuttering children about their parenting practices and concluded that mothers of stuttering children tended to be more critical, more protective, and more domineering toward their children than the mothers of nonstuttering children. Not long afterwards, Frederick Darley, a student of Wendell Johnson at the University of Iowa, investigated the attitudes of stutterers' parents in more detail. Using interview techniques based on Alfred Kinsey's studies of sexual behavior, Darley (1955) questioned the parents of 50 stutterers and 50 nonstutterers. Although there was a great deal of overlap in the attitudes of both groups of parents, the parents of children who stuttered had significantly higher standards and expectations, particularly with regard to speech. They had greater sensitivity to speech deviations and believed in early intervention for nonfluencies; their overall drive and need for domination was greater as well.

Darley's study was expanded by Wendell Johnson and his research associates (1959) to the parents of 150 stuttering and 150 nonstuttering children. Again, there was much overlap between parents of stutterers and parents of nonstutterers, but parents of children who stutter were reported to be more perfectionistic and to have higher standards of behavior than the parents of children who did not stutter. These studies by Moncur, Darley, Johnson, and others were largely responsible for the widespread belief that parents are a key factor in precipitating the onset of stuttering. Parents could transmit a culture's "competitive pressure for achievement or conformity," which may be the environmental factor most likely to be linked with stuttering (Bloodstein, 1987).

I should emphasize that there are many conflicting findings in the literature and that parents of stutterers, if they do differ from parents of nonstutterers, differ only slightly. Because these studies have not used additional control groups of parents of children with other disorders, we can't dismiss the possibility that, rather than causing stuttering, these differences may be the result of stuttering. This possibility is all the more likely given that these parents were interviewed more than a year after the onset of their child's stuttering. Perhaps any parent of a child with a disorder would appear to have high standards for him. We note, also, that these are group differences and that many parents of stuttering children are more accepting and less competitive than many parents of nonstuttering children.

Even if parents of children who stutter do have high standards and are perfectionistic, this alone would not be sufficient to produce stuttering. After all, the brothers and sisters of a child who stutters may thrive under these circumstances. And, as I have suggested before, most children of demanding parents do not stutter. However, for a child who is constitutionally predisposed to stutter, this may be just the straw that breaks the camel's back. One can imagine a child feeling self-conscious in a family that strives for perfection, especially in speech. Such a child could become so concerned about minor disfluencies that she tries too hard to be perfectly fluent and begins to labor and struggle when her speech is disfluent. Some children who begin to stutter may have only slight constitutional predispositions but are subjected to overwhelming environmental pressures. For example, a child with few noticeable disfluencies may gradually develop stuttering under relentless pressure to perform at higher levels socially, academically, or athletically.

Let us digress for a moment from the Iowa studies that found competitive pressures to be common in the homes of stutterers. Different results were found in England. Gavin Andrews and Mary Ann Harris (1964), whose work was described in Chapter 2, collected and analyzed data from families in Newcastle, England. Andrews and Harris compared the medical and home visit records of parents of stutterers with those of nonstuttering children and concluded that both groups of parents, most of whom were mothers, were generally similar in personality but differed in some key traits. The parents of stutterers were lower in intelligence, had poorer school records when they were younger, had poorer work histories, and provided poorer housing for their children. There was no evidence, however, that they criticized or pressured their children. This finding is a far cry from the reports of excessively high standards in the homes of children who stutter in Iowa.

Why are these researchers' results so different from those of the Iowa studies? There may be many reasons, but two come readily to mind. First, stuttering may emerge in children under many types of stress. In industrial England, the greatest stress may have come from social and economic disadvantages, but the greatest stress in Iowa may have been the high standards of upwardly mobile parents. Second, these different results may reflect differences in these researchers' expectations and theoretical biases of two decades ago. Americans tend to believe that everyone is created equal, and American researchers, especially those conducting studies in the heartland of the United States during the 1950s, would be predisposed to look for causes of stuttering in the environment rather than the child's heredity. In contrast, many Britons believe that inheritance plays a major role in determining one's life outcomes, and researchers in the United Kingdom would be inclined to consider parents' intelligence and social class as likely causes of stuttering.

The hypothesis that lower class homes provide stress that may precipitate stuttering did not originate in Great Britain. John Morgenstern (1956), who investigated stuttering in Scottish children, found that stuttering was more prevalent in the lower class homes of skilled manual, weekly wage earners compared with the homes in the Iowa studies. However, this was a social stratum in Scotland that was upwardly mobile and may have expressed families' ambitions through high speech standards for their children. Here we have a combination of forces if Morgenstern's hypothesis was correct. The stress of lower class homes lies not in their deprivation but in the cultural pressure to perform well and rise above humble beginnings.

More recent studies of parents of children who stutter present mixed results. Some have reported that they are more rejecting or anxious than are parents of children who do not stutter (Flugel, 1979; Zenner et al, 1978), but others have found either small or no differences between the two groups of parents (Goodstein, 1956; Goodstein and Dahlstrom, 1956). In his thorough review of the home environments of children who stutter, Yairi (1997b) concluded that the mix of diverse findings boils down to the likelihood that children who stutter grow up in unfavorable environments. But he also noted that, even though many studies suggest that parents of children who stutter may be somewhat anxious, overprotective, socially withdrawn, and prone to negatively evaluate their children, there is no evidence that these parental tendencies cause stuttering. Yairi went on to point out that, because a child's risk for stuttering is often inherited, the parents of these children may themselves stutter, have stuttered in the past, or had contact with other family members who stuttered. Thus, their negative traits may be a result of their own experiences with this disability.

My own view is in accord with Yairi's, but I would add that at least some of the children with persistent stuttering may have vulnerable temperaments (Oyler and Ramig, 1995), which may be inherited. Their parents, the genetic source of these temperaments, may be the anxious, overprotective mothers or fathers that have been described in the literature on parents of stutterers. Therefore, such children are in double jeopardy for persistent stuttering because of their own temperaments and because one or both parents are overly concerned about the child's stuttering because of their own temperament. On the other hand, some parents may have an ameliorating effect on a child's vulnerable temperament, making it possible for a child who begins to stutter and who is emotionally reactive to recover from stuttering. In a discussion of environmental influences on biological predispositions of children who do not stutter, Calkins and Fox (1994, p. 209) said that "the child's interactions with a parent provide the context for learning skills and strategies for managing emotional reactivity."

Once again, we see that influences on stuttering are numerous and complex, coming from both the child and the environment. Some of these influences may precipitate stuttering, others may interact to make remission difficult, and still others may provide the kinds of support that make remission possible.

Speech and Language Environment

Because every preschool-age child is tuned in to the speech and language around her, especially that of her parents, the communication style surrounding her may be an important influence on the child who stutters. Writers have hypothesized that, as a child tries to emulate adult models of speech and language, to use longer words and longer sentences, to try less familiar words, and to pack more meaning into her utterances, she will be more likely to stutter. Van Riper (1973, p. 381) expressed it this way: "Stuttering usually begins at the very time that great advances in sentence construction occur, and it seems tenable that, when the speech models provided by the parents or siblings of the child are too difficult for him to follow, some faltering will ensue." Later, in the same volume, Van Riper goes on to cite nine references in which clinicians point to parental speech models as a major source of stress on a child's fluency (pp. 380–383). This stress includes not only the parents' speech and language, but also the conditions under which the child tries to speak.

Following in Van Riper's footsteps, many other clinicians have speculated that speech and language environments are a potential source of stress for children who stutter (e.g., Conture, 2001; Shapiro, 1999; Starkweather, Gottwald, and Halfond, 1990; Zebrowski and Kelly, 2002). Table 3–1 lists a variety of sources of possible communicative stress.

Two writers have moved beyond clinical speculation to develop informal theories about the influence of adult models on a child's fluency. Crystal (1987) proposed an "interactive" view of many speech and language disorders, which suggested that demands at one level of language production (e.g., syntax) may deplete resources for other levels (e.g., prosody or phonology) and result in breakdown. His supporting data nicely illustrate how stuttering may be exacerbated by a child's use of advanced language. He presented evidence that the more complex the syntax and semantics that a child used, the more he stuttered. Starkweather (1987), describing a demands and capacities view of stuttering, commented that: "the production of speech and the formulation of language

Table 3–1 Possible Speech and Language Stresses	
Stressful Adult Speech Models	
Rapid speech rate	Complex syntax
Polysyllabic vocabulary	Use of two languages in home
Stressful Speaking Situations for Child	
Competition for speaking	Hurried when speaking
Frequent interruptions	Frequent questions
Demand for display speech	Excited when speaking
Loss of listener attention	Many things to say

place a simultaneous demand on the young person. If the demands in either of these two dimensions are excessive, performance in the other dimension may be reduced." These two views imply that stuttering may increase when an individual uses longer words, less frequently occurring words, more information-bearing words, and longer sentences. Stuttering may also increase when the individual is uttering a more linguistically complex sentence.

What do we know about the speech and language of parents of stutterers? Several clinical researchers have examined parent-child conversational interactions, seeking to determine if parents of children who stutter talk to their children differently than parents of nonstuttering children. A review of many such studies was conducted by Nippold and Rudzinski (1995). In the following paragraphs, we highlight some of the important studies in this area. Susan Meyers and Frances Freeman (1985a,b) compared the speech of mothers of stuttering children with that of mothers of nonstutterers. They found that mothers of stutterers spoke more rapidly than the mothers of nonstutterers. This may be critical because a mother's high speech rate may encourage a child to try to speak faster than his optimal speed (e.g., Jaffe and Anderson, 1979). The possibility that rapid speech rates may lead to stuttering is consistent with Johnson and Rosen's (1937) finding that adult stutterers were more likely to stutter when they spoke more rapidly than their habitual rate. Children who stutter may be even more vulnerable to fluency breakdowns during rapid speech than adults who stutter by virtue of the fact that children's natural rates of speech are slower and their temporal coordination less than that of adults (e.g., Kent, 1981).

Several studies subsequent to those of Meyers and Freeman (1985a,b) failed to find speech rate differences between parents of children who stutter and parents of children who do not stutter. For example, Kelly and Conture (1992) found no differences in the speaking rates of mothers of these two groups of children; Kelly (1994) found no differences in the rates of fathers of the two groups; and Yaruss and Conture (1995) found no differences in the articulatory rates (the rate at which each individual phrase is spoken, in contrast to speaking rate, which includes pauses between phrases) between mothers of stuttering children and mothers of nonstuttering children. However, the latter researchers did find a significant correlation between children's severity of stuttering and parent-child differences in speaking rate; greater differences in parent-child speech rates were associated with more severe stuttering in the children. These results could have been obtained if more severely stuttering children talk more slowly than other children and their parents have speech rates similar to other parents in the study. It is also possible that greater parent-child differences in rate make the stutteing in a child who already stutters more severe.

In general, earlier studies found differences between parents' speaking rate, but later ones did not. Why might this be so? Zebrowski (1995) discussed this disparity in her review of the conversational patterns of families of children who stutter. She suggested that differences in measurement techniques and the fact that Meyers and Freeman (1985a,b) had a larger number of severe stutterers in their sample might account for the differences in the studies. I think it is possible, also, that parents of children just beginning to stutter have become increasingly aware of the importance of speaking slowly because of publicity aimed at stuttering prevention. Such parents may try to speak slower than usual while under the scrutiny of clinical researchers, thus adding to the likelihood that more recent studies may not find differences in the speaking rates of parents of stutterers and nonstutterers.

Another suspected parental stress, in addition to rapid speech rates, is the frequency with which they interrupt their children. One of Meyers and Freeman's reports (1985a) presented some unexpected evidence about interruptions. The mothers of both stuttering and nonstuttering children interrupted most frequently when a child was disfluent. It seems possible that such parental interruptions, some of which may have been elicited by the child's disfluencies, may, in turn, elicit changes in the child's speech. Some children might increase tension and rate and, thereby, develop the struggled behaviors of stuttering. Others might suppress disfluencies to avoid interruptions and eventually be "taught" by parents not to be disfluent.

In a later study, Kelly and Conture (1992) found no significant differences in the interruptions of mothers of stuttering children and those of mothers of nonstuttering children. However, a closer inspection of their data revealed a correlation between the duration of "simultalk" (one person talking at the same time another is talking) of the mothers of children who stutter and the severity of their stuttering. Thus, mothers of more severe stutterers did more simultalk when their children were talking than mothers whose children stuttered less severely. In a later study of fathers, Kelly (1994) found no differences in the interruptions of fathers of children who stutter and those of fathers whose children do not stutter. Moreover, the correlation between these fathers' simultalk and severity of stuttering was not significant.

Another variable of children's speech and language environments that has been studied is the extent to which parents ask questions. Meyers and Freeman (1985a) found no significant difference in the number of questions asked by mothers of children who stutter compared with mothers of children who do not stutter. Langlois, Hanrahan, and Inouye (1986), however, did find significant differences when making a similar comparison. Langlois and Long (1988) then conducted an experimental treatment of a 4-year old who stuttered, in which the mother was taught to reduce the number of questions she asked, among other changes. After 16 treatment sessions in which the mother had markedly reduced her number of questions and given her child more speaking turns, the child no longer stuttered. This finding is especially interesting because it is tempting to assume that asking questions results in more stuttering. However, subsequent studies tested this assumption. In a study of eight stuttering children in conversations with their parents, Weiss and Zebrowski (1992) found that the children stuttered less when they answered questions than when they made assertions. This appeared to be related to the fact that questions were often answered with brief responses, but assertions were often longer responses. A more direct test of the effect of parents asking questions was carried out by Wilkenfeld and Curlee (1997), who used a single-subject ABAB (baseline-treatment-baseline-treatment) design to vary an adult's verbal behavior (questions vs. comments) in conversations with a child who stuttered. Their results with three children who stuttered demonstrated that stuttering did not appear to be related to whether the adult asked questions or commented, but stuttering was more likely to occur in either condition when the child's utterances were longer.

It is becoming evident that findings about speech rates, interruptions, and questions in the conversations of parents with their children who stutter are equivocal. But what about the linguistic complexity of their speech? A recent study of the overall complexity of the langauge of parents of children who stutter was conducted by Miles and Ratner

(2001), who gathered samples of conversations from 12 mother-child dyads involving stuttering children and 12 involving fluent children. All children were between 27 and 48 months of age, and the stuttering children were within 3 months of the onset of their stuttering. Mothers' utterances were assessed for syntactic complexity, lexical diversity and rarity, and mean number of utterances per turn. No significant differences between the mothers of the stuttering children and the mothers of the fluent children were found.

Two recent studies have taken a different approach to examining the effects of parents' verbal behavior on children's stuttering. The complexity of mothers' language was examined in relationship to whether or not their child recovered from stuttering. Kloth et al (1999) studied 23 children who stuttered, 16 of whom had recovered after 4 years and seven of whom had not. The complexity of the mothers' language was measured in terms of mean length of utterances in words in conversations with their child, both before and immediately after the onset of stuttering. They found that the language of the mothers of children who persisted in stuttering was significantly more complex than that of the mothers of children who recovered both before their children began to stutter and again after stuttering began. In another study of persistent and recovered stutterers, Rommel et al (2000) assessed the complexity of 71 mothers' language soon after their child had begun to stutter, rather than before stuttering began. They followed these children for 3 years and found that one of the more powerful predictors of whether or not a child would recover were "the linguistic demands to which the child is exposed" (p. 181). More specifically, these researchers found that the more complex the mother's syntax (mean length of utterance or MLU) and the greater number of different words she used in talking to her child, the more likely that her child would not recover over the following 3 years. The language abilities of the children had no predictive value (Rommel et al, 2000). The findings of these two studies support the hypothesis that the language environment of a child who stutters may influence recovery.

Nippold and Rudzinski's (1995) review of research on parents' speech and children's stuttering through the mid-1990s makes it clear that there was only weak support for the hypothesis that parents of children who stutter have more demanding verbal interaction styles than other parents. However, the studies by Kloth et al (1999) and Rommel et al (2000) suggest that earlier researchers were asking the wrong questions. Asking whether the parents of children who stutter talk faster, interrupt more, ask more questions, or use more complex language than other parents suggests that earlier studies had assumed that such parent behaviors create stuttering in otherwise normal children. However, given the strong evidence cited in Chapter 2 that stuttering has a neurophysiological basis, assuming that the verbal behaviors of parents of stuttering children are unusually demanding seems unnecessary. Rather, parents may have normal verbal behaviors that may precipitate stuttering in those children whose neurophysiological makeup has delayed their ability to produce long, rapid, complex fluent utterances.

What are the clinical implications of this view? Even the most cautious researchers examining the parent-child interactions of stuttering children are hopeful about the possible therapeutic value of changing some parents' verbal behaviors. They advocate clinical research on the therapeutic effects of reducing parents' speech rates (Nippold and Rudzinski, 1995), changing their language patterns (Miles and Ratner, 2001), or even combining these approaches with direct treatment of children's fluency.

Life Events

Certain events in life can deliver a blow to a child's stability and security. When this happens, stuttering may suddenly appear out of nowhere, or previously easy repetitions may be transformed into hard, struggled blocks. To have someone close to you die, to be hospitalized for an operation, or to have parents divorce is difficult for any of us, but it is especially difficult for children. Obviously, many children go through such events and adapt to them without major problems. But children who are predisposed to stuttering often show the effects of such events in their speech. Kagan (1994a) noted that some children who begin life with a relaxed temperament may even become shy and fearful under the onslaught of stressful events. This may well set the stage for stuttering if other constitutional factors predispose the child for it.

There is little research on the relationship that difficult life events may have on stuttering, but many authors have observed the connection. Starkweather (1987), for example, wrote, "All children speak more disfluently during periods of tension—when moving or changing schools, when their parents divorce, or after the death of a family member" (pp. 146–147). These increases in disfluency could easily result in the onset of stuttering or in increased stuttering in children who are vulnerable to such stresses. Johnson et al (1959) noted that the following events were among the 16 situations in which parents first noticed their child's stuttering: (1) child's physical environment changed (e.g., moving to new house), (2) child became ill, (3) child realized his mother was pregnant, and (4) a new baby arrived. In discussing the onset of stuttering, Van Riper (1982) acknowledged that various studies have found no differences in the amount of emotional conflict in the homes of children who developed stuttering versus those who did not. However, he went on to note, "Nevertheless, we have studied individual cases in which stuttering did seem [to be] triggered by such conflicts, and it is difficult for us to ignore these experiences" (p. 79).

My own clinical experience is similar. In the past several years, for example, during which I've evaluated about 20 children who stutter, I've encountered four children in four different families who began to stutter when their parents were in the early stages of divorce. However, this turmoil was not the only factor in their stuttering. Three of the children had relatives who stuttered, and the father of the fourth child was a stutterer. Moreover, all four were preschoolers and were likely experiencing various growth and development pressures. But for all of them, their parents' divorce appeared to us to be a factor that pushed them from normal speech to stuttering.

In another case of a life event precipitating stuttering, I evaluated a 9-year-old girl who began to stutter when her classroom teacher had an emotional breakdown. The teacher's outbursts of anger and crying, interspersed with high demands for rapid performance on frequent examinations, were apparently extremely stressful for this student. Under this stress, she developed tight blocks, with physical tension at the level of the larynx and abdomen, a pattern that Van Riper (1982) described as "Track III" stuttering. Even though I was convinced through extensive interviews with the family that the child had no prior stuttering, I noted several predisposing factors for stuttering. First, her younger sister had significant learning disabilities, including auditory processing problems. Second, her mother described herself and her daughter who stuttered as shy and emotionally reactive. These two factors—a family history of learning disability and a

Table 3–2 Stressful Life Events That May Increase a Child's Disfluency
1. The child's family moves to a new house, a new neighborhood, or a new city.
2. The child's parents separate or divorce.
3. A family member dies.
4. A family member is hospitalized.
5. The child is hospitalized.
6. A parent loses his or her job.
7. A baby is born or a child is adopted.
8. An additional person comes to live in the house.
9. One or both parents go away frequently or for a long period of time.
10. Holidays or visits occur, which cause a change in routine, excitement, or anxiety.

vulnerable temperament—may have provided a fertile matrix for the sudden germination of stuttering when a stressful life event occurred.

In a few cases, traumatic life events appear to precipitate stuttering in children and adults who appear to have no predisposition to stuttering. These unusual onsets are discussed in Chapter 13 when I explore "psychogenic stuttering." Such individuals often stutter in unusual ways, which differ from the "garden variety" stuttering of those who begin stuttering when a stressful life event interacts with various predisposing conditions. Table 3–2 lists some of the life events that I have found to be stressful to children's fluency.

Learning Factors

When I was in high school, I stuttered severely. If I had to make a phone call, I dreaded it for hours beforehand. When I finally got up the courage to pick up the phone and dial, an invisible hand seemed to tighten around my throat. When someone answered, all I could get out was a series of "um's" punctuated by the listener's repeated "Hello? Hello? Hello?" Finally, I could say, "Is Mmmmmm" and there I was, stuck fast, until, with a huge head jerk, I would blurt out, "Is Molly there?" And the listener would say, typically, "What?"

I had gone downhill a long way since my stuttering began at age 3 with simple repetitions of words like "I-I-I ...." So, how did this change take place? The answer is learning; that is, the change that takes place in a person or animal as a result of their experiences in the environment (Lefton, 1997). Not only did learning create my more severe stuttering symptoms, it also helped me, with the guidance of a good stuttering therapist, to reduce those symptoms to the mild form of stuttering that I have today. In this section, you will learn more about how learning works so that you will understand your client's stuttering behaviors and then can help him or her change them. The different components of my stuttering were created by different types of learning. Specific types of learning are often referred to as different kinds of conditioning. These include **classical conditioning**, **operant conditioning**, and **avoidance conditioning**.

Classical Conditioning

The feelings of dread I had before making a phone call and the tightening of my throat were the products of classical conditioning. This type of learning takes place when there is a repeated association between a neutral stimulus, like the phone, and another stimulus, such as stuttering, that naturally and consistently evokes a response, which in my case were feelings of dread and throat tightening. Such emotional responses often come from the reactions of someone in the environment, such as an impatient listener. I learned this association because I repeatedly stuttered severely on the phone, which made me frustrated, embarrassed, and afraid. These feelings naturally elicited muscle tightening, as we discussed in Chapter 2 in the section on temperament. After repeated pairings of the telephone and stuttering, I began to experience the emotions associated with stuttering whenever I had to make a phone call, even before I picked up the phone.

An everyday example of this type of learning is the classically conditioned response your cat has learned when she hears you open a can of cat food. When she was a new kitten, she made no particular association to the whir of an electric can opener. But when you repeatedly whirred open a can of tuna-flavored Kitty Delight just before feeding her, she began to associate the sound of the can opener with eating. Now she meows, trips you, and becomes a general pest whenever she hears the electric can opener, because she associates the sound of the opener with food.

How can you use the principles of classical conditioning to help someone who stutters talk more fluently? One way is to associate a previously neutral stimulus, like the telephone, with more positive speaking experiences. Once you've used various therapy techniques to help a client become more fluent while talking to you in the therapy room, you can then have her take a series of small steps toward talking fluently on the telephone. For example, you might first have her talk fluently to you with the phone resting on a nearby table. Then, have her talk fluently to you while holding the disconnected phone up to her ear. Once she feels comfortable and is fluent doing this, she can talk to you on the phone while you're in another room. Repeated experiences of fluent speech like this have the potential to erase the client's association between the telephone and stuttering, which, in turn, can eliminate or reduce her emotional response and muscle tension as she prepares to make a phone call. You are undoing the client's initial association between the telephone and bad experiences with stuttering by making a new association between the telephone and her more fluent speech.

Another way to de-condition a client's classically conditioned response is by having her associate experiences of stuttering on the phone with positive responses from the environment. One way to accomplish this is by teaching the client to stutter on purpose, while staying relaxed and feeling comfortable during the stutter. (I'll talk more about stuttering on purpose in Chapters 11 and 12.) Your praise and calm words when she is stuttering will help her reduce her fear and tension. You would begin this de-conditioning in the safe environment of the therapy room without a telephone nearby and have her make a series of small steps, as in the previous example, that would gradually move her toward making real phone calls with listeners whose responses might be less than warm and accepting. The outcome of this procedure is to help the client learn that, although she may stutter, she need not be embarrassed or afraid of stuttering. In turn, her muscle tension responses to these emotions will be drastically reduced, and she will find her more relaxed stuttering that results quite acceptable. Repeated work of this type can change severe stuttering to fluency or to very mild stuttering.

Operant Conditioning

When I stuttered severely in high school, I would often end stutters by jerking my head just as I made a big push that finally got the word out. Operant conditioning was responsible for my learning this behavior and for the fact that it remained part of my stuttering pattern for many years. In this type of learning, the frequency at which a behavior occurs is related to the consequences that follow. If a behavior is followed by a reward, it increases; if it is followed by an aversive consequence, it decreases. Like many operant behaviors, my head nod had begun as random struggles when I was jammed on a word. Several times, the word I was stuck on popped out of my mouth just as I jerked my head up. The relief I felt in freeing myself of the stutter and being able to finish my sentence caused my head jerking to increase whenever I stuttered. The escape behaviors we described in Chapter 1, such as eye blinks, are learned through operant conditioning. They begin as part of random struggle efforts to escape from a stutter, and they are rewarded by the release of the word.

A common type of operant conditioning is called *positive reinforcement.* The next time you are in a public building with an elevator, watch what happens when people are waiting for the elevator to arrive and it's delayed. One person will usually keep pressing the elevator button several times even though the button is illuminated and the elevator is on its way. Like everyone else, this person has been reinforced many times by the prompt arrival of the elevator after pushing the button. At some later time, however, he must have encountered a delayed elevator, and after pressing the button repeatedly, he was rewarded by the eventual arrival of the elevator. Thus, positive reinforcement conditioned him to repeat this behavior even though he had to have known that it wasn't necessary. The same is true if you have a "lucky shirt" to wear to an exam. If you do well, you will probably be more likely to wear the same shirt, even if it is in need of a wash, to your next exam, despite knowing, intellectually, that it doesn't actually affect the outcome.

Another kind of operant conditioning is *punishment.* It probably has shaped your behavior if you've ever gotten a ticket for speeding. The punishing effect of an expensive fine makes you drive more cautiously when you are on the same section of road. You can appreciate the disadvantage of punishment, however, if you can remember referring to the police officer as a "weasel" when you described the incident to your friends and family. Unless it is mild and delivered with good humor, punishment usually is not beneficial to clinical relationships.

A third kind of operant conditioning, *negative reinforcement,* is the mechanism behind the escape behaviors, like eye blinks and head nods, that are part of many stuttering patterns. The head jerks that were part of my own stuttering pattern were the result of just this type of conditioning. Negative reinforcement occurs whenever a behavior is followed by the termination of an unpleasant situation. In stuttering, a sudden movement may terminate a moment of stuttering, which means that behavior is reinforced and is likely to occur more frequently in the future when the stutterer is jammed up. All of us can develop habits through negative reinforcement in our daily routines. For instance, if you are trapped in a long line at the cash register in the bookstore, you may bail out and discover that the register upstairs in the compact disk section has no line at all. If so, your escape behavior is reinforced, making it more likely that you will again go upstairs to the other register the next time you are stuck in the long line.

The principles of operant conditioning are a major part of every stuttering clinician's tool kit. When you are working with a preschool-age child who stutters, you first arrange a situation in which she is fluent and use praise or tangible rewards to reinforce her fluency. The environment in which operant conditioning takes place is where the child will speak most fluently, so it is important to teach parents how to use operant conditioning at home. Punishment is rarely used, but sometimes you can effectively use mild self-punishment, coupled with negative reinforcement, to change the behavior of adults or older children. A classic example is called "cancellation." In this procedure, persons who stutter are taught to mildly punish *themselves* with a few seconds of silence immediately after a hard, effortful block. After the silent pause, they say the word again, but slightly slower and with less muscle tension. The escape from silence and saying the word more easily reinforces them for a milder form of stuttering, which gradually approximates normal speech. Negative reinforcement is also used in a technique called a "pullout." This technique teaches a person who stutters to escape from a hard block, not by pushing or squeezing with excess tension, but by reducing the tension of the stutter and finishing the word with a relaxed, nearly normal-sounding production.

Avoidance Conditioning

My stuttering in high school, described earlier, was peppered with dozens of "ums." I usually said "um" three or four times before I even tried to say a word I expected trouble on. Sometimes my classmates, in a curious and friendly way, would count the number of "ums" I had in a row and tell me later what my record was. Once they counted 17 "ums" as I was trying to say, "Yugoslavia." These "ums" were the result of avoidance conditioning. I first learned to use "um" as an escape behavior. When I was hopelessly stuck on a word, I could sometimes release it by quickly saying "um" and trying the word again. Then I began to say "um" even before starting a word I expected to be difficult. This sometimes prevented a stutter from occurring, and I was on my way to a serious case of avoidance conditioning. Because I rarely tried to say a difficult word without saying "um," I never learned that I might do better without it.

There are many types of avoidance behaviors that people who stutter learn. They include avoiding speaking situations, avoiding certain words and substituting easy words for hard ones, and using extra sounds, words, or phrases, such as "um," "well," and "you know," to get a running start on a difficult word. One political activist I worked with cringed every time he'd see himself on television hemming and hawing and dodging difficult words, looking like a caricature of a politician. He successfully learned to be open about his difficulty and stutter mildly on words he really wanted to use.

Avoidance conditioning is a big part of every day life. The example I presented earlier, in which you learned to escape from a long line in the bookstore by going to a register in the CD section, can also be used to describe how avoidance conditioning may be common in your life. Perhaps after escaping from long lines at the front register several times, you might have started to avoid that register altogether and just go straight to the register in the CD section. Although many avoidance behaviors are first learned as escape behaviors, many are not. Think about why you put on your seat belt when you drive or wear a helmet when you get on a motorcycle or snowboard. You may never have had an accident, but public safety spots on TV make us imagine what can happen if you don't take these precautions to avoid brain damage or worse.

Clinically, you will need to help people who stutter to reduce their avoidance behaviors using a number of approaches. It is often difficult to get rid of avoidance behaviors because the person doesn't dare to find out what would happen if he didn't do them. It's like the man who was referred to a psychiatrist for habitually snapping his fingers. "Why do you do that?" the psychiatrist asked. "Because it keeps the elephants away," the man replied. The psychiatrist then said, "But you don't need to. There are no elephants for miles around." "Well, then," the man replied, "it works, doesn't it!"

This patient might be helped if the psychiatrist could convince him to stop snapping his fingers in the office where the psychiatrist could give him protection and reassurance. This would enable the patient to see that no elephants came even though he didn't snap his fingers for at least an hour. You can use similar techniques to help a high school student learn to tackle difficult words without saying "um." For example, you could praise him highly for starting a feared word without saying "um," but beginning it slowly and deliberately instead and using a pullout if stuttering occurs. I have always found it important to teach a client what *to do* when she is afraid she will stutter before teaching her what avoidance behaviors *not to do.*

Fortunately, some individuals who stutter will stop using avoidance behaviors without having to work directly on them. Directly improving fluency, for example, will often decrease avoidances. This is particularly true for children, who may be avoiding a few words or speaking situations but have not developed a widespread pattern of avoidance. For them, learning how to speak more fluently will reduce their fear of stuttering enough so that they are motivated to approach all the speaking opportunities presented to them.

Summary

- During the preschool years, rapid and differential changes in a child's body, especially in speech structures, may make it difficult for a child to coordinate the rapid movements necessary for fluency.

- A child's cognitive development may not only compete with speech production for resources, but may also provide the intellectual ability for a child to compare herself with others, which may lead to embarassment and shame about stuttering.

- In younger children with immature brains, speech pathways may not be buffered from the effects of emotional arousal, resulting in more disfluency. Some children may be especially vulnerable to the effects of emotion on speech because they can be easily emotionally aroused. Self-conscious emotions develop soon after age 2, and the emotional distress of these children in reaction to stuttering may produce increased physical tension, particularly in the larynx.

■ As language develops rapidly, the increasing length and compexity of children's utterances may sometimes exceed their speech production abilities. Selecting words, encoding phonology, planning syntax, and working out the complex prosody for an entire utterance all occur just as the child is starting to speak. It is no wonder, then, that most early stuttering occurs on the first words of sentences.

■ There is some evidence that delays in language acquisition and, especially, phonological development may be associated with increased risk of persistent stuttering.

■ Parents of children who stutter may, as a group, show slight tendencies to be demanding and perfectionistic. This may be the result of having a child with a speech difficulty or a manifestation of the genetic background that also results in a child having a vulnerable temperament. Research in this area is equivocal, however, with many studies finding no differences between the parents of children who stutter and those of children who do not.

■ There is no clear evidence that parents of children who stutter converse using faster rates, more questions, more interruptions, and more long, complex utterances than parents of nonstuttering children. Several studies have found differences between these groups of parents, but many have not. Despite the lack of research support, many clinicians believe that it is helpful therapeutically for parents to slow their speech rate and speak in shorter sentences when talking to their children who stutter.

■ There is a wealth of clinical anecdotes suggesting that difficult events in a child's life, such as parents' divorce or the arrival of a new baby in the family, may trigger stuttering. However, there is little empirical support for these anecdotes.

■ Classical conditioning may cause stuttering to spread to many different contexts and to be consistently present rather than episodic. Operant conditioning can increase the frequency of escape behaviors. Avoidance conditioning can increase the frequency of behaviors that stutterers use to postpone or evade expected stutters. All three types of conditioning are important contributors to the establishment of secondary stuttering behaviors and are also critical to the treatment of stuttering.

Study Questions

1. The effect of a child's development on fluency has been likened to the effect of multiple tasks for a computer. Explain this analogy.

2. It has been said that children usually do not learn to walk and talk at the same time. What does this suggest about how motor development might affect fluency?

3. There is a high incidence of stuttering among retarded individuals. What might this suggest about the relationship between cognition and fluency?

4. What aspects of social and emotional development might threaten fluency?

5. What evidence is there that emotional arousal might increase disfluency?

6. What is the possible connection between atypical hemispheric localization and the effects of emotion on fluency?

7. Why would children's speech and language development be likely to put greater pressure on fluency than their physical or cognitive development?

8. What aspects of parents' behavior might put pressure on a child who is disfluent?

9. Identify several characteristics of parents' speech that may create difficult models for a disfluent child to emulate.

10. Name several life events that have been suggested to increase a child's disfluency.

11. What is the central hypothesis of the diagnosogenic view?

SUGGESTED PROJECTS

(1) Record a natural speech sample from someone who stutters, and analyze the relationship between the occurrences of stuttering and the linguistic level of the utterances in which they occur.

(2) Develop an experimental protocol to assess the relationship between linguistic variables and stuttering. For example, compare the variables of length of utterance, syntactic level of utterance, and phonological complexity of utterance on the liklihood of the utterance being stuttered.

(3) Design a therapy activity for someone who has a classically conditioned fear of dogs. One way to do this would be to develop a hierarchy of situations that progress from easy and non-threatening to gradually more realistic encounters with dogs. At each level of the hierarchy, have the client engage in some "approach" behavior (like talking to the dog) that will counteract their old tendency to avoid dogs.

(4) Study the effect of your speech rate on other people by designing and carrying out an experiment in which you vary the speed at which you talk. Tape record conversations in which you talk slowly for several minutes and then talk rapidly for several minutes. Measure the effect on your conversational partners' speed of talking. You will need to practice varying your rate beforehand.

(5) In the section on Speech and Language Development, research on language abilities of children who stutter is reviewed. Some studies found that children who stutter have poorer langauge abilities and other studies did not. Review these studies and suggest what might be causing this disagreement in the literature.

Suggested Readings

Andrews, G., and Harris, M. (1964). *The Syndrome of Stuttering.* **London: W. Heinemann Medical Books.**

These authors present data from longitudinal studies of a thousand families in Newcastle, England. The interpretation of results presents evidence that both genetic and environmental influences are at work to create stuttering. This book gives an early version of the "capacities and demands" view that stuttering is due to a lack of capacity for some aspect of speech and language processing.

Ayres, J.J.B. (1998). Fear conditioning and avoidance. In W. O'Donohue (Ed), *Learning and Behavior Therapy.* **Boston: Allyn and Bacon.**

This chapter provides a good update of the animal learning literature on fear conditioning. Several findings appear to be relevant to stuttering. First, some responses to fear may be part of an animal's hard-wiring (perhaps laryngeal tension is a natural response to fear of speaking in some individuals). Second, some individual animals freeze in response to fear rather than learn an effective coping response (are some children who begin to stutter more predisposed to tense blockages than others?). Third, for a fear-conditioned response, reducing fear without teaching a new response to fear leaves the animal vulnerable to relapse (it may be important to reduce stutterers' fear of stuttering as well as teaching them a coping skill they can use when fear is present).

Bernstein Ratner, N. (1997). Stuttering: A psycholinguistic perspective. In R. Curlee and G. Siegel (Eds), *Nature and Treatment of Stuttering: New Directions* **(ed 2). Boston: Allyn and Bacon.**

This is an insightful review of the many connections between language to stuttering. The author's background allows her to use linguistic theories and evidence from child language studies to discuss how language influences the loci of stuttering in speech, how parent-child interactions may affect stuttering, how language development may be important in stuttering onset, and the role of feedback on speech, language, and stuttering development.

Bloodstein, O. (1995). Inferences and conclusions. In, *A Handbook on Stuttering.* **San Diego: Singular Publishing Group, Inc.**

This chapter presents the communicative failure and anticipatory struggle view of stuttering onset. Bloodstein musters the evidence he has summarized in earlier chapters of this handbook to argue convincingly that stuttering develops from an interaction between the child and his environment.

Crystal, D. (1987). Towards a "bucket" theory of language disability: Taking account of interaction between linguistic levels. *Clinical Linguistics and Phonetics,* **1:7–22.**

A theoretical discussion of interaction among levels of speech and language, with an illustrative case of a child whose stuttering increases when language demands are greater. The article makes a clear argument for the influence of speech and language development on stuttering.

Johnson, W., et al. (1959). *The Onset of Stuttering.* **Minneapolis: University of Minnesota Press.**

This book presents extensive data on parents' perceptions of the onset of their child's stuttering compared with other parents' perceptions of their child's normal disfluency. Johnson eloquently lays out his view of stuttering as the product of an interaction between the child's disfluency, his sensitivity, and the listener's reactions.

Kagan, J., Reznick, J.S., and Snidman, N. (1987). The physiology and psychology of behavioral inhibition in children. *Child Development,* **58:1459–1473.**

This article discusses the findings of Kagan and his colleagues that behaviorally inhibited children show high levels of laryngeal tension. Neurophysiological mechanisms are also discussed, as well as possible genetic and environmental contributions. This article is recommended for those interested in the hypothesis that behavioral inhibition may be a component in some stuttering.

Paden, E.P. (2005). Development of phonological ability. In E. Yairi, and N. Ambrose (Eds), *Early Childhood Stuttering.* **Austin, TX: Pro-Ed.**

This chapter focuses on the phonological development of children who stutter, with particular emphasis on comparisons between children who recover without intervention and those who persist in stuttering. The author brings to light several aspects of her research that are intriguing puzzles for future researchers to solve.

Watkins, R.V. (2005). Language abilities of young children who stutter. In E. Yairi and N. Ambrose (Eds), *Early Childhood Stuttering.* **Austin, TX: Pro-Ed.**

Although current evidence reviewed in this chapter suggests that language abilities of children who stutter and those who do not stutter are similar, language factors appear to play an important role in stuttering. The author discusses several interesting relationships between language and stuttering, including the role of language factors in the occurrence of stuttering in an utterance and the finding that early onset of stuttering is often associated with advanced language skills.

Chapter 4

Theories About Stuttering

What are theories and what can we learn from them? Theories are a way of putting together the bits and pieces of what is known about something to understand it better. A theory puts together findings in a systematic way so that a past phenomenon is explained and a future one is predicted. A theory about tsunamis explains how they are caused by earthquakes on the ocean floor and predicts that when a large undersea earthquake occurs again, another tsunami will occur. A theory about stuttering would take the many facts, findings, and observations that you have been reading about in the first three chapters and put them together to explain why one person stutters and another does not. A complete theory would also explain why a person stutters on some words and not others or in some situations and not others, and why stutterers do the things they do when they stutter. When a theory can explain these things well, it can lead to effective treatment. When we know what causes stuttering, we will have a better chance of being able to modify it and perhaps even prevent it.

Scientists often use the word "theory" to mean a formal set of hypotheses that explain the important causal relationships in a phenomenon. These hypotheses are then tested, and the theory may be thrown out, improved, or confirmed as a result. The field of stuttering research and treatment hasn't developed far enough to have a formal theory of stuttering, although there are a number of informal theories that might be called theoretical perspectives or theoretical models. Just to simplify my writing, I'll use the term theory to refer to these perspectives or models, acknowledging they are far from formal theories.

In this chapter, I present several theories of stuttering as well as my own attempt to integrate research and clinical findings. I have organized the theories by the areas covered in chapters 2 and 3—constitutional, developmental, and environmental factors. These models change every few years as more data are gathered on stuttering and new information is generated in related areas. Without a doubt, the explanations of stuttering I summarize in this chapter, including my own, will be superseded by others in a few years.

Theoretical Perspectives About Constitutional Factors in Stuttering

I have chosen several contemporary views of constitutional factors to discuss in the following sections. Although the views differ, they are not mutually exclusive. If linked together, they provide us with some interesting notions about what factors might be inherited or acquired and how that might result in stuttering.

Stuttering as a Disorder of Brain Organization

Many studies of both normal speakers and brain-damaged patients have demonstrated that the left hemisphere is dominant for language in most people. One early theory of stuttering suggested that it is caused by lack of hemispheric dominance (the Orton-Travis theory of stuttering referred to in Chapter 2). The theory came about in this way. In an atmosphere of intense scientific curiosity and collaboration among researchers at the University of Iowa in the 1920s, Samuel Orton, a neurologist, and Lee Edward Travis, a psychologist and speech pathologist, observed that many stutterers seemed to have been left-handers whose parents changed them into being right-handed (Travis, 1931). They suspected that this change led to conflicts in the control of speech in which neither hemisphere was fully in charge of the movements of the structures used for speech. The lack of a dominant hemisphere, they reasoned, created neuromotor disorganization and mistiming of speech, which resulted in stuttering. Their treatment was simply to switch stutterers back to being left-handed. This approach, as you might guess, turned out to be fruitless. Furthermore, there was never convincing evidence that high numbers of stutterers were originally left-handed. Consequently, the original cerebral dominance theory of stuttering languished for many years. But in the 1960s, evidence began to accumulate that stutterers may not, after all, have normal left hemisphere dominance for language. In the 1970s and early 1980s, more published studies supported this finding.

In 1985, a new version of the cerebral dominance theory of stuttering was proposed. Two neurologists, Norman Geschwind and Albert Galaburda, proposed that many disorders, including stuttering, dyslexia, and autism, resulted from delays in left hemisphere growth during fetal development that led subsequently to right hemisphere dominance for speech and language (Geschwind and Galaburda, 1985). The delay in left hemisphere growth that resulted in these predominantly male disorders was thought to be caused by a male-related factor. Geschwind and Galaburda hypothesized that these delays might result from fetal exposure to excess testosterone during embryonic development. So far, however, no evidence has been found to support their hypothesis about testosterone. In fact, Neilson, Howie, and Andrews (1987) provided some evidence against this hypothesis, but the idea of a delay in left hemisphere development continues to be of great interest.

Geschwind and Galaburda's theory suggests that a delay in left hemisphere growth and development may affect speech and language for the following reasons. Various left hemisphere structures that evolve during embryonic development appear to be especially suited for speech and language functions. As these structures develop, specialized nerve cells, which are genetically programmed to sprout the neural connections for speech and language processes, disperse from their point of origin in the "neural tube," where the central nervous system is formed. These nerve cells normally migrate to previously developed structures in the left hemisphere that are appropriate for their specialized functions. But if development of left hemisphere structures is delayed, cells migrating from the neural tube may not receive the "homing beacon" they need to reach the left hemisphere. Instead, these specialized cells receive signals from the more developed right hemisphere and migrate there instead. These specialized cells then organize themselves as "networks" of neural activity in the right hemisphere for processing of speech and language. However, because the right hemisphere is not designed—by its architecture and interconnections—for this function, speech and language operate inefficiently there, like the internet search engine Google trying to access information through the postal service.

Although speculation about atypical cerebral localization in stutterers has received some support from research, especially from the recent brain imaging studies reviewed in Chapter 2, details of how stuttering behaviors result from abnormal localization is another issue, requiring other theories that will be described in a later section of this chapter.

Another version of the view that stuttering results from anomalous cerebral organization has been proposed by William Webster. As I noted in the discussion of studies of nonspeech motor control in Chapter 2, Webster (1993) studied the effect of interference on one task (sequential finger tapping) caused by another task (turning a knob in response to an auditory signal) done simultaneously by the other hand. He concluded that people who stutter have normal localization of speech and language in the left hemisphere but that their left hemisphere structure for speech planning and sequencing (the supplementary motor area [SMA]) is especially vulnerable to disruption by activities in other areas of the brain. Webster suspected the SMA because it is strongly connected to the motor cortex as well as to subcortical motor areas and is known to be involved in the initiation, planning, and sequencing of motor activities. The left SMA is located near the corpus callosum and receives input coming across this bridge from the right hemisphere, as well as input from the left hemisphere, and might be highly susceptible to disruption by excess activity from either hemisphere. Webster further suggested that individuals who stutter often may have overactive right hemispheres and speculated that overflow of right hemishere activation, especially from right hemisphere emotions (e.g., fear), would disrupt SMA functions in planning, initiating, and sequencing speech motor output.

Stuttering as a Disorder of Timing

Several authors believe that the known facts about stuttering point toward a disorder of timing. For example, Van Riper (1982, p. 415) stated that, "when a person stutters on a word, there is a temporal disruption of the simultaneous and successive programming of muscular movements required to produce one of the word's integrated sounds...." Building on Van Riper's view, Kent (1984) marshalled several lines of evidence to support a hypothesis that stuttering arises from a deficit in temporal programming. He speculated that this deficit reflects the inappropriate localization of speech and language functions to the right hemisphere that results in an inability to create the precise timing patterns needed to perceive and produce speech efficiently. Like a conductor of a symphony orchestra who determines when each section plays, as well as their speed or tempo, mechanisms in the brain control the rate at which we speak and the order of movements for producing sequential sounds. Just as a conductor integrates the timing of an orchestra's several sections, the brain must coordinate complex timing relationships for phonemes, syllables, and phrases of speech.

Kent (1994) suggested that the inability to perform precise timing functions consistently may stem from a stutterer's left hemisphere being less well developed than the right hemisphere (cf., Geshwind and Galaburda, 1985). Because the left hemisphere is specialized for processing brief, rapidly changing events, such as those needed for fine motor control of verbal output, a person who stutters may be disadvantaged when trying to process at the speed required for normal speech. This central timing function, Kent points out, must not only regulate left hemisphere aspects of speech production, but must also integrate the production of rapid, left hemisphere–generated speech segments with the slower prosodic elements of speech.

Kent also noted that emotion may play an important role in disrupting the timing of the speech of someone who stutters. As I indicated earlier, the right hemisphere is believed to be heavily involved in the regulation of certain negative emotions. The stutterer's deficit, then, may be that his timing functions for speech are arranged so that they are (1) less efficient than those of nonstutterers and (2) vulnerable to interference by right hemisphere activity during increased emotion. How this deficit causes the repetitions, prolongations, and blocks we hear in stutterers' speech is not explained in this theory.

Stuttering as Reduced Capacity for Internal Modeling

Another view of constitutional factors in stuttering has been advanced by Megan and Peter Neilson, whose research on stutterers' tracking abilities was reviewed in Chapter 2. The Neilsons proposed that the repetitions of beginning stutterers are the result of a deficit in their ability to create and use "inverse internal models of the speech production system" (Neilson and Neilson, 1987). This rather complicated sounding model can be easily understood if we go back to an assumption about how children learn to speak.

During the first year of life, infants store up perceptions of the speech sounds they hear around them and begin to play with speech sounds, trying to imitate what they hear. Gradually, as they grow older, children learn how to make these sounds accurately. Some scientists, like the Neilsons, believe that too much of the brain's neural resources would be required if children had to remember each of the movements needed to produce each sound of their language in every possible phonetic context. Instead, children are thought to develop a mental "model" of the relationship between their speech movements and sounds they hear. Just as someone beginning to play a trombone must learn the relationship between the movements of the trombone "slide" and the sounds that result, experienced trombonists have established mental models of the relationship of their arm movements to the sounds produced and are able to move the slide to produce a desired sound without having to think about it in any deliberate way.

A child, then, develops a mental model of the relationship between speech sounds and motor commands, as if speaking and playing a trombone have similar roots. The mental model in the brain might be called a sensory-motor model for speech, which the Neilsons call an "inverse internal model" of how speech is produced. It is an "inverse" model because it transforms or inverts sensory targets (i.e., speech sounds) into the motor commands needed to produce them. As infants learn to produce the sounds they hear, they constantly use and refine their sensory-motor model for speech. They plan a word or sentence in terms of what it should sound like (the target) and then rely on their sensory-motor model to generate the motor movement commands that will produce the speech targets they are trying to hit.

The process of learning to speak is something like learning to drive a car. At first, keeping the car on the road requires constant vigilance. But as we learn the relationships between turning the wheel, stepping on the accelerator, and going where we want, the linkage becomes automatic, even when driving a stick-shift vehicle in stop-and-go traffic. Moreover, the linkage is refined as we encounter different driving conditions and different cars (e.g., cars with loose steering wheels and sticky accelerators). Just as drivers establish sensory-motor models for driving, children develop sensory-motor models for speaking.

Figure 4–1 is a schematic depiction of how the brain may transform desired sensory (perceptual) targets into motor commands for speech. In the figure, the desired output (the word or phrase, for example, that a child intends a listener to hear) is fed into the internal inverse model of the speech production system. Here, the desired output is entered as sensory code of its expected auditory and kinesthetic results, which is "inverted" by the model to generate its output as movement codes or motor commands. Experience, practice, and vocal play help the child to acquire these inversions or transformations. Moreover, this internal model is continually updated as a child's speech and language skills mature and the speech production system changes with age. The internal model's motor commands are sent to the muscles of the speech production system, whose coordinated contractions produce the acoustic output that result in a planned utterance. Concurrently, ongoing planning and feedback of this process are fed into the modeling circuitry. Let us retrace our steps for a moment; when motor commands are sent to muscles, a copy of these commands, which is called the "efference copy" by

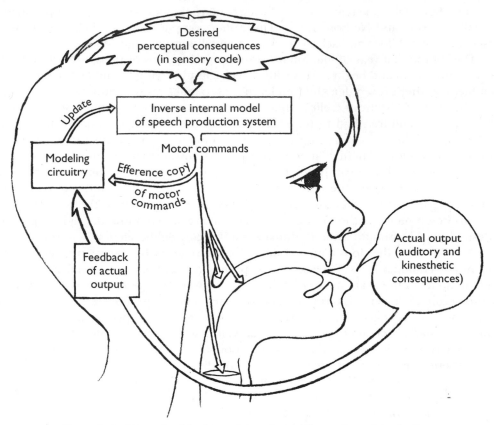

Figure 4–1   *Schematic of the inverse internal model theory of speech production.*

motor physiologists, is also sent to the modeling circuitry. Here, efference copy is transformed into its hypothetical output, which is a model, or template, of the output that should be produced based on the motor commands. This hypothetical output is continuously compared with feedback on the current positions and movements of the speech mechanism so that the inverse internal model can update its ongoing motor commands, if necessary, to produce the desired output more accurately. These components of the speech production process are assumed to involve the corticocerebellar structures and pathways that are commonly described in neural models of speech output (e.g, Neilson and Neilson, 1987; Neilson, Neilson, and O'Dwyer, 1992; Neilson and Neilson, 2000).

The Neilsons and their coworkers have used the inverse internal model of the speech production system to understand the performance of stutterers in experiments (Neilson, Quinn, and Neilson, 1976) that tested their ability to track an auditory tone that changed unpredictably. The subjects heard an unpredictably changing "target" tone in one ear and a "cursor" tone, which they could control with a hand-held device, in the other ear. Their task was to track the pitch of the target tone with the cursor tone as accurately as possible. The Neilsons' experiments found that stutterers were poorer than nonstutterers in tracking auditory tones that went up and down in pitch. Stutterers were still poorer than nonstutterers even after practicing the task. These findings suggested to the Neilsons that if stutterers had difficulty learning the relationships between the sounds they want to say and the movements required to produce them as young children, they would also, therefore, have difficulty making the sensory-to-motor and motor-to-sensory transformations required by the tracking tasks. However, this difficulty would not always result in stuttering. When circumstances don't call for much of the brain's functional capacities in speech and language areas, stutterers should be able to compensate for their slight weakness. On the other hand, when large portions of the brain's functional capacity are allocated for language tasks, such as choosing new or unfamiliar words or constructing complex sentences, the diminished neural capacity cannot be accommodated, and more repetitions would result. As these researchers put it, "whether one will become a stutterer depends on one's neurological capacity for these sensory-to-motor and motor-to-sensory transformations and the demands posed by the speech act" (Andrews et al, 1983).

How do these intermittent deficits in available functional neural capacity result in the symptoms of stuttering? This theory attempts to account only for the core behaviors of early stuttering, that is, repetitions and prolongations. According to the theory, repetitions and prolongations result from inadequate transformations of sensory targets, transformations that should generate the motor commands for speech. A speaker with reduced functional neural capacity may begin to speak but be unable to plan and carry out the rest of his utterance without disruption. Repetitions or prolongations may occur if a speaker is attempting to push ahead with speech, while his brain is still planning the syllables that follow and how to link them with the initial sound.

Recently, other researchers have also used the concept of internal models to explain the behaviors of stuttering. Max et al (2004) proposed a theoretical model of stuttering based on unstable or insufficiently activated internal models. One of their hypotheses parallels the Neilsons' proposition, that some children are predisposed to stutter because of the difficulty learning the relationships between their motor commands and the desired acoustic output. This difficulty would result in an inaccurate inverse internal model of the speech production system (Fig. 4–1), which would generate output that would not match the desired perceptual consequences. The speech production system would then "reset" itself to try again, producing repetitions. This resetting process would continue until the child's error correction process could update the model sufficiently to make the output match the consequences. If this could be done quickly, only one or two repetitions would occur; if not, many repetitions would occur. Max et al's proposal has other hypotheses and an extensive review of the literature to support them. Their proposal is particularly effective in relating various stuttering phenomena to aspects of the model. For example, the findings that stutterers' movements are slower during fluent speech (see Chapter 2) and the evidence that slow speech can induce fluency are both explained by the possibility that a slower rate of speech production would allow the stutterer more time for feedback to update the internal model so that it becomes more accurate as the movements are being produced, thus avoiding the need for resetting the system and its consequent repetitions. In other words, slower speech makes corrections possible while a syllable is being produced rather than after it is completed. Note that if this hypothesis is accurate, errors would be found in the stutterer's unsuccessful repetitions.

Stuttering as a Language Production Deficit

Many researchers have been intrigued by the influence of linguistic factors on stuttering. For example, stuttering often begins when a child enters a period of intense language development. Similarly, stuttering is most frequent when the load on language functions is heaviest (e.g., in longer utterances, at the beginnings of sentences, and on longer, less familiar words) (Bloodstein, 2002). These factors have prompted several theorists to propose that stuttering reflects an impairment in some aspect of spoken language. I use the term "spoken language" because these theorists believe the major problem is not in the motor execution of speech, but rather in the planning and assembly of language units, such as phonemes, that occur before speech is produced.

Herman Kolk and Albert Postma (1997) developed the "Covert Repair" hypothesis to explain stuttering from a language production point of view. They believe that both stuttering and normal disfluencies result from an internal monitoring process that we all use to check whether what we are about to articulate is exactly what we mean to say. Perhaps this may be clearer if we imagine for a moment that language production is like a factory making bicycles (Fig. 4–2). The factory must monitor the quality of its bicycles by checking them at different stages. Some quality control checks occur after the bicycles leave the factory, when factory workers themselves ride the bicycles and tell the factory about any defects they find. In speech and language production, this is like a speaker's auditory feedback (the sound of your own words as you are speaking them).

The bicycle factory might also use another quality control process, one that occurs inside the factory before the bicycles are shipped out. This is like our internal monitoring process of speech and language. Without being aware of it, we check the "phonetic plan" for what we are about to say before we articulate it. This allows us to detect potential semantic, syntactic, lexical, and phonological errors before they are produced. Just as the production line in a bicycle factory would have to be halted when a defect is detected, speech production is interrupted when our internal monitor detects an error in our phonetic plans. Repairs need to be made before production can continue. Kolk and Postma (1997) believe that the halting of production and the repair process cause the disfluencies of both normal speakers and individuals who stutter.

To Kolk and Postma (1997), the most common stuttering disfluencies (repetitions, prolongations, and blocks) are the result of correcting or "repairing" the phonological (rather than semantic, syntactic, or lexical) errors detected in the phonetic plan before they are spoken. In the case of part-word repetitions, if a speaker detects an error in the final part of a syllable (e.g., the /p/ in "cup"), he restarts the phonological encoding process ("cu-cu-") and keeps going until the phoneme is encoded correctly and the entire syllable can be produced. In contrast, prolongations are thought to occur when the phoneme of a word or syllable preceding the error is a continuant (e.g., the /l/ in the word "lip" when the error involves the vowel). In this case, the continuant, /l/, is prolonged until the speaker successfully encodes the vowel, /i/, following /l/. Blocks are thought to result from errors in the initial sounds of words or syllables. When an error is detected, speech production is halted for repairs, but the speaker may try to plunge ahead, building up muscle tension and unaware of the automatic error detection and repair that is in progress. Kolk and Postma (1997) suggest that stutterers are prone to have more phonological encoding errors because they are constitutionally slower in

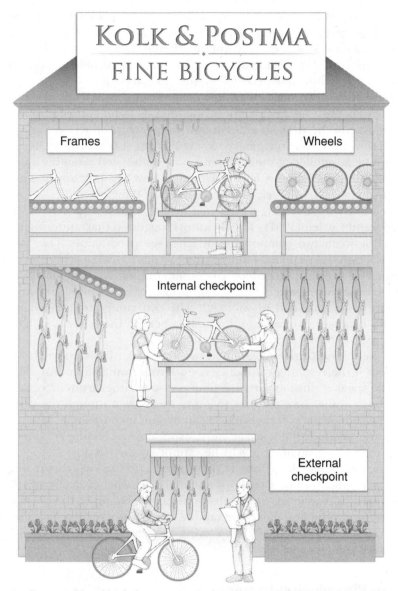

Figure 4–2 *Quality control in a bicycle factory as an analogy for part of the language production system in the brain.*

encoding and need more time than a typical conversational rate gives them. In various articles, Kolk and Postma lay out the evidence supporting their views and suggest, among other things, that the benefits of a slower speech rate on stuttering are derived from the greater amount of time that stutterers have for phonological encoding.

Several years before Kolk and Postma (1997) published their covert repair hypothesis, an innovative language production view of stuttering was published by Wingate in *The*

Structure of Stuttering: A Psycholinguistic Approach (1988). In this book, he reviewed linguistic and neurological research on stuttering and hypothesized that stuttering results from a dyssynchrony of functions in the left and right hemispheres, as well as subcortical structures. These different areas, Wingate suggested, are responsible for different components of language planning and production, such as consonants, vowels, and prosody. He theorized that, when speakers produce the initial portion of a syllable, the consonant and vowel and prosody must be synchronously blended. If some component lags behind at this critical moment, the result is a disruption in speech production that we observe as stuttering. Returning to our imaginary bicycle factory, it is as if the wheels, gears, and frame all must be assembled at the same time on a high-speed assembly line. If one component is delayed, production is halted. However, how this halt appears in speech as a repetition, prolongation, or block is not explained by Wingate.

Another theory of stuttering as a deficit in language production was proposed by Perkins, Kent, and Curlee (1991). These authors suggested that stuttering results from a dyssynchrony between two components of language production. The "paralinguistic" component is a right hemisphere–controlled social-emotional process that is responsible for vocal tone and prosodic functions. The other component is linguistic and involves a left hemisphere segmental system that is responsible for the content and structure of language (semantics, syntax, and phonology). The two components must be integrated before spoken language is produced. If one lags behind the other for whatever reason, the resulting dyssynchrony produces disfluency.

Perkins, Kent, and Curlee (1991) add two elements to this dyssynchrony that must also be present if the resulting disfluency is stuttering, rather than just a normal disfluency. First, the speaker must experience time pressure either from an outside source or an inner feeling, so that he continues trying to speak even though the dyssynchrony in paralinguistic or linguistic processes has resulted in an incomplete or anomalous speech motor program. Second, the speaker must experience a feeling of "loss of control," which arises from being unaware of why he cannot say the word.

In our imaginary bicycle factory, Perkins, Kent, and Curlee's theory might be characterized as a production line that stops automatically whenever one of the two major subcomponents of a bicycle are not ready for assembly. However, the boss in this factory demands that the production line move rapidly, and the workers panic if the production line grinds to a halt and frantically keep trying to restart production even though they don't know what the problem is or how to fix it.

Stuttering as Physiological Tremor

One of the mysteries of stuttering is how it changes from brief, easy repetitions or prolongations of words and syllables that are hardly noticed by the child or listeners to the long, tense blockages that frustrate, embarrass, and upset both the speaker and, often, his audience. The previously described constitutional theories focused on mechanisms resulting in the beginning repetitions and prolongations of stuttering children. Now, I will turn to a theory that may account for some of the more severe disfluencies of stuttering—the tense blockages of sound and airflow.

For amost 25 years, Anne Smith has been carrying out a systematic program of research on stuttering, developing a theory that at the core of stuttering is an unstable neuromuscular system that is influenced by a wide variety of cognitive, linguistic, and psychosocial factors (e.g., Zimmerman, Smith, and Hanley, 1981; Smith and Goffman, 2004). Some of this research has indicated that some stutters are characterized by rapid (5-12 Hz), rhythmic, oscillatory neural input to the muscles of speech so that they are contracting in a rapid, tremor-like way (Smith, 1989). Not every stutterer's muscles show these tremors during stuttering, and they may not appear in younger stutterers but may appear only after stuttering has persisted for some time. In one study, Kelly, Smith, and Goffman (1995) found that these neural oscillations were present in the stutters of the three older children in their study (ages 10 to 14 years) but were absent in the stutters of the seven younger children (ages 2 to 7 years). The researchers noted that such tremors may appear in the stuttering of only those individuals who have stuttered for some time and have developed maladative reactions. As Kelly et al (1995) pointed out, it is also possible that these tremors are evoked or magnified by autonomic arousal or the emotion that arises in response to the expectation or occurrence of speech difficulties.

Several writers have linked stress with stuttering and suggested that the tiny tremors that appear in everyone's muscles may be amplified by emotion to a level that interferes with talking (Fibiger, 1971, 1972; Weber and Smith, 1990; Van Riper, 1982). The effects of emotion on tremor may provide a physiological explanation of how the mild disfluencies of young children become the more severe blockages we see as beginning stuttering evolves into advanced stuttering. Even mild disfluencies may trigger emotional responses in some children that result in increased tremors that block speech. Emotional responses may also explain the unusual cases of severe blocks at the onset of stuttering, especially when stuttering begins during conditions of stress and strong emotion. The interaction of very strong emotion with a child's vulnerable speech motor system may create sudden severe stuttering because it amplifies tremors in the speech musculature. Such tremors may be analagous to the quivering lip of a toddler who is about to burst into tears when frightened by a barking dog or a screaming parent. Just how magnified tremors block or slow the forward movement of speech is not known, but Van Riper's (1982, p. 126) description of tension and tremor may give us some clues. He suggested:

> What usually seems to happen is that tremors begin when the stutterer creates a fixed closure, invests its antagonistic musculatures with tension, and then suddenly produces an increase of air pressure behind or below the closure. At the moment this increase occurs, the antagonistic musculatures become suffused with a sudden burst of further tension and the stuttering tremor comes into being. Then it persists...

Why stutterers would create fixed closures is a mystery. Perhaps it is one of the body's responses to fear that Gray (1987) described as a behavioral inhibition system, which I will discuss later in the section on secondary stuttering and temperament.

Theoretical Perspectives on Developmental and Environmental Factors

The three views presented in this section represent three different conceptualizations of how developmental or environmental stresses (or both) result in stuttering. One view is called the "diagnosogenic" view because it proposes that stuttering begins when parents mistakenly diagnose normal disfluency as stuttering. The other two views look more broadly at circumstances under which stuttering might arise. For example, the communicative failure and anticipatory struggle view assumes that some form of communication difficulty precipitates stuttering, whereas the capacities and demands view presumes that almost any developmental or environmental pressure may precipitate it. As you read this section, keep in mind that these three views differ not only in their concept of the roles that development and the environment play but also in their specificity. The first view (i.e., diagnosogenic) proposes that specific factors create stuttering; the last view (i.e., capacities and demands) describes how many different variables may interact to produce stuttering. The specificity of the remaining view (i.e., communicative failure) lies somewhere in between the others.

Diagnosogenic Theory

In the 1930s, Wendell Johnson and other researchers at the University of Iowa began studying the onset of stuttering in children. As Johnson examined the speech of young stutterers and nonstutterers, he noticed a similarity. The most common disfluencies of both groups were repetitions. As Johnson contemplated this observation, he was struck by the possibility that all of these children may have had the same disfluencies to begin with but that those who became stutterers developed more serious disfluencies by overreacting to their repetitions. But why? Perhaps their parents or other listeners mislabeled their repetitions as stuttering, and in so doing, made the children so self-conscious that they tried to speak without any disfluencies. Their efforts to avoid all disfluencies may have become, with the help of listeners' further negative reactions, what is generally regarded as stuttering (Johnson et al, 1942).

Johnson's hypothesis, which came to be called the diagnosogenic theory, meaning that stuttering begins with its diagnosis or, in this case, misdiagnosis, was the most widely accepted explanation of stuttering throughout the 1940s and 1950s. It pinpointed environmental factors as the sole cause of stuttering by placing the blame on the negative reactions of parents and other listeners.

Johnson and his associates continued gathering data on the disfluencies of stuttering children and their nonstuttering peers to further support the diagnosogenic theory. The results of several studies were summarized in a landmark book, *The Onset of Stuttering* (Johnson et al, 1959). Table 4–1, taken from Johnson's book, gives an overview of the similarities and differences in the disfluencies reported by stutterers' and nonstutterers' parents. Johnson interpreted these data as showing similarity between the disfluencies of stuttering and nonstuttering children; both groups of children were reported to show at least some of each type of disfluency. He suggested that the same disfluency types that parents of nonstuttering children considered normal were reported by parents of stuttering children as the earliest signs of stuttering. Johnson used this as evidence to support the diagnosogenic hypothesis that the problem was parents' interpretation of their child's disfluencies, or as some often put it, "the problem was not in the child's mouth but in the parent's ear."

It should be noted that later authors interpreted the data in Table 4–1 quite differently than Johnson did. The data were seen as evidence that the two groups of children were different at the onset of stuttering. McDearmon (1968), for example, argued that these findings showed that the disfluencies of normal children were significantly different from those in the stuttering children. Syllable repetitions, sound prolongations, and complete blocks were recalled to have occurred much more frequently in the stuttering children,

Table 4–1	Percentage of Parents of Stutterers and Nonstutterers Who Reported Child Was Performing Each Speech Behavior When They First Thought Child Was Stuttering

		Repetition		Sound Prolonga-tion	Other Nonfluency		
Group	Syllable	Word	Phrase		Silent Intervals	Interjec-tions	Complete Blocks
Control (nonstutterers)							
Fathers	4	59	23	3	36	30	0
Mothers	10	41	24	4	41	21	0
Experimental (stutterers)							
Fathers	57	48	8	15	7	8	3
Mothers	59	50	8	12	3	9	3

From Johnson, W., et al. (1959). The onset of stuttering. Minneapolis: University of Minnesota Press. Copyright © 1959 by the University of Minnesota. © 1987 Edna Johnson. Reprinted by permission of the University of Minnesota Press.

whereas phrase repetitions, pauses, and interjections were reported more frequently in the nonstuttering control group. This evidence and new findings about genetic and constitutional factors in stuttering have caused the diagnosogenic view of stuttering to be largely abandoned.

To illustrate the diagnosogenic view, I take an example from a master's thesis that Johnson directed (Tudor, 1939). At that time, the diagnosogenic theory had not been formally proposed, but undoubtedly, Johnson and others must have entertained the possibility that labeling a child as a stutterer would create more hesitancy in his speech. This thesis was an exploration of that idea. Johnson's student, Mary Tudor, screened all the children at a nearby orphanage for speech and language disorders. Tudor selected six children who were normal speakers, but she told these children that they should speak more carefully because they were making errors when they talked. She warned them that they were showing signs of stuttering. She also cautioned caregivers that these children should be watched closely for speech errors and corrected when they slipped up. After several months, Tudor went back to the orphanage and found that a number of these childen showed stuttering-like behaviors. Although she tried to treat them, at least one child was reported to have continued stuttering for some time thereafter (Silverman, 1988). Tudor was remorseful about these results and regretted conducting this experiment (Zebrowski, personal communication). Nonetheless, it reinforced Johnson's strong conviction, which he held throughout his career, that if a child is made self-conscious about his normal disfluencies, he may begin to stutter.

Communicative Failure and Anticipatory Struggle

This theoretical view, developed by Oliver Bloodstein (1987, 1997), proposes that stuttering emerges from a child's experiences of frustration and failure when trying to talk. The child's original difficulty in talking need not be disfluency. Many types of communication

> **Table 4–2**   Experiences That May Make Some Children Believe That Speaking Is Difficult
>
> 1. Normal disfluencies criticized by significant listeners
> 2. Delay in speech or language development
> 3. Speech or language disorders, including articulation problems, word finding difficulty, cerebral palsy, and voice problems
> 4. Difficult or traumatic experience reading aloud in school
> 5. Cluttering, especially if listeners frequently say, "Slow down" or "What?"
> 6. Emotionally traumatic events during which child tries to speak

failure may lead the child to anticipate future difficulty with speech. It is common, Bloodstein noted, to find delays in the development of articulation and language, cluttering, and other speech problems in the histories of children who begin to stutter. Table 4–2 lists some of the circumstances that Bloodstein suggested might cause some children to believe that speaking is difficult. If a child cannot make himself understood or is penalized for the way he talks, he may begin to tense his speech muscles and fragment his speech, reactions that become the core behaviors of the child's stuttering. And these behaviors, in turn, result in more frustration and failure in communication, which the child anticipates with dread.

Other aspects of the child's "internal" and "external" environments and his development also play important parts. The child's personality may be perfectionistic, or he may harbor needs to live up to parental expectations. His family may have high standards for speech, find any speech abnormality unacceptable, or otherwise pressure the child to conform to standards beyond his reach. The presence or absence of these sorts of developmental and environmental pressures may cause some children to interpret an articulation difficulty, language problem, or disfluency as a failure, whereas other children only shrug it off.

This perspective on stuttering accounts for the wide variability of disfluency among children. Most normal children experience temporary frustration when learning to talk as they produce the mild fragmentations of speech we associate with normal disfluency. Children who stutter for just a few weeks may encounter unusual difficulty when first learning to talk but soon master the fundamentals and feel successful. Children who become chronic stutterers may be those who repeatedly experience communication failure and grow up in an environment fraught with communicative pressure.

Here is a case that illustrates some of the environmental pressures that some children who begin to stutter may experience. Susan grew up in the oil fields of Oklahoma, where her parents set themselves apart from the rest of the community by their aloof manner and precision of speech. They raised their children to feel that they were more cultured than their neighbors; in fact, Susan's father would often say, "We speak better than other people." Unfortunately, Susan's speech development was delayed. When she did begin talking in sentences, at about age 3, she began to stutter with mild repetitions. When she started school, she worried that her father was embarrassed by her speech.

Then she tried to speak better and began to push out the words instead of repeating the first parts of them. She soon developed severe secondary stuttering.

Although we have no way of knowing for sure, Susan's critical father may have been a major factor in the onset of her stuttering. However, many children grow up in families that are critical of speech but don't develop stuttering. Perhaps both a constitutional deficit, which led to her delayed speech development, and family pressure for perfect speech were necessary to produce Susan's stutterng. Neither may have been sufficient by itself to create stuttering, but together, they may have been enough to tip the balance.

Capacities and Demands

A third interactional view of stuttering onset is proposed by the capacities and demands theory. Others have called this a "demands and capacities" view, but I prefer to put capacities first, because they exist in the child before demands are placed on them. This view suggests that disfluencies, as well as real stuttering, emerge when a child's capacities for fluency are not equal to speech performance demands. Earlier in this chapter, I briefly discussed a narrow version of this view in describing the reduced capacity for internal modeling theory of stuttering. Andrews et al (1983) stated that, "whether one will become a stutterer depends on one's neurological capacity...and the demand posed by the speech act." These authors indicated that some demands come from the rapid development of language between ages 3 and 7 years. Other demands may come from fast-talking parents, whose speech rates may be hard for a child to keep up with. Demands for speech performance sometimes come from within the child, sometimes from outside stimuli, and sometimes from both.

Joseph Sheehan (1970, 1975) expressed an early variation of the capacities and demands view when he wrote that, "a child who has begun to stutter is probably a child who has had too many demands placed on him while receiving too little support" (Sheehan, 1975, p. 175). The demands that Sheehan pinpointed were primarily those of parents who have high standards and high expectations for their child's behavior. The support he refers to appears to be the environment's capacity to provide love, care, and encouragement. In addition, he believed that, "there are persisting reasons for retaining the possibility that some kind of physiological predisposition for stuttering exists" (Sheehan, 1975, p. 144). Thus, Sheehan, who is best known for a theory that stuttering is learned, professed the view that stuttering is precipitated by the demands of the environment interacting with a predisposition to stutter.

Starkweather (1987) added considerable detail to the concept of capacities and demands as an explanation of stuttering onset and development. The normal child's capacities, he points out, include the potential for rapid movement of speech structures in well-planned sequences that are coordinated with the rhythms of his language. Demands on the child include those of his internal environment, such as the demand of his increasingly complex thoughts to be expressed, which require more sophisticated phonology, syntax, semantics, and pragmatic skills. The external environment often places demands on the child's fluency through parents' interactions. Parents may ask questions rapidly, interrupt frequently, and use complex sentences choked with big words. They may show impatience about the child's normal disfluencies and may make the child feel that he meets their expectations only when he performs at high levels.

These kinds of interactions can stress any child but are likely to push a slowly developing child to try to speak beyond his capacity for fluency.

Because a child's capacities develop in spurts and environmental demands fluctuate, stuttering may wax and wane in rapid cycles. A child may be highly fluent for a day or a week when he has mastered new speech and language skills and when external demands are low. But his stuttering may suddenly flare up if his capacities become strained by his efforts to use more advanced syntax or if the demands of the external environment suddenly increase when his fast-talking, interrupting, big-city cousins arrive for the Fourth of July holiday weekend.

The capacities and demands view provides a way to account not only for the day-to-day variability of stuttering within an individual, but also the great differences between one individual who stutters and another. As Adams (1990) pointed out, some children may grow up in an environment with normal levels of demand but have limited speech production capacities. Others may have normal capacities for speech production but grow up with excessive demands for rapid, fluent speech.

Treatment based on this model would begin with a careful evaluation of the child's capacities and the demands in his environment. Therapy would be designed to enhance capacities, decrease demands, and provide support for the child and his family while these changes are taking place. Starkweather and his colleagues have used this approach to formulate a sensible and effective program of stuttering prevention (Gottwald and Starkweather, 1984, 1985; Starkweather and Gottwald, 1990; Starkweather, Gottwald, and Halfond, 1990). Figure 4–3 depicts the ratios of capacities and demands in a child predisposed to stutter. In one view, the demands are greater than the child's capacities and stuttering appears. In the second, the demands are lessened, and although capacities stay the same, stuttering is diminished.

To illustrate the capacities and demands view more fully, the following case is from my own experience. Gina was a bright, happy 7 year old. Her mother had been a severe stutterer as a child, but through treatment and her own perseverance, she had largely recovered. When Gina began the second grade, she had no history of stuttering or any problem with school. Some time before Christmas that year, however, when her class was learning to read, Gina began to dislike school, and her mother soon discovered that she was having problems academically. After some testing, it was discovered that she had a learning disability, which had not been apparent before; however, once reading was required, it became obvious. As Gina struggled to cope with her reading problem throughout the rest of the second grade, she began to stutter. Over the course of the next 2 years, she stuttered noticeably but did not receive therapy. She was, however, given extra help for her reading disability. By the fourth grade, Gina was making headway with reading, and her stuttering had diminished to an inconsequential level without treatment.

Although there are various ways to account for the onset of Gina's stuttering and recovery, a capacities and demands view would see it this way: Gina was predisposed to stutter, but it lay dormant until she was faced with the challenge of reading. Reading, at least when first learned, involves highly conscious use of linguistic processes, in contrast to the more automatic linguistic processing used in listening and speaking. Consequently, learning to read puts a heavy demand on the pool of available resources that are also used for speech and language processing. Such demands may result in a reduced capacity (i.e., fewer available resources) for speech production, which may result in

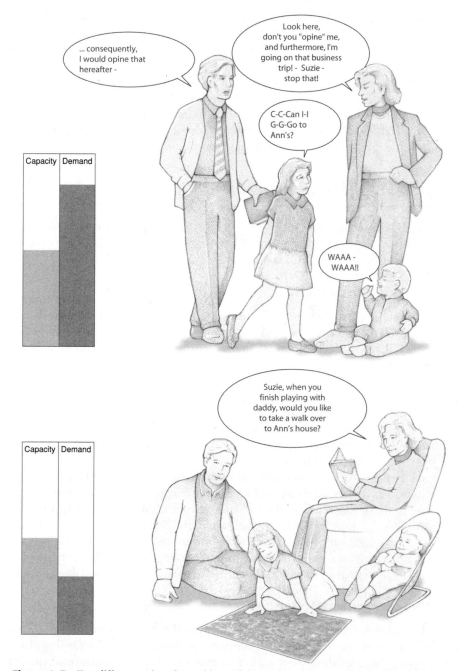

Figure 4–3 *Two different ratios of capacities and demands and their hypothesized effect on fluency.*

disfluency for a vulnerable child. In this case, Gina did not seem to develop a persistent fear of speaking as a result of her stuttering. Thus, when she overcame her initial reading difficulty and reading became more automatic (i.e., demanded fewer resources), her available capacity for speech processes increased, and she "outgrew" her stuttering.

Once again, the reader is reminded that the capacities and demands view is a model for describing relationships that appear again and again but are not well understood. As such, its major function is to help students and clinicians organize the complex interrelationships of variables associated with stuttering into a set of principles that may guide its treatment and suggest research hypotheses for its study.

An Integration of Perspectives on Stuttering

In this section, I will try to draw together some of the theoretical views just described, coupled with my own speculations, to provide a description of the etiology of stuttering that may guide your assessment and treatment.

A Two-Stage Model of Stuttering

Many years ago, a child psychiatrist who stuttered, Charles Bluemel, observed that stuttering begins in most children as repetitions, which they are hardly aware of. Over time, many of these children increase the tension and tempo of their disfluencies and develop fears and other reactions to their stuttering. He called the beginning behaviors "primary" stuttering and the later reactions "secondary" stuttering (Bluemel, 1932). Recently, Bloodstein (2001) concluded that this division of stuttering into primary and secondary phases is an appropriate description of the early development of stuttering. This view of stuttering as having two separate stages or components seems useful to me also and suggests the possibility that each component may have a different etiology. In fact, I think each may have a constitutional basis.

There are reasons to be cautious about embracing this apparently simple view. For example, primary and secondary stages of stuttering may overlap in children because the forces that create these stages wax and wane and make it hard to place them in one phase or another. Moreover, there is evidence that some children begin stuttering in the secondary phase (Yairi and Ambrose, 2005). Despite these exceptions, I will lay out an integrated view of stuttering on the presumption that there are, for most children, two stages of stuttering, and I will describe how the exceptions themselves can be explained in this view.

A Perspective on Primary Stuttering

In Chapter 2, I reviewed studies of brain structures and functions, sensory-motor coordination, central auditory processing, and hemispheric dominance. The findings from this research support theories described earlier in this chapter that stutterers' speech and language functions are not as left hemisphere dominant or as efficient as those of non-stutterers. These findings, plus evidence that a predisposition to stutter is genetically transmitted or associated with perinatal brain damage and that stuttering typically emerges in early childhood, all point toward some deficits or differences in the left hemisphere's neural circuitry for perception and production of spoken language as likely constitutional bases of stuttering. These deficits may not be exactly the same in every person who stutters, but there is enough similarity in the effect on spoken language that the symptoms most often begin as repetitions of single-syllable words or parts of words.

Before I describe how I think these neurophysiological differences might result in stuttering, I will briefly review how such differences might be created during embryonic and neonatal growth. The development of language and speech neural networks begins soon after conception, with the proliferation, migration, and differentiation of neural cells, a process guided by genetic predisposition and affected by external events, such as experience, injury, and disease (Chase, 1996). As neural cells continue to proliferate and differentiate, millions of synapses are formed, and pathways of communication emerge when clusters of cells send information back and forth in response to stimulation. Cells that communicate readily among themselves become self-organized, functional neural circuits that perform various tasks. For example, after birth, as an infant interacts with the outside world, groups of circuits in the infant's brain bind together to form "maps" to process information and produce motor responses (Edelman, 1992).

There is good reason to suspect that brain development in individuals who stutter is in some way atypical due to genes, environment, or both. Research on the genetics, perinatal brain injury, neuroanatomy, and neurophysiology of stuttering, reviewed in Chapter 2, suggests that stutterers have anomalies in left hemisphere structures and functions. The developing brain responds to such anomalies in a number of different ways, most commonly by extensive anatomical reorganization, including growth of new fibers, new synapses, and entire new cortical tracts (Hadders-Algra and Forssberg, 2002, p. 491). This reorganization would attempt to establish the functional circuits necessary for the development of spoken language in whatever structures are available. It seems to me that if reorganization involves relocation of these circuits to areas that have not naturally evolved to serve these circuits or if reorganization entails neuronal groups being placed at some distance from each other, these circuits will be both inefficient and vulnerable to disruption by other brain activities occurring in nearby areas.

Which neural circuits underlying spoken language may be displaced? One of the functions that often seems to be atypical in stuttering is sensorimotor processing, particularly auditory-motor processing. Because auditory processing plays a major role in infants' use of the sounds of adult speech and the sounds of their own babbling, a dysfunction in this area would obviously have an influence on the development of interacting neuronal circuits for speech and language production. The sounds of adult speech give infants auditory targets to aim for when they are able to speak. The sensorimotor activity in babbling helps a child develop internal models that specify what articulatory gestures are needed to produce desired auditory targets (see the discussion of Neilson and Neilson's theory earlier in this chapter). Moreover, the auditory information from babbling allows the child to adapt his internal auditory-articulatory model to his rapidly growing speech production mechanism (Callan et al, 2000). Because these circuits are self-organizing, they may develop a variety of solutions to the auditory processing problem. Some individuals may use homologous right hemisphere structures for auditory processing, others may continue to use inefficient areas of the left hemisphere, and still others may try to do both. Whatever an individual's solution, brain imaging studies suggest that adults who stutter activate widely distributed areas in both right and left hemispheres when they speak and especially when they stutter. Such widespread distribution of neural circuitry would make communication and timing among the subcomponents of speech and language production less efficient.

Imagine, for example, that a group of musicians meets spontaneously without a leader and tries to learn to play together. If this musical group's evolution were to parallel the normal, self-organizing development of the brain's neuronal circuitry, all of them would need to be equally capable musicians who would seat themselves in the same room where they can hear and see each other. Over a period of several months of regular practice, they would gradually meld into a synchronous group, easily communicating their tempo to each other and effectively signaling when each would join the others and when small subgroups would play while others would wait. Now imagine that one member, for example, the drummer, is not as musical as the others and cannot play in sync with them. In a real band, of course, they'd toss him out, like the Beatles did to Ringo's predecessor, Pete Best. But our imaginary band can't find a replacement and has to keep the dyssynchronous drummer. When conditions are good and the music is simple, the drummer can keep the tempo, but when the music gets complex or the drummer is tired or hungover, he seems unable to start out right, and the band falls out of beat and has to stop and start again. Let's go back to our neuronal groups of speech and language production; if one component or circuit is inefficient, this may prevent the development of a coordinated, well-timed speech production process.

Theories of Dyssynchrony

Several authors have proposed that mistiming or dyssynchrony in the assembly of components for speech and language output causes stuttering. Van Riper (1971, 1982) suggested that the dyssynchrony occurs in the assembly of sequential motor movements; Neilson and Neilson (1987) suggested that it occurs during execution of the phonetic plan; Kolk and Postma (1997) suggested that it occurs during the covert repair of phonological segments; and Kent (1984), Perkins, Kent, and Curlee (1991), and Wingate (1988) all argued that it results from failures to integrate linguistic with paralinguistic components. Stuttering, according to these views, emerges when the components required for speech production are not assembled in a timely, synchronous way. The impulse to press ahead with normally rapid speech, even though all the components are not ready, results in the disfluencies that are perceived as stuttering.

Webster (1993, 1997) has a somewhat similar perspective, but his view is very specific about where the dyssynchrony occurs. He lays the problem squarely on the left supplementary motor area (SMA), a structure involved in the planning of complex sequential motor movements. In that role, the SMA coordinates activity from many circuits in both the left and right hemispheres. The SMA may be one of the locations that theorists have implicated in their speculations about inefficient assembly of the components of speech.

This description of dyssynchrony in the assembly of components of speech and language production is intended only as a possible explanation of primary stuttering, which is a stage of stuttering characterized by relatively relaxed repetitions and occasional prolongations that typically occur, as Bloodstein (2001, 2002) has suggested, at the beginnings of phrases or sentences. Most children who begin to stutter outgrow their primary disfluencies as their speech and language systems mature or as they develop effective ways to work around the problem. Other children, however, react to their primary stuttering by increasing the speed and tension of their disfluencies. They go on to develop the characteristics of secondary stuttering: blocks, escape behaviors, and avoidance reactions. Why? And why do some children begin to stutter with blocks rather than repetitions? The answer, I think, can be found in the temperament of these children, interacting with the processes of learning.

A Perspective on Secondary Stuttering

Temperament

This section focuses on the personality or temperament of children and uses both "sensitive" and "reactive" to refer to the same thing: a behavioral and emotional style characterized by being easily aroused by stimuli, as well as a tendency to withdraw when confronted by unfamiliar people or situations. Kagan (1994) often uses "inhibited" to describe the same traits. There is evidence, which was discussed in Chapter 2, that individuals who stutter tend to have more sensitive or reactive temperaments (Anderson, Pellowski, and Conture, 2001; Fowlie and Cooper, 1978; Embrechts and Ebben, 1999; Guitar, 2003; LaSalle, 1999; Oyler and Ramig, 1995; Wakaba, 1998). If so, such reactivity may explain why some children who stutter eventually respond to their disfluencies by tightening their muscles. Research on normal children who have sensitive temperaments indicates that they respond to novel, threatening, or unfamiliar events by increasing their physical tension, particularly in the larynx (Kagan, Reznick, and Snidman, 1987). If children who stutter have more sensitive temperaments than their peers, they may be more likely to increase their laryngeal tension in response to primary stuttering, which they experience as threatening because it seems out of their control. This may be the mechanism that causes the disfluencies of some children who stutter to change from easy, relaxed repetitions to tense repetitions, which become progressively higher in pitch, and to evidence other manifestations of secondary stuttering.

Such increases in physical tension may be part of a larger defensive response that is triggered more easily in individuals with reactive temperaments. In describing his Behavioral Inhibition System, Gray (1987) proposes that when individuals experience frustration or fear, their innate response is freezing (i.e., widespread muscular contractions that produce tense and silent immobility), flight (i.e., speeded up activity to escape), or avoidance. Gray (1987) indicates that these unconditioned responses may occur rapidly, without intervening autonomic arousal, arising from the central nervous system substrate underlying the increased muscle tension, increased tempo, and escape behaviors and avoidance behaviors that characterize secondary stuttering. It is notable, also, that Gray suggests that how individuals' Behavioral Inhibition Systems affect behavior is influenced by temperament. The more reactive individuals are, the more they will engage in freezing, flight, or avoidance responses when experiencing fear.

Further evidence of a neurological substrate underlying the characteristics of secondary behavior is provided by the research of Davidson (1984), Kinsbourne (1989), and Kinsbourne and Bemporad (1984), which was described in Chapter 2. They propose that the right hemisphere is specialized for emotions that accompany avoidance, withdrawal, and arrest of ongoing behavior, whereas the left hemisphere is specialized for emotions that are associated with approach, exploration, and release of ongoing behavior. Thus, it can be argued that individuals who stutter and are more reactive are more prone to behaviors regulated by right hemisphere emotions. This argument is supported by the findings of Calkins and Fox (1994) and Davidson (1995) who reported that sensitive children are right hemisphere dominant for emotion. Their research may also explain why secondary behaviors develop in the forms they do in many stutterers. Those beginning stutterers who develop secondary behaviors may be more sensitive individuals whose innate defensive mechanisms, the Behavioral Inhibition System of Gray (1987), are triggered more easily because of their right hemisphere dominance for emotions. These stutterers, especially those whose behaviors at onset are characterized by tension and struggle, do not outgrow their stuttering.

Learning

It has been evident for some time that learning plays a major role in persistent stuttering, which is the variant of the disorder that continues beyond the primary stage and usually grows more severe. In the last section of Chapter 3, I described the major types of learning involved in stuttering, but I did not deal with the question of why some children seem more vulnerable to this learning than others. One answer to this puzzle was given by Brutten and Shoemaker (1967) in their influential book, *The Modification of Stuttering*. They proposed that individual differences in conditionability and in autonomic reactivity are a constitutional predisposition in stuttering. My own understanding of the role of learning, described in the following paragraph, is in agreement with theirs and adds some detail from recent literature about emotional learning.

The perspective given earlier that some children who stutter are more temperamentally reactive and thus are more prone to physical tension, rapid escape behaviors, and avoidance suggests that these children will also be more emotionally conditionable. That is, the physiology that predisposes these children to be temperamentally reactive involves the limbic system, especially the amygdala, which is that part of the limbic system that stores emotional memories. This is what makes learning for them so indelible.

Emotional events are etched into the brain more strongly than neutral ones. Think about how well you can remember what you were doing when you found out about a very exciting or upsetting event. Many people can remember vividly what they were doing when they heard about the planes crashing into the Twin Towers on September 11, 2001. The strength of emotional memories is enhanced even further in persons having a more reactive limbic system, which may account for why some people suffer post-traumatic stress syndrome and others do not. Children with reactive limbic systems are more likely to react to the multiple repetitions of primary stuttering with tension, escape, and avoidance and are also much more likely to store their memory strongly (e.g., LeDoux, 2002). Such reactions and memories can snowball. The child's natural fear response to a repetition that feels out of control is to tense his muscles. This increased tension soon makes the stutter last longer, which increases his feeling that he is helpless and triggers a bigger fear response. Stuttering experiences become even more traumatic as the child increases physical tension because of his initial negative emotion, which causes repetitions to become tense prolongations or blocks. These new, tense forms of stuttering can be more unpleasant to the child and can provoke expressions of anxiety and alarm by his parents. The child's stronger feelings of "stuckness" and his concern about his parents' alarm are likely to generate more activity in the limbic system, thereby creating stronger memories that will trigger these more tense forms of stuttering more quickly whenever he experiences primary stuttering. The child's reactive amygdala mediates the storage of unpleasant memories of stuttering, largely on an unconscious level. At the same time, another part of the limbic system, the hippocampus, stores information about the situations in which stuttering occurs (e.g., who the child was talking to, what word was being said, where it happened). These contextual cues cause stuttering to spread rapidly from isolated experiences to more and more repeated experiences in similar contexts and, eventually, to many other situations.

Children with reactive temperaments are not only more likely to learn to increase tension when they anticipate or experience stuttering, but are also more likely to engage in other components of the Behavioral Inhibition System. These include increases in tempo, other aspects of escape behaviors, and a wide array of avoidances. Thus, these children quickly develop secondary symptoms, such as eye blinks and changing words, to avoid or escape stuttering.

Emotional conditioning occurs rapidly in these children, but unlearning is a much slower and more difficult process. There is evidence that emotional memories are stored permanently, and even when new behaviors replace them, the original emotions and learned behaviors may reappear under stress (Ayres, 1998). When clinicians work with individuals who have secondary stuttering, they need to keep in mind the strength and persistence of behaviors learned through fear conditioning. New behaviors will have to be learned as new responses to the stimuli that elicited the old responses. Because emotional conditioning may produce cortical as well as subcortical changes in the brain, cognitive therapy may be a useful adjunct to behavioral therapy in older children and adults.

Two Predispositions for Stuttering

This view of primary and secondary stuttering proposes that there are two constitutional predispositions: one for primary stuttering and one for secondary stuttering. As may be evident, the most common occurrence is for a child to have a predisposition for primary stuttering that is resolved through neural maturation or reorganization. It is also possible for a child's primary stuttering to continue into adulthood and for secondary behaviors never to emerge; these adults may simply be considered highly disfluent, rather than stutterers. Some children, of course, do acquire secondary behaviors in response to their primary stuttering, and I would hypothesize that these children have the second predisposition, a reactive temperament, which predisposes them to the tension, escape, and avoidance behaviors that characterize secondary stuttering. I believe that neither of these predispositions is "all or nothing"; that is, a child may have a little or a lot of either. For instance, an adolescent may have a substantial amount of repetitions in his speech but only occasionally show tension, escape, or avoidance behaviors. Or a child may start stuttering suddenly at age 3, with severe stutters marked by struggle, tension, escape, and avoidance. Perhaps the child has only a little predisposition for primary stuttering but a substantial predisposition for secondary stuttering. This continuum for stuttering agrees with most clinicians' observations that we see a wide range of severity, from mild to very severe, with some stutterers having little avoidance and others having a great deal. I also notice that, outside the clinic, there are many individuals whose "stuttering" is so mild that they don't recognize it in themselves and other lay persons don't notice it either.

The possibility of two predispositions for stuttering may also shed light on such phenomena as neurogenic stuttering, which are the disfluencies that sometimes appear in persons with neurological diseases or injuries. The changes in the brain that may occur as part of a neurological problem may give rise to a dyssynchrony in speech and language production processing that is similar to that of primary stuttering. On the other hand, the changes in temperament that sometimes occur with brain injury (e.g., Kinsbourne, 1989) may, in a few cases, give rise to disfluencies that are more characteristic of secondary stuttering.

There is support in genetic research for two (or more) predispositions in individuals who do not naturally recover from stuttering. After an analysis of many children who stuttered for some period of time in their lives, Ambrose, Cox, and Yairi (1997) concluded that persistent and recovered stuttering are not two different forms of the disorder. Those children who persisted in stuttering (i.e., continued to stutter for more than 3 years) have additional genetic factors, beyond those that created the emergence of their stuttering in both the persistent and recovered groups. There may be much overlap between the designations I have used (i.e., secondary stuttering and persistent stuttering). It seems plausible that many of the persistent stutterers are children who react to their stuttering and thus develop secondary stuttering. This connection between a child reacting to his stuttering and the persistence of the stuttering is reflected in Van Riper's beliefs that "...most children who begin to stutter become fluent perhaps because of maturation or because they do not react to their...repetitions, or prolongations by struggle and avoidance...those who struggle or avoid because of frustration or penalties will probably continue to stutter all the rest of their lives no matter what kind of therapy they receive" (Van Riper, 1990).

Indeed, as Ambrose, Cox, and Yairi (1997) suggest, there may be more than two predispositions in stuttering. The factors that cause a child to react with frustration and fear to primary stuttering may also cause another child to react the same way to lack of intelligibility or difficulties in word finding, for example. Communicative failures may lead to anticipatory struggle, as described earlier in this chapter. However, no matter how many predispositions a child may have, the chance of his actually developing primary or secondary stuttering is enhanced or diminished by both developmental and environmental factors.

Interactions with Developmental Factors

In this section, I describe three ways in which aspects of children's development may interact with the two predispositions to trigger or exacerbate stuttering. In Chapter 3, I argued that children's physical, cognitive, emotional, and linguistic development may provide the extra demands on resources that precipitate stuttering or worsen it. Now I want to relate these demands to the two predispositions described earlier. You will see elements of the capacities and demands theory of stuttering in this section.

The first interaction is with the demands of language development and a predisposition for primary stuttering. Consider a child who begins to acquire speech with dysfunctional or inefficient speech and language networks. The functional plasticity of the child's brain may allow these pathways to reorganize or repair themselves so that the child processes spoken language more efficiently as he strives to communicate. However, the exponential growth of the child's speech and language at this very time may compete for cerebral resources, straining or exceeding the child's capacity to handle both the demands of reorganization and advancing language at the same time. To see what this may be like, imagine yourself as a student who has let part of the semester slip by without studying. After bombing the first two exams, you resolve to reorganize your study habits and catch up, but just then, your professors decide to pile on even more work than before. Like the child, you may or may not be able to accommodate the professors' increasing demands at the same time you are spending energy to reorganize.

A second interaction will be the maturation of the brain with a predisposition for primary stuttering. Some individuals will have an earlier maturation of the brain or a natural flexibility to respond to anomalies in the wiring for spoken language. Girls, for example, are more likely to recover from early stuttering, probably because of their inherently greater organizational plasticity and their more widely distributed language centers (Shaywitz et al, 1995). Some males may also be genetically endowed with more flexibility than average for reorganizing their cerebral circuitry and thus may recover more readily than others.

The third type of interaction will occur when a child has normal neural circuitry for spoken language but has a constitutionally inhibited temperament. Typical developmental challenges for most children include some frustration at not being able to speak as fast or with the same complexity as adults and older children in the family. The child may not only be frustrated but embarrassed at his inability to produce more advanced speech and language. Social-emotional development takes the child through some stressful times. All of these typical experiences may produce increased tension and avoidance behaviors associated with speech. Based on my clinical experience, I suspect that some children fitting this description might be hesitant to speak and may be referred for a stuttering evaluation but would not manifest the typical signs of stuttering. Their hesitancies may consist of long pauses, phrase repetitions, or both when their right hemisphere proclivity toward avoidance, withdrawal, and arrest of ongoing behavior manifests itself while they are speaking. Such hesitancies may diminish in time as myelinization of connections between the hemispheres progresses and the left hemisphere has increasingly modulating effects on right hemisphere–modulated emotions.

Interactions with Environmental Factors

Here I would like to consider the influence of the environment on anomalous speech and language neural networks (predisposition for primary stuttering) and on constitutional predispositions for inhibited temperaments (predisposition for secondary stuttering).

Interactions of Anomalous Neural Networks with Environmental Factors

As a child's developing central nervous system adapts to the inherited or acquired differences in his neural substrates for speech and language, the environment plays a role through various listeners' responses to the child's emerging speech and language skills. Obviously, a child's family will have the most opportunities to provide acceptance and support. The accommodations they can provide, such as slower speech rates, fewer interruptions, and dedicated one-on-one listening time, may foster adaptations of the child's inefficient, dyssynchronous neural networks. At least this environment will not stress the child's speech and language production system and will probably enable the child to develop his own adapted rate of speech and language output. In contrast, an environment with many interruptions, rapid conversational give and take, demands for recitations, and little time for the child to talk may "overdrive" the child's immature speech and language production system, produce an excess of disfluencies, and inhibit the successful adaptation of the child's system to its original anomalous wiring.

Interactions of Temperament with Environmental Factors

The work of Calkins (1994), Kagan and Snidman (1991), and others suggests that families can have a strong influence on temperament. As Calkins and Fox (1994) expressed it, "the child's interactions with a parent provide the context for learning skills and strategies for managing emotional reactivity." In addition, the environmental factors that I have called "life events" can also influence the development of temperament. As noted earlier, Kagan (1994b) suggested that certain life events could cause a child who is not particularly reactive to become more reactive and inhibited.

Implications for Treatment

The conditions that I have just been describing may be ameliorated by a supportive environment and specific therapy approaches. By judicious control of speech and language processing demands, the environment may support a child's adaptive neuroplasticity, enabling him to improve the efficiency of his speech and language neural networks. Equally important is the family's fostering of the child's adaptation of inefficient neural networks. With appropriate models of slower speaking rates and pausing, the child may develop a rate of speech and language processing that allows him to synchronize the various components of spoken language. This is analogous to the spontaneously formed band example I described earlier that had a dyssynchronous drummer. When the band played slowly, the drummer could keep up a synchronized beat.

Families may also help a child develop a less inhibited temperament by encouraging positive, assertive behaviors. Therapy, too, can help a child respond to disfluencies with fewer inhibitory responses. Active, positive treatment sessions often lead to improvements in a child's confidence. Training in fluency skills can provide a child with many satisfying speaking experiences, thereby reducing fear of talking. Development of a slower speaking style and the use of proprioception (conscious awareness of movement) may help a child make the best of an inefficient speech production system. Confronting feared words and situations, reducing tension in stutters, and improving eye contact during speech may help shift a child's characteristic emotional valence from "avoidance" (right hemisphere) to "approach" (left hemisphere). In the chapters on treating stuttering, I expand on this theme and suggest a variety of other ways to help individuals overcome or compensate for factors that predispose them to stutter.

Some recent research indicates another way in which treatment may affect the two predispositions for persistent stuttering. Brain imaging studies of adults before and after treatment (DeNil et al, 2003; Neumann et al, 2003; in press) suggest that successful treatment is associated with activation of left hemisphere areas that had not been active before treatment and reductions in activations of right hemisphere areas that were highly active. These findings parallel evidence from treatment of nonfluent aphasic patients whose recovery was associated with the same pattern (M. Naeser, personal communication, January 5, 2005). Because this relocation of circuitry serving spoken language places it in areas very near to those used by nonstutterers in the left hemisphere (Neumann et al, in press), activity may be less vulnerable to disruption by right hemisphere emotions, thus affecting the mechanisms for both primary and secondary stuttering.

Accounting for the Evidence

Let us now turn to the research findings and clinical observations that these views of stuttering must account for. The fact that stuttering is universal should not be unexpected because it depends less on culture than on basic biological variations of the human brain. Many other disorders, such as dyslexia and specific language impairment, as well as such personality differences as sensitive temperament, are associated with atypical activity of the central nervous system and are also universal. The fact that the prevalence of stuttering is relatively low may be a consequence of chronic stuttering resulting from a combination of at least two biological predispositions, the co-occurrence of which does not happen frequently.

Evidence about Stuttering at Onset

Why does stuttering usually begin only after fluency at the one- and two-word stage has been achieved? My view is that stuttering emerges first from disruptions caused by a child's inefficient neural networks for speech and language processing. Perhaps the task of coordinating all the phonetic, phonological, syntactic, and semantic components of longer utterances is too much for inefficient neural circuitry under stress. Just like normal disfluency, the neural processing circuitry of children who stutter may be adequate to handle one-word utterances. But once children begin to reorganize their language functions from a lexical to a grammatical-rules basis and try out more complicated syntax, their inefficient neural organization breaks down. An added demand on their planning system is that the shift from one- to two-word utterances requires the use of a more complex prosody. Remember that Kent (1984), Perkins, Kent, and Curlee (1991), and Wingate (1988) suggested that a major source of breakdown is in timing linguistic and paralinguistic components. This demand for complex prosody at the multiword stage at the same time that phonological, syntactical, and lexical demands are added is likely to be a time when an inefficient speech and language system cannot keep up with the demands for rapid and complex speech production. It is as if our imaginary bicycle factory had been producing old style bikes with pedal brakes and no gears (the one-word stage) but is now being asked to produce bicycles with hand brakes and two sets of gears (multi-word stage), even as customer demand is requiring faster work on the production line (speech rate increases with longer utterances).

Why doesn't a child's sensitive temperament affect speech before the multiple repetitions and prolongations of early stuttering emerge? It may, in a few cases. There are children who begin to stutter with tense blocks that did not follow a period of repetitions and occasional prolongations. I have recently been working with a 2-year-old girl who showed excessive squeezing and tension in her stutters after only a few hours of stuttering in a repetitive pattern. For most children who stutter, however, tension responses, as well as escape and avoidance reactions, are elicited by the frustration and fear provoked by early stuttering. Speech itself is not threatening, but when a long repetition occurs as a result of the dyssynchrony in the speech and language production system, the child feels that his speech mechanism is out of control. This triggers his tension, escape, and avoidance responses, and as this happens more frequently, learning takes place, and his tension, escape, and avoidance responses are soon triggered without "runaway" repetitions.

So, how do we account for both the genetic transmission of stuttering and that evidence of genetic transmission is lacking in some cases? Genetic transmission of stuttering in many cases may be through the two factors I just described: anomalous neural organization for speech and sensitive temperament. In some cases of childhood stuttering, genetic transmission may be suspect because no other family members seem to be affected. This may occur because persistent stuttering appears to require both predisposing factors. Some family members may inherit one factor and some the other, but unless both factors are inherited by the same individual, persistent stuttering does not develop. Another reason for the absence of stuttering in other family members may be that the predisposing factors were the result not of genetic inheritance, but of environmental factors affecting fetal development that created the neural substrate for stuttering. Moreover, such anomalous speech and language circuitry may create language, learning, or phonological problems in other family members. Remember that the unfolding of the genetic blueprint is extensively influenced by environmental factors and by chance. Thus, the anomalous circuitry in one child may result in stuttering, but it an uncle or grandmother, it may have resulted in an articulation disorder or learning problem.

How does this view of stuttering explain its most common signs: part-word repetitions, prolongations, and blocks? The immediate causes of the core behaviors of stuttering are not entirely clear in my view. All of them reflect an inability to move forward in speech, but the effortless sound and syllable repetitions of many stutterers at onset seem somewhat different from later tension-filled repetitions, prolongations, and blocks. The sound and syllable repetitions of early stuttering more closely resemble the disfluencies resulting from nervous system damage or "neurogenic stuttering" (Rosenbek, 1984). Thus, these early signs of childhood stuttering (less tense repetitions and prolongations) may arise from a breakdown in the inefficient function of neural circuits, perhaps from causes similar to those of neurogenic stuttering. Repetitions may occur simply because there is a lag in the readiness of the next part of a word or sentence, although the impulse or pressure to continue speaking is strong. Signs of stuttering with tension that emerge later than effortless repetitions in many stutterers likely stem from the frustration and fear elicited by a child's difficulty in speaking. In those cases in which the earliest signs of stuttering are characterized by tension and blocking (Van Riper, 1982), an emotional response may be primary. As Van Riper (1982) suggested, these may be children whose onset is very sudden, resulting usually after an emotionally difficult period or traumatic emotional stress.

Any view of stuttering should explain its more common recovery in girls than boys. I suspect that the reason more boys stutter than girls is that their genetic blueprints for neural organization of speech and language differ and may be more flexible in females (Shaywitz et al, 1995). Neuroplasticity of the human brain is greatest in the first few years of life, and this neuroplasticity probably diminishes after puberty. Neuroplasticity permits reorganization of neural pathways and, in many cases, recovery. An important additional predictor of recovery, I believe, is an uninhibited temperament. I have met several siblings of stutterers who have gone blithely through periods of stuttering but were so unconcerned that tension and struggle never occurred, and they recovered.

Evidence about Stuttering as It Develops

Does this view account for the development of stuttering? The course of development of stuttering seems to us to be determined in part by the biological responses of the child to fear and frustration and to autonomic conditioning, to which a child prone to chronic stuttering may be particularly sensitive. Details on the development of stuttering are discussed in Chapter 5.

How do we account for conditions that reduce stuttering? Conditions that temporarily ameliorate stuttering, such as singing or speaking in a rhythm, probably improve fluency by giving speech and language processes more time or an external organizing stimulus to aid speech production. They may also involve other parts of the brain and not those anomalous networks used inefficiently for typically spoken language. Other conditions, such as speaking when alone or when relaxed, often reduce stuttering but do not necessarily eliminate it. Such conditions may calm a person, thereby diminishing the reactivity of limbic circuits, whereas some conditions, such as speaking more slowly, both provide more time and diminish reactivity.

Evidence about Deficits in Stutterers' Performance

How about differences in performance between groups of stutterers and nonstutterers? As intimated earlier in this chapter, it seems to me that the wide range of performance on IQ tests, school achievement tests, and tests of sensory-motor ability by groups of stutterers may reflect the wide range of delays and deviations in the neural substrates for these abilities that led to their inefficient processing of speech and language. Among groups of individuals who stutter, there are likely to be some whose neural organization for sensory-motor processing is deviant enough to depress the group mean. In highly selected groups of stutterers, however, such as all males with no medical, neurological, or psychiatric diagnoses and complete right-body dominance (Ingham, Fox, and Ingham, 1996), the chance of finding significant differences between this group and a group of nonstutterers is decreased. In this regard, it is interesting that two independent studies have shown that children whose stuttering is their only disorder show no speech reaction time differences from nonstutterers, whereas children who stutter and have other language or articulation disorders show significantly poorer reaction time scores than children who only stutter and children with typical speech (Cullinan and Springer, 1980; Maske-Cash and Curlee, 1995). Perhaps the coexistence of poorer sensory-motor integration performance and speech and language disorders reflects additional anomalies in neural organization and function in this subgroup of stuttering children. In other words, I propose that children who stutter have at least some degree of inefficient organization of their neural circuitry for speech and language production; those children who stutter and have poorer sensory-motor skills or other speech and language disorders may simply have greater anomalies in their neural circuitry functions, which affect fluency, articulation, language, or other sensory-motor tasks.

Other characteristics of stuttering that I have said should be explained by any view of stuttering, such as the influence of developmental and environmental factors, are explicitly addressed in earlier parts of this chapter. Some characteristics, findings, and observations are explained more easily than others. However, those that are not accounted for satisfactorily are important. They are a reality and are hard facts that should mold and shape any theoretical view until it is more fully explanatory.

Summary

- Several theoretical perspectives have been proposed to account for constitutional factors in stuttering. They include views of stuttering (1) as an anomaly of how the brain is organized for speech and language, (2) as a disorder of timing of the sequential movements for speech, (3) as a result of deficits in the internal modelling process used to control speech production, (4) as a disorder of spoken language production, and (5) as a result of physiological tremor in speech musculature. The first four of these views (1-4) focus on dysfunctions of cortical and subcortical mechanisms that control the planning and production of speech and language to produce the initial repetitions and prolongations of early stuttering; the last view (5) targets neuromuscular malfunctions that may explain the tension and tremors of secondary stuttering.

- Theories concerning developmental and environmental factors include (1) the diagnosogenic theory, which implicates the listener's response to the disfluencies of the child, (2) the anticipatory struggle theory, which suggests that a child may develop stuttering as a result of negative anticipation of speaking after he has had frustrating or embarrassing experiences in communicating, and (3) the capacities and demands theory, which postulated that stuttering arises when the child's capacities for rapid, fluent utterances are unequal to the demands within the child himself or within the environment.

- A two-stage etiological model of stuttering is proposed. The first stage is primary stuttering, which involves repetitions and prolongations that are frequently the first signs of stuttering. These signs are thought to be the result of a constitutional factor: a dyssynchrony at some level of the speech and language production process. The second stage is secondary stuttering, which involves the tension, struggle, escape, and avoidance behaviors that are often present in persistent stuttering. These behaviors are proposed to be the result of a separate constitutional factor: a reactive temperament that triggers a defense response from the Behavioral Inhibition System and that makes the individual more emotionally conditionable than the average speaker.

Study Questions

1. What are the differences between the Geswind and Galaburda theory of stuttering and the view of Webster?

2. Compare Kent's view of stuttering as a disorder of timing with the Geshwind and Galaburda theory.

3. Both Neilson and Neilson's view of stuttering and one of Max et al's hypotheses about stuttering suggest that repetitions occur because of a problem with the internal models used for speech production. What is the difference between the cause of repetitions in each view?

4. The study by Kelly, Smith, and Goffman (1995) reviewed in this chapter suggested that tremors don't appear in younger children who stutter but do appear older children. Why would this be?

5. Table 4–2 lists experiences that may generate stuttering in some children because the experiences have led children to believe speaking is difficult. Add as many other hypothetical experiences as you can to this list.

6. A capacities and demands view of stuttering in children would lead to a therapy strategy of enhancing a child's capacities. What are some examples of what capacities in a child you could strengthen to reduce stuttering? Describe how you would do this.

7. What is the relationship between a sensitive temperament and a high level of conditionability?

8. I have suggested there may be two predispositions for persistent stuttering—one for primary stuttering and one for secondary stuttering. How, according to this view, would primary stuttering lead to secondary stuttering?

9. There is strong evidence that girls are more likely than boys to recover from stuttering and are, therefore, less likely to become persistent stutterers. Is this because girls recover quickly from primary stuttering or because their primary stuttering is less likely to trigger secondary stuttering?

10. In this chapter, I have suggested that there are two stages of stuttering—primary and secondary. What are the signs and symptoms of each, and what is the suggested etiology of each?

SUGGESTED PROJECTS

(1) The view of stuttering as a problem of the "internal modelling" process in speech production is a complex idea. Read the article by Max et al (2004) and make a class presentation about their full theoretical model, explaining it in as clear and simple a way as possible.

(2) Read the article entitled "Resources—A theoretical stone soup" (Navon, 1984) and use the arguments in it to evaluate the capacities and demands theory in this chapter.

(3) Wendell Johnson's "diagnosogenic" view of stuttering led to a master's thesis that tried to create stuttering in orphans in 1939. In 2003, this thesis was the topic of a controversy that centered on the ethics of trying to induce stuttering in children. Using the internet, research this controversy, using "Monster Study" as a keyword. Make a presentation or write a paper on the ethics of this research, given the fact that it was conducted more than 50 years ago when the ethical climate was markedly different than it is now.

(4) Pick a theory of stuttering—either one described in this first two sections of this chapter or one you have found elsewhere—and evaluate how it can account for the basic facts about stuttering enumerated in Chapter 1.

Suggested Readings

Brutten, E.J., and Shoemaker, D.J. (1967). *The Modification of Stuttering.* **Englewood Cliffs, NJ: Prentice-Hall, Inc.**

This is a classic book in the field of stuttering. It describes a theory of stuttering that ascribes the initial symptoms of childhood stuttering to the effect of anxiety on fluency and ascribes the later symptoms to learning. The authors go on to suggest therapeutic approaches that derive from their model.

Gray, J.A. (1987). *The Psychology of Fear and Stress* **(ed 2). Cambridge: Cambridge University Press.**

Gray's experimental work and his theoretical model of a behavioral inhibition system are clearly described here. Some of the book (those parts dealing with the effects of pharmacological agents on the brain) is for specialized readers. Much of it, however, is a readable exposition on the biological basis of learning, stress, and fear. Because this is the second edition of a popular book, I hope a new edition will be available soon.

Kagan, J., Reznick, J.S., and Snidman, N. (1987). The physiology and psychology of behavioral inhibition in children. *Child Development,* **58:1459–1473.**

This article discusses the findings of Kagan and his colleagues that behaviorally inhibited children show high levels of laryngeal tension. Neurophysiological mechanisms are also discussed, as well as possible genetic and environmental contributions. This book is recommended for those interested in the hypothesis that behavioral inhibition may be a component in some stuttering.

LeDoux, J. (1996). *The Emotional Brain: The Mysterious Underpinnings of Emotional Life.* **New York: Simon & Schuster.**

LeDoux, a highly respected brain researcher, brings together a great deal of evidence about how the brain processes experiences that we consider emotional. His explanations of emotional learning are very clear and relevant to stuttering.

Packman, A., and Attanasio, J. (2004). *Theoretical Issues in Stuttering.* **New York: Psychology Press.**

The authors review current and past theories of stuttering and evaluate them in terms of testability, explanatory power, parsimony, and heuristic power. This book effectively teaches the reader what a theory should be expected to do.

Chapter 5

Normal Disfluency and the Development of Stuttering

Overview

This chapter describes the evolution of stuttering. It is designed to help you understand why stuttering often (but not always) progresses from a few relaxed repetitions in preschool children to frequent stuttering accompanied by tension, avoidance, and many negative feelings and beliefs in older children or adults. This chapter will also help you understand how to match treatment procedures to the underlying dynamics of stuttering, as well as to the age of the client. To accomplish these goals, I have organized the material into five levels that reflect not only the stages of evolution of stuttering but also important landmarks to guide your selection of a therapy approach.

The five levels are shown in Table 5–1, along with the age ranges typically associated with each. I have also divided the characteristics of stuttering at each level into four subcategories. The first three subcategories—*core behaviors, secondary behaviors,* and *feelings and attitudes*—were described in a general way in Chapter 1. The fourth subcategory, *underlying processes,* is introduced to explain why symptoms change from level to level. These explanations are hypotheses, based on evidence from studies of animal and human behavior, about how stuttering behaviors become more severe and complex. This subcategory should help you understand the nature of the symptoms, as well as the rationales for the treatments presented in the second section of the book.

The developmental/treatment levels are divided into age ranges because age is often more important than frequency of stuttering in selecting the appropriate treatment. Let me give two examples. No matter how severely a preschool child stutters, treatment should always involve his parents, and, in my experience, should focus primarily on increasing fluency rather than modifying stutters. Conversely, a school-age child, whether stuttering is mild or severe, needs an approach that involves teachers and classmates, as well as parents. Also, children of this age can be helped by discussing their stuttering and their feelings about it. In general, the cognitive-emotional level associated with different ages needs to be considered when choosing a therapy strategy.

Exceptions and Variations

The developmental/treatment levels presented in this chapter do not characterize everyone who stutters. Some won't fit neatly into any one of the levels I've constructed. Some behaviors of the same individual will suggest one level; other behaviors will suggest another level.

Table 5–1 Developmental/Treatment Levels of Stuttering	
Developmental/Treatment Level	**Typical Age Range**
Normal disfluency	1.5–6 years, although a small amount of normal disfluency continues in mature speech
Borderline stuttering	1.5–6 years
Beginning stuttering	2–8 years
Intermediate stuttering	6–13 years
Advanced stuttering	14 years and above

However, most individuals who stutter will fit reasonably well within a single level. Moreover, even though all behaviors of a person may not reflect a single level of stuttering, deciding on a treatment need not be a problem; when some aspects of a person's stuttering seem more advanced than others, strategies can be borrowed from other levels to treat them.

Another qualification of the hierarchy presented here concerns the implication that all individuals who stutter pass through each stage in sequence. This is generally true, but there are exceptions. A child may show only normal disfluencies one day and beginning or intermediate stuttering on another day. He may stop stuttering, without apparent reason, a week later, or he may continue stuttering unless treated. One 3-year-old boy I knew changed overnight from borderline to severe beginning stuttering after a change in his allergy medication. As soon as he resumed taking the original prescription, he became a borderline stutterer again and then recovered completely without treatment. There are many unsolved mysteries in stuttering.

Two clinical researchers who wrote extensively about the development of stuttering, Van Riper (1982) and Bloodstein (1960a,b; 1961a), agreed that a simple sequence of stages could never capture every stutterer's pattern. Bloodstein (1960b) proposed a series of four phases of stuttering development, which he described as "typical, but not universal" (Bloodstein, 1995, p. 53). He also cautioned that, although stuttering near onset is often characterized by repetitions without awareness or by a lack of concern, some children show considerable effort and strain in their stuttering as well as crying from frustration at their inability to produce speech easily (1960a).

Van Riper (1982) also noted the presence of forcing and struggle in some children at the onset of stuttering, and like Bloodstein, he was struck by the fact that most children, especially in their early years, oscillate between remissions and recurrences of their stuttering, between mild stuttering and normal disfluency, or between more advanced and less advanced stages of development.

In addition to such swings in the course of stuttering development, there may also be different paths of development, which different stutterers may follow. After searching his clinical files on many individuals whom he had followed for several years, Van Riper (1982) found that his data suggested there are subgroups of stutterers who are characterized by different onsets and different trajectories of development. He proposed that there are four distinctive "tracks" that an individual may follow. The most common consists of children whose stuttering begins as repetitions between 2 and 4 years of age, progresses to include prolongations, then gradually develops into blocks with more and more tension, as well as fears and avoidances. The next most common track comprises children whose onset is a little later and is sometimes accompanied by delayed speech development, articulation problems, or very rapid speech. An interesting aspect of this track is that these children seem to have had difficulty hearing their own speech, perhaps as a result of auditory processing problems. This is particularly interesting in light of recent findings from brain imaging studies of adults who stutter (e.g., Foundas et al, 2001), indicating that some have anatomical anomalies might produce difficulty with higher level auditory processing. A third, less common, track includes children who have sudden onsets of stuttering with a great deal of tension that results in tight, laryngeal blocks. Finally, a fourth track consists of individuals whose disfluency appears to have psychogenic components. (An expanded discussion of psychogenic disfluency is presented in Chapter 13). This track is characterized by late onset, a stereotyped pattern of stuttering that changes very little with age, and few avoidances. Van Riper's four tracks serve as a warning to us that there is much diversity in the evolution of stuttering.

Keeping these variations, exceptions, and limitations in mind, I now begin a detailed description of the levels of stuttering development and treatment, starting with a behavior that is really not stuttering at all, but part of normal speech.

Normal Disfluency

Children vary a great deal in how disfluent they are as they learn to communicate. Some pass their milestones of speech and language development with relatively few disfluencies. Others stumble along, repeating, interjecting, and revising, as they try to master new forms of speech and language, on their way to adult competence. Most are somewhere between the extremes of exceptional fluency and excessive disfluency, such as the 2-year-old shown in Figure 5–1.

Children also swing back and forth in the degree of their disfluency. Some days they are more fluent and other days they are less fluent. Such swings in disfluency may be associated with language development, motor learning, or other developmental or environmental influences mentioned in the preceding chapters. In the following sections, I discuss factors that may influence disfluency, specific behaviors that I categorize as normal disfluency, and the reactions that some children may have to their disfluency. I also highlight aspects of normal disfluency that distinguish it from early stuttering, because one of my aims in this chapter is to prepare you to make this differentiation.

Core Behaviors

Normal disfluencies have been cataloged by several authors, and there is general agreement among them about what constitutes disfluency (Bloodstein, 1987; Colburn and Mysak, 1982a,b; Williams, Silverman, and Kools, 1968; Yairi, 1982, 1983, 1997a;

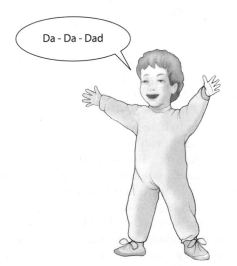

Figure 5–1 *Child who may be normally disfluent.*

Table 5–2	Categories of Normal Disfluencies
Type of Normal Disfluency	**Example**
Part-word repetition	"mi-milk"
Single-syllable word repetition	"I...I want that."
Multisyllabic word repetition	"Lassie...Lassie is a good dog."
Phrase repetition	"I want a...I want a ice-ceem comb."
Interjection	"He went to the...uh...circus."
Revision-incomplete phrase	"I lost my...Where's Mommy going?"
Prolongation	"I'm Tiiiiiiiimmy Thompson."
Tense Pause	"Can I have some more (lips together; no sound) milk?"

Yairi and Ambrose, 2005). Table 5–2 lists eight commonly used categories of disfluency.

Some of the major distinguishing features of normal disfluency—features that differentiate it from stuttering—are the amount of disfluency, the number of units of repetitions and interjections, and the type of disfluency, especially in relation to the age of the child.

Let's begin with the amount of disfluency. This is often measured as the number of disfluencies per 100 words or syllables, rather than "percent disfluencies." Percent disfluencies implies that the disfluencies are associated with the production of particular words. For example, if you said that a child had 10% disfluent words, it would be assumed that 10% of the words spoken were spoken disfluently. However, many disfluencies, such as revisions, interjections, or phrase repetitions, are associated with several words or occur between words. For example, a child may say "Mommy, can you . . . can you . . . um . . . can you buy me that?" It's inaccurate to say that some of these words were spoken disfluently, because the disfluencies were the repetition of the phrase "can you" and the interjection of "um." Were the disfluencies on the words spoken or did they occur because the child was having trouble formulating the remainder of the sentence? In this case, we say that the child spoke six words ("Mommy can you buy me that?") and had two disfluencies (a phrase repetition and an interjection). Hence, we calculate the number of disfluencies that occur when the child speaks 100 words. More details on counting disfluencies are given in Chapter 7.

Although many researchers have measured disfluencies per number of words spoken, a good argument can be made for measuring disfluencies per number of *syllables* spoken. Andrews and Ingham (1971) first recommended the practice of assessing frequency of stuttering in relation to syllables spoken because some multisyllable words may have more than one disfluency, like "s-s-s-sept-t-t-tember" or "di-dinosa-sa-saur." These examples would be one disfluency each if disfluent words were counted but would be two disfluencies if disfluent syllables were counted. In line with this, Yairi (1997a) noted that, as children get older, they are more likely to use multisyllable words. To keep the count equitable between younger and older children, Yairi has assessed disfluencies in children as the number per 100 syllables attempted (Hubbard and Yairi, 1988; Yairi and Lewis, 1984; Yairi and Ambrose, 1996).

When the frequency of all of a child's disfluencies is measured, we need to know how many of these disfluencies are normal. Some of the earliest research on disfluency was conducted by Wendell Johnson at the University of Iowa. He assembled a team of researchers in the 1950s to examine the evidence for his "diagnosogenic" theory of stuttering. As indicated in Chapter 4, Johnson hypothesized that, at the time a child is first "diagnosed" a stutterer by his parents, the child's disfluencies do not differ from those of nonstuttering children. One of the research team's projects was to record children identified by their parents as stutterers and compare the disfluency in their speech with that of nonstuttering children (Johnson et al, 1959). One part of this study compared 68 male children who stuttered with 68 male children who did not stutter. The results showed that, although there was some overlap, the stuttering children had more than twice the amount of disfluency (on average, 18 disfluencies per 100 words) than the nonstuttering children (only seven disfluencies per 100 words). Johnson interpreted the findings as showing that the two groups were essentially the same, because there was so much overlap in both the amount and type of disfluency. Other researchers have reinterpreted these data as indicating that there are two different groups, as I discussed in the last chapter.

Other researchers who have examined the disfluencies in nonstuttering children put the amount of their disfluencies at about the same level (DeJoy and Gregory, 1985; Hubbard and Yairi, 1988; Wexler and Mysak, 1982; Yairi, 1981; Yairi and Ambrose, 1996; Yairi and Lewis, 1984; Zebrowski, 1991). Bringing all these studies together, we can estimate that normally speaking preschool children have, on average, about seven disfluencies for every 100 words spoken. If measured in terms of syllables, it would be closer to six disfluencies per 100 syllables. This figure may be a little high if children are examined throughout their preschool years (Yairi, 1997a); however, many children at age 2 or 3 years go through a period of increased disfluency, which will reach this level.

The range in frequency of normal disfluency is important to note also, especially if the frequency of disfluency is used to make clinical decisions. Johnson et al (1959) and Yairi (1981) found that, although many nonstuttering children have only one or two disfluencies per 100 words, at least one child in their samples had slightly more than 25 disfluencies per 100 words. Thus, the frequency of disfluencies is not, by itself, a definitive clinical measure.

Another distinguishing characteristic of normal disfluency is the number of units that occur in each repetition or interjection. Yairi's (1981) data suggest that normal repetitions typically consist of only one extra unit. For example, a child might say "That my-my ball." Interjections are likely to be just a single unit, such as "I want some . . . uh . . . juice." Instances of multiple repetitions were occasionally observed in these children, but they were the exception. The rule is one and sometimes two units per repetition or interjection, which agrees with Johnson et al's (1959) findings that average nonstuttering children have one- or two-unit repetitions.

Another major characteristic of normal disfluency is the type of disfluency that is most common. Johnson et al (1959) found that interjections, revisions, and whole-word repetitions were the most common disfluency types among the 68 nonstuttering males, who ranged in age from 2½ to 8 years of age. Yairi's (1981) study of 33 2-year-old normal subjects found that there were two clusters of common disfluency types. One cluster involved repetitions of speech segments of one syllable or less (one-syllable words or parts of words were repeated). The second cluster consisted of interjections and revisions.

Table 5–3 Characteristics of Normal Disfluency in the Average Nonstuttering Child

1. No more than 10 disfluencies per 100 words.
2. Typically one-unit repetitions, occasionally two.
3. Most common disfluency types are interjections, revisions, and word repetitions. As children mature past age 3 years, they will show a decline in part-word repetitions.

The most common disfluency type seems to change as a child grows older. In a follow-up to his earlier study, Yairi (1982) found that children between 2 and 3½ years showed an increase in revisions and phrase repetitions, together with a decrease in part-word repetitions and interjections. He suggested that these data indicate that, as non-stuttering children mature, part-word repetitions decline, even if other disfluency types increase. Thus, an increase in part-word repetitions as a child is observed longitudinally may be a sign that warrants concern.

Although the research is far from complete, we can characterize normal disfluency types as follows. Revisions are common in normal children and may continue to account for a major portion of their disfluencies as they grow older. Interjections are also common, but usually decline after 3 years of age. Repetitions may also be a frequent type of disfluency around 2 to 3 years of age, especially single-syllable word repetitions having fewer than two extra units. Repetitions are also more likely to involve longer segments (e.g., phrases) as a child grows older. Table 5–3 summarizes the major characteristics of normal disfluency.

Secondary Behaviors

A normally disfluent child generally has no secondary behaviors. He has not developed any reactions to his disfluencies, such as escape or avoidance behaviors. Although research suggests that some normal children occasionally display "tense pauses," such tension does not appear to be a reaction to their disfluency. If a child shows what appears to be normal disfluencies, such as single-word repetitions, but consistently displays pauses or interjections of "uh" immediately before or during disfluencies, he should be carefully evaluated as possibly stuttering.

Feelings and Attitudes

A normally disfluent child rarely notices his disfluencies, even though they may be apparent to others. Just as a child may stumble when walking but regains his balance and keeps walking without complaint, a normal child who repeats or interjects or revises usually continues talking after a disfluency without evidence of frustration or embarrassment.

Underlying Processes

First, let's review the behaviors we are trying to account for. Normal disfluency occurs throughout childhood and adulthood. It may begin earlier than 18 months of age and peak between ages 2 and 3½ years. It slowly diminishes, thereafter, but also changes in form. Some types of disfluency, such as repetitions, decrease after 3½ years, but other types, such as revisions, may increase. Episodic increases and decreases in disfluency are also common throughout childhood. What causes these changes; why are there ups and downs and changes in form? Like most natural phenomena, multiple forces probably have an impact on fluency at any given moment, but some may predominate at certain times. In Chapter 3, I talked about developmental and environmental influences on stuttering and normal disfluency, and I will review these influences as we discuss studies of normally disfluent children.

Certainly, the development of language is likely to be one major influence on fluency. As my earlier review showed, children tend to be most disfluent at the beginning of syntactic units (Bernstein, 1981; Bloodstein, 1974, 1995; Silverman, 1974) and when the length or complexity of their utterances increase (DeJoy and Gregory, 1973; Gordon, Luper, and Peterson, 1986; Pearl and Bernthal, 1980). These findings suggest that disfluency is greatest when a child is busy planning long or complex language structures and must, at the same time as he is planning, begin to produce them, putting a heavy load on cerebral resources. It seems likely that producing newly learned language structures would be hardest of all and result in more frequent disfluencies on a child's most recently acquired forms. However, evidence gathered from four children between 2 and 4 years of age suggests that normal disfluency may be greatest on structures that have been learned but perhaps not fully automatized, thereby requiring more cerebral resources than are allocated to their production (Colburn and Mysak, 1982a,b).

Pragmatics may influence disfluency, too. Studies by Davis (1940) and Meyers and Freeman (1985a,b) indicate that children's disfluency increases under certain pragmatic conditions, such as when interrupting, when directing another's activity, or when responding to requests/demands to change their own activity. Mastering such pragmatic skills, especially those involving more complex social interactions, creates yet another challenge for a developing child. The pressures of language acquisition, interacting with other factors, can be seen as competing for cerebral resources, which leaves fewer remaining resources available for fluent speech production.

Another likely influence on disfluency, in addition to language acquisition, is speech motor control. Between 2 and 5 years of age, most children begin to produce almost all the segmental and supersegmental targets of their native language, as well as increase their speech rate as they produce longer and longer utterances. These maturational changes must keep the average child fairly busy, although it may not be obvious. He is continually scanning his parents' and older siblings' speech, acquiring information about talking. He is also continuously modifying his own productions to make them more and more like the speech he hears. This period, from 2 to 5 years, also encompasses an intensive refinement of nonspeech motor skills. Children are mastering a myriad of other motor tasks at the same time they are acquiring the ability to speak in rapid, complex, fluent sequences.

In general, the view of stuttering described earlier, which suggests that a breakdown may occur when cerebral resources of the motor control system are reassigned for use elsewhere, may fit a nonstuttering child as well as the child who stutterers (Andrews et al, 1983; Starkweather, 1987). Some of the upswings in disfluency may occur when a normal child is occupied with spoken language planning and production, as well motor control for other things besides speech fluency. Remember the dyssynchrony hypotheses we discussed in Chapter 4? Even normal disfluencies may be the product of a child learning to integrate all the subcomponents of spoken language at increasingly faster rates with increasingly greater options for vocabulary, syntax, and prosody.

Besides the continuing demands of normal development, there are also episodic stresses in a child's environment that may temporarily increase normal disfluency. An experiment by Hill (1954) demonstrated that conditioned fear could elicit disfluency in normal adults' speech. It is easy to imagine, therefore, that there are many psychological stresses in a child's life that would also increase disfluency. Clinically, I have observed many situations that seem to increase normal disfluency. Among them are the stress of a move from one home to another, parents' separation or divorce, the birth of a sibling, and other events that decrease a child's security.

We have also seen increases in normal disfluency during periods of excitement, such as holidays, vacations, and visits by relatives. Disfluency increases especially when excitement is combined with competition to be heard, such as during dinner table conversations when everyone is talking at once or after school when several children are competing to tell Mom what happened during the day. As we speculated in Chapter 4, emotions may have an especially strong influence on fluency in young children. This happens after interactions between right and left hemispheres develop during the child's first 2 years (Fox and Davidson, 1984), and overflow activity from emotional arousal in the right hemisphere may disrupt vulnerable, immature language production networks in the left hemisphere.

Summary

1. Between ages 2 and 5 years, many children pass through periods of disfluency. Repetitions, interjections, revisions, prolongations, and pauses are commonly heard during this period.

2. When the average child is between 2 and 3½ years, disfluencies reach seven per 100 words spoken and may occur even more frequently in some normally disfluent children.

3. Repetitions are probably most common in younger children, whereas revisions are more common in older children.

4. Despite the fact that children's disfluencies may occasionally attract some adult attention, normally disfluent children seem generally unaware of the disfluencies in their own speech and don't react to them or engage in secondary behaviors to escape or avoid them as a consequence.

5. Some factors thought to contribute to increases in normal disfluencies include the demands of language acquisition, lagging speech-motor control skills, interpersonal stress associated with growing up in a typical family, and threats to security from such events as relocation, family breakup, or hospitalization. Disfluencies may also increase under the ordinary daily pressures of competition and excitement while speaking.

Borderline Stuttering

Borderline stuttering has most of the characteristics of normal disfluency (Fig. 5–2); however, more disfluencies occur, and they often differ from normal ones in several ways. Diagnosis of borderline stuttering is sometimes difficult because a child may drift back

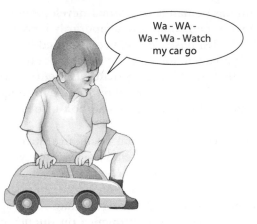

Figure 5–2   *Child who may be a borderline stutterer.*

and forth between normal disfluency and borderline stuttering over a period of weeks or months. Some children with borderline stuttering gradually lose their stuttering and grow up without a trace of it. Others develop more stuttering symptoms and progress through levels of beginning, intermediate, and advanced stuttering. Still others may continue to show borderline stuttering throughout their lives but may never seek treatment because their disfluency is so mild.

In describing the behaviors of borderline stuttering, I will begin to define my view of how stuttering differs from normal disfluency. The distinction between stuttering and normal disfluency has been of great interest to theorists for many years. Some theorists (e.g., Wendell Johnson et al, 1942, 1959) suggested, as was noted previously, that a stuttering child developed symptoms only after his parents mislabeled his normal disfluencies as stuttering. That is, a child's first "stuttering" symptoms were actually just normal speech disfluencies.

An opposing view maintains that there are objective differences between the speech of a normal child and the speech of a child who is stuttering, even before a parent or someone else labels the behaviors as stuttering. Although I hold this latter view, I also agree that there is much overlap between the disfluencies of stuttering children and the disfluencies of normally disfluent children. Moreover, as previously stated, these children often go back and forth between stuttering and normal disfluency over a period of months. For this reason, we use the term "borderline" to indicate that these children are neither entirely normally disfluent nor definitely stuttering.

Core Behaviors

There is no single core behavior that distinguishes borderline stuttering from normal disfluency. However, many researchers and clinicians have suggested a few guidelines. The *frequency of disfluencies* is one important aspect to consider. As we indicated in our description of normal disfluencies, nonstuttering children between 2 and 5 years may go through periods of increased disfluency. Even so, their level of disfluency averages about seven per 100 words. Typically, if children have many more disfluencies per 100 words (e.g., more than 10), we consider them borderline.

Another feature that can help identify borderline stuttering rather than normal disfluency is *the proportion of certain types of disfluencies*. The study we cited earlier by Johnson (Johnson et al, 1959) suggested that, compared to nonstuttering children, those who stutter had significantly more sound and syllable repetitions, word repetitions, phrase repetitions, broken words (i.e., phonation or airflow is abnormally stopped within a word), and prolonged sounds. There were no significant differences between the groups in their number of interjections, revisions, or incomplete phrases.

More information on types of disfluencies was provided by Young (1984), who reviewed a large number of studies that had assessed which types of disfluencies were identified as stuttering and which were not. His summary impression was that repetitions of parts of words and, to a lesser extent, prolongations are the disfluency types that are likely to be classified as stuttering. Bloodstein (1987) and Conture (1982, 1990, 2001) generally concurred with other writers, suggesting that "within-word" disfluencies (i.e., part-word repetitions, single-syllable word repetitions, and audible and inaudible prolongations including blocks) and broken words are the types of disfluencies most frequently heard in stuttering children.

Yairi and colleagues (Yairi and Ambrose, 1996; Yairi, 1997a,b) proposed that children who stutter can be distinguished from normally disfluent children using a grouping of "stuttering-like" disfluencies. Included in this grouping were short-segment repetitions (i.e., part-word and monosyllabic word repetitions), tense pauses (i.e., stoppage of speech with evident muscular tightening both within and between words), and a category introduced by Williams, Silverman, and Kools (1968) called "dysrhythmic phonations" (i.e., any distortion, prolongation, or break in phonation within a word that is not included in another category). Yairi (1997a,b) notes that, when many previous studies of stuttering and nonstuttering children are reanalyzed using this grouping, the proportion of stuttering-like disfluencies in nonstuttering children is always less than 50% of the total number of disfluencies. Thus, if a child has more than 50% stuttering-like disfluencies, he might be considered to be stuttering.

In summary, we can say that one measure that will help us distinguish a child with borderline stuttering from a normally disfluent child is a higher proportion of part-word and monosyllabic whole-word repetitions and prolongations, compared with multisyllabic word and phrase repetitions. In the next section, we will see that children who show the types of tension in their disfluencies that have been labeled blocks, broken words, and dysrhythmic phonations are beginning rather than borderline stutterers.

The *number of times a word or sound is repeated* in a part-word or monosyllabic word (repetitive disfluency) appears to be another sign that distinguishes children who stutter from their normally disfluent peers. In Yairi's (1981) sample of 33 nonstuttering children, repetitions typically involved only one or two extra units of repetition (e.g., one extra unit would be li-like this). Other studies comparing stuttering and nonstuttering children (Ambrose and Yairi, 1995; Johnson et al, 1959; Yairi and Lewis, 1984; Zebrowski, 1991) have found that the repetitive disfluencies of nonstuttering children average 1.13 extra units and the repetitive disfluencies of stuttering children average 1.51 extra units. Thus, the frequent occurrence of repetitions having more than one extra unit is a warning sign of borderline stuttering.

We have said that borderline stuttering consists primarily of effortless repetitions and occasional prolongations. However, as Van Riper (1971, 1982) and Bloodstein (1995) have noted, these young children are often highly variable in their stuttering. Although they usually show the core behaviors of borderline stuttering, they may have brief periods of normal fluency, as well as days when they show signs of more advanced stuttering.

Secondary Behaviors

A child with borderline stuttering has few, if any, secondary behaviors. The degree of tension may sometimes seem to be slightly greater than normal, but repetitions and prolongations generally look and sound relaxed. The child does not exhibit accessory movements before, during, or after stutters. In fact, there is usually nothing in his behavior to indicate that he is aware of his stutters. Some children with predominantly borderline stuttering may go through periods when their stuttering suddenly escalates to the level of beginning stuttering, with tension and some other secondary behaviors, but then it falls back again to the borderline level.

Feelings and Attitudes

Because a child with borderline stuttering seems to have little awareness of his stutters, he does not show concern or embarrassment. When he repeats a sound or a syllable, even five or six times, he usually goes on talking as though nothing has happened. One exception, however, is that once in a while a child with borderline stuttering might appear surprised or frustrated when he is repeating a syllable several times and is unable to finish a word. Then, he may stop and cry out, "Mommy, I can't say that word!" or otherwise demonstrate brief alarm or surprise. But, in general, a borderline stutterer shows little or no evidence of awareness that he has disfluencies that are different from those of his peers. Table 5–4 summarizes the major characteristics of the borderline stutterer.

Underlying Processes

I hypothesize that the symptoms of borderline stuttering result from the constitutional, developmental, and environmental factors described in Chapters 2, 3, and 4. The constitutional factors associated with borderline stuttering often first show their effects as an excess of normal disfluencies. As previously stated, environmental and developmental

Table 5–4 Characteristics of Borderline Stutterer
1. More than 10 disfluencies per 100 words
2. Often more than 2 units in repetition
3. More repetitions and prolongations than revisions or incomplete phrases
4. Disfluencies loose and relaxed
5. Rare reaction of child to his disfluencies

pressures may be great between 2 and 4 years of age, and it is during this period that borderline stuttering typically emerges. The converging demands of expressive language and motor speech development ordinarily peak between ages 2 and 4 years, "when an explosive growth in language ability outstrips a still-immature speech motor apparatus" (Andrews et al, 1983, p. 239). This age is also filled with psychosocial conflicts, as a child copes with security needs as an infant while striving to become more independent as a toddler. The child may be ready to explore but also fearful. The birth of a new brother or sister may trigger the child's insecurity with the threat of being replaced. Or, an older sibling may turn belligerent toward the child because of the older child's own need to express aggression as a prelude to puberty. Just as these stresses wax and wane in strength during preschool years, so does the child's stuttering.

After age 4½ or 5 years, developmental stresses taper off for most children. Some of the parent-child conflicts are resolved, and children may feel more integrated within themselves and within their families. Articulation and language skills, although still not at adult levels, have been mastered sufficiently for most children to say what's on their mind and to be understood. They have also mastered other motor skills, such as walking and running, as well as riding a tricycle or a bike with training wheels. They may also have adjusted to a new, younger sibling as well and made at least temporary peace with an older one.

By now, the capacities of many of the children who had modest predispositions to stutter can easily meet most environmental demands. Therefore, many of those who were borderline stutterers will have acquired normal fluency skills by the time they are 4½ or 5 years old. Other children may still have many disfluencies at this age but will eventually outgrow them, perhaps because they are not frustrated by them and do not respond with tension or by rushing. In general, they are functioning well, feel accepted, and can use their resources to compensate for whatever difficulties in speaking remain.

Some children, of course, do not outgrow borderline stuttering. They may continue to stutter, and their symptoms may worsen. They may be children who have substantial predispositions to stutter, which cannot be offset by a "good enough" environment (Winnicott, 1971). Their ability to produce speech and language at the rate and level of complexity used by parents and peers and their own desires to express their thoughts may be insufficient. Their continuing efforts to meet advanced speech and language targets may result in excess disfluency that does not diminish as they pass their third and fourth birthdays. Their frustration tolerance for the repetitions that 2- and 3-year-olds exhibit may be low. Rather than shrugging them off, they may begin struggling to produce flawless speech, thereby placing greater demands on their speech production and emotional resources. Still other children may continue to stutter because environmental and developmental stresses do not diminish. Their insecurity may continue from sibling rivalry, breakup of their family, or a parent's death. They may have language or articulation problems, as well as stuttering, which limit their communication abilities throughout their preschool years.

Deficits in the processes underlying speech and language development, plus the frustration of being unable to communicate easily, may be devastating to fluency. This may result in the increased tension of beginning stuttering. A child in this situation is unlikely to outgrow stuttering unless parents and professionals provide extensive support.

Summary

1. Children with borderline stuttering usually exhibit a greater amount of disfluency than normal children (i.e., more than seven disfluencies per 100 words).

2. Using another measure of frequency, the proportion of stuttering-like disfluencies may be greater than half of all disfluences.

3. Children with borderline stuttering are also likely to repeat units more than once in many of their part-word and monosyllabic word repetitions and to have many more part-word and monosyllabic word repetitions and prolongations than multisyllabic word and phrase repetitions, revisions, and interjections.

4. At the same time, the disfluencies of borderline stutterers, like those of nonstuttering children, are usually loose and relaxed-appearing. Also, like nonstuttering children, children with borderline stuttering show little or no awareness of their speaking difficulty. Only rarely do they express frustration about it.

5. Among the underlying processes behind borderline stuttering are probably some of the speech and language-processing anomalies described in Chapter 2 on constitutional origins of stuttering. Such deficits in resources may interact with the demands of speech and language development and the pressure from higher rates of speech, more complex language, competitive speaking situations, and other attributes of a normal home. In addition, some of the psychosocial conflicts described earlier that increase normal disfluency are likely to be active in creating borderline stuttering.

Beginning Stuttering

When stuttering persists, a child who has had borderline stuttering often begins to increase muscle tension and speaking rate during repetitions, like the child in Figure 5–3 appears to be doing. At first, the child may do this only occasionally, when he's excited or stressed. But tension and hurry may gradually become a regular part of his stuttering. The child's borderline stuttering is now becoming beginning stuttering. He is stuttering more often and is less tolerant of it. He is impatient with his stuttering and begins to use a variety of escape behaviors as a consequence. For example, he may try to end long repetitions by using an eye blink or head nod. These signs, and his stuttering in general, may still come and go, as they would in a the child with borderline stuttering. In beginning stuttering, however, periods of increased stuttering may last for several months, but periods of fluency may last only a few days. As these signs occur more consistently, tension increases, and struggle is more evident. Instrumental and classical conditioning processes increase the frequency of struggle behaviors, complicate the child's pattern of stuttering, and spread the symptoms to many more situations.

It should be noted that some children exhibit beginning stuttering at onset, without passing through a stage of borderline stuttering. Van Riper (1971, 1982) described several different profiles of stuttering with tense blockages at onset. Many of the children he depicted as more severe at onset were relatively older (e.g., 4, 5, or 6 years old) when their stuttering first appeared. Onset in these children seemed to be related to one of two

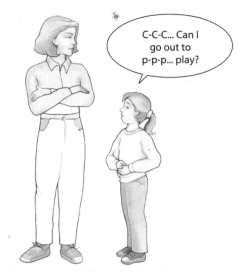

Figure 5–3 Child who may be a beginning stutterer.

factors: delayed language development or emotional events. In a study of the onset of stuttering, Yairi and Ambrose (1992b) described onsets of stuttering that were characterized by the signs I described for beginning stuttering in 28% of their sample of 87 children. Many of these children had relatively sudden onsets, with normal fluency changing to beginning stuttering within 1 day or, at most, 1 week.

Core Behaviors

The core behaviors of beginning stuttering differ from those of borderline stuttering in several ways. Repetitions begin to sound rapid and irregular. The final segment of a repeated syllable often sounds abrupt; if it is a vowel, it will sound as if it were suddenly cut off or were a neutral or schwa vowel ("uh") that had been substituted for the appropriate one, as in "luh-luh-luh-like" instead of "li-li-li-like." Repetitions are also produced more rapidly, sometimes with an irregular rhythm. Rather than patiently repeating a syllable as a borderline stutterer does, a child with beginning stuttering hurries through repetitive stutters, as though juggling a hot potato.

As symptoms progress, a beginning stutterer increases tension throughout the speech mechanism. Stuttering is often accompanied by a rise in vocal pitch, resulting from increased tension in the vocal folds. Rising pitch may first appear toward the end of a string of repeated syllables, but, over time, will appear earlier in the repetitions. A child with beginning stuttering sometimes prolongs sounds that he would have previously repeated. Initially, he may prolong the first sounds of syllables, but as stuttering grows more severe, he may also prolong middle sounds, and they, too, may be accompanied by an increase in pitch.

As beginning stuttering progresses, the first signs of blockages appear. These are significant landmarks, which indicate that a child is stopping the flow of air or voice at one or more places (Van Riper, 1982). He may inappropriately jam his vocal folds closed or wide open, interrupting or possibly delaying the onset of phonation (Conture, 1990). Shutting off the airway is usually heard as a momentary stoppage of sound in a child's speech and is sometimes accompanied by visual cues: the child may seem momentarily unable to move his mouth or may make groping movements as he tries to get air or get his voice going again. When the stoppage of movement, voice, or airflow first begins, it may be so fleeting that we don't notice it unless we are listening and watching carefully. As these blocks worsen, they become so obvious that they may overshadow the repetitions and prolongations that may remain.

Secondary Behaviors

As beginning stutterers' symptoms progress, secondary behaviors are added. They are called secondary because they appear to be responses to the muscle tension that has emerged. In addition, although hard evidence is lacking, the core behaviors of tension and speeding-up seem to be "involuntary," to have begun as a reaction that is beyond the stutterer's ability to control. In contrast, the secondary behaviors we are describing seem to have begun "voluntarily." They are, at least initially, deliberate. Among the earliest are escape behaviors, which are maneuvers used to end a stutter and finish a word. Children with beginning stuttering often show escape behaviors after several repetitions of a syllable. They may nod their head or squint their eyes just as they try to push a word out. This extra effort often seems to help in the short run. They escape, for the moment, from the punishing repetition, prolongation, or block. Alternatively, they may insert a filler, such as "uh" or "um," after a string of fruitless repetitions. The "um" seems to release the word, perhaps by relaxing the tightly squeezed larynx or by unlocking the lips. The "um" can always be said fluently, and once uttered, phonation and movement for the word often begin. The fillers work like a little push you might give your sled if it were stuck in the snow as you start down a hill; the "um" gets the child going again when he is stuck in a stutter.

A beginning stutterer starts to use escape behaviors earlier and earlier in stutters. The first appearance of these behaviors is usually after a child has repeated a sound quite a few times and is thoroughly frustrated about it. It may sound this way: "Luh-Luh-Luh-Luh-Luh-umLet's go!" Soon, however, the child will not wait until he has tried to say the sound five times. He finds himself about to say a word, feels convinced it won't come out, and then, perhaps instinctively, uses escape behaviors when he is first starting to stutter: "L-umLet's go!" Such "starters" may even appear before the first sound of the word, in this fashion: "umLet's go!" This is more common, however, among children with intermediate stuttering, even though it occasionally appears in the speech of a child with beginning stuttering.

Feelings and Attitudes

A child with beginning stuttering has stuttered many times. He is aware of stuttering when it happens. The feelings a beginning stutterer has just before, during, and after stutters are often strong. Frequently, frustration is a major feeling. The child may stop in the middle of a stutter and say, "Mom, why can't I talk?" However, such momentary frustration grows into momentary fear when a word or sound is stuck for several seconds, and the child feels helpless and out of control.

Table 5–5   Characteristics of Beginning Stutterers
1. Signs of muscle tension and hurry appear in stuttering. Repetitions are rapid and irregular, with abrupt terminations of each element.
2. Pitch rise may be present toward the end of a repetition or prolongation.
3. Fixed articulatory postures are sometimes evident when the child is momentarily unable to begin a word, apparently as a result of tension in speech musculature.
4. Escape behaviors are sometimes present in stutterers. These include, among other things, eye blinks, head nods, and "um's."
5. Awareness of difficulty and feelings of frustration are present, but there are no strong negative feelings about self as speaker.

Although a child with beginning stuttering is conscious that he has some "trouble" when he talks, he has not yet developed a belief that he is a defective speaker. This lack of a negative self-image may be attributed, as Bloodstein (1987) and Van Riper (1982) have suggested, to the "episodic" nature of stuttering. Some days it's there; some days it's not. Sometimes a child feels that he has problems when he talks; other times he forgets about it. The essential characteristics of beginning stutterers are presented in Table 5–5.

Underlying Processes

The signs and symptoms of beginning stuttering that I described can be observed by any experienced clinician. We have seen them in hundreds of children who stutter. But the processes underlying these behaviors are not so easy to see. In Chapter 3, we suggested that beginning stuttering may result from the interplay between constitutional and environmental factors, especially in a child with a reactive temperament. I will review my hypotheses about the core behaviors of beginning stuttering, as well as the learning processes that are likely to perpetuate the core behaviors and a child's secondary reactions.

Increases in Muscle Tension and Tempo

One of the first signs of beginning stuttering is the appearance of extra muscular tension in repetitions and prolongations and increased tempo or rate in repetitive stutters (Van Riper, 1982). Why do these changes occur? Oliver Bloodstein (1987) suggests that facial tension and strained glottal attacks in the speech of young children who stutter may reflect the extra muscular effort that emerges when they anticipate difficulty. Edward Conture (1990) offers a related view. He sees the increased articulatory and laryngeal muscle tension as a child's attempt to control sound-syllable repetitions, which are so distressing to him and his listeners. I have described such tension as a child's effort to control a frustrating and scary behavior of his own body, an attempt to stiffen the speech muscles and brace himself against the perturbations of seemingly involuntary, runaway repetitions (Guitar et al, 1988). One can imagine this taking place in the same way that a child who is attempting to ice skate may, in response to rough spots in the ice, stiffen and assume a less than ideal stance for continued, forward movement.

The other early sign of beginning stuttering, increases in the rate of repetitive stutters, is cited by a number of authors as an indication that stuttering is worsening. Van Riper (1982), in describing the developmental course of the majority of children whose stuttering persists, stated that, "the tempo changes as the disorder develops. The repetitive syllables become irregular and are often spoken more rapidly than other fluent syllables." Starkweather (1987) explained this increase in the speed of repetitions as a product of the pressure that children feel as they become more aware of the extra time it takes them to produce an utterance.

But why are these increases in tension and tempo so common in the development of stuttering, and why are they so difficult to change in therapy? In Chapter 4, I described my view that children in whom stuttering persists may be especially sensitive to certain kinds of experiences. Faced with frustration or fear, I hypothesized, they would react with elements of their biologically based freezing or flight responses. The signs of beginning stuttering appear to have similarities with such reactions. The excessive muscle tension in beginning stuttering can be viewed as a way that the limbic system can cause a child to freeze in the face of his frustrating or frightening repetitive disfluencies, transforming them into abrupt, tense repetitions, blocks, or prolongations. As I have mentioned, some children appear to show tense blocks at the onset of their stuttering. These may be children who have a high degree of emotional sensitivity and whose very first manifestation of stuttering may result from fear-based responses to speaking experiences.

Research bears out the speculation that at least some adults who stutter contract their muscles in such a way that movement and phonation are immobilized. Studies by Freeman and Ushijima (1978) and Shapiro and DeCicco (1982) indicate that stuttering is associated with abnormal muscle co-contraction of adductor and abductor muscles in the larynx. Such co-contraction could produce stiffening of the phonatory structures and silencing of vocal output. Other studies of stuttering have demonstrated co-contraction in articulatory structures (Fibiger, 1971; Guitar et al, 1988; Platt and Basili, 1973), which could also produce immobility and silence.

Unfortunately, little research directly supports the notion that the increased rate of repetitions reflects the flight response. We have some preliminary evidence that stutterers have more rapid productions during repetitions than nonstutterers. An unpublished study (Allen, 1988) carried out in our clinic indicated that the durations of beginning stutterers' repeated segments and the silences between them were shorter than the durations in similar disfluencies of nonstuttering children matched for age. This finding has been confirmed in the work of Throneburg and Yairi (1994), who found that the silent intervals and the total durations of repetition disfluencies were significantly shorter in stuttering children compared with those of nonstuttering children controls. Such shortening of segments results in a faster speech rate, at least for the stuttered elements, and may reflect the "great increase in activity" seen in the flight response, although these particular data do not exclude the possibility that stuttering children were more rapid speakers to begin with. It may be relevant at this point to note that Kloth et al (1995) found that rapid speaking rate was a predictor of which young children with a family history of stuttering and who were fluent at the time of testing would eventually stutter. The rapid rate in these children might be related to a reactive limbic system, although there is no evidence that speech rate is related to such reactivity.

The possibility that increased muscle tension and rapid repetitions are a result of biologically based freezing or flight responses is highly speculative at this time. If these responses are part of humans' neural wiring designed for survival, then this may be a potential explanation of why some children develop stuttering so rapidly and why tension responses are so difficult to change.

Effects of Learning on Stuttering

It is not clear whether the increases in tension and rate are voluntary, involuntary, or both, but I have observed repeatedly that these reactions increase with persistent stuttering. This is likely to be the result of classical and instrumental conditioning, which are the forces at work when stuttering escalates from an occasional tense and hurried repetition to speech that is riddled with tense and hurried repetitions. Learning also turns occasional eye blinks or head nods during stutters into stereotyped patterns of blinking and nodding that transform innocuous disfluencies into something so obvious that listeners gape in surprise and parents look away. Let us examine these learning processes more closely, so that we can better understand those who come to us for help.

Classical conditioning, I surmise, is responsible for previously "neutral" experiences and situations becoming able to elicit tense and hurried stuttering in a child's speech. This occurs after many experiences in which a child's repetitive stutters have brought on emotions that trigger increases in tension and hurry. Classical conditioning spreads this change in stuttering behaviors to more and more situations. In a few children, tension appears at the onset of the disorder because these children experience a high degree of emotion during a speaking situation. Many children whose stuttering persists may be highly susceptible to classical conditioning because of their reactive nervous systems.

Instrumental conditioning is responsible for the increase in frequency of escape behaviors in beginning stuttering because the child is reinforced for such things as head nods or eye blinks when they are followed by gratifying releases of the words that a child is stuttering on. Instrumental conditioning generalizes escape behaviors to more and more situations and causes escape behaviors to occur earlier and earlier in stutters, so that escape behaviors may eventually become "starters."

Summary

The principal differences between borderline and beginning stuttering are as follows:

1. The child with beginning stuttering shows more tension and "hurry" in his stuttering. This is often manifested in abruptly ended syllable repetitions, irregular rhythms of repetitions, evident stoppages of phonation, and momentarily fixated articulatory postures. Beginning stutterers also evidence such secondary behaviors as escape devices and starters. In addition, beginning stutterers see themselves as persons who sometimes have trouble talking.

2. A major factor underlying beginning stuttering appears to be a child's sensitivity to stress, which may result in the emotion of frustration, triggering tension responses.

3. Classical conditioning then links such unconditioned response sensitivity to disfluency (i.e., when the child is disfluent, he feels threatened, frustrated, or afraid), which leads to the rapid, tense disfluencies that begin to appear in beginning

stutterers. After repeated pairings, disfluency itself, rather than the emotion, elicits increased tension and rate. Classical conditioning also links a child's disfluency to more and more people and places.

4. A third factor in beginning stuttering is instrumental conditioning, which increases and then maintains the use of escape devices. These behaviors are negatively reinforced when a stutterers' frustration is terminated by an escape behavior and are positively reinforced when the stutterer completes his communication.

Intermediate Stuttering

The youngster with intermediate-level stuttering, who is typically between ages 6 and 13 years (Fig. 5–4), has two major characteristics that distinguish him from a child with beginning stuttering. First, he is starting to *fear* stuttering, whereas beginning stutterers are usually only frustrated, surprised, or annoyed by it. Second, he reacts to his fear of stuttering by appearing to *avoid* it, something beginning stutterers don't do with any regularity. These new symptoms emerge gradually as a young stutterer experiences negative emotion more frequently during stuttering. For example, he blocks and feels helpless, listeners respond with discomfort or pity, and after this has happened frequently, he becomes afraid.

This fear may be attached first to the sounds and words on which he stutters most, and he starts to believe that these sounds are harder for him. Then, he begins to scan ahead to see whether he might have to say them. When he anticipates that he will, he tries to avoid them. For example, he may say, "I don't know," to questions or substitute "my sister" for his sister's name when talking about her. Sometimes, he may start a sentence, realize a feared word is coming up, then switch the sentence around to avoid stuttering, and end up producing a maze of half-finished sentences. With tactful questioning, the clinician can verify these avoidances.

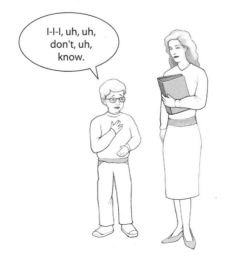

Figure 5–4   *Child who may be an intermediate stutterer.*

An intermediate stutterer's fear of stuttering may be associated with situations as well as words. The youngster may find that he stutters more in some situations than in others. At first, he approaches these situations with dread, but later, he may go to great lengths to avoid them. Van Riper (1982) suggested that the development of such situational fears and avoidances depends on listener reactions. Consequently, counseling or advice for key listeners in a stutterer's environment may help prevent them.

Core Behaviors

What are intermediate stutterers' moments of stuttering like when they don't avoid them? What are the core behaviors? Although they still repeat and prolong, their most notable core behaviors are now blocks. The blocks of children with intermediate stuttering seem to grow out of the increasing tension seen initially in beginning stuttering. A child at the intermediate level usually stutters by stopping airflow, voicing, movement, or all three and then struggling to get his speech going again. His stutters seem to surprise him less than when he was a beginning stutterer. Instead, as evidenced by his voice and manner in certain situations, he anticipates stutters.

I have the impression that the intermediate stutterer's blocks are frequently characterized by excessive laryngeal tension, but he often blocks elsewhere, as well. He may squeeze his lips together, jam his tongue against the roof of his mouth, or hold his breath. Even though he is not highly conscious of just what he's doing during a block, he has a vivid awareness that he is stuck, that he feels helpless, and that the word he wants to say won't come out.

A school-age child described his feeling of being blocked as like "a rock stuck in my throat." When he was lucky, he said, a little army of men would come into his throat and break the rock into little pieces, breaking the block so that sounds would come out. He was describing the experience of first being totally stuck, and then rapidly repeating the first segment of the sound as he fought his way out of the block. A common example is the "...uh-uh-uh-I" that you will hear when someone is blocked on "I" and tries to push through it. At first, there is a moment of silence and then the rapid, staccato first segment of the sound as the stutterer gets his larynx vibrating while maintaining a static articulatory posture. The larynx is still very tense; vibration stops and starts again and again. The vowel—either at the beginning or end of the syllable—is often what Van Riper (1982) called the "schwa" or neutral vowel. In fact, it is only the first, brief segment of the intended vowel, which is cut off too abruptly to be perceived as the sound normally used in the word. Inexperienced clinicians sometimes mistakenly categorize these repeated parts of blocks as repetitions.

In addition to repetitions of parts of sounds, blocks can have prolongations in them. Sometimes, as he is pushing through a block, a stutterer will momentarily prolong a continuent sound, as in "...mmm...mmmm.....my." Again; this probably results from the stutterer's larynx vibrating momentarily, then seizing up again, and then vibrating again. I catalog such events as blocks rather than prolongations because I think the core behavior is a complete stoppage of speech, even though it is mixed with momentary releases of laryngeal vibration. This confusing situation probably results from the fact that the sequence of repetitions, prolongations, and blocks reflect basically similar behaviors along a continuum of increasing tension, particularly in the larynx, as stuttering progresses.

Secondary Behaviors

The blocks just described can be devastating to a child who stutters. He is frustrated not only with his inability to make a sound, but he is often faced with surprised and uncomfortable listeners, as well. Even patient listeners may not know what to do. They may interrupt, look away, or fidget, leaving the child or adolescent to conclude that he is doing something wrong and should try to escape or avoid these painful moments.

The escape behaviors that a speaker uses to free himself from stutters are present in children with beginning stuttering, but they occur far more frequently in children with intermediate stuttering. They are often more complex, too. An intermediate stutterer may blink his eyes and nod his head in an effort to escape a block. Sometimes he may do both, and if he is still unable to say the word, he may resort to yet another device, such as slapping his leg. As these patterns grow more complex, they also may become disguised to look like natural movements and are performed more rapidly.

In addition to escape behaviors, a child at the intermediate level develops both word and situation avoidances, as previously mentioned. Word avoidances appear after he has had repeated difficulty with a particular word or sound and has discovered how to take evasive action before he has to say it. For example, a young stutterer in our clinic had been asked his name by a particularly stern teacher. He blocked severely on it and subsequently became fearful of saying his name, as well as other words starting with the same sound. He could usually think up synonyms for other words but found it awkward to substitute anything different for his name. So, he learned to get a running start in saying his name by beginning with "My name is . . ." whenever he was asked his name. This permitted him to avoid stuttering about half of the time. It is a subtle form of avoidance that many clinicians call "starters." More obvious examples of avoidances are given in the following paragraph.

Van Riper's (1982) catalog of word avoidance techniques included *substitutions* (substituting a word or phrase for another when stuttering is expected, as in "he's my unc-unc-unc . . . my father's brother"), *circumlocutions* (talking all around a word or phrase when expecting stuttering, as in "well, I went to . . . yes, I really had a good time there, I saw the Empire State Building."), *postponements* (waiting a few beats or putting in filler words before starting a word on which stuttering is expected, as in "My name is. . . . . .Bill"), and *anti-expectancy devices* (using an odd manner or funny voice to avoid stuttering when it's anticipated).

Like escape behaviors, word avoidance techniques often become more rapid and more subtle with time. Indeed, some stutterers can disguise word avoidances to look like normal behavior. For example, they may put on a pensive facial expression and appear to search for a word while postponing their attempt to say a feared sound. Experienced clinicians learn to pick up subtle cues in the rate and manner of speaking that tip them off to the use of such avoidances. Such avoidances can be explored by the clinician and client at the appropriate moment in treatment.

Situational fears and avoidances are also beginning to appear in the intermediate stutterer. Past stuttering in specific places or with specific people are the seeds from which situation fears grow. In school, stutterers usually have more trouble reading aloud or giving oral reports. Most people who stutter, and many nonstutterers, dread those classes in which teachers call on students by going up and down the rows. As in an earlier example, the students' fears steadily mount as a teacher goes down the row, getting closer and closer to calling on them. Then, if called on, they may take a failing grade rather than give the oral report. In contrast, other school situations, especially casual ones like gym class or lunch period, are likely to hold little fear or expectation of stuttering for them.

Situational fears quickly generate situation avoidances. The student who fears giving answers in class may try to slouch low in his seat in hopes of being overlooked. A stutterer who is afraid of making introductions will contrive ways of having other people make them. As a teenager, I coped with my fear of ordering in restaurants by ducking into the bathroom when the waitress approached our table, leaving my friends to order for me. Every stutterer has his own pattern of situation avoidances, which may provide an important focus for therapy in many cases.

Feelings and Attitudes

Youngsters with intermediate stuttering have gone well beyond the momentary frustration and mild embarrassment experienced by those with beginning stuttering. They have felt the helplessness of being caught in many blocks and runaway repetitions. The anticipation of stuttering and subsequent listener penalties have been fulfilled many times. These experiences pile up like cars in a demolition derby to create an entanglement of fear, embarrassment, and shame that accompanies stuttering. These feelings may not be pervasive or dog a stutterer all the time. But stuttering has now changed from an annoyance to a serious problem.

A major influence on such youngsters' feelings is the cognitive development, which started at age 3 or 4 years, that enables him to compare himself with his peers. Once he begins school, peers have a greater and greater influence on him. He may stutter more as he encounters new people and new situations, and as he does, peers may begin to ask him why he talks the way he does and to make comments about his stuttering or tease him about it. As a result, increasingly negative self-awareness about his speech leads to feelings of embarrassment, shame, and guilt.

A child with intermediate stuttering shows his increasingly negative feelings about stuttering in many ways. He may look away from listeners when he is stuttering and flush with embarrassment afterward. He may become stiff and uneasy at the prospect of speaking. His stuttering pattern includes an increasing number of avoidance devices, and he is beginning to evade situations in which he feels he may stutter. These are all signs that his feelings and attitudes are becoming suffused with fear. Table 5–6 lists the characteristics of intermediate stutterers.

Table 5–6   Characteristics of Intermediate Stutterers

1. Most frequent core behaviors are blocks in which the stutterer shuts off sound or voice. He may also have repetitions and prolongations.
2. Stutterer uses escape behaviors to terminate blocks.
3. Stutterer appears to anticipate blocks and often uses avoidance behaviors prior to feared words. He also anticipates difficult situations and sometimes avoids them.
4. Fear before stuttering, embarrassment during stuttering, and shame after stuttering characterize this level, especially fear.

Underlying Processes

Many of an intermediate stutterer's symptoms result from the same processes that underlie those of beginning stutterers. There are major differences, however. In the intermediate stutterer, classically conditioned tension responses are more evident, conditioned frustration is now becoming a more intense fear reaction, and avoidance conditioning has become a factor in shaping stuttering behaviors.

Avoidance conditioning transforms *escape* behaviors, such as the use of "um" to escape from a stuttering block, into *avoidances,* such as saying "um" before saying a word on which stuttering is expected. This learning process also leads individuals with intermediate stuttering to avoid words, to change sentences around, and to avoid speaking situations entirely. Avoidance learning also generalizes from one word to another and from one situation to another.

Avoidance conditioning may proceed very quickly in people with persistent stuttering because they may have a genetic or congenital bias toward right-hemisphere, emotionally based behaviors, as I described in Chapters 2 and 3. The threat of stuttering may elicit "prepared" defensive reactions, such as avoidances of words or situations. Such avoidances are strongly maintained because individuals who have developed them use them when they anticipate stuttering, which decreases or eliminates the fear. Thus, avoidances are maintained by negative reinforcement. By avoiding the stuttering, they never have the opportunity to discover that stuttering is not so painful after all. Therapy must structure situations to help stutterers learn this and must give them new behaviors to substitute for the old avoidances.

Summary

Intermediate stuttering is differentiated from beginning stuttering by the following:

1. There are increasingly tense blocks, repetitions, and prolongations; the increased tension results from feelings of frustration, fear, and helplessness. These feelings trigger tension responses, which interfere with fluency and, in turn, produce more frustration, fear, and feelings of helplessness. As tension mounts, this vicious cycle continues; blocks are longer and more noticeable, more listeners react with surprise and impatience, and the child's fear increases in response to these reactions.

2. The increasing presence of fear and anticipation of bad experiences spurs the child to develop avoidance behaviors in addition to the escape behaviors he is already using. Avoidance conditioning is difficult to undo.

3. The child with intermediate stuttering increasingly feels embarrassment, shame, and guilt as he realizes that his speech is markedly different from that of his peers.

Advanced Stuttering

The last developmental/treatment level, advanced stuttering, is characterized more by the age of a stutterer than by differences in stuttering pattern or underlying processes. The advanced level pertains to older adolescents and adults (Fig. 5–5), but it is important to remember that some adolescents and adults who stutter will not progress to this level.

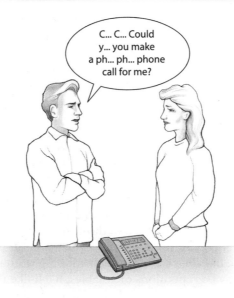

Figure 5–5   *Individual who may be an advanced stutterer.*

Treatment at the advanced level differs from treatment of younger stutterers because the client can take much of the responsibility for therapy, including substantial work outside the clinic.

An advanced stutterer's increased capacity for independent work may compensate for another characteristic of this level: a long history of stuttering. Patterns of stuttering with tension, escape, and avoidance behaviors are now firmly established. Emotions like frustration, fear, guilt, and hostility have built up over many years of being unable to speak like other people and after many bad experiences with thoughtless or uninformed listeners. Beliefs are usually distorted by the conviction that other people are impatient or disgusted by the speaker's stuttering.

After many years of stuttering, adults and adolescents who stutter increasingly think of themselves as stutterers, rather than as persons who have occasional difficulty speaking. Except for a few safe situations, in which they may be relatively fluent, most speaking situations hold some fear for them, and they shape their lives accordingly. Their friends, social activities, and jobs are often influenced by this view of themselves as a stutterer. They may believe that their stuttering is as noticeable to others as having two heads and nearly as unacceptable.

Core Behaviors

Core behaviors in advanced stuttering are typically blocks, that is, stoppages of sound and movement. Advanced stutterers may block, then release a little sound, only to fall back into the block again. It might sound like this: "(silence)...m-m-m...(silence)...m-m-muh... (silence)...my (said with a sudden effort)...name is Barry." Such behaviors may be longer and more struggled in clients with advanced stuttering than in clients with intermediate stuttering, but they are essentially the same. Blocks may be associated with tremors. During blocks, tremors of lips, jaw, or tongue may be apparent. As you may remember from the discussion of tremors in Chapters 2 and 4, tremors appear in those who have been stuttering for many years and may occur when stuttering is accompanied by strong emotion.

In a few advanced stutterers, blocks are hardly evident at all. They may have honed their avoidance devices to such a fine edge that core behaviors are scarcely noticeable. If stuttering does become evident, it usually devastates them. Consequently, much of their energy is spent anticipating blocks that often don't occur and mustering avoidances to keep anxiety at bay. One such individual, a delightful woman I knew and whom I'll call Lenore, said she had stuttered since childhood. Yet, she almost never had a repetition, prolongation, or block that I could see. She was highly competent at everything she did but severely limited her life because of her fear that she would stutter. In particular, she often felt she came across as far less articulate than she otherwise might have because of the frequency with which she substituted words to avoid stuttering.

Individuals with advanced stuttering, like those at the intermediate level, have repetitions as well as blocks. These are not the easy, regular repetitions of borderline stuttering but, instead, are more like the repetitions of beginning stuttering: tense, with a rapid, irregular tempo. They may be repetitions of syllables, li-li-li-like this, or mixed with fixed articulatory postures of tense blocks, l...l...li-li-li...like this. The latter repetitions look as if the speaker recoils from a momentary fixation and then gets stuck again.

Secondary Behaviors

Advanced stuttering involves many of the same word and situational avoidances that are seen in intermediate stuttering, but the avoidances are likely to be more extensive. Some behaviors are more obvious than others. When I was in high school, I used several avoidance devices that often didn't work, such as "uh...well...you see" and a gasp of air, followed by a block of long duration, filled with unsuccessful escape attempts before I finally released the blocked word with great effort. Other advanced stutterers may approach feared words cautiously and use subtle mannerisms, such as appearing to think just before saying them, so that most listeners don't realize they were stuttering. These stutterers are usually on guard much of the time, scanning ahead with their verbal early-warning systems.

Many advanced stutterers also control their environments carefully so that they can avoid situations in which they are likely to stutter. They may feign sickness when they have to give a speech, use answering machines rather than answering the telephone, or arrange to have their spouses or children deal with store clerks. Often, with careful questioning of advanced stutterers who use avoidances a great deal, you can learn what occurs when avoidances don't work. Even the most skillful avoiders are sometimes caught with their defenses down and become stuck in a block. Core behaviors may also be elicited by asking some stutterers to stutter openly, without using secondary behaviors. Stutterers who can do this, especially those who can do it without excessive discomfort, are more amenable to change.

Feelings and Attitudes

The feelings and attitudes of advanced stutterers, like their stuttering patterns, have been shaped by years of conditioning. Over and over, they have learned that much of their stuttering is unpredictable. When it is predictable, it comes when they want it least—when they want more than anything to be fluent. As a result, they often feel out of control. Figure 5–6 reflects one individual's depictions of his own feelings of being out of control when stuttering.

These uncomfortable feelings are often buttressed by a stutterer's perceptions of how others see him. Listeners' reactions look overwhelmingly negative to him. Even when listeners say nothing, their faces appear to say everything. It is as though stuttering is a rattletrap car that always stalls in heavy traffic amid honking drivers. Such experiences gradually shape advanced stutterers' attitudes toward feelings of helplessness, frustration, anger, and hopelessness.

Of course, individuals' responses to stuttering vary greatly. If a person who stutters has many talents and abilities for which he is recognized and has an assertive personality, he may be less devastated by stuttering. But if he has many other problems and a highly sensitive nature, his feelings and attitudes about stuttering may be an important component of his problem.

The point is that, by the time a stutterer is an adult, he has had years of experiencing stuttering and feeling frustrated and helpless and has developed techniques to minimize pain. Unless he has strong attributes to compensate, such as a superb athletic ability, he is likely to feel that stuttering is a big part of who he is to other people. It is a part that he hates, a part on which he blames many other troubles, and a part he wants to eliminate.

On the other hand, some stutterers who reach the advanced level have become reconciled to their stuttering. If they are in their 20s or 30s or beyond, there may be some natural resistance to treatment, because stuttering has become part of their identity. After years of doubt and turmoil, they've grown accustomed to themselves as stutterers. To consider treatment is to reject part of themselves, to open old wounds. Those who risk change, enter treatment, and succeed will find the risk to have been worthwhile. But those who enter treatment and do not succeed may suffer twice, from the pain of failure as well as the loss of what had been gained before but was given up.

Table 5–7 lists the major characteristics of advanced stutterers.

Underlying Processes

Advanced stuttering, unlike lower levels of stuttering, is influenced only minimally by its original constitutional, developmental, and environmental factors. The effects of home environments, developmental pressures of speech and language, and maybe even some

---

Table 5–7   Characteristics of Advanced Stutterers

1. Most frequent core behaviors are longer, tense blocks, often with tremors of lips, tongue, or jaw. Individual will also probably have repetitions and prolongations.
2. Stuttering may be suppressed in some individuals through extensive avoidance behaviors.
3. Complex patterns of avoidance and escape behaviors characterize the stutterer. These may be very rapid and so well habituated that the stutterer may not be aware of what he does.
4. Emotions of fear, embarrassment, and shame are very strong. Stutterer has negative feelings about himself as a person who is helpless and inept when he stutters. This self-concept may be pervasive.

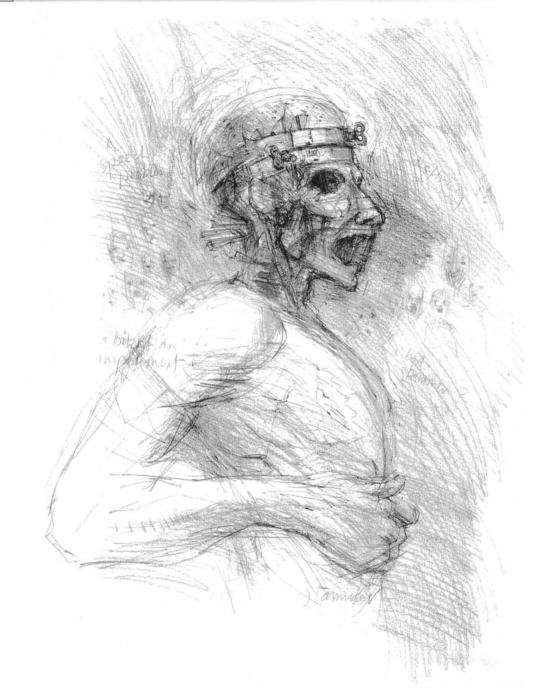

Figure 5–6 *"How I feel when I stutter" by Mike Peace. (Courtesy of Dr. Trudy Stewart.)*

differences in central nervous system function have been diminished by maturation and learning. However, conditioned habits that were learned in response to these early factors are stronger than ever. Their effects have been magnified by years of experience, and the way the brain operates in speech has been modified as a consequence. Moreover, an individual's characteristic patterns of tension, escape behaviors, and word and situation avoidances have become almost automatic through years of practice. For example, he may exhibit a string of avoidance and escape behaviors but only remember that "the word got stuck."

The advanced stutterer's disorder is affected by higher-level, explicit learning, as well. He has developed a self-concept as an impaired speaker, which carries highly negative connotations for most. Self-concepts begin to be formed during preschool years and are based initially on what one can do, rather than what one is (Clarke-Stewart and Friedman, 1987). More enduring traits are added as a result of social interactions in later childhood, adolescence, and beyond (Roessler and Bolton, 1978). Thus, a stutterer's self-concept at the earliest levels of development is determined, in part, by his perception of how he talks. It may be a fleeting notion, not necessarily negative, that he has difficulty talking sometimes. At later levels of development, the reactions of significant listeners, such as parents, peer group, and other adults, have a major impact. Now his self-concept may become filled with relatively enduring negative perceptions as a result of listeners' impatience and rejection. A negative self-concept is formed not only by perceptions of listeners' reactions, but it, in turn, also affects those perceptions.

Researchers studying the psychology of disability suggest that "one's perception of self influences one's perception of others' views of oneself, rendering social interaction more difficult" (Roessler and Bolton, 1978). Applied to clients with advanced stuttering, this suggests that they are likely to project their own rejections of stuttering onto listeners, thereby inhibiting interactions with them. This vicious cycle can only be stopped when an outsider helps a stutterer test the reality of his perceptions.

In addition to working on cognitive aspects of the problem, therapy for advanced stuttering also deals directly with avoidances such clients have learned so well. As mentioned in the discussion of intermediate stuttering, as avoidance conditioning progresses, individuals fear not only words and situations, but also stuttering itself. By deconditioning this fear and changing such responses, treatment enables stutterers to stutter with less fear by associating the clinician's approval with a calmer, more relaxed way of stuttering. Gradually, tension and hurry fade from disfluencies, and stutterers feel more in control, and their fears diminish even further as a result.

Summary

The diagnosis of advanced stuttering describes a developmental level and implies a particular treatment orientation, as characterized by the following:

1. Treatment may be easier because the client can assume much of the responsibility for generalization beyond the clinic.

2. On the other hand, treatment is more challenging because the client with advanced stuttering has habituated patterns of behavior more deeply than at earlier levels. The advanced stutterer's core behaviors often consist of long blocks

with considerable tension and, at times, visible tremors. Secondary behaviors may consist of long chains of word avoidance and escape behaviors. Situational avoidance is common.

3. Some advanced stutterers may hide and disguise their stuttering well enough to avoid detection by many listeners, but this is at the cost of constant vigilance.

4. Feelings of frustration and helplessness usually accumulate over the years, leading to coping behaviors and a lifestyle that may be highly constraining. Such responses create a self-concept of an inept speaker whose stuttering is unacceptable to listeners. This, in turn, affects the stutterer's perceptions of the listener's reactions.

Overall Summary

Table 5–8 summarizes the characteristics of the five developmental/treatment levels described in this chapter. Each individual who stutters will have his own course of development, influenced by the interaction of constitutional and environmental factors. The clinician needs to use his or her understanding of the underlying processes to design procedures to treat each individual's core behaviors, secondary behaviors, and feelings and attitudes.

Study Questions

1. In the "exceptions and variations" section of the overview, different types of stuttering onset and development are described. What factors might cause these differences?

2. In discussing normal disfluency, it is suggested that, "If a child shows what appears to be normal disfluencies, such as single-word repetitions, but consistently displays pauses or interjections of 'uh' immediately before or during disfluencies, he should be carefully evaluated as possibly stuttering." What might be going on? What might these pauses or interjections signify?

3. The idea of a dyssynchrony in the spoken language production process is suggested as an underlying process of normal disfluency. It is also used to account for primary stuttering. How can both types of disfluency be accounted for by the same process?

4. What is the difference between core behaviors and secondary behaviors?

5. At what ages is normal disfluency likely to be most frequent?

6. Name three influences that may cause normal disfluency to increase.

7. What are three ways in which core behaviors of normal disfluency differ from those of borderline stuttering?

8. Describe the core behaviors of the beginning stutterer.

9. What causes the beginning stutterer's increase in tension in his disfluencies?

10. Describe why an escape behavior is used by a stutterer. Give examples.

Table 5–8 Characteristics of Five Developmental/Treatment Levels

Developmental/ Treatment Level	Core Behaviors	Secondary Behaviors	Feelings and Attitudes	Underlying Processes
Normal disfluency	10 or fewer disfluencies per 100 words; one-unit repetitions; mostly repetitions, interjections, and revisions	None	Not aware, no concern	Stresses of speech/language and psychosocial development
Borderline stuttering	11 or more disfluencies per 100 words; more than 2 units in repetitions; more repetitions and prolongations than revisions or interjections	None	Generally not aware; may occasionally show momentary surprise or mild frustration	Stresses of speech/language and psychosocial development interacting with constitutional predisposition
Beginning stuttering	Rapid, irregular, and tense repetitions may have fixed articulatory posture in blocks	Escape behaviors, such as eye blinks, increases in pitch, or loudness as dysfluency progresses	Aware of disfluency, may express frustration	Conditioned emotional reactions causing excess tension; instrumental conditioning resulting in escape behaviors
Intermediate stuttering	Blocks in which sound and airflow are shut off	Escape and avoidance behaviors	Fear, frustration, embarrassment, and shame	Above processes, plus avoidance conditioning
Advanced stuttering	Long tense blocks; some with tremor	Escape and avoidance behaviors	Fear, frustration, embarrassment, and shame; negative self-concept	Above processes, plus cognitive learning

11. What is the major secondary behavior that differentiates the intermediate from the beginning stutterer?

12. Compare the feelings and attitudes of the borderline, beginning, and intermediate stutterer.

13. Describe the role of the listener in the development of the advanced stutterer's self-concept.

SUGGESTED PROJECTS

(1) Create videotape clips of speakers who are representative of each level of stuttering (normal disfluency, borderline, beginning, intermediate, and advanced) and play them in random order for your class and see how many of your fellow students can correctly identify each level.

(2) Make audio or video recordings of 20 to 30 nonstuttering students in a class and determine which of them are more disfluent and which are less disfluent. Is there a gradual continuum between more disfluent and less disfluent, or are there two distinct groups? Are any of the more "normally disfluent" students actually borderline stutterers? Should the term "borderline stutterer" be used only for preschoolers?

(3) Read Yairi and Ambrose's (2005) chapter on the development of stuttering (see Suggested Readings) and compare that perspective with the view presented in this chapter.

Suggested Readings

Bloodstein, O. (1995). Symptomatology. In *A Handbook on Stuttering* **(ed 5). San Diego: Singular Publishing Group, Inc.**

The subsection titled "Developmental Changes in Stuttering" in this chapter describes four stages similar to our levels of stuttering development. Other schemas of developmental changes are also discussed in a clear and logical style.

Gray, J.A. (1987). *The Psychology of Fear and Stress.* **Cambridge: Cambridge University Press.**

This is a very readable exposition of relatively recent findings about innate fears, conditioning, and brain processes involved with escape and avoidance learning. Gray also describes his concept of the "behavioral inhibition system," a model of the role of conditioning, language, the limbic system, and anxiety on behavior.

Luper, H.L., and Mulder, R.L. (1964). *Stuttering: Therapy for Children.* **Englewood Cliffs, NJ: Prentice-Hall.**

An excellent treatment text that describes four developmental levels of stuttering similar to our own. Although out of print, this book is available at most university libraries.

Starkweather, C.W. (1983). *Speech and Language: Principles and Processes of Behavior Change.* **Englewood Cliffs, NJ: Prentice-Hall.**

This book describes the principles of instrumental, classical, and avoidance conditioning that underlie much of stuttering behavior. It gives a clear account of how these principles create stuttering behavior and how conditioning is used in treatment.

Van Riper, C. (1982). The development of stuttering. In *The Nature of Stuttering.* **Englewood Cliffs, NJ: Prentice-Hall.**

In this chapter, Van Riper describes four developmental tracks of stuttering, three of which depart substantially from our stages of stuttering development. This chapter will give the reader a good sense of individual variability in stuttering.

Yairi, E., and Ambrose, N.G. (2005). The development of stuttering. In *Early Childhood Stuttering: For Clinicians by Clinicians.* **Austin, TX: Pro-Ed, pp. 141–195.**

This chapter reviews other authors' descriptions of the development of stuttering and presents a different perspective on the changes that occur in stuttering from onset to recovery or persistence. The data provided support the view that 75% to 85% of childen who begin to stutter will recover without treatment and that stuttering typically decreases in severity and frequency after onset.

Assessment and Treatment of Stuttering

Chapter 6

Preliminaries to Assessment

Assessment operates on many levels, like most satisfying endeavors. On one level, there is information gathering, such as interviewing, measuring speech, and administering tests and questionnaires. This requires careful planning, good observation, and thorough analysis. It begins with clients seeking help and often ends with a plan for treatment. On another level, assessment is a personal encounter. It involves getting to know another person or a family, trying to understand them, and tuning your antennae to pick up the subtle signals they may be sending out about their needs and how you might help them. On this more subjective level, you are becoming aware of the entire person or family, not just the stuttering. Your clients are also getting to know you and sizing up your ability to help them; thus, this first meeting may be the most critical. Although you will want to show an individual client or family that you know about stuttering and understand its treatment, you will want to spend most of your time listening to their concerns and demonstrating your desire to understand them. The two hats you will wear, that of the humanist and that of the scientist, will become a natural part of your wardrobe as you gain more experience.

The Client's Needs

It is easy to say we must always consider a client's needs, but it's hard to put this into practice. One reason is that we can develop expectations that function as blinders. Such expectations affect our perceptions of what our clients want, what caused or precipitated their stuttering, what their priorities are, and many other things. Although I know intellectually that every client is different, I have found a tendency in myself, as I have become more experienced, to jump to conclusions. I sometimes think, "Ah, yes, I understand this kiddo. So much like that child I saw last month." You will find this true for yourself too, as you work with more and more clients. We must try to listen carefully to what each client says and see each person with fresh eyes.

We also must be cautious about letting referral information, past experience, and biases cloud our ability to see all aspects of the person clearly. Also, we must be wary of simple explanations and quick judgments about which factors are critical for a client. For instance, if parents tell us that they often ask their child to stop and start again when she stutters, that both parents work long hours outside the home, and that dinner is a noisy and confusing time, we should try not to assume that these pressures at home are a major problem for the child. They may be, but other things may be even more critical. We need to ask more questions and explore how the child responds in these and other situations before we decide how to begin helping the child and her family.

Sometimes individuals' or families' requests differ from what we think they need. An adult may say that she wants "completely fluent speech," but we know this is not attainable by even the most fluent nonstutterer. Or, a family may want us to treat their 3-year-old child without their having to take part in therapy, although our preferred approach for a child this age involves parent participation. I have found it best not to feel I have to resolve such issues during an assessment session. I make no promises but do make a concerted effort to understand what clients and families want and why. My experience has been that, after I work with a family or individual for several sessions, we build up enough trust to work together to make the changes that we mutually decide are appropriate.

I remember seeing a young man who came to our clinic from some distance away for intensive therapy. During the evaluation, he made it quite clear that he didn't want to be treated like a rat in a cage; in other words, he wanted no talk of conditioning, reinforcement, or shaping. In responding to his concerns, I discussed his stuttering with him in terms of cognitions, perceptions, and beliefs. Together, we designed an intensive treatment program for him that included plenty of "fluency shaping" and "maintenance" but that made him feel respected as a human and not treated like a rat. In the process, I also explored with him his concerns about being controlled by others.

In trying to meet a client's needs, I consider the person as well as the problem. The client, no matter what age, will sense quickly whether a clinician is seeing her as an individual or is only seeing her stuttering. An effective clinician is genuinely interested and empathetic; he accepts failures and backsliding as well as victories and progress. The initial evaluation session is a clinician's first opportunity to show the client that he accepts her just as she is, without rejection or fear of her stuttering. This atmosphere helps the client to begin accepting herself and her stuttering and to take the first critical steps toward more fluent speech and effective communication.

The Client's Right to Privacy

All clients should feel they can trust you to protect their privacy and confidentiality. Trust is a vital element of client-clinician relationships. It enables the client to feel that she can safely reveal personal information to you that will help you plan and carry out appropriate treatment. In many cases, the act of expressing feelings in an accepting, secure environment can be therapeutic. For example, a mother whose school-age child was not making progress told her clinician that she was feeling resentment and impatience about her child's stuttering. Once she had released these feelings, her child made remarkable progress. Although this example is more about creating an accepting atmosphere for the child, this parent had to trust the clinician not to share this information inappropriately with other family members or the child.

Federal and State legislation, such as the Health Insurance Portability and Accountability Act of 1996 (HIPAA), helps clinicians follow guidelines for protecting clients' privacy. Clinicians should familiarize themselves with these laws and guidelines and ensure that clients give their consent for videotaping and observation and for sharing information about them. When clients perceive that we are scrupulous in guarding their privacy and confidentiality, we gain a level of trust that enhances therapy. This confidentiality extends to children as well. The bond between a child and clinician will be enhanced if the clinician discusses what information the child is willing to have shared with her parent and what not to share. This is especially relevant for school-age children, who should also be consulted about the extent to which they would be comfortable having their parents involved in treatment.

Cultural Considerations

I have been discussing the need to understand and accept as unique everyone who comes to us for treatment. When people who stutter are from other cultures, our task of really understanding them can be more difficult. The 21st century will be a time of more and more migration among cultures and countries. Even tiny Burlington, Vermont has recently become home to immigrants from Vietnam, Cambodia, Croatia, Bosnia, and Somalia. Clinicians need to develop a multicultural perspective on assessment and therapy. An underlying principle of this perspective is becoming sensitive to differences in communicative style in other cultures and learning how other cultures view speech and language disorders. You can improve your multicultural sensitivity by reading about cultural issues related to communication disorders in general (Coleman, 2000; Goldstein, 2000; Taylor, 1994) and to stuttering in particular (Conrad, 1996; Cooper and Cooper, 1993; Culatta and Goldberg, 1995; Watson and Kayser, 1994).

Multicultural and interpersonal issues relevant to stuttering include:

1. Most treatments for stuttering encourage clients to improve their eye contact when speaking. A major reason for this is that many people who stutter look away from their listener when they stutter, increasing the perceived abnormality of the symptom and further disrupting communication. In some cultures, however, eye contact with a listener may be inappropriate, depending on the status of the listener

and the context. Among some Native Americans, for example, not looking at the listener is a sign of respect. Thus, a person who stutters from such a culture may look away from listeners but not necessarily because of shame or embarrassment. The clinician should become aware of situations when eye contact while speaking is appropriate and when it is not.

2. During an evaluation or in treatment, many clinicians may touch clients to help them identify points of tension or to signal them to make a change in their stuttering as it is happening. However, many individuals may regard being touched during an evaluation as an invasion of their personal space. It is important to ask permission before touching someone. You might say, for example, "I'd like you to try to catch a stutter and keep it going without finishing the word. Is it okay if I touch your arm to signal you to stay in the stutter?"

3. Some approaches to treatment use praise as a reinforcer that is given immediately after a child has spoken fluently. Cultures differ in the amount and type of praise they give children. A clinician I know working in a suburb of Sydney, Australia, which is a city rich in new immigrants, adapts her treatment contingencies to fit many different cultures. One family from the Middle East was adamantly against giving verbal praise to their child. Instead, they developed a special signal that the father gave to his son to reinforce fluent speech.

4. Children with borderline stuttering are often helped when families change their interaction patterns. One such change that families can make is to speak more slowly and pause between conversational turns when speaking with the child (e.g., Stephanson-Opsal and Bernstein Ratner, 1988). However, in some cultures, particularly in urban areas of the eastern U.S., families speak quickly and often overlap each other while talking. For these families, slowing speaking rate and not interrupting each other may seem so unnatural that they are unable to sustain this new interaction pattern. For their children, an operant conditioning approach in daily one-on-one conversations with a parent may be more appropriate.

5. Sometimes I ask the person I am working with in therapy to stutter on purpose, thereby decreasing her tendency to avoid and be afraid of stuttering. But, in some cultures, stuttering is regarded so negatively that stuttering on purpose would be unthinkable, at least in the early stages of treatment. It is important for you to become aware of how stuttering is viewed in different cultures and to understand when and where voluntary stuttering might be helpful and acceptable to your clients. Sometimes, the cultural stigma of stuttering makes it difficult for individuals and families even to discuss it.

   Our clinic recently treated a young man from China because he wanted to reduce his accent. Only after months of accent reduction treatment was he willing to talk about his greater problem, stuttering. Until we discussed it, he thought he had been successful in disguising it, even though his stuttering was obvious to most of his listeners.

6. Sensitive evaluations and treatment take into consideration not only the culture's view of stuttering but also the culture's style of verbal and nonverbal interaction.

Orlando Taylor (1986) described a number of cultural differences in communication style that are relevant to evaluations of stuttering. For example, interruptions of one speaker by another may be expected among African Americans, so trying to change that style of interaction in a family may meet with resistance. In addition, persons from African American and Native American cultures may feel uncomfortable responding to the personal questions often asked in an initial interview, and persons from an Hispanic culture may feel it is rude to get down to business before greetings and pleasantries are exchanged.

It may not be possible for a clinician to know all relevant aspects of each new client's culture. But clinicians can be aware of the importance of culture in a person's response to stuttering, as well as the differences in communication styles between their own culture and those of their clients. Such awareness can come from reading about a client's culture and discussing it with the client, if appropriate.

Similar sensitivity should be extended to different social classes within the clinician's own culture. Understanding and respecting class differences in such areas as vocabulary and values are crucial. Sometimes working with people from other cultures increases our respect for class differences within our own culture. When I worked in Australia, I often attended grand rounds in a Sydney hospital. One particular case presentation involved a white working-class Australian woman who had been mutilating herself with needles. Some of the staff and medical residents were highly unsympathetic to her condition, but a psychiatrist, renowned for his work in Aboriginal culture, shifted their attitudes. He spoke passionately about how we fail to understand people when we are blinded by our own values and beliefs and that trying to learn about this woman's circumstances would go a lot farther in helping her than our simple condemnations of her self-mutilating behavior.

Some clients will not only be from a different culture or different social class, but they will also speak a different language, and one that the clinician may not understand. In this case, an interpreter is necessary. Because interpreters are often from the same culture as that of the client, they may help not only in translating, but also in providing information about important aspects of the culture to aid the clinician's understanding. In the process of translating sensitive or complex messages, interpreters sometimes need to change the clinician's message to the client. When a message is rephrased by an interpreter to a more culturally appropriate style, therapeutic interaction will be facilitated. However, if an interpreter doesn't understand the intent of a question or statement, he or she may inadvertently convey wrong information. A friend of mine who was working with non-English-speaking Haitian immigrants in Boston understood just enough French to realize that wrong information was being given to a client by an interpreter. She rectified the situation by giving the interpreter a brief overview of what she wanted to discuss with the Haitian family and why certain elements were vital, which immediately improved communication.

Special considerations apply when clients are both bicultural and bilingual. Bilingual clients, in fact, are not uncommon; there is evidence of an increased risk for stuttering in bilingual individuals (Karniol, 1992; Mattes and Omark, 1991; Van Borsel, Maes, and Foulon, 2001). In these cases, one challenge for clinicians is to determine if the "stuttering" is really stuttering or is simply an increase in disfluency as a result of limited proficiency in a second language. Making this determination may be aided by careful observation of whether there are secondary symptoms (such as eye blinks or signs of increased tension) and cognitive or emotional responses to the suspected stuttering. For example, does the client feel ashamed of her disfluencies? Does she anticipate them? Are they consistently on the same words or same sounds? Another clue is that the disfluencies may be stuttering is if there is a history of stuttering in the client's family.

There is some debate in the literature about the extent to which stuttering occurs in one or more languages of a bilingual speaker. The excellent review of stuttering and bilingualism by Van Borsel et al (2001) discusses the evidence on this issue, concluding that, although stuttering may occur in one or both languages, it is more likely to occur in both. In some speakers, stuttering may be more severe in one language than another, so that careful analysis of stuttering in both languages will enable the clinician to decide whether to apply treatment to both. Analysis of stuttering in a language not spoken by the clinician is likely to be more accurate if a native speaker of that language, such as a family member or friend of the client, can work with the clinician to identify stutters. In adults, the client herself will be able to help identify stuttering in the language unfamiliar to the clinician.

The Clinician's Expertise

During an assessment, the clinician has a chance to demonstrate not only her empathy with a client's feelings but also her mastery of evaluating and treating stuttering. Adolescents and adults who stutter, and their family members, often come with feelings of frustration, fear, and helplessness. They are looking for someone they can trust and someone who can successfully guide them through the often difficult process of recovery. One of the first things a clinician can do to establish trust and credibility is to show that she not only knows about stuttering, but is comfortable asking questions about it, duplicating it in her own speech, and exploring it empathically. This provides both clients and family members with an ally, someone who is unafraid of "the thing" that is so troubling to them.

In the process of trying to understand an adult's or adolescent's stuttering, the clinician can ask the client to teach her how to stutter the way she does. As she interviews the family of a preschooler, she can emulate repetitions, prolongations, and blocks as she asks about the types of stuttering the child exhibits at various times and in various situations.

The clinician's statements and questions also convey her expertise. For example, as she interviews an older child, she can show that she knows about stuttering by making empathetic comments, such as "Giving reports in front of class can sometimes be hard for kids who stutter." This allows the child to respond without the pressure of a direct question but also lets the child appreciate that the clinician is someone who has experience with stuttering. When talking with families, the clinician can intersperse questions with such statements as "When children keep repeating a sound that won't come out, their voices sometimes rise in pitch as the repetition continues." The family can then confirm whether or not they have noticed this in their child's speech and, at the same time, recognize that the clinician is knowledgeable about children's stuttering. Obviously, these kinds of comments and questions are easier for experienced clinicians, but even beginning clinicians can rely on their reading, their all-too-brief practicum experiences, and their intuition to convey their interest and understanding.

Because it has risks as well as rewards, the approach to interviewing clients and families that was just described should be used carefully. By making comments based on past experience, we may inhibit some individuals and families from telling us about experiences that differ from those offered by the clinician. It is an art to find the balance between showing understanding and "leading the witness." As your clinical judgment develops, you will learn which clients will be helped by this approach and when.

I would also caution that demonstrating your expertise should be secondary to acquiring an understanding of clients' needs. A clinician's first task is to discern what an individual or family would like from the clinician. The second task is to understand the stuttering problem. In the normal course of accomplishing these two tasks—with attentive listening, empathetic comments, and perceptive questions—the clinician's expertise will emerge naturally.

Assessment of Stuttering Behavior

Assessment of stuttering behaviors is a broad topic that can be divided into several different targets, such as frequency, type, duration, and severity. In some situations, it may also be important to assess speech naturalness, speech rate, and concomitant or associated behaviors. The importance of each of these is slightly different, depending on the age of the client and the type of treatment you expect to use. Before describing how to assess stuttering, I will clarify what behaviors are considered stuttering. As I discussed in Chapter 5, a number of authors (e.g., Conture, 2001; Yairi and Ambrose, 1992a) have discussed which types of disfluencies distinguish stuttering from nonstuttering children. Borrowing from their discussions, I have concluded that the following behaviors should be counted as stutters: part-word repetitions, monosyllabic whole-word repetitions, sound prolongations, and blockages of sound or airflow. The latter category (blockages of sound or airflow) can sometimes be quite subtle, occurring in the middle of a word (as in "co-ookie" in which a glottal stop appears to break the word in half) or before a word. I also count successful avoidance behaviors as stutters if they are, unequivocally, an avoidance.

Reliability

Whenever a procedure is used to assess a behavior or a trait, it is important to know how reliable the procedure is. For example, if a police officer pulls you over for speeding because her radar gun has clocked you going 40 mph in a 25-mile an hour zone, you might want to know how reliable her radar gun was. When this happened to me several years ago, I went to court to contest the ticket. Many factors, I figured, could affect the accuracy of the radar gun's measurement of my speed: the weather, the age of the gun, and whether it was adjusted properly. Fortunately, the judge asked the officer for evidence of reliability of the radar gun to prove that it could repeatedly, dependably, and consistently measure the speed of a car. Unfortunately, the officer was able to provide the judge with evidence of her radar gun's recent reliability check, and I shelled out $85 for the fine.

Reliability is obviously an important characteristic of a procedure to measure stuttering. Many factors affect the measurement process, and some of these influences may result in data that are not representative of a client's true performance. In addition, it appears that stuttering is a particularly changeable behavior, making it difficult to measure. This phenomenon and its consequences are described by Cordes (1994) in her seminal article about reliability:

> *Perceptions, judgements, and observations are affected by variables attributed to the observers, to the instrumentation or coding procedures, to the situation or conditions of observation, to the subjects being observed, and to interactions among all of these. Consequently, researchers using direct observation methods are currently expected to provide evidence that their findings are not simply the results of situational influences or observer idiosyncrasies. They are expected, in other words, to provide evidence that their data are reliable. (p. 264).*

The same caveat is true for clinicial work. Observations of clients' stuttering before treatment and after may be influenced, despite our good intentions, by our desires to see them improve. Measurements may also be affected by random fluctuations in stuttering apart from treatment effects, by the setting in which the client is assessed, by length and type of sample taken, and by the particular dimension of stuttering, such as frequency, severity, duration, or type, that is chosen for assessment. It is important for clinicians to learn to assess stuttering reliably and to provide evidence that they have done so. It is also part of clinicians' responsibilities to know the reliability of the standardized measures they use to assess stuttering and to choose those measures that are most reliable.

When human judgement is involved, as it always is with measures of stuttering, reliability is checked first by demonstrating that the observer makes the same judgement when observing the same behavior a second time from a videorecording, usually several weeks later so that the second observation is fresh and not affected by memories of the earlier judgement. This is called intra-rater reliability. Reliability is also checked by comparing the original judgement with the judgement of a second observer, who rates the sample independently of the first observer. This is called inter-rater reliability.

Remeasurement of the data does not have to include the entire sample that is used, although doing so would certainly be the most rigorous approach (eg., O'Brian, Packman, and Onslow, 2004). It is common for clinical researchers in stuttering to remeasure a randomly selected portion (10% to 25%) of samples taken (e.g., Hakim and Ratner, 2004; O'Brian et al, 2003). When reliability of judgements is to be established for measurements made on clients who increase their fluency over the course of a treatment regimin, samples should be randomly selected from various points in therapy to include both less fluent and more fluent samples.

Measures of reliability are usually selected according to what behavior is being measured. In situations where evaluation and treatment depend on accurate identification of stuttering moments (such as whether a word or syllable is stuttered or not), reliability can be measured using what is commonly called "point-by-point agreement." A videotaped sample (for example, 400 syllables of conversational speech) can be transcribed, and each stutter can be identified and marked on the transcript by an original judge or rater. Some time later, the rater can return to the sample and again identify stutters by marking a fresh copy of the transcript. The two transcripts are then compared syllable by syllable, and the rater determines how many syllables are agreed upon as stuttered and how many are agreed upon as fluent. This total is termed "number of agreements." The number of disagreements (syllables that were determined to be stuttered in the first rating but not stuttered in the second rating or vice versa) are totalled and termed "number of disagreements." The reliability measure is then the number of agreements divided by the total number of agreements plus disagreements, multiplied by 100. Cordes (1994) notes that 80% agreement is commonly thought of as the lower limit for a sample to be considered reliable. Figure 6–1 gives an example of a point-by-point assessment of reliability.

When clinical research is carried out, some authors (e.g., Cordes, 1994) are concerned that point-by-point agreement can be affected by the fact that some agreements might happen by pure chance. To deal with this, it may be useful to report both

---

Observer 1:

<u>You</u> <u>wish</u> to know all about my <u>grand</u>father. Well, he is <u>nearly</u> <u>nine</u>ty-three years old; yet he still thinks as <u>swift</u>ly as ever. He dresses himself in an old <u>black</u> frock <u>coat</u>, usually several <u>but</u>tons missing. A long <u>beard</u> clings to his chin, giving those who <u>ob</u>serve him a pronounced feeling of the utmost respect. When he <u>speaks</u> his voice is just a bit cracked and quivers a <u>tri</u>fle. <u>Twice</u> each day he <u>plays</u> skillfully and with <u>zest</u> upon our small organ. <u>Ex</u>cept in the winter when the <u>snow</u> or ice prevents, he <u>slow</u>ly takes a short walk in the open air each day. We have often urged him to walk more and <u>smoke</u> less, but he always answers, "<u>Ba</u>nana oil!" Grandfather likes to be modern in his language.

Observer 2:

<u>You</u> <u>wish</u> to know all about my <u>grand</u>father. Well, he is nearly <u>nine</u>ty-three years old; yet he still thinks as <u>swift</u>ly as ever. He dresses himself in an old black frock coat, usually several <u>but</u>tons missing. <u>A</u> long <u>beard</u> clings to his chin, giving those who observe him a pronounced feeling of the utmost respect. <u>When</u> he speaks his voice is just a bit cracked and quivers a trifle. <u>Twice</u> each day he plays skillfully and with zest upon our small organ. Except in the winter when the snow or ice prevents, he <u>slow</u>ly takes a short walk in the open air each day. We have often urged him to walk more and smoke less, but he always answers, "<u>Ba</u>nana oil!" Grandfather likes to be modern in his language.

There are approximately 14 syllables upon which the observers did not agree. There are approximately 156 syllables upon which they agreed were either stuttered or were fluent. The simple point-by-point agreement (rather than the kappa statistic) would be calculated as agreements (156) divided by agreements plus disagreements (170), or 92%.

Figure 6–1 *An example of point-by-point agreement. An initial observer has marked the reading passage by underlining syllables on which stuttering was judged to occur. A second observer has marked the second passage. Point-by-point agreement can be calculated by comparing the total number of agreements with the agreements plus disagreements.*

percentage of agreement for stutters and percentage of agreement for fluent syllables or words. Alternatively, the agreement·calculation can be corrected by a procedure that takes into account the effects of chance, such as the kappa statistic (Cohen, 1960; Cordes, 1994).

Point-by-point agreement is appropriate when it is important to judge whether stuttering is present or absent on each syllable. It is also a good tool for new clinicians to use to assess their ability to accurately judge stuttering. However, other procedures are called for when assessment requires quantification rather than presence or absence. An example would be measurement of the duration of stutters. An appropriate measure of reliability would be percent error, obtained by remeasuring at least 10% of the data. In this case, it is appropriate to begin by (1) obtaining the absolute differences between each first judgement and each second judgement (change all negative numbers to positive), (2) summing those absolute differences together, (3) dividing by the total number of them to get the average, and finally (4) dividing the average absolute difference by the average of the first judgements. Table 6–1 shows an example.

A third method of assessing reliability can be used when measuring the amount of stuttering in cases when point-by-point agreement is not critical. One example would be when you are assessing frequency of stuttering as a measure of week-by-week progress. This procedure involves calculating both the correlation between the first rating and a second rating for multiple samples, as well as test of significant differences between the means of the ratings, such as a paired samples t test. Correlations and t tests should be done for both intra-rater and inter-rater reliability. Correlations should be above 80%, and t tests should show no significant difference between the samples. Table 6–2 depicts correlations and t tests for a sample of 12 original and re-rated samples.

As a final comment about reliability, I would suggest that, although different measures of reliability can be used for different purposes, beginning clinicians should establish their reliability using a point-by-point agreeement procedure, both during their initial training and to recheck their reliability periodically as they gain more experience. This may help them develop relatively consistent and agreed upon definitions of what a stutter is and is not.

Table 6–1   An Example of Assessment of Reliability by Calculating Percent Error of Duration Measurements

	Time 1	Time 2	Absolute Difference
	3.5	3.0	0.5
	4.0	4.0	0.0
	0.5	0.7	0.2
	0.4	0.3	0.1
	___		___
Mean	2.1		0.2

Duration of stuttering (in seconds) measured by an observer at Time 1 and remeasured at Time 2. Percent error = 0.2/2.1 = 9.5%.

Table 6–2	Assessing Inter-Rater Reliability by Calculating Correlations and t Tests	
Observer 1		**Observer 2**
12		11
10		9
15		10
4		6
8		5
2		2
14		12
7		9
3		4
6		6
5		3
1		3

Measures are percentage of syllables stuttered measured by Observer 1 and Observer 2.

Pearson $r = 0.90$; paired $t = 0.92$; $df = 11$; $P = .38$.

These calculations suggest that there is substantial inter-rater reliability because the ratings are highly correlated and there is no significant difference between the means.

Speech Sample

The size and number of samples depend on the purpose of the assessment. In a first assessment, it would be wise to have at least two samples: one recorded in the clinic and one recorded in the client's typical environment. Before I see a preschool child for an evaluation, I ask parents to send in a videotape of the child in conversation at home. Videotaping is so common in some homes so that the presence of a video camera will probably not make most children self-conscious. I sometimes ask parents to leave the camera on a tripod in a familiar place for several days so the child is used to it when the videotaping is actually done. When videotaping is not possible, audiotaping is still useful. With a school-age child, a sample collected in the school would be important; practically speaking, a sample could be most easily recorded in the therapy room. A second sample from home would also be very helpful, but it is not always obtainable. When evaluating an adolescent or adult, I recommend that a sample be taken in the treatment room and a sample be taken from work or home. It is often convenient for adolescents or adults to audiotape telephone conversations.

An important consideration in obtaining samples is how much stuttering varies. It differs in frequency and severity from month to month, week to week, day to day, and from situation to situation within the same day. Such variability affects both children and adults but is most apparent with younger stutterers. Sometimes a preschool child is stuttering severely, then 3 weeks later, during the evaluation, the child is entirely fluent. Therefore, it is important to discuss with the client or family whether the sample you have obtained is representive of the stuttering and, if not, whether more samples should be taken, maybe in other situations and at other times.

After the initial sample, when further assessment is done to measure progress in therapy, it is crucial to ensure that any reduction in stuttering is not confined to the therapy room. Thus, ongoing assessments should include measures taken in the client's real world, outside the treatment situation.

For any sample in which severity of stuttering is to be rated or any sample for research purposes, videotaping is essential. Many subtleties of stuttering would be missed if only an audiotape were used, thus videotaping allows better assessment of observer reliability than audiotaping. Sometimes on-line (while the client is talking) scoring can be done without either videotaping or audiotaping. For example, on-line scoring is appropriate when the clinician samples frequency of stuttering at the beginning of every session for clinical rather than research purposes.

The length of the sample must be long enough for it to be representative of the speaker's typical stuttering. Too short of a sample won't include enough stuttering to see the range of severity and types of stuttering, and too long of a sample would take time away from other assessment activities and would be tedious to score. I usually like to take a sample of 300 to 400 syllables of conversational speech (where there is likely to be more variability) and 200 syllables of a reading passage (where there is likely to be less variability). Using a typical figure of 1.5 syllables per word (Williams, Darley, and Spriestersbach, 1978), these samples would be equivalent to approximately 200 to 265 words and 130 words, respectively.

When obtaining a reading sample, it is important to ensure that the reading passage is at or below the client's reading level. A client's stuttering is likely to worsen when reading a passage that is difficult, giving a false impression of typical stuttering during reading. Reading passages in the *Stuttering Severity Instrument-3* (Riley, 1994) are designed for third, fifth, and seventh grade levels, as well as for an adult reading level. You can also write your own passages and check them for grade level using the Tools option on Microsoft Word, which uses the Klesch-Kincaid Reading Level statistics, or you can use the Fry Readability Graph available on the Internet at http://school.discovery.com/schrockguide/fry/fry.html.

When obtaining a speaking sample, it would be wise to select topics that are not emotional unless it is desirable to elicit a maximal amount of stuttering, as you might do with a client who says she stutters but is not demonstrating any during the evaluation. I usually ask children and adolescents to talk about their favorite activities over the weekend or after school, sports, hobbies, or pets. With adults, I ask them to talk about their favorite activities, sports, hobbies, work, or school.

When making a formal assessment or when first learning to assess stuttering, it is very useful to make a written transcript of the spoken material, including all words and even those nonmeaningful utterances, such as "uh." However, you should not indicate on the transcript which syllables are stuttered, so that you, at a later date, or another rater can rescore a copy of the transcript to check for reliability without being influenced by the notations indicating which syllables were stuttered. Using your recording of the spoken material and an unmarked transcript, you can note where the stutters are, with details of how the individual stuttered. Write out each element of a repeated sound or syllable, the sounds that were prolonged, and the sounds on which blocks occurred. Describe escape and avoidance behaviors accompanying each moment of stuttering. Mark those moments of stuttering that seem longer than most. For a complete assessment, you will want to return to the longer stutters and time how long each one was to deter-mine the average length of the three longest stutters. You will also want to count the words or syllables spoken, although it is often most accurate to count syllables from recordings because some speakers omit syllables in longer words.

Assessing Frequency

Frequency of stuttering is a simple, reliable measure (Andrews and Ingham, 1971) that can be used for a variety of purposes. It is important in an initial assessment to help dis-tinguish a normally disfluent child from a child with borderline stuttering. It is a vital part of composite ratings, such as the *Stuttering Severity Instrument-3* (Riley, 1994), that provide a multidimensional view of stuttering. Frequency of stuttering is also useful as a "snap-shot" measure of progress during treatment. In the first place, it is highly correlated with severity (Young, 1961). If used alone, however, frequency has the limitation that it does-n't reflect the duration of stutters or physical tension associated with stuttering. Decreases in these variables are often signs of improvement.

Frequency of stuttering is most commonly reported as percentage of syllables stuttered, although some use percentage of words stuttered or number of stutters per 100 words. I prefer to use percentage of syllables stuttered, following the logic of Minifie and Cooker (1964), because it can capture instances when a speaker stutters on more than one sylla-ble of a multisyllable word. Moreover, when counting syllables and stutters on-line, sylla-bles can be counted more easily than words, by counting the syllable beats as the client talks. When counting stutters, I assume that each syllable can be stuttered only once. Thus, multiple repetitions, like "Where is my ba-ba-ba-basketball?" are counted as only one stutter. "Where is my...my...uh...well ba-ba-ba-ba-basketball?" is also one stutter, because I assume that the repetition of "my" and interjections of "uh" and "well" are posponements associated with the stutter that was anticipated and actually occurred on "basketball." If a speaker appears to have a habit of using a particular word or sound as an avoidance behavior, I will count a word as stuttered even if no overt stuttering occurred. For example, a speaker may say "Where is my...uh...uh...uhbasketball?" In this case, the speaker appears to be using "uh" to postpone starting the word "basketball" on which he anticipates stuttering. And he keeps saying "uh" until he feels he can say "bas-ketball" fluently, then rushes to say "basketball" after saying the last "uh." When I am fairly certain that a speaker has used a sound or word as a (successful) avoidance behav-ior like this, I count the word as stuttered. When I am in doubt, I count it as fluent.

When assessing the speech of someone who can read, I find it helpful to compare the frequency of stuttering in reading to that in speaking. If stuttering is markedly greater in the reading task, this may be because the speaker is avoiding words he expects to stutter on in the speaking task, but he can't do this when reading. In most cases, I talk about my hypothesis with the client to see if he agrees.

Assessing Types of Stutters

When assessing the speech of preschool children, it is often useful to count the total num-ber of disfluencies, both those that are considered stutters and those considered normal. As you will remember from Chapter 5, disfluencies that are not considered stutter-like include multi-syllable word repetitions, phrase repetitions, interjections, and revisions in which a phrase is incomplete. When both types of disfluencies are counted, you can use the proportion of total disfluencies that are stutter-like to help you decide whether a child is stuttering or normally disfluent. As I indicated in Chapter 5, Yairi (1997a,b) surveyed a number of studies and proposed that, if less than 50% of a child's disfluencies are stutter-like, the child is more likely to be normally disfluent. Caution must be used with any single measure used alone. Conture (2001) noted that a child he had recently evaluated was, in his opinion, stuttering severely, even though the child's proportion of stutter-like disfluencies was only 34% of the total disfluencies. Clearly, Conture had relied on several other measures of stuttering in concluding that the child was a severe stutterer.

Another measure involving the type of disfluencies a child produces is the number of stutter-like disfluencies per 100 words. In summarizing his findings on disfluencies in stuttering and nonstuttering children, Yairi (1997b) noted that children who stutter have more than three stutter-like disfluencies per 100 words, whereas normally disfluent children have fewer. In this same chapter, Yari reviewed research about the gradual decline in some types of disfluencies as children grow older. Perhaps the most important finding is that part-word repetitions show a steady decline in normally disfluent children by age 4 years and thereafter. Thus, if a child shows a plateau or increase in part-word repetitions in later preschool years, the child may be showing stuttering rather than normal disfluency.

Assessing Duration

In a thorough assessment, measures of the duration of a client's longest blocks can give us important information about how much stuttering may be interfering with communication. Van Riper (1982, p. 208) noted, in his inimitable prose, that: "The duration of the individual moments of stuttering is one of the basic components of any adequate index of severity. Like tapeworms, longer stutterings are worse than shorter ones."

A common practice is to average the duration of the three longest stutters in a speech sample (Myers, 1978; Preus, 1981; Riley, 1994; Van Riper, 1982). Typically, I use a digital stopwatch while watching a videotape of the client speaking. With a little practice, you can turn on the stopwatch at the moment the stutter begins and turn it off when it ends and measure the moment of stuttering to the nearest half-second. Any delays in starting the stopwatch at the beginning of stutters are compensated for by similar delays when you stop it at the end. I recommend using duration as part of a more complete assessment of severity, such as the *Stuttering Severity Instrument-3* (Riley, 1994), when making an initial assessment of a client's progress and when you want to give a detailed description of a client's stuttering in a report.

Assessing Secondary Behaviors

Stuttering feels like the grip of an unseen hand damming up the flow of speech or, as one of my young clients said, a rock jammed in your throat. You struggle to keep going, squeezing your lips, blinking your eyes, or twisting your shoulders in the process. Such behaviors add to the abnormality of stuttering and reflect an important aspect of its development. Reducing or eliminating these behaviors may be a vital goal for therapy.

Secondary behaviors are also referred to as "concomitant," "associated," or "accessory" behaviors. They are most often escape behaviors that are used to break out of a stutter once it has started, but secondary behaviors may also be avoidance behaviors that are used in an attempt to keep from stuttering (see Chapters 1, 3, and 5 for further discussion of these terms). These behaviors may be physical movements (e.g., eye blink), extra sounds (e.g., "uh"), or changes in the way speech is produced (e.g., pitch rise). They are often signs that stuttering has progressed to a more advanced stage (i.e., escape behaviors distinguish beginning from borderline stuttering) but may, in a few cases, appear very close to the onset of stuttering.

Conture (2001) briefly reviewed the limited research on secondary behaviors and noted that most are just more frequent and more exaggerated versions of behaviors seen in normal speakers. Zebrowski and Kelly (2002) suggested that the most common behaviors involve the eyes, particularly blinking, squeezing, lateral and vertical eye movements, and loss of eye contact. These authors and Shapiro (1999) also pointed out that the presence of secondary behaviors can be an important diagnostic sign that may distinguish normally disfluent children from those who are beginning to stutter.

Some clinicians enumerate these secondary behaviors as part of their assessment, particularly when they will use a treatment approach that helps the client gradually modify her stuttering behaviors. Standardized measures, such as the *Stuttering Severity Instrument-3* (Riley, 1994), include ratings of these behaviors as part of an overall severity assessment. We will consider this assessment next.

Assessing Severity

Measures of severity may be the most clinically relevant assessment of overt stuttering behaviors. Severity reflects an overall impression that listeners may have when they listen to an individual who stutters. Thus, it is an important measure for assessing the outcome of treatment. It is also an important yardstick of progress during therapy because many treatments gradually reduce the abnormality of stuttering rather than eliminate it.

The most commonly used measure of severity is the *Stuttering Severity Instrument (SSI)*, which was first published in the *Journal of Speech and Hearing Disorders* (Riley, 1972). Its most current version, SSI-3, which is illustrated in Figure 6–2, is available with forms and a manual from Pro-Ed (this publisher can be found by searching for "stuttering severity instrument" on the internet). In my mind it is the best measure of severity available, but like its predecessors, the SSI-3 has some drawbacks. The sample of children and adults on which it was normed is not well described, its reliability is not strong, and its validity has not been convincingly demonstrated (McCauley, 1996). Despite these limitations, the SSI is easy to use and captures the severity of overt stuttering behaviors as a composite of three important dimensions: frequency, duration, and physical concomitants. The SSI-3 is one of the few measures of stuttering that has standardized procedures for gathering and scoring speech samples and is the only measure that includes the three dimensions just cited.

The total overall score for the SSI is the sum of the three subcomponents measured. (1) Frequency is assessed as the percentages of syllables stuttered on a speaking task and a reading task. For nonreaders, the speaking task is given twice the weight in the scoring procedures. Riley originally used percentage of words stuttered but currently uses the percentage of syllables stuttered, which is converted to a "task score" on the form. (2) Duration is assessed by measuring the length of the three longest stutters, calculating their mean duration, and finding the appropriate "scale score" on the form. (3) Physical

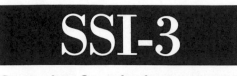

Stuttering Severity Instrument-3
TEST RECORD AND FREQUENCY COMPUTATION FORM

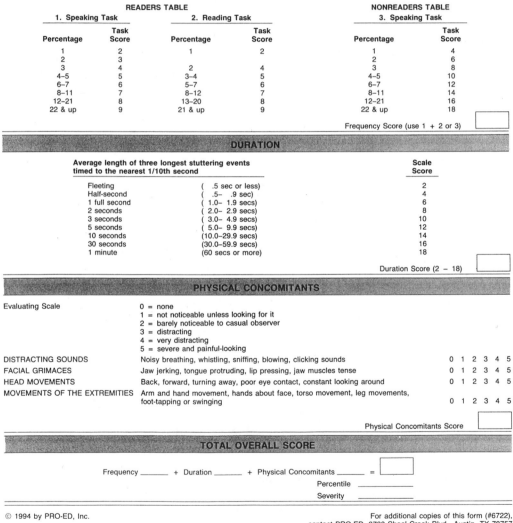

Identifying Information

Name _____

Sex M F   Grade _____   Age _____

Date _____   Date of Birth _____

School _____

Examiner _____

Preschool ___ School Age ___ Adult ___ Reader ___ Nonreader ___

FREQUENCY Use Readers Table or Nonreaders Table, not both.

READERS TABLE

1. Speaking Task		2. Reading Task	
Percentage	Task Score	Percentage	Task Score
1	2	1	2
2	3		
3	4	2	4
4–5	5	3–4	5
6–7	6	5–7	6
8–11	7	8–12	7
12–21	8	13–20	8
22 & up	9	21 & up	9

NONREADERS TABLE

3. Speaking Task	
Percentage	Task Score
1	4
2	6
3	8
4–5	10
6–7	12
8–11	14
12–21	16
22 & up	18

Frequency Score (use 1 + 2 or 3) _____

DURATION

Average length of three longest stuttering events timed to the nearest 1/10th second		Scale Score
Fleeting	(.5 sec or less)	2
Half-second	(.5– .9 sec)	4
1 full second	(1.0– 1.9 secs)	6
2 seconds	(2.0– 2.9 secs)	8
3 seconds	(3.0– 4.9 secs)	10
5 seconds	(5.0– 9.9 secs)	12
10 seconds	(10.0–29.9 secs)	14
30 seconds	(30.0–59.9 secs)	16
1 minute	(60 secs or more)	18

Duration Score (2 – 18) _____

PHYSICAL CONCOMITANTS

Evaluating Scale
0 = none
1 = not noticeable unless looking for it
2 = barely noticeable to casual observer
3 = distracting
4 = very distracting
5 = severe and painful-looking

DISTRACTING SOUNDS	Noisy breathing, whistling, sniffing, blowing, clicking sounds	0 1 2 3 4 5
FACIAL GRIMACES	Jaw jerking, tongue protruding, lip pressing, jaw muscles tense	0 1 2 3 4 5
HEAD MOVEMENTS	Back, forward, turning away, poor eye contact, constant looking around	0 1 2 3 4 5
MOVEMENTS OF THE EXTREMITIES	Arm and hand movement, hands about face, torso movement, leg movements, foot-tapping or swinging	0 1 2 3 4 5

Physical Concomitants Score _____

TOTAL OVERALL SCORE

Frequency _____ + Duration _____ + Physical Concomitants _____ = _____

Percentile _____

Severity _____

© 1994 by PRO-ED, Inc.

10 9 8 7 6 5 4 3 2 1   98 97 96 95 94

For additional copies of this form (#6722),
contact PRO-ED, 8700 Shoal Creek Blvd., Austin, TX 78757

Figure 6–2 *The Stuttering Severity Instrument–3.*

**Percentile and Severity Equivalents of
SSI-3 Total Overall Scores for Preschool Children ($N = 72$)**

Total Overall Score	Percentile	Severity
0– 8	1– 4	Very Mild
9–10	5–11	
11–12	12–23	Mild
13–16	24–40	
17–23	41–60	Moderate
24–26	61–77	
27–28	78–88	Severe
29–31	89–95	
32 and up	96–99	Very Severe

**Percentile and Severity Equivalents of SSI-3
Total Overall Scores for School-Age Children ($N = 139$)**

Total Overall Score	Percentile	Severity
6– 8	1– 4	Very Mild
9–10	5–11	
11–15	12–23	Mild
16–20	24–40	
21–23	41–60	Moderate
24–27	61–77	
28–31	78–88	Severe
32–35	89–95	
36 and up	96–99	Very Severe

**Percentile and Severity Equivalents of
SSI-3 Total Overall Scores for Adults ($N = 60$)**

Total Overall Score	Percentile	Severity
10–12	1– 4	Very Mild
13–17	5–11	
18–20	12–23	Mild
21-24	24–40	
25–27	41–60	Moderate
28–31	61–77	
32–34	78–88	Severe
35–36	89–95	
37–46	96–99	Very Severe

Figure 6–2 *(Continued)*

concomitants are assessed by adding the scale values of each subcomponent (i.e., distracting sounds, facial grimaces, head movements, and movements of the extremities) and deriving a total score. The values for frequency, duration, and physical concomitants are then added together to provide a Total Overall Score. Percentiles and severity ratings (e.g., mild, moderate, and severe) based on total overall scores are given on the form. Clinicians should carefully read Riley's directions on administering this measure in the manual of the SSI-3 before using it.

Clients should be videotaped, and the SSI should be calculated from the tape because duration measures and assessment of physical concomitants cannot be done easily on-line and the frequency count will be more accurate if equivocal stutters are replayed repeatedly until a decision can be reached.

Another measure of severity, which captures frequency, duration, and perhaps secondary behaviors, is the *Scale for Rating Severity of Stuttering* (Johnson, Darley, and Spriestersbach, 1952, 1963; Williams, 1978). This early scale, shown in Figure 6–3, is more subjective than the SSI, relying on an overall impression of a speech sample to rate the sample with one of eight values (0-7). Raters are encouraged to treat each of the eight intervals between the scale values as equal, although there is some debate about whether this is truly an equal-interval scale (Berry and Silverman, 1972). Although it has been shown to be reliable when a group of raters is used, the reliability of the Scale for Rating Severity of Stuttering for use with single raters is questionable. Williams (1978) cautions that the scale gives only a rough measure of severity because of its limitations. But he also notes that it has clinical utility because it captures the listener's impression of a client's speech and may, therefore, convey information about what the client faces every day when he is speaking. Ratings by a number of real listeners in the client's environment, as well as the client herself, would increase the value of this information. Any scale, including this one, has real risks if used as a single measure of therapeutic progress by a clinician. Unconscious bias and familiarity with the client may lead to improved ratings in the absence of change. Progress should be assessed with a variety of tools, including the SSI-3.

A third measure of severity is the Lidcombe Program's Severity Rating Scale, which was developed by Onslow, Costa, and Rue (1990) as part of an operant treatment program for preschool children. This is simply a 1 to 10 scale that parents use to make daily ratings of their child's stuttering (1 = no stuttering, 2 = extremely mild stuttering, and 10 = extremely severe stuttering). The scale, in a format that allows for a week's ratings, is shown in Figure 6–4. At the beginning of treatment, parents are trained to accurately rate their child's severity using videotaped samples or observations of the child's speech in the clinic. The clinician and parent compare their ratings and discuss any differences between them until the parent's ratings are essentially the same as the clinician's. Throughout treatment, the parent's severity ratings are compared with the clinician's measures of percent syllables stuttered in a 2-minute speech sample at the beginning of each session. If substantial differences occur between a parent's severity ratings at home and the clinician's percentage of syllables stuttered (%SS) measures in the clinic, the clinician works with the parent to resolve the differences. The clinician may, for example, explore possible causes for the disparity and ask the parent to measure stuttering at home by counting stutters per minute of speaking time or total stutters in a 5- or 10-minute period. These data are then used to explore whether the child is actually stuttering more or less at home than in the clinic or whether the parent needs further help in making severity ratings.

This severity rating scale has also been used with school-age children who stutter. These older children often rate themselves, in a version of the Lidcombe Program developed for older children. Research on this severity rating scale has shown it to be a valid and reliable tool for conveniently obtaining information on a child's stuttering outside of the treatment environment (Onslow, Andrews, and Costa, 1990; Onslow et al, 2002).

Scale for Rating Severity of Stuttering

Speaker_____   Age ____   Sex____   Date_____
Rater _____   Identification _____

Instructions:
Indicate your identification by some such term as "speaker's clinician," "clinical observer," "clinical student," or "friend," "mother," "classmate," et cetera. Rate the severity of the speaker's stuttering on a scale from 0 to 7, as follows:

0   No Stuttering

1   Very mild–stuttering on less than 1 percent of words; very little relevant tension; disfluencies generally less than one second in duration; patterns of disfluency simple; no apparent associated movements of body, arms, legs, or head.

2   Mild–stuttering on 1 to 2 percent of words; tension scarcely perceptible; very few, if any, disfluencies last as long as a full second; patterns of disfluency simple; no conspicuous associated movements of body, arms, legs, or head.

3   Mild to moderate–stuttering on about 2 to 5 percent of words; tension noticeable but not very distracting; most disfluencies do not last longer than a full second; patterns of disfluencies mostly simple; no distracting associated movements.

4   Moderate–stuttering on about 5 to 8 percent of words; tension occasionally distracting; disfluencies average about one second in duration; disfluency patterns characterized by an occasional complicating sound or facial grimace; an occasional distracting associated movement.

5   Moderate to severe–stuttering on about 8 to 12 percent of words; consistently noticeable tension; disfluencies average about 2 seconds in duration; a few distracting sounds and facial grimaces; a few distracting associated movements.

6   Severe–stuttering on about 12 to 25 percent of words; conspicuous tension; disfluencies average 3 to 4 seconds in duration; conspicuous distracting sounds and facial grimaces; conspicuous distracting associated movements.

7   Very severe–stuttering on more than 25 percent of words; very conspicuous tension; disfluencies average more than 4 seconds in duration; very conspicuous distracting sounds and facial grimaces; very conspicuous distracting associated movements.

Figure 6–3 *Scale for Rating Severity of Stuttering.*

10							
9							
8							
7							
6							
5							
4							
3							
2							
1							
	Date_____	Date_____	Date_____	Date_____	Date_____	Date_____	Date_____

Figure 6–4　*The Severity Rating Scale. Rate the speaker on a 10-point scale, where 1 = no stuttering and 10 = extremely severe stuttering (the worst stuttering the speaker has produced) for the entire day. Put an X in the appropriate box at the end of each day.*

Assessing Speech Naturalness

In recent years, clinical scientists have been concerned that treatments that produce fluency may not always result in natural-sounding speech. As Schiavetti and Metz (1997) warned, "Some stutterers may reduce their number of stutters at the expense of a speech pattern that is stutter free but not really fluent." Thus, some stuttering treatments may get rid of stuttering but leave an individual with speech that sounds odd, unusual, or unnatural. Martin, Haroldson, and Triden (1984), one of the first investigative teams to report on this problem, found that unsophisticated listeners rated the stutter-free speech of individuals who stutter speaking under DAF (delayed auditory feedback) as significantly more unnatural than the general speech of nonstutterers. Ingham, Gow, and Costello (1985) used the same rating scale and found that the fluent speech of treated stutterers was judged to be more unnatural than that of nonstutterers. Both investigations used a 9-point, equal-appearing intervals scale to rate speakers based on judges' intuitive sense of what sounded "natural." The judges in these and most subsequent studies exhibited satisfactory levels of inter-rater reliability and agreement, although individual rater reliability was only marginally satisfactory.

Clinically, we need to be sure that clients sound as natural as possible after treatment. Otherwise, they are likely to abandon their fluency skills in favor of old, familiar stuttering patterns because of their own and listeners' negative reactions to their posttreatment speech. Can we rate our clients' naturalness reliably? Schiavetti and Metz (1997) indicated that clinicians who have learned to be consistent raters of speech naturalness may rely on the relative values of their ratings. Thus, they can judge when a client sounds less natural than other clients they have treated and take appropriate steps to improve that client's naturalness before releasing her from treatment.

Assessing Speaking and Reading Rate

Many clinicians believe that speaking rate often reflects the severity of stuttering (e.g., Shapiro, 1999; Starkweather, 1985, 1987). Van Riper (1982) described studies that found correlations that ranged from 0.68 to 0.88 between reading rate and severity. If a client's speaking rate is well below average for her age, communication will be affected; listeners may become impatient or lose the thread of what the speaker is saying. Speech rates that are too fast will also affect communication. A subgroup of individuals who stutter also have the disorder of cluttering, which is rapid, often unintelligible speech (see Chapter 13). Thus, it is useful to measure the client's rate in standard speaking and reading tasks. Table 6–3 gives average speaking rates for children and adults.

Rate can be measured as either words or syllables per minute, depending on the clinician's preference. Some clinicians find it easier to calculate rate by using words per minute because words are easily observable units on the page. Others note that syllables per minute can be calculated more rapidly than words because clinicians can use the "beat" of syllables to count them on-line (i.e., while a speaker is talking). The syllables-per-minute approach also accounts for the fact that some speakers use more multi-syllabic words than others and might be penalized because such words take longer to produce than one-syllable words. I recommend using syllables for these reasons.

No matter which method is used, the following rules can be used for counting words or syllables. Count only those words or syllables that would have been said if the person

Table 6–3 Speaking Rates for Children and Adults

Age (yr)	Range in Syllables per Minute	Reference
3	116–163	Pindzola, Jenkins, and Lokken (1989)
4	117–183	"
5	109–183	"
6	140–175	Davis and Guitar (1976)
8	150–180	"
10	165–215	"
12	165–220	"
Adult	162–230	Andrews and Ingham (1971)

*add reading rates.

had not stuttered. Thus, if a person says, "My-my-my, uh, well my name is Peter," this should be counted as four words or five syllables because it is apparent that the extra "my's" and the "uh" are part of the stuttering. If a person says, "When I went to Boston, I mean when I went to New York . . .," and it does not appear that the person was postponing or using a "trick" to avoid stuttering, this would be counted as 13 words or 14 syllables because stuttering did not interfere with the utterance. Only words (or syllables in words) are counted: "uh" or "um" are not counted. "Oh" or "well" are counted, unless they are used as a postponement, starter, or other component of stuttering. These distinctions may seem difficult to remember, but the main rule of thumb you should use is that you are counting syllables or words that convey information to the listener.

When syllables per minute are calculated, it is often easiest to use an inexpensive calculator to count syllables cumulatively as they are spoken, although this takes some practice. Before the speaker begins, push the "1" key, then the "+". When the speaker starts speaking, press the "=" key for each syllable spoken or read, and the cumulative total will appear in the readout window. It is easier to count syllables by reading a transcript of the conversational sample aloud slowly and pushing the "=" key for each syllable spoken; inexperienced raters should learn to count syllables first from a transcript. Experienced raters can assess conversational speech rate directly from tape recordings by pressing the "=" key for each syllable spoken. Some calculators will count cumulatively when the "1" is pressed, followed by repeated presses of the "+" button; some expensive calculators will not count cumulatively.

Some clinicians have found that they are able, with practice, to count syllables per minute as the client is speaking by using graph paper with small boxes. As the client is talking, they put a dot in each box for each syllable spoken. They also use this method to assess frequency of stuttering, by putting a check instead of a dot for each syllable stuttered.

When words per minute are calculated, a transcript is made of a client's 5-minute sample of conversational speech, and her 5-minute reading sample is marked to indicate where she finished. The total number of words is counted, and this figure is divided by five to give a per-minute conversation or reading rate.

It is important to measure these samples accurately with a stopwatch. In measuring the amount of speaking time in a conversational sample, I stop the watch whenever the client is not talking but allow it to run during moments of stuttering. Short pauses of less than 2 seconds are incorporated into the 5 minutes, but formulation pauses longer than 2 seconds are excluded. With a little practice, starting and stopping a stopwatch during pauses and turn-switching become easy and natural.

Assessing Feelings and Attitudes

The feelings or emotions of individuals who stutter, as well as their beliefs and attitudes about themselves, about communication, and about stuttering are all components of stuttering. For most people who stutter, the experience of stuttering and the reactions of others to their stuttering have a notable effect on their behavior and on their response to therapy. Therefore, assessment of these aspects of stuttering is important. In this section, I focus on formal measures of feelings and attitudes that can be administered throughout therapy to assess progress. As clinicians gain more experience, they will develop informal procedures to supplement formal measures. I will describe these in the next chapter, as well as in appropriate treatment chapters.

Assessment of Preschool Children

Several assessment tools are being developed for preschool children who stutter, but none are available for use at this time. One example is the KiddyCAT, which was designed to assess communication attitudes of preschool children (Vanryckegham, 2002).

A number of clinicians have suggested that a preschool child's sensitivity or reactivity to new situations may be an important consideration in therapy and possibly predictive of chronicity (Conture, 2001; Guitar, 1998). I have found that the *Behavioral Style Questionnaire* (BSQ; McDevitt and Carey, 1978, 1995), which is administered to parents, provides some information on this dimension. Some research indicates that the BSQ may be able to identify those children who have a more inhibited, more sensitive temperament (Anderson et al, 2003; Conture, 2001). The BSQ has relatively high mean test-retest reliability for the 3 to 7 years scales (0.81) and a moderate internal consistency for this age range (0.70) (McDevitt and Carey, 1995).

School-Age Children

There are two formal tools available for assessing attitudes about speaking in children. Figure 6–5 depicts a scale that a graduate student and I developed many years ago, called the A-19 Scale (Guitar and Grims, 1977). It consists of questions that we have found will distinguish between children who stutter and children who do not. Thus, if treatment is effective, a child's attitude about communication may change, although this has not been established by research.

In addition to the A-19, the Communication Attitude Test (CAT) (Fig. 6–6), which was developed by Brutten and his students, was first tested on normal children (Brutten and Dunham, 1989) and has been shown to differentiate nonstuttering children from children who stutter (De Nil and Brutten, 1991). The CAT has been extensively researched and has been shown to have good inter-item reliability and substantial test-retest reliability (Vanryckeghem and Brutten, 1992). It is important that a trusting relationship with the child has been developed before administering either the A-19 or the CAT.

Although not strictly a measure of attitude, the Teachers Assessment of Student Communicative Competence (TASCC) (Smith, McCauley, and Guitar, 2000), which is depicted in Figure 6–7, is useful in assessing a child's communicative functioning in the classroom. I have listed it here because one of the subscales purports to measure approach/avoidance in the classroom based on questions about the child's class participation and volunteering to talk. Other areas that the teacher rates the child on include intelligibility, comprehension, appropriateness of communication, and pragmatic/nonverbal communication skills. I have found the TASCC to be helpful in getting information about how a child's communication is changing over the course of treatment. Although still in the development stage, it has been tested on 69 students in grades 1 through 5 in Maine, Vermont, Texas, Virginia, and Idaho and was found to have high internal consistency. Assessment of its reliability with groups of childen who stutter compared to those who do not is under way.

Establish rapport with the child, and make sure that he or she is physically comfortable before beginning administration. Explain the task to the child and make sure he or she understands what is required. Some simple directions might be used: "I am going to ask you some questions. Listen carefully and then tell me what you think: True or False. There is no right or wrong answer. I just want to know what you think." To begin the scale, ask the questions in a natural manner. Do not urge the child to respond before he or she is ready, and repeat the question if the child did not hear it or you feel that he or she did not understand it. Do not re-word the question unless you feel it is absolutely necessary, and then write the question you asked under that item.

Circle the answer that corresponds to the child's response. Be accepting of the child's response because there is no right or wrong answer. If all the child will say is "I don't know," even after prompting, record that response next to the question. For the younger children (kindergarten and first grade), it might be necessary to give a few simple examples to ensure comprehension of the requited task:

a. Are you a boy?   Yes   No

b. Do you have black hair?   Yes   No

Similar, obvious questions may be inserted, if necessary, to reassure the examiner that the child is actively cooperating at all times. Adequately praise the child for listening and assure him or her that a good job is being done.

It is important to be familiar with the questions so that they can be read in a natural manner.

The child is given 1 point for each answer that matches those given below. The higher a child's score, the more probable it is that he or she has developed negative attitudes toward communication. In our study, the mean score of the K through 4th grade stutterers (N = 28) was 9.07 (S.D. = 2.44), and for the 28 matched controls, it was 8.17 (S.D. = 1.80).

Score 1 point for each answer that matches these:

1. Yes	10. No
2. Yes	11. No
3. No	12. No
4. No	13. Yes
5. No	14. Yes
6. Yes	15. Yes
7. No	16. No
8. Yes	17. No
9. Yes	18. Yes
	19. Yes

Figure 6–5 *A-19 Scale of Children's Attitudes by Susan Andre and Barry Guitar (University of Vermont; reprinted with permission from Susan Andre).*

A-19 SCALE

Name_____   Date _____

1. Is it best to keep your mouth shut when you are in trouble?   Yes   No
2. When the teacher calls on you, do you get nervous?   Yes   No
3. Do you ask a lot of questions in class?   Yes   No
4. Do you like to talk on the phone?   Yes   No
5. If you did not know a person, would you tell your name?   Yes   No
6. Is it hard to talk to your teacher?   Yes   No
7. Would you go up to a new boy or girl in your class?   Yes   No
8. Is it hard to keep control of your voice when talking?   Yes   No
9. Even when you know the right answer, are you afraid to say it?   Yes   No
10. Do you like to tell other children what to do?   Yes   No
11. Is it fun to talk to your dad?   Yes   No
12. Do you like to tell stories to your classmates?   Yes   No
13. Do you wish you could say things as clearly as the other kids do?   Yes   No
14. Would you rather look at a comic book than talk to a friend?   Yes   No
15. Are you upset when someone interrupts you?   Yes   No
16. When you want to say something, do you just say it?   Yes   No
17. Is talking to your friends more fun than playing by yourself?   Yes   No
18. Are you sometimes unhappy?   Yes   No
19. Are you a little afraid to talk on the phone?   Yes   No

Figure 6–5   *(Continued)*

Adolescents and Adults

A variety of questionnaires can be used to assess various aspects of a stutterer's feelings and attitudes about communication and stuttering. I typically use the Modified Erickson Scale of Communication Attitudes (S-24) (Andrews and Cutler, 1974) to obtain information about a client's communication attitudes (Fig. 6–8). This questionnaire has been normed on both stutterers and nonstutterers. A colleague and I (Guitar and Bass, 1978) studied a sample of 20 individuals treated by a fluency-shaping program and found that, if communication attitude, as measured by the S-24, does not change during treatment, the likelihood of relapse within 12 to 18 months increases. Ingham (1979) disputed this finding, but Young (1981) confirmed it using a reanalysis of the original data. Later data by Andrews and Craig (1988) also supported the relationship between normalizing attitudes on the S-24 and long-term treatment outcome.

Read each sentence carefully so you can say if it is true or false for you. The sentences are about talking. If you feel that the sentence is right, circle true. If you think the sentence about your talking is not right, circle false. Remember, circle false if you think the sentence is wrong and true if you think it is right.

1.	I don't talk right	True	False
2.	I don't mind asking the teacher a question in class.	True	False
3.	Sometimes words stick in my mouth when I talk.	True	False
4.	People worry about the way I talk.	True	False
5.	It is harder for me to give a report in class than it is for most of the other kids.	True	False
6.	My classmates don't think I talk funny.	True	False
7.	I like the way I talk.	True	False
8.	People sometimes finish words for me.	True	False
9.	My parents like the way I talk.	True	False
10.	I find it easy to talk to most everyone.	True	False
11.	I talk well most of the time.	True	False
12.	It is hard for me to talk to people.	True	False
13.	I don't talk like other children.	True	False
14.	I don't worry about the way I talk.	True	False
15.	I don't find it easy to talk.	True	False
16.	My words come out easily.	True	False
17.	It is hard for me to talk to strangers.	True	False
18.	The other kids wish they could talk like me.	True	False
19.	Some kids make fun of the way I talk.	True	False
20.	Talking is easy for me.	True	False
21.	Telling someone my name is hard for me.	True	False
22.	Words are hard for me to say.	True	False
23.	I talk well with most everyone.	True	False
24.	Sometimes I have trouble talking.	True	False
25.	I would rather talk than write.	True	False
26.	I like to talk.	True	False
27.	I am not a good talker.	True	False
28.	I wish I could talk like other children.	True	False
29.	I am afraid the words won't come out when I talk.	True	False
30.	My friends don't talk as well as I do.	True	False
31.	I don't worry about talking on the phone.	True	False

Figure 6–6 *Communication Attitude Test (Gene J. Brutten, Ph.D., Southern Illinois University).*

32. I talk better with a friend.   True   False

33. People don't seem to like the way I talk.   True   False

34. I let others talk for me.   True   False

35. Reading aloud in class is easy   True   False

Score 1 point for each answer that matches these:

1. True	9. False	17. True	25. False	33. True
2. False	10. False	18. False	26. False	34. True
3. True	11. False	19. True	27. True	35. False
4. True	12. True	20. False	28. True	
5. True	13. True	21. True	29. True	
6. False	14. False	22. True	30. False	
7. False	15. True	23. False	31. False	
8. True	16. False	24. True	32. True	

In a study using this scale on Belgian children (De Nil and Brutten, 1990), mean score of a group of children who stutter (N = 70) was 16.7; mean score of a group of children who do not stutter (N = 271) was 8.71.

Figure 6–6   (Continued)

TEACHER ASSESSMENT OF STUDENT COMMUNICATIVE COMPETENCE (TASCC)

Student's: Name _____ **Age** ____ **Gender** _____ **Ethnicity** _____

Below are a series of items that describe a student's communicative competency. Use the following scale to rate a student in your grade whom you consider to have communication competency issues. For each item, circle the number that best describes the student's communication. Please answer each item as well as you can, even if the item does not seem to apply to the student.

1 = Never   2 = Seldom   3 = Sometimes   4 = Often   5 = Always

1) Student remains attentive when others   1   2   3   4   5
   communicate with him/her

2) Student verbally relates thoughts in an age   1   2   3   4   5
   appropriate meaningful manner to adults

Figure 6–7   *Teacher Assessment of Student Communicative Competence.*

3) Student adjusts style and content of speech according to communication partner and situation   1   2   3   4   5

4) Student appears to nonverbally relate feelings in an age appropriate meaningful manner (e.g., facial glare, smile)   1   2   3   4   5

5) Student demonstrates age appropriate nonverbal requests for message repetition (e.g., makes a "puzzled" face)   1   2   3   4   5

6) Student participates in age appropriate turn-taking in conversations and class discussions   1   2   3   4   5

7) Student demonstrates age appropriate verbal requests for message repetition (e.g., "Could you say that again?" or "What?")   1   2   3   4   5

8) Student uses appropriate voice inflection when speaking (e.g., intonation with questions)   1   2   3   4   5

9) Student uses appropriate eye contact when speaking to adults   1   2   3   4   5

10) Student gets the listener's attention before the student introduces a topic   1   2   3   4   5

11) Student uses age appropriate opening and closing communication comments in conversations with peers (e.g., "Hello, See you later")   1   2   3   4   5

12) Student's speech is understandable even when the topic is unknown   1   2   3   4   5

13) Student participates in story-description/retell interactions   1   2   3   4   5

14) Student verbally relates thoughts in an age appropriate meaningful manner to peers   1   2   3   4   5

15) Student sticks up for his/her own views when confronted by group pressure   1   2   3   4   5

16) Student's overall speech is understandable (e.g., clear voice, clear articulation)   1   2   3   4   5

17) Student nonverbally expresses frustration towards peers when appropriate   1   2   3   4   5

18) Student responds within an appropriate time frame to remarks, questions, requests   1   2   3   4   5

19) Student joins into conversations with peers easily   1   2   3   4   5

20) Student uses vocabulary that is relevant to the conversation   1   2   3   4   5

21) Student appropriately engages in group discussions   1   2   3   4   5

Figure 6–7   *(Continued)*

22) Student uses appropriate rate of speech for situation	1	2	3	4	5
23) Student initiates topics of conversation in one-to-one situations with adults	1	2	3	4	5
24) Student initiates topics of conversation in one-to-one situations with peers	1	2	3	4	5
25) Student adjusts vocal intensity to account for distance and noise variables	1	2	3	4	5
26) Student freely volunteers answers to questions in class	1	2	3	4	5
27) Student uses speech effectively in directing peer's actions when intended	1	2	3	4	5
28) Student's speech is understood by unfamiliar listeners	1	2	3	4	5
29) Student uses appropriate eye contact when speaking to peers	1	2	3	4	5
30) Student uses age appropriate humor within peer conversations	1	2	3	4	5
31) Student uses age appropriate verbal communication to gain attention	1	2	3	4	5
32) Student nonverbally expresses frustration towards adults when appropriate	1	2	3	4	5
33) Student uses a variety of age appropriate (or better) vocabulary	1	2	3	4	5
34) Student seems to understand age appropriate humor within peer conversations	1	2	3	4	5
35) Student clarifies and/or rephrases when verbal communication is not understood by the listener	1	2	3	4	5
36) Student uses age appropriate (or better) sentence length when answering questions in class	1	2	3	4	5
37) Student is able to shift to different topics within conversations	1	2	3	4	5
38) Student links his/her words together with age appropriate (or better) grammatical structures	1	2	3	4	5
39) Student follows 3-step instructions with minimal need for repetitions or visual cues	1	2	3	4	5
40) Student's speech is understood even when the speech becomes more complex (e.g., longer sentences, change in topic)	1	2	3	4	5

Figure 6–7 *(Continued)*

41) Student verbally or nonverbally indicates that he/she understands the speaker's message	1	2	3	4	5
42) Student is able to integrate information presented auditorily (e.g., lessons, stories, a sequence of directions) and comprehend the meaning	1	2	3	4	5
43) Student identifies characters/people in conversations	1	2	3	4	5
44) Student uses age appropriate (or better) sentence length when having a conversation	1	2	3	4	5
45) Student uses the environment to get a message across when the student's verbal communication is not understood (e.g., points to relevant objects or people)	1	2	3	4	5
46) Student seems to understand nonverbal communication (e.g., gestures)	1	2	3	4	5
47) Student uses age appropriate nonverbal communication to gain the attention of adults	1	2	3	4	5
48) Peers and adults seem to understand the student says to them	1	2	3	4	5
49) Student interacts with a variety of peers what and adults	1	2	3	4	5
50) Student uses age appropriate nonverbal communication to gain the attention of peers (e.g., wave, gentle tap)	1	2	3	4	5

TASCC SUBSCALES

The TASCC is divided into 5 subscales. The following information indicates which items, distributed randomly, belong to which subscales.

Subscale	Item #'s
I. Intelligibility	8, 12, 16, 22, 25, 40, 48
II. Appropriateness of Communication	2, 3, 6, 10, 11, 13, 14, 18, 20, 27, 30, 31, 33, 36, 37, 38, 44
III. Comprehension (of input) and Clarification or Repair (of output)	7, 34, 35, 39, 41, 42, 43, 46
IV. Pragmatic/Nonverbal	1, 4, 5, 9, 17, 29, 32, 45, 47, 50
V. Approach/Avoidance Attitude	15, 19, 21, 23, 24, 26, 49

Figure 6–7   (Continued)

MODIFIED ERICKSON SCALE OF COMMUNICATION ATTITUDES (S-24)

Name: _____ Date: _____ Score: _____

Directions: Mark the "true column with a check () for each statement that is true or mostly true for you and mark the "false" column with a check () for each statement which is false or not usually true for you.

	TRUE	FALSE
1. I usually feel that I am making a favorable impression when I talk.		
2. I find it easy to talk with almost anyone.		
3. I find it very easy to look at my audience while speaking to a group.		
4. A person who is my teacher or my boss is hard to talk to.		
5. Even the idea of giving a talk in public makes me afraid.		
6. Some words are harder than others for me to say.		
7. I forget all about myself shortly after I begin a speech.		
8. I am a good mixer.		
9. People sometimes seem uncomfortable when I am talking to them.		
10. I dislike introducing one person to another.		
11. I often ask questions in group discussions.		
12. I find it easy to keep control of my voice when speaking.		
13. I do not mind speaking in front of a group.		
14. I do not talk well enough to do the kind of work I'd really like to do.		
15. My speaking voice is rather pleasant and easy to listen to.		
16. I am sometimes embarrassed by the way I talk.		
17. I face most speaking situations with complete confidence.		
18. There are few people I can talk with easily.		

Figure 6–8 *Erickson S-24 Scale of Communication Attitudes. (Reprinted with permission from Andrews, G., and Cutler, J. [1974]. Stuttering therapy: The relation between changes in symptom level and attitudes. Journal of Speech and Hearing Disorders, 39:312–319. Copyright 1974, American Speech-Language-Hearing Association.)*

19.	I talk better than I write.
20.	I often feel nervous while talking.
21.	I find it hard to talk when I meet new people.
22.	I feel pretty confident about my speaking ability.
23.	I wish that I could say things as clearly as others do.
24.	Even though I knew the right answer, I have often failed to give it because I was afraid to speak out.

Data on the "Modified Erickson Scale of Communication Attitudes"
I. Answers (Andrews and Cutler, 1974)
Score 1 point for each answer that matches this:

1. False	13. False
2. False	14. True
3. False	15. False
4. True	16. True
5. True	17. False
6. True	18. True
7. False	19. False
8. False	20. True
9. True	21. True
10. True	22. False
11. False	23. True
12. False	24. True

II. Adult Norms (Andrews and Cutler, 1974)

	Mean	Range
Stutterers	19.22	9–24
Nonstutterers	9.14	1–21

Figure 6–8   *(Continued)*

I also use a questionnaire to assess a client's tendency to avoid stuttering, which is the avoidance scale of the Stutterer's Self-Rating of Reactions to Speech Situations (SSRSS) (Johnson, Darley, and Spriestersbach, 1952); this questionnaire assesses a client's tendency to avoid specific speaking situations (Fig. 6–9). Research suggests that clients with avoidance scale scores higher than 2.56 before treatment may be more likely to have appreciable levels of stuttering 1 year after treatment with fluency-shaping therapy than clients with lower scores (Guitar, 1976). Thus, I suggest that clinicians use a client's avoidance scale score to guide them in choosing whether to focus more on ways

STUTTERER'S SELF-RATING OF REACTIONS TO SPEECH SITUATIONS

Name_____ Age_____ Sex _____
Examiner _____ Date _____

After each item put a number from I to 5 in each of the four columns.

Start with the right-hand column headed Frequency. Study the five possible answers to be made in responding to each item, and write the number of the answer that best fits the situation for you in each case. Thus, if you habitually take your meals at home and seldom eat in a restaurant, certainly not as often as once a week, write number 5 in the Frequency column opposite item No. 1 "Ordering in a restaurant." In like manner respond to each of the other 39 items by writing the most appropriate number in the Frequency column.

Now, write the number of the response that best indicates how much you stutter in each situation. For example, if in ordering meals in a restaurant you stutter mildly (for you), write number 2 in the Stuttering column.

Following the same procedure, write your responses in the Reaction column and, finally, write your responses in the Avoidance column.

Numbers for each of the columns are to be interpreted as follows:

A. Avoidance

1. I never try to avoid this situation and have no desire to avoid it.
2. I don't try to avoid this situation, but sometimes I would like to.
3. More often than not I <u>do not</u> try to avoid this situation, but sometimes I do try to avoid it.
4. More often than not I <u>do</u> try to avoid this situation.
5. I avoid this situation every time I possibly can.

B. Reaction

1. I definitely enjoy speaking in this situation.
2. I would rather speak in this situation than not speak.
3. It's hard to say whether I'd rather speak in this situation or not.
4. I would rather not speak in this situation.
5. 1 very much dislike speaking in this situation.

C. Stuttering

1. I don't stutter at all (or only very rarely) in this situation.
2. I stutter mildly (for me) in this situation.
3. I stutter with average severity (for me) in this situation.
4. I stutter more than average (for me) in this situation.
5. I stutter severely (for me) in this situation.

Figure 6–9 *Stutterer's Self-rating of Reactions to Speech Situations.* (Reprinted with permission frm Johnson, W., Darley, F., & Spriestersbach, D.C. (1952). *Diagnostic manual in speech correction.* New York: Harper & Row. Copyright 1952 by Harper & Row. Copyright renewed 1980 by Edna B. Johnson, Frederick L. Darley, and Duane C. Spriestersbach.)

D. Frequency

1. This is a situation I meet very often, two or three times a day or even more, on the average.
2. I meet this situation at least once a day with rare exceptions (except Sunday perhaps).
3. I meet this situation from three to five times a week on the average.
4. I meet this situation once a week, with few exceptions, and occasionally I meet it twice a week.
5. I rarely meet this situation—certainly not as often as once a week.

	Avoidance	Reaction	Stuttering	Frequency
1. Ordering in a restaurant.	____	____	____	____
2. Introducing myself (face to face).	____	____	____	____
3. Telephoning to ask price, train fare, etc.	____	____	____	____
4. Buying plane, train, or bus ticket.	____	____	____	____
5. Short class recitation (10 words or less).	____	____	____	____
6. Telephoning for taxi.	____	____	____	____
7. Introducing one person to another.	____	____	____	____
8. Buying something from a store clerk.	____	____	____	____
9. Conversation with a good friend.	____	____	____	____
10. Talking with an instructor after class or in his or her office.	____	____	____	____
11. Long-distance phone call to someone I know.	____	____	____	____
12. Conversation with my father.	____	____	____	____
13. Asking girl for date (or talking to a man who asks me for date.	____	____	____	____
14. Making short speech (1–2 minutes).	____	____	____	____
15. Giving my name over telephone.	____	____	____	____
16. Conversation with my mother.	____	____	____	____
17. Asking a secretary if I can see the employer.	____	____	____	____
18. Going to house and asking for someone.	____	____	____	____
19. Making a speech to unfamiliar audience.	____	____	____	____
20. Participating in committee meeting.	____	____	____	____
21. Asking the instructor a question in class.	____	____	____	____
22. Saying hello to friend passing by.	____	____	____	____
23. Asking for a job.	____	____	____	____
24. Telling a person a message from someone else.	____	____	____	____
25. Telling a funny story with one stranger in a crowd.	____	____	____	____
26. Parlor game requiring speech.	____	____	____	____

Figure 6–9   *(Continued)*

27. Reading aloud to friends. _____ _____ _____ _____
28. Participating in a bull session. _____ _____ _____ _____
29. Dinner conversation with strangers. _____ _____ _____ _____
30. Talking with my barber/hairdresser. _____ _____ _____ _____
31. Telephoning to make appointment
    or to arrange to meet someone. _____ _____ _____ _____
32. Answering roll call in class. _____ _____ _____ _____
33. Asking at a desk for book or card
    to be filled out, etc. _____ _____ _____ _____
34. Talking with someone I don't know well
    while waiting for bus, class, etc. _____ _____ _____ _____
35. Talking with other players during game. _____ _____ _____ _____
36. Taking leave of a host or hostess. _____ _____ _____ _____
37. Conversation with friend while walking. _____ _____ _____ _____
38. Buying stamps at post office. _____ _____ _____ _____
39. Giving directions to a stranger. _____ _____ _____ _____
40. Taking leave of a girl/boy after date. _____ _____ _____ _____

Totals _____ _____ _____ _____

Averages (divide total by # of answers) _____ _____ _____ _____

Figure 6–9 (Continued)

of enhancing fluent speech or to combine shaping fluency with an approach that modifies stuttering as well as the fears and avoidances associated with stuttering.

I also may use the Perceptions of Stuttering Inventory (PSI) (Woolf, 1967) to examine a stutterer's perception of the presence of struggle, avoidance, and expectancy of stuttering (Fig. 6–10). Woolf suggests that the PSI can be used to help a stutterer view her problem more objectively, to develop treatment goals, and to assess progress. I find that the avoidance section of the PSI complements the avoidance scale of the SRSS because the SRSS focuses more on situations, whereas the PSI deals more with stuttering behaviors.

Another measure of attitude that has been shown to predict long-term outcome is the Locus of Control of Behavior Scale (Craig, Franklin, and Andrews, 1984), which assesses the extent to which a client believes he controls his own behavior (i.e., whether the control is "internal" or "external") (Fig. 6–11). Scoring adds the points for each item, and higher scores reflect greater perceived "externality" of control. Because the values of items 1, 5, 7, 8, 13, 15, and 16 are reversed to minimize the effect of social desirability in responding, the scores on these items are transposed (e.g., you change a 5 to a 0, a 4 to a 1, and so on) before totaling the score. This scale is given just before treatment and again immediately after treatment. Studies have shown that clients who did not decrease their locus of control scores more than 5% from pre-treatment to post-treatment are in danger of relapse (Craig and Andrews, 1985; Craig, Franklin, and Andrews, 1984).

PERCEPTIONS OF STUTTERING INVENTORY (PSI)

The symbols S, A, and E after each item denote struggle (S), avoidance (A), and expectancy (E). In practice, these symbols are not included in the Inventory, but are listed on a separate scoring key.

<u>S</u> <u>A</u> <u>E</u>

Name _____ Age _____ #_____

Examiner _____ Date _____ %_____

Directions

Here are 60 statements about stuttering. Some of these may be characteristic of <u>your</u> stuttering. Read each item carefully and respond as in the examples below.

Characteristic
of me

_____   Repeating sounds

Put a check mark (✓) under "characteristic of me" if <u>repeating sounds</u> is part of your stuttering; if it is not characteristic, leave the space blank.

"Characteristic of me" refers only to what you do <u>now</u>, not to what was true of <u>your</u> stuttering in the past and which you no longer do, and not what you think you should or should not be doing. Even if the behavior described occurs only occasionally or only in some speaking situations, if you regard it as characteristic of your stuttering, check the space under "characteristic of me."

Characteristic
of me

_____   I. Avoiding talking to people in authority (e.g., a teacher, employer, or clergyman). (A).

_____   2. Feeling that interruptions in your speech (e.g., pauses, hesitations, or repetitions) will lead to stuttering. (E).

_____   3. Making the pitch of your voice higher or lower when you expect to get "stuck" on words. (E).

_____   4. Having extra and unnecessary facial movement (e.g., flaring your nostrils during speech attempts). (S).

_____   5. Using gestures as a substitute for speaking (e.g., nodding your head instead of saying "yes" or smiling to acknowledge a greeting). (A).

_____   6. Avoiding asking for information (e.g., asking for directions or inquiring about a train schedule). (A).

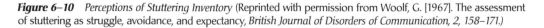

Figure 6–10 *Perceptions of Stuttering Inventory* (Reprinted with permission from Woolf, G. [1967]. The assessment of stuttering as struggle, avoidance, and expectancy, *British Journal of Disorders of Communication, 2, 158–171.*)

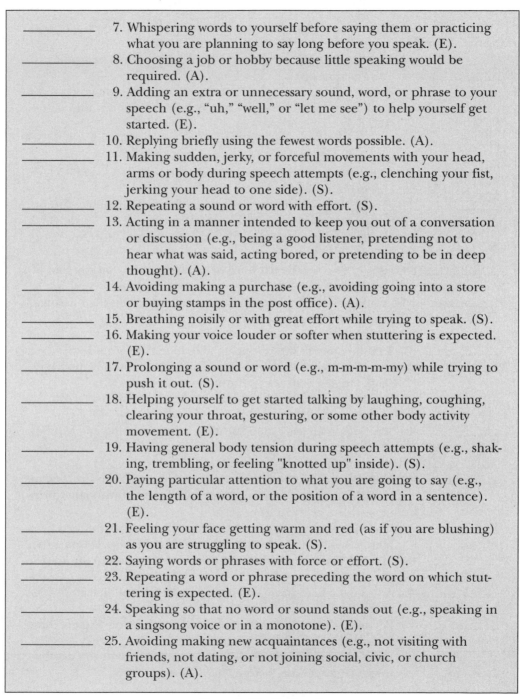

_____ 7. Whispering words to yourself before saying them or practicing what you are planning to say long before you speak. (E).

_____ 8. Choosing a job or hobby because little speaking would be required. (A).

_____ 9. Adding an extra or unnecessary sound, word, or phrase to your speech (e.g., "uh," "well," or "let me see") to help yourself get started. (E).

_____ 10. Replying briefly using the fewest words possible. (A).

_____ 11. Making sudden, jerky, or forceful movements with your head, arms or body during speech attempts (e.g., clenching your fist, jerking your head to one side). (S).

_____ 12. Repeating a sound or word with effort. (S).

_____ 13. Acting in a manner intended to keep you out of a conversation or discussion (e.g., being a good listener, pretending not to hear what was said, acting bored, or pretending to be in deep thought). (A).

_____ 14. Avoiding making a purchase (e.g., avoiding going into a store or buying stamps in the post office). (A).

_____ 15. Breathing noisily or with great effort while trying to speak. (S).

_____ 16. Making your voice louder or softer when stuttering is expected. (E).

_____ 17. Prolonging a sound or word (e.g., m-m-m-m-my) while trying to push it out. (S).

_____ 18. Helping yourself to get started talking by laughing, coughing, clearing your throat, gesturing, or some other body activity movement. (E).

_____ 19. Having general body tension during speech attempts (e.g., shaking, trembling, or feeling "knotted up" inside). (S).

_____ 20. Paying particular attention to what you are going to say (e.g., the length of a word, or the position of a word in a sentence). (E).

_____ 21. Feeling your face getting warm and red (as if you are blushing) as you are struggling to speak. (S).

_____ 22. Saying words or phrases with force or effort. (S).

_____ 23. Repeating a word or phrase preceding the word on which stuttering is expected. (E).

_____ 24. Speaking so that no word or sound stands out (e.g., speaking in a singsong voice or in a monotone). (E).

_____ 25. Avoiding making new acquaintances (e.g., not visiting with friends, not dating, or not joining social, civic, or church groups). (A).

Figure 6–10 _(Continued)_

26. Making unusual noises with your teeth during speech attempts (e.g., grinding or clicking your teeth), (S).

27. Avoiding introducing yourself, giving your name, or making introductions. (A).

28. Expecting that certain sounds, letters, or words are going to be particularly "hard" to say (e.g., words beginning with the letter "s"). (E).

29. Giving excuses to avoid talking (e.g., pretending to be tired or pretending lack of interest in a topic). (A).

30. "Running out of breath" while speaking. (S).

31. Forcing out sounds. (S).

32. Feeling that your fluent periods are unusual, that they cannot last, and that sooner or later you will stutter. (E).

33. Concentrating on relaxing or not being tense before speaking. (E).

34. Substituting a different word or phrase for the one you had intended to say. (A).

35. Prolonging or emphasizing the sound preceding the one on which stuttering is expected. (E).

36. Avoiding speaking before an audience. (A).

37. Straining to talk without being able to make a sound. (S).

38. Coordinating or timing your speech with a rhythmic movement (e.g., tapping your foot or swinging your arm). (E).

39. Rearranging what you had planned to say to avoid a "hard" sound or word. (A).

40. "Putting on an act" when speaking (e.g., adopting an attitude of confidence or pretending to be angry). (E).

41. Avoiding the use of the telephone. (A).

42. Making forceful and strained movements with your lips, tongue, jaw, or throat (e.g., moving your jaw in an uncoordinated manner). (S).

43. Omitting a word, part of a word, or a phrase that you had planned to say (e.g., words with certain sounds or letters). (A).

44. Making "uncontrollable" sounds while struggling to say a word. (S).

45. Adopting a foreign accent, assuming a regional dialect, or imitating another person's speech. (E).

46. Perspiring much more than usual while speaking (e.g., feeling the palms of your hands getting clammy). (S).

47. Postponing speaking for a short time until certain you can be fluent (e.g., pausing before "hard" words). (E).

Figure 6–10   *(Continued)*

_____ 48. Having extra and unnecessary eye movements while speaking (e.g., blinking your eyes or shutting your eyes tightly). (S).

_____ 49. Breathing forcefully while struggling to speak. (S).

_____ 50. Avoiding talking to others of your own age group (your own or opposite sex). (A).

_____ 51. Giving up the speech attempt completely after getting "stuck" or if stuttering is anticipated. (A).

_____ 52. Straining the muscles of your chest or abdomen during speech attempts. (S).

53. Wondering whether you will stutter or how you will speak if you do stutter. (E).

54. Holding your lips, tongue, or jaw in a rigid position before speaking or when getting "stuck" on a word. (S).

_____ 55. Avoiding talking to one or both of your parents. (A).

_____ 56. Having another person speak for you in a difficult situation (e.g., having someone make a telephone call for you or order for you in a restaurant). (A).

_____ 57. Holding your breath before speaking. (S).

_____ 58. Saying words slowly or rapidly preceding the word on which stuttering is expected. (E).

_____ 59. Concentrating on <u>how</u> you are going to speak (e.g., thinking about where to put your tongue or how to breath). (E).

_____ 60. Using your stuttering as the reason to avoid a speaking activity. (A).

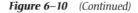

Figure 6–10   *(Continued)*

Andrews and Craig (1988) reported that two measures of attitude, combined with a measure of stuttering behavior, are useful in predicting relapse after fluency-shaping treatment. They found little relapse among those stutterers who met the following three goals by the end of treatment: (1) no stuttering on telephone calls to strangers, (2) a score of 9 or below on the Modified Erickson Scale of Communication Attitudes, and (3) locus of control score reductions greater than 5%. Their assessment of relapse was based on a single telephone call with a stranger 10 to 18 months after treatment, and relapse was considered to be more than 2% of syllables stuttered during the call.

Continuing Assessment

Assessment is an ongoing process. As treatment progresses, the clinician should continue to ask herself, "Am I using the best approach with this person? Is there something else or something different I should be doing?" She should also decide what measures of progress are important for a client and apply these measures at regular intervals. My own approach is to assess stuttering behavior at the beginning and the end of each semester. In other settings, I often assess a client after every 10 hours of treatment. In these periodic assessments,

LOCUS OF CONTROL OF BEHAVIOR SCALE

Directions: Below are a number of statements about how various topics affect your personal beliefs. There are no right or wrong answers. For every item there are a large number of people who agree and disagree. Could you please put in the appropriate bracket the choice you believe to be true? Answer all the questions.

0	1	2	3	4	5
Strongly disagree	Generally disagree	Somewhat disagree	Somewhat agree	Generally agree	Strongly agree

1. I can anticipate difficulties and take action to avoid them................................( )
2. A great deal of what happens to me is probably just a matter of chance.........( )
3. Everyone knows that luck or chance determines one's future.........................( )
4. 1 can control my problem(s) only if I have outside support.............................( )
5. When I make plans, I am almost certain that I can make them work..............( )
6. My problem(s) will dominate me all my life...( )
7. My mistakes and problems are my responsibility to deal with.........................( )
8. Becoming a success is a matter of hard work; luck has little or nothing
   to do with it...( )
9. My life is controlled by outside actions and events...( )
10. People are victims of circumstance beyond their control.................................( )
11. To continually manage my problems I need professional help ....( )
12. When I am under stress, the tightness in my muscles is due to things
    outside my control..( )
13. 1 believe a person can really be the master of his fate....................................( )
14. It is impossible to control my irregular and fast breathing when I am having
    difficulties...( )
15. I understand why my problem(s) varies so much from one occasion
    to the next...( )
16. 1 am confident of being able to deal successfully with future problems ....( )
17. In my case, maintaining control over my problem(s) is due mostly to luck....( )

Figure 6–11   *Locus of Control of Behavior Scale.*

I try, but don't always succeed, to obtain samples of my clients' speech in nonclinical situations, such as in the classroom or at work. I also assess their stuttering when I bring them in for maintenance checkups at increasingly longer intervals after formal treatment is over.

In addition, I assess clients' feelings and attitudes at the beginning and end of treatment and may assess them at other times if I am concerned about progress. If I am working on changing attitudes and feelings, change should be reflected in my measures, or I should try a different approach. Decreases in negative attitudes and feelings should be accompanied by decreases in stuttering severity, and my measures should show this.

Summary

- In an assessment, the clinician has a variety of tasks. These include
  1. Gathering data from the client
  2. Getting to know the client as an individual
  3. Showing an understanding of the client's point of view
  4. Demonstrating an understanding of stuttering

- Clinicians must develop skills and sensitivities in working with clients from cultures other than their own.

- Building a relationship with a client begins in the very first meeting, which is usually the assessment. A clinician must take this opportunity to demonstrate that she knows about the disorder of stuttering, is unafraid of it, and is accepting of it. At the same time, she must show that she expects change.

- Behaviors counted as stutters include: part-word repetitions, single-syllable whole-word repetitions, prolongations, blocks, and unequivocal avoidance behaviors.

- Samples for assessing stuttering should include a variety of situations. The initial sample and samples assessing outcome should be videotaped for more accurate scoring and measurement of reliability. These samples should include speaking and, when appropriate, reading.

- Frequency of stuttering is commonly assessed as the percentage of syllables or words stuttered.

- Different types of disfluencies can be assessed to reveal the percentage of stutter-like disfluencies or number of these disfluencies per 100 words. This information may be particularly useful in helping to decide if a preschool child needs treatment.

- Durations of moments of stuttering are useful in quantifying an aspect of the abnormality of a client's stuttering and the extent to which it may interfere with communication. Speaking and reading rates will also help to quantify this aspect.

- Frequency and severity of secondary or concomitant behaviors associated with stuttering can be important measures of how much these behaviors call attention to themselves and distract listeners.

- Three severity scales are the *Stuttering Severity Instrument,* the *Scale for Rating Severity,* and the Lidcombe Program's Severity Rating Scale. The commonly used *Stuttering Severity Instrument* combines an assessment of frequency of stuttering, mean duration of three longest stutters, and physical concomitants accompanying stuttering.

- Speech naturalness can be reliably and easily assessed. It is thought to be an especially important measure when evaluating treatment outcomes.

- Various instruments have been created to assess emotions and attitudes associated with stuttering. Added to measures of stuttering behavior, these measures provide a multi-dimensional view of the disorder. In some cases, they can aid the clinician in selecting appropriate treatment and in assessing whether a client is ready for dismissal.

- Assessment is an ongoing activity. Measures of progress are important indicators of whether ongoing treatment is effective and should be continued. Measures of outcome are critical for our knowledge of how effective a treatment has been, in the long term, with each client.

Study Questions

1. What does it mean to suggest that a clinician must play two different roles during an evaluation?

2. Which types of disfluencies are counted as stutters, and which are considered normal?

3. What factors can affect the process of measuring stuttering?

4. Describe the procedures for the two measures of reliability called "point-by-point agreement" and "percent error."

5. Why is it important to obtain several samples of speech from a client when assessing stuttering, whereas a single sample might be adequate for assessing a phonological disorder.

6. Give two reasons why assessment of reliability of measurements of stuttering is important. In doing so, give an example in each case in which errors are likely to occur in measuring stuttering.

7. Describe five dimensions or aspects of stuttering that may be assessed in an evaluation of a client who stutters.

8. To you, what is the most important aspect of stuttering? Defend your choice. How do you measure it?

9. Why is it relevant to assess speech rate for a person who stutters?

10. Discuss the pros and cons of keeping conversations between yourself and a teenage client private and not shared with parents.

SUGGESTED PROJECTS   ABC

(1) Research how different cultures react to stuttering and suggest how evaluation procedures in this chapter need to be changed for individuals from a culture that has very different beliefs about stuttering than those suggested in this text.

(2) Make or obtain a videotape of a conversational and a reading sample of a person who stutters. Use two different methods of measuring the stuttering and obtain intra-observer and inter-observer reliability assessments for each method and discuss why one measurement procedure is more reliable than the other.

(3) Obtain a videotaped conversational sample of one or more individuals who stutter and identify moments when you think the client has used an avoidance behavior to prevent stuttering. Discuss whether these avoidances should be counted as stutters.

(4) Obtain samples of repetitive stutters from normally fluent children and from children who stutter. Compare the repetitions from both groups in terms of length of silent periods between iterations, pitch, and other acoustic variables.

(5) Search the literature on assessment of stuttering to determine whether reliable methods have been developed for clients to assess their own stuttering during the progress of treatment.

Suggested Readings

Conture, E. (2001). Assessment and Evaluation. In *Stuttering: Its Nature, Diagnosis, and Treatment.* **Boston: Allyn & Bacon.**

This chapter is rich with many ideas for assessment of children, adolescents, and adults who stutter. It is particularly good in the breadth of coverage of evaluation of children who stutter, reflecting the years of experience the author has had in working with this age group.

Cordes, A.K. (1994). The reliability of observational data: I. Theories and methods for speech-language pathology. *Journal of Speech and Hearing Research,* **37:264–278.**

This article provides an excellent tutorial on the problems associated with establishing reliability of observational data in stuttering.

Rosenberry-McKibbin, C. (2002). Multicultural Students With Special Language Needs: Practical Strategies for Assessment and Intervention (ed 2). Oceanside, CA: Academic Communication Associates, Inc.

This book provides many insights into evaluation of multicultural students.

Wright, L., and Ayre, A. (2000). *The Wright & Ayre Stuttering Self-Rating Profile.* **United Kingdom: Winslow Press Ltd. (www.winslow-press.co.uk)**

This assessment tool was designed to be used by clinicians working with adolescent and adult clients who can participate in assessing their own behaviors and feelings. It is intended to go beyond traditional clinician-based assessments to obtain indications of how clients observe themselves.

Chapter 7

Assessment and Diagnosis

This chapter and the preceding one are bridges between chapters on the nature of stuttering and chapters on treatment. My aim is to show you how to understand a client and his stuttering problem and then use the information you have gathered to determine a treatment approach. Figure 7–1 illustrates the components of assessment and diagnosis.

I've organized the assessment procedures in this chapter by age levels: preschool, school age, and adolescent/adult. I've done this, in part, because in preparing to evaluate a client, you often know little about him except his age, so you will at least know what section of this chapter to turn to as you plan an evaluation. Another reason for this organization is because each age level requires a different approach and quite different procedures. When evaluating preschool children, for example, the clinician must plan to determine whether they are stuttering or normally disfluent and then whether treatment should be direct or indirect. With school-age children, a clinician often follows procedures that will allow her to develop an Individualized Education Program (IEP) for children who are eligible for services. With adolescents and adults, a clinician may do more extensive assessment of emotions and attitudes as well as core and secondary behaviors to determine appropriate treatment.

Within each age level, I have created subdivisions for the sequence of activities you will typically engage in when you evaluate a client. First, under Preassessment, I describe the clinical questions to be answered in the evalution, as well as preliminary information-

Components of Assessment and Diagnosis

Background information

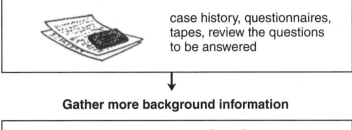

case history, questionnaires, tapes, review the questions to be answered

Gather more background information

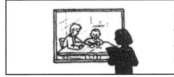

parent interviews, teacher interviews, student/adolescent/adult interviews

Observation of present behavior and feelings

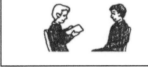

parent-child interaction, clinician-child interaction, structured conversation, and reading sample

Diagnosis

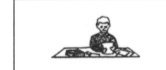

data interpretation, developmental/treatment level determination

Meet with client or family to review options for treatment

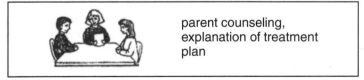

parent counseling, explanation of treatment plan

Figure 7–1 *Sequence of assessment and diagnosis.*

gathering activities. Under Assessment, I have described the observations, interviews, and measurements at the heart of the evaluation. Under Diagnosis, I discuss how to integrate the information you have gathered to decide on a course of action (whether to recommend treatment and, if so, the type of treatment). Last, under Summary and Recommendations, are the closing interviews, assignments, and the means to assess progress and outcome.

Preschool Child

Preassessment

Clinical Questions

When you assess a preschool child, you first want to answer the question, is this child stuttering or is he normally disfluent? In the process of trying to answer this, I have found that certain other information is critical: What are the amounts and types of disfluency this child shows in various situations? What kinds of risk factors for stuttering does the child have? Is the child reacting to his speech with frustration, fear, or other emotion? This information will also help you answer the question: What is the developmental/treatment level of the child's disfluency? To respond to the family's needs and to involve them fully in planning treatment, you need to know the answers to questions like: What are the family's concerns about the child and his stuttering and their preferences, expectations, and availability for treatment? Once you have gathered this information, you will need to decide among several options for the child and family: no treatment, watchful waiting, parent-delivered treatment, or clinic-based treatment. You will also want to answer the question: Is the child within the normal range for language, articulation, and voice? Last, you should answer the question: Is a referral to another professional (for example, a family counselor or a learning specialist) warranted?

Initial Contact

In your initial contact, the family member who has contacted you is forming their first impression of you. In many cases, this is the beginning of a helping relationship. Focus on understanding the other person's point of view, their concerns, and their hopes. When you can, give reassurance about the prospect of recovery, but in all cases, convey that you are ready to work with them as part of a team who will, together, help the child.

Your initial contact is likely to be on the telephone. If it is, listen to the parent's voice and pay attention to their level of concern. Often, the most helpful thing you can do in this conversation is to listen. As you listen carefully, you may need to ask an occasional question to get clarification. When you think you have an initial understanding of the problem, set up an appointment, if appropriate. If you cannot meet with them for several days or longer, it is important to give the family some suggestions to get started. For example, you may want a parent to rate their child's stuttering using the Severity Rating Scale described in Chapter 6. It may be helpful also to have the family set aside a few minutes every day in which one parent can play alone with the child and give him special attention. I think it is helpful also to let the family know that they can contact you before the first formal meeting if they have new concerns.

Case History Form

The case history form, shown in Figure 7–2, is sent to parents several weeks before their child's assessment. The case history form informs the clinician about the parents' perception of the problem, at present, as well as its onset and development, and the child's medical and family history and school history. This information is used as a starting place for further questions during the parent interview.

Audio-Video Recording

I ask parents of a preschool child to send me an audio recording or, preferably, a video recording of their child speaking in a typical home situation, along with the case history form. I encourage parents to videotape 5 or 10 minutes of themselves playing with their child. This allows me to preview the child's speech soon after the parents have contacted me. In cases in which several weeks go by between the parents' contact and the evaluation, the child's stuttering may have diminished substantially, and I may observe only a fluent cycle of the child's speech. In addition to previewing the child's stuttering, the tape often gives me a chance to learn a little about parent-child interactions.

Assessment

Parent-Child Interaction

When possible, I observe one or both parents interacting with their child. I prefer to do this at the beginning of the evaluation for several reasons. First, parents may be less affected by my orientation toward stuttering, which they would learn during the parent interview. So observing the parent-child interaction first gives me a more natural sample. Second, this interaction gives me an opportunity to see the child's stuttering first-hand. I can note, for example, how much the child seems aware of his stuttering, whether or not there are escape and avoidance reactions, and to what extent the child is reacting emotionally to his stuttering. Third, I can observe how the parents interact with their child. Do they interrupt? Do they correct? Do they talk at a fast rate or use complex vocabulary or advanced syntax? Such observations add to what I have learned from the audio-video sample that the parents have sent before the assessment. Together, the observation of the sample from home and the sample observed live provide a basis for planning the parent interview and developing recommendations for treatment.

The parent-child interaction can be done formally or informally. Some clinicians observe these interactions in the waiting room. Others who work in preschool or early intervention programs may visit a child's home and arrange to observe parent-child interactions while they sit quietly in the same room. Still others, myself included, videotape the parents and child in a play-style interaction in a treatment room supplied with toys and games. When recording these interactions is possible, this sample of a child's speech can be assessed for severity and types of stuttering behavior, as described in Chapter 6.

Parent Interview

In the last few years, I have talked more freely about stuttering directly with preschoolers, as well as with their parents when their child is within earshot. I think this directness may reduce parents' distress about their child's stuttering; perhaps talking about stuttering

Note: Please complete and return this form before your appointment. Thank you.

Speech Clinic
Stuttering Case History Form—Child and Preteen

Date: _____

Child's name: _____

Address: _____

_____ Tel: _____

Date of birth: _____   Place of birth: _____

Medicaid # _____   Referring physician: _____

Child lives with: Own parents: _____   Other relative: _____

Foster parents: _____   Institution: _____

(If other than own parents, give name/s): _____

_____

Referred by: _____

Teacher's name: _____

School (if applicable): _____   Age: _____

School placement or grade level _____

Name of person completing this form: _____

Relationship to child: _____

FAMILY

Father:
  Name: _____   Age: _____
  Living with the family? _____   Occupation: _____
  Employed by: _____
  Educational level _____
  Telephone (home): _____   (Work): _____
  Social Security #: _____

Mother:
  Name: _____   Age: _____
  Living with the family? _____   Occupation: _____
  Employed by: _____
  Educational level _____
  Telephone (home): _____   (Work): _____
  Social Security #: _____

Brothers and sisters:
  (Name)   (Age)   (Name)   (Age)

  _____   _____   _____   _____

  _____   _____   _____   _____

  _____   _____   _____   _____

Figure 7–2   *Case history form for preschool and school-age children.*

History of Stuttering

Give approximate age at which stuttering was first noticed. _____

Who first noticed or mentioned the stuttering? _____

In what situation was the stuttering first noticed? _____

Describe any situations or conditions that might be associated with the onset of stuttering. _____

Under what circumstances did the stuttering occur after initial onset?

_____

Were the first signs of stuttering (check all that apply):

    A. Repetitions of the whole word? (boy-boy-boy) _____

    B. Repetitions of the first letter? (b-b-b-boy) _____

    C. Repetitions of the first syllable? (ca-ca-cat) _____

    D. Complete blocks on the first letter? (b. . .oy) _____

    E. Prolongations of the vowel? (caaaaaaat) _____

    F. Visible attempt to speak (e.g., mouth movement) but no sound forthcoming? _____

Was the stuttering always the same, or did it occur in several different ways? _____

If it occurred in different ways, how were they different from one another? Describe.

_____

Approximately how long did each block (on one word) seem to last? _____

Was the stuttering easy or was there force at the time when the stuttering was first noticed?_____

Were the words that were stuttered at the beginning of sentences, or were they scattered throughout the sentence being said? _____

_____

When stuttering first began, was there any avoidance of speaking because of it? Give examples, If any. _____

_____

At the time when stuttering was first noticed, what was the child's reaction?

    Awareness that speech was different? _____   Surprise? _____

    Indifference? _____   Anger or frustration? _____

    Fear of stuttering again? _____   Shame? _____

    Other? Describe. _____

What attempts have been made to treat the stuttering problem (either formally or informally)? _____

_____

Does the child have articulation or pronunciation problems in addition to stuttering? If so, please describe. _____

_____

Development of Stuttering

Since the onset of stuttering, has there been any change in stuttering symptoms? Check those that are appropriate.

Figure 7–2   (Continued)

Increase in number of repetitions per word _____

Change in amount of force used _____ (Increased? _____ Decreased? _____

Increase in amount of stuttering _____

Increase in length of block _____

Periods of no stuttering _____; longer periods of stuttering? _____

More precise in speech attempts _____

Lowered voice _____

Slower speech rate _____

Change in location of force when stuttering (if voice has been present) _____

Looking away from the listener _____

Describe any of the above that apply _____

_____

_____

Were there any periods (weeks/months) when the stuttering disappeared? _____

_____

Were there any periods (weeks/months) when stuttering increased? _____

_____

Can you give any explanation for these "worse" periods? _____

_____

Are there any situations that are particularly difficult? If so, describe. _____

_____

List any situations that never cause difficulty. _____

_____

Answer "yes" or "no" to the following as they apply to your (your child's) stuttering.

Do you stutter when you—

Talk to young children?_____	Say your name? _____
Answer direct questions_____	Talk to adults, teachers? _____
Use new words that are unfamiliar?_____	Use the telephone? _____
Read out loud? _____	Recite memorized material? _____
Ask questions? _____	Talk to strangers? _____
Speak when tired? _____	Speak when excited? _____
Talk to family members? _____	Talk to friends? _____
Do you know any stutterers? _____	Describe your relationship. _____

_____

Do you feel that stuttering interferes with your (your child's) daily life? _____

Social relationships? _____ Success in school? _____

Medical, Developmental, and Family History

Describe mother's health during pregnancy and birth history (i.e., complications).

_____

Describe any development problems during infancy or early childhood (i.e., late in walking, feeding problems, food allergies, late in talking). _____

_____

Figure 7–2   *(Continued)*

Do you think the child's speech and language development was unusually rapid or delayed? If so, please describe. _____
_____

List all illnesses, injuries, and operations:

Name	Date	Fever	Complications	Treatment	Name of Physician

List all present physical disabilities. _____
Any chronic illnesses, allergies, or physical conditions? _____
Vision normal? _____ Hearing normal? _____
Do other members of the family have speech, language, or reading problems or learning disabilities? If so, please describe. _____
_____
_____
_____

Are any family members left-handed, or do they use both right and left hands equally well? _____
Does the child or other family members show artistic talent or interest? _____
_____
Do any family members talk very rapidly? If so, who? _____
_____

School and Social History
Favorite subjects or activities in school _____
Difficult subjects _____
Hobbies _____ Sports _____
Leisure time activities _____
What specific questions do you have about your child that you would like us to try to answer? (Use back of sheet if necessary.) _____
_____
_____
What goals would you like to see accomplished as a result of this evaluation?
_____

If, in order to help your child, it is appropriate to send reports to other agencies or professional persons, or to contact other agencies or professional persons, please indicate your permission by signing below.
I authorize and request [fill in name of clinician or clinic] to obtain or exchange pertinent medical/educational information. I understand that all information will be kept confidential.

Figure 7–2   (Continued)

Name: _____

Relationship to child: _____

Date: _____

Return this completed form at least 2 weeks before your evaluation. You may mail it to [fill in name of clinician or clinic].

Figure 7–2   (*Continued*)

openly reduces everyone's fear of it. When I first meet a child and his parents, however, I hold back a little until I have had a chance to discuss this openness with the parents. The child may be only normally disfluent or the parents may be reluctant to talk about stuttering in front of the child. The parent interview gives me a chance to suggest how, in my experience, openness about stuttering decreases some of the shame a child (and parents) may feel about stuttering. Thus, I talk to parents without the child present in the initial interview, giving them an opportunity to talk about matters that they feel they would like to share in confidence, at this time. If I'm working with another clinician or a student, she or he plays with the child while I talk to the parents. If I'm working alone and both parents have come to the evaluation, I talk to each parent separately, while the other is with the child. If only one parent is present, I often arrange to have the child playing by himself in a nearby room with the door open.

I begin the interview by letting parents know what I will be doing with them and their child during the remainder of the evaluation. I assure them there will be a time for me to share my assessment and recommendations with them at the end. Sometimes, during an initial interview, parents ask direct questions about things they think they may be doing wrong. I let them know that, in my view, stuttering is often the result of many factors acting together and that parents do not cause it (see Chapters 2 and 3 for evidence). I rarely give advice about what they should change or what they should do until after I have interviewed the parents and assessed the child directly. It has been my experience that I am more accurate and parents are more receptive to my recommendations if I delay a discussion of what to do until after all available information has been pulled together in a closing interview. On the other hand, there may be "clinical moments" during an initial interview when parents might be most receptive to suggestions. Many times, for example, parents have asked me whether it's a good idea for them to tell their child to slow down whenever the child stutters when excited. My response is usually to ask them how the child responds to this and to build upon their answer so that we can, together, brainstorm the best way to help the child.

I begin initial interviews by asking parents to describe the problem their child is having. I ask open-ended questions, such as "Tell me about Justin's speech" or "Please describe Justin's speech and tell me what concerns you." Open-ended questions allow parents to describe their concerns in their own words. This is then an opportunity for me to listen carefully, to be nonjudgmental, and to be comfortable with silence so that parents can express themselves fully. When parents have had a chance to describe the problem and appear to have no more to say at that moment, I ask about the first stages of the child's life (the child's birth and development) and then work up toward the present time. In the ensuing conversation, I try to be sure I get information indicated by the questions in the following paragraphs. This interview is not a strict question-and-answer format, but rather a discussion that is punctuated by both their questions and mine.

1. **Were there any problems with your pregnancy or the birth of this child?**

   Although there is little evidence that stutterers, as a group, have difficult birth histories, there is an increased incidence of stuttering among brain-damaged individuals (Boehme, 1968; Poulos and Webster, 1991). Thus, I am seeking to determine whether there is the possibility of congenital brain damage. If a difficult pregnancy or birth is reported, I might examine the child's motor and cognitive development more closely. The case history form, which is completed before the evaluation, provides preliminary information about birth history that may or may not need to be followed up.

2. **What was the child's speech and language development like? How did it compare with siblings' development and with your expectations?**

   The first appearance of stuttering may be influenced by the "processing load" that language acquisition has on a child's speech production, as described in the section on speech and language development in Chapter 3. Thus, it is important to understand the course of a child's overall speech and language development. I explore the possibility that a child's language acquisition is proceeding so rapidly that his developing motor system cannot keep up. I also examine the possibility that a child's speech and language development are delayed, and he is frustrated and finding it hard to talk. As mentioned in Chapter 2, there is some evidence that poorer speech and language skills may be predictive of persistent stuttering (Yairi et al, 1996).

3. **Describe the child's motor development compared with that of his brothers, sisters, or other children.**

   I am interested in parents' general impressions. Does their child seem to be developing motor skills like other children his age, or do they think he may be delayed? Some indicators of the normal range of children's gross and fine motor development, as well as their personal-social and speech-language development, can be found in the Denver Developmental Screening Test (Frankenburg and Dodds, 1967) and is shown in Figure 3–2 (Child development in the first 5 years).

   In my experience, many children who stutter appear to be slightly advanced in their language and, to a lesser extent, slightly delayed in their motor skills. Or, they may be well advanced in language but with completely normal motor skills. In either case, these children seem to benefit from models of speech produced at a slow rate (Guitar et al, 1992; also see the section in Chapter 9 on Indirect Treatment). Other children who stutter may be delayed in several areas and may need treatment for language and articulation that is integrated with therapy for stuttering (see the section of Chapter 10 on Treatment of Concomitant Speech and Language Problems).

4. **Have any other members of your family had speech or language disorders?**

I ask this general question and then ask more specifically whether family members or other relatives have ever stuttered, had articulation or language disorders, or have been clutterers (see Chapter 13 for a description of cluttering). To confirm that a disorder was a problem, I ask if the person ever received treatment. I use this information when we discuss stuttering as a disorder that may have predisposing factors. Handled tactfully, a discussion of predisposing factors may help parents realize that their child's stuttering was not something they caused. This, in turn, can help them be more effective in facilitating their child's fluency because they do not feel guilty or anxious about his stuttering.

If a parent stutters or used to stutter, he or she may have strong negative feelings about the disorder, including guilt that they have passed it on to their child. Such feelings need to be discussed in the initial interview and throughout any treatment the child receives. The ways in which a parent handles stuttering are also important, because these behaviors serve as a model for the child. It is my observation that a parent who avoids words or otherwise tries to hide his stuttering is communicating an attitude that may move the child to the intermediate level faster than if the parent accepts his stuttering, comments neutrally about it in front of the child, and uses facilitating techniques to handle it.

If any of the child's relatives stutter, it is important to find out whether or not they recovered. Research cited earlier found that, among children who were identified within 6 months of the onset of stuttering, those with relatives who did not recover from stuttering were more likely to have persistent stuttering than were those with relatives who did recover (Yairi et al, 1996). After obtaining this background information, I turn to the onset and development of the child's stuttering.

5. **When did you first notice the child's disfluency?**

I have found that, if treatment is begun relatively soon after a child starts to stutter (within 18 months, rather than after several years), we have a better chance of preventing negative feelings from building up, for both the parents and the child. Therefore, I praise parents for bringing a child in promptly for an evaluation, if they did so relatively soon after they first realized there may be a problem. Another reason I want to know how much time has passed since onset is that most of the predictive information on chronicity of stuttering is based on children identified within 6 months of onset. For example, Yairi et al (1996) found that children who naturally recovered began to show a steady decline in their stuttering within 12 months of stuttering onset, whereas children whose stuttering persisted for at least 3 years did not show such a decline. Therefore, knowing how long a child has been stuttering helps me make treatment decisions based on findings that some children are likely to recover without therapy.

6. **Was anything special going on in the child's life when the stuttering started?**

This may provide some leads about the kinds of pressures to which a child may be vulnerable, which can help clinicians determine what changes parents can make to reduce stuttering. Events that may precipitate the onset of stuttering include the birth of a sibling, moving to a new home, family travel, prolonged periods of anxiety or excitement, and growth spurts in a child's language or cognition (see Chapter 3). Many times, no special circumstances have occurred at the onset of stuttering. Events surrounding the onset of stuttering should be discussed in a way that helps parents feel they are not to blame for the stuttering.

7. **What was the disfluency like when it was first noticed?**

Most stuttering begins with easy repetitions, although some children exhibit prolongations and blocks, as well. Some preliminary information suggests that when repetitions sound quite rapid (i.e., when the pause between repetition units is brief), a child is more likely to be stuttering rather than normally disfluent (Allen, 1988; Throneburg and Yairi, 1994). Rapid-sounding repetitions may be predictive of persistent stuttering (Yairi et al, 1996). However, the length of pauses between repetition units cannot be determined accurately without instrumentation, even though a practiced ear can help clinicians perceive the brevity of pauses between repetition units. This information should be used only to support an overall pattern of findings that will help the clinician decide whether or not to recommend treatment.

8. **What changes, if any, have been observed in the child's speech since stuttering was first noticed?**

The changes I am most interested in include the frequency and types of disfluencies and whether and for how long the stuttering diminished greatly or disappered altogether. As indicated in the discussion of question 5, children whose frequency of core stuttering behaviors (i.e., part-word and single-syllable whole-word repetitions, prolongations, and blocks) does not decrease during the 12 months after onset are at risk for becoming persistent stutterers. In my clinical experience, if a child's physical tension and struggle during stuttering are increasing or if stuttering is becoming more consistent and less intermittent, the child is not exhibiting a borderline level of stuttering, and direct treatment should be considered. I now turn to current observations of the disorder:

9. **Does the child appear to be aware of his disfluency?**

If a child appears to have no awareness of his disfluencies, I am more likely to categorize him as normally disfluent or as a borderline stutterer than if he notices or seems concerned about his disfluencies. If he shows negative awareness, such as expressing frustration, he may be a beginning stutterer. Note that a child may be aware of his stuttering but not particularly bothered by it; some children are even amused by it. Indicators of a child's awareness include such things as his commenting about his stuttering, either when it occurs or at some other time, and responses to the fact that people have brought it to his attention. Awareness is also indicated if a child stops when he is disfluent and starts again or laughs, cries, or hits himself when he stutters. Even without any of these signs, a child may still be aware of his stuttering.

In some cases, preschool children may show more than just signs of frustration. They may show negative feelings about talking and may fear using certain words and may even comment that they wish they could speak like someone else. These signs of awareness are indications that treatment is warrented.

10. **Does the child sometimes appear to change a word because he expects to be disfluent on it?**

Parents are usually able to guess this is happening because they can sense the child's apprehension about saying a word. I also may ask them if the child changes words in midstream; that is, does he start a word, get stuck on it, and then change it? Such behaviors are warning signs; they may indicate that the child is moving toward a more serious problem.

11. **Does the child seem to avoid talking in some situations, when he expects to be disfluent?**

Again, this is something that most parents know because they sense the child's fear of talking, and like the word avoidances discussed in question 9, this behavior may indicate a need for direct treatment.

12. **What do the parents believe caused the problem?**

In some cases, parents may express ideas about the possible cause of their child's stuttering that I believe are appropriate and accurate. In other cases, parents' beliefs about causal factors appear to be incorrect, and I respond by providing more accurate information. I am particularly sensitive to whether or not parents blame themselves or each other for their child's stuttering. This is usually a good time to let parents know that they are not to blame. I tell them that some children may have slight differences in their neurological organization for speech, which may emerge as stuttering during the normal stresses and strains of growing up and learning to talk (see Chapters 2 and 3). Parents should know that they didn't cause their child's stuttering, but they should also know that they can play a key role in their child's learning to deal with it appropriately.

13. **How do the parents feel about the child's disfluency problem?**

The kinds of feelings and attitudes we are looking for are: Do they feel concern? Guilt? Do they assume the child will outgrow it? Parental emotions and attitudes are contagious and will obviously influence the child, particularly a sensitive child. If parents feel guilty or highly anxious, it is important to engage them in positive treatment activities as soon as possible, and I will suggest some beginning activities you can use in the Summary and Recommendations section.

14. **What, if anything, have the parents done about the child's disfluency problem?**

This question is aimed at finding out how the parents have responded to the child's disfluencies. For example, have they asked the child to slow down or stop and say the word again? Knowing this will help me to decide what to do in counseling them. If parents are correcting the child, I may get them involved in therapeutic activities immediately, so that they may develop appropriate ways of responding.

15. **Has the child been seen elsewhere for the problem? If so, what were the outcomes?**

This information can be important in planning therapy and counseling parents. For example, if their family doctor told them, several years ago, the child will outgrow stuttering, this needs to be addressed, since they may now be convinced he will not outgrow it. It is wise to comment positively or neutrally on what other professionals may have said or done. So many children appear to overcome stuttering without treatment that most doctors and nurses believe that their advice to parents to ignore the stuttering will have a good outcome. Increasingly, however, doctors and nurses are being educated to distinguish between children who are likely to recover without treatment and those who are not.

   If the child has been in other treatment previously, it is important to know what advice the parents were given. Sometimes, parents have been given excellent advice but were not able to follow it. If so, we need to find out why and help them change their response. Sometimes parents have had their child in successful therapy but have moved away and sought me out to continue the same kind of treatment. In these cases, I try to contact the previous therapist, as well as explore with the parents what was done, so that we can continue to work in the same direction as before. In some cases, parents come to me seeking a second opinion, and I am able to reinforce what others have said, if I agree. In other cases, they may have been advised to ignore the child's stuttering, which may lead me to tactfully discuss the possibility of taking an entirely different direction.

16. **When and in which situations does the child exhibit the most disfluency? The least disfluency?**

This information helps to identify fluency disrupters and fluency facilitators that I will use to help parents facilitate their child's fluency. I have also found it effective to point out, whenever possible, all of the helpful things the parents are already doing. Just the awareness that their child's stuttering responds to environmental cues and thereby has some logic to it helps most parents feel more competent to manage it. After I think I understand a child's current stuttering behavior, I ask about social and emotional development.

17. **How does the child get along with his brothers and sisters and other children?**

I usually find that children who stutter relate fairly well to others, but I want to find out if a child's stuttering may be interfering with his relationships. Sometimes, when asking this question, I learn about pressure and competition from siblings or teasing by a neighborhood bully.

18. **What is the child's personality and temperament like?**

Some children who stutter are more sensitive and fearful than most other children. More senstive children would be more likely to respond negatively to parents' anxieties about their speech. A child with this temperament may benefit from extra help in developing self-confidence. There is good evidence that families can help a child develop a more resilient temperament.

19. **What is a typical day like for your child?**

    It can be helpful to get an idea of how busy and rushed a family is. For one thing, it has been my experience that many children who stutter and their families benefit from having less hectic schedules. You can add this information to what the parents told you about when their child stutters most to develop a hypothesis about how much the family's schedule may be affecting the child's fluency. If the child stutters more when things are busy, hectic, and stressed, it may be appropriate to brainstorm with the parents about how everyone can have a little more "down time." Knowledge of the family's schedule will also help you begin to consider treatment recommendations. Some treatments are demanding of parents' time and attention, and their schedule must be considered in working with them to determine the most appropriate treatment approach for their child.

    I then finish with an open-ended question, such as the following question.

20. **Is there anything else you can think of to tell me that will help me better understand your child's stuttering?**

    Sometimes, it is not possible to direct questions to all areas of concern, and this question provides parents an opportunity to provide information that I have not thought of asking about.

Clinician-Child Interaction

One of the most important parts of a preschool child's evaluation is the interaction between the clinician and the child. Here, the clinician can see first-hand what the child's speech is like, how he responds to various cues, and how well he can modify his disfluency. I always record this interaction for later analysis because it is difficult to make notes as we interact. If videotape is available, it is preferable to videotape because visual cues are often critical in determining a child's developmental and treatment level. If audiotape must be used, the clinician should make notes on visual aspects of the child's disfluencies.

I focus my interactions on toys or games that are suitable to the child's age. The Playskool® farm or airport are good examples. I play alongside the child, letting him direct the action, commenting on what he's doing or playing with. I refrain from questions when I first start and talk in an easy, relaxed manner, much like I advise parents to do.

If a child is stuttering similarly to the way the parents described, I maintain the same speech style throughout the interaction. However, if a child is entirely fluent or normally disfluent and the parents have described behaviors typical of stuttering, I speak more rapidly and ask many questions. Occasionally, I interrupt the child to elicit disfluent speech, which may be more characteristic. I do this to avoid misdiagnosing a child who is stuttering as a normally fluent speaker.

An adult client of mine described an experience that illustrates my concern. When she was 5 years old, she stuttered quite severely, and her parents were understandably concerned. Seeking the best help, her mother took her to a famous Midwestern university speech clinic for an evaluation. For reasons she never understood, she was relatively fluent throughout the entire evaluation. The clinicians observed her temporary fluency and, despite her mother's protestations that her daughter stuttered at home, labeled her as a normal-speaking child and advised her mother to ignore any disfluency. Her disfluency gradually worsened, and she became a severe, chronic stutterer.

I realize that, even by putting pressure on the child, I may not elicit stuttering that the child displays in other settings. Thus, the parents' report and the recording they made before the evaluation are of vital importance for a full understanding of a child's speech.

Talking About Stuttering

Before interacting with a child, I try to determine from talking with a child's parents whether the child is aware of his stuttering. If I think he isn't, I use observations of the child's speech while he and I play to assess his speech. If it seems clear from earlier information or our own observations that he is aware of his stuttering, I then try to determine how comfortable the child is in talking about his stuttering. Sometimes, I ask if he knows why he has come to see me. Most children answer noncommittally, but some say something like, "Because I don't talk right." This gives me an opening to discuss the stuttering. It is also an important opportunity to let the child know that he isn't alone and that I know other children who get stuck on words and am usually able to help them.

Some clinicians help a child talk about his stuttering by first talking about another child who stutters (Bloodstein, personal communication, 1990). In discussing stuttering with a child, I usually try to use their vocabulary, such as "getting stuck" or "having trouble on words." If a child seems reluctant to talk about stuttering, I drop the issue for the moment and return to playing. Then, later, I will insert a few natural-sounding disfluencies in my speech and comment that I sometimes have trouble getting words out. I might play some more and then insert a few more disfluencies and ask the child if he ever has trouble like this. As before, the child's response will indicate that either he remains unwilling to discuss stuttering or he will give the clinician an opening to discuss, little by little, his disfluency problem. In summary, the goals of these attempts to discuss a child's disfluency are (1) to see if he accepts himself and his disfluencies enough to discuss them and (2) to assure him that he is not alone with the problem and that his parents and I may be able to help him.

A Child Who Won't Talk

At times, I encounter a preschooler who is reluctant to separate from his parents. A shy child may start to cry and cling to his parents. I don't force the child to separate, of course. It is more important to have him positively inclined toward therapy than to try to extract a few stutters. In this situation, I sit quietly while the parent and child play together. After a few minutes, I join in the play, without focusing on the child, and after a few more minutes, I'll comment on what the parent and child are doing or what I'm doing with a tractor or a farm animal or whatever I'm playing with. In most cases, the child will soon say something to me or include me in the play. This interaction, leading to at least a little speech from the child, gives me an opportunity to observe, at close range, any stuttering the child may have. Only after a child gets comfortable with me do I attempt to discuss his trouble talking, and then only if I'm sure he is aware of his stuttering.

With some children, I do not attempt to discuss stuttering, and I always take my cue from the child and go slowly in this area. A very shy child, who gets even more shy if I produce a few easy disfluencies, may be quite turned off to therapy if I invade his space by asking about his stuttering at this point. You can infer many things about a child's feelings from observations rather than direct questions.

A Child Who Is Entirely Fluent

Some preschool children who stutter may be entirely fluent during an evaluation. In such cases, there are several options. First, the recording I asked the parent to send me may include enough stuttering to provide a good sample for analysis. Second, if a child is in a particularly fluent period, I may reschedule his evaluation for a later time. If my recommendations to the parents enable them to change the home environment enough in the meantime so that the child remains fluent, the parents may wish to postpone the evaluation until and if the child's stuttering returns.

Speech Sample

The following sections describe how to analyze samples of a preschool child's speech. You should have more than one speech sample to analyze from the recordings that the parents sent in, the parent-child interaction, and the clinician-child interaction. Because you will want to use the SSI-3 (Riley, 1994) as part of your assessment, you need to follow the procedures it recommends for this analysis. Thus, the sample obtained from the clinician-child interaction should include conversation using the pictures in the SSI-3. Riley recommends that, as the child talks, the clinician should "interject questions, interruptions, and mild disagreements to simulate the pressures of normal conversation at home and elsewhere" (Riley, 1994, p. 7). The samples should include at least 200 syllables; samples this long or longer make it more likely that you will have an accurate picture of the child's speech. By making transcripts of the samples, you can more easily quantify the variables described in the following section.

Pattern of Disfluencies

By analyzing the child's speech sample, I can try to determine whether or not the child truly stutters and, if so, his developmental/treatment level. I analyze the following six variables to begin this determination. The choice of variables owes much to four individuals who have written about the differential diagnosis of preschool stuttering (Adams, 1977; Curlee, 1984; Riley and Riley, 1979).

1. Frequency of disfluencies. This is calculated from the entire sample and is expressed as the number of disfluencies per 100 words (see Chapters 5 and 6 for details). Both normal disfluencies and those associated with stuttering are included in this count. Normally disfluent children usually have fewer than 10 disfluencies per 100 words.

2. Types of disfluencies. I described the following eight types of disfluencies in Chapter 5: part-word repetitions, single-syllable word repetitions, multisyllable word repetitions, phrase repetitions, interjections, revisions-incomplete phrases, prolongations, and tense pauses. Children who are normally disfluent are likely to have more revisions and multisyllable whole-word repetitions, as well as many interjections when they are younger than 3½ years old. Part-word repetitions, single-syllable word repetitions, prolongations, and tense pauses occur more frequently in stuttering children. Another distinguishing measure is the proportion of total disfluencies that are stutter-like disfluencies (SLDs) (i.e., part-word repetitions and single-syllable repetitions, prolongations, and blocks). Less than half of the disfluencies of normally disfluent children are SLDs, but about two-thirds of the disfluencies of children who stutter will be SLDs (Yairi, 1997a).

3. Nature of repetitions and prolongations. This variable has several dimensions. First, normally disfluent children usually have only one extra unit in their repetitions, li-like this, but sometimes they may have two. As the number of repetition units increase, however, so does the likelihood that the child is stuttering. Second, I listen to the tempo of repetitions. If they are slow and regular, a child is more likely to be categorized appropriately as a normally disfluent speaker. If they are rapid or irregular, it is more likely that the child is stuttering. Third, I look for signs of tension in both repetitions and prolongations. Both visual and auditory cues can help here; tension can be seen in the child's facial expression and heard in his increased pitch or loudness and more staccato voice quality. Children who I would label as normally disfluent seldom exhibit tension in their disfluencies.

4. Starting and sustaining airflow and phonation. The child who we usually categorize as stuttering often has difficulty here. You may observe abrupt onsets and offsets of words, especially repeated words, or momentary pauses with fixed articulator positions at the onset of words. Moreover, transitions between words may seem abrupt, jerky, or broken much of the time.

5. Physical concomitants. I look for physical gestures that accompany a child's disfluencies, such as head nods, eye blinks, and hand or finger movements, especially gestures that coincide with the release of a disfluent sound. I also include such extra noises as a child gritting his teeth or clicking his tongue during disfluencies.

6. Word avoidances. Another sign I sometimes see in a disfluent preschool child, which suggests that he stutters, is word avoidance. This can be blatant, as when a child starts a word and then changes it, as in "pu-pu-pu. . . . dog," or it may be more subtle, as when he says, "I don't know," when it's clear that he does know. I also ask about word avoidances when I interview a child's parents. When a clinician interacts with a child, she may sometimes miss avoidances in a live interaction, and it may take a viewing of the videotape to pick them up. For example, a few years ago I noted on the videotape I watched after an evaluation a very subtle avoidance that I had completely missed during the face-to-face interaction. I had asked the child what he was going to dress as for Halloween. He pursed his lips for a "B," but when he couldn't say the word, he used an avoidance by singing the Batman theme, "Na-na-na-na-na-na-na-nah! Batman!"

In my experience, if a child shows any of the characteristics of stuttering just described, he should be considered at least a borderline stutterer. The presence of tension, stoppage of airflow or phonation, physical concomitants, or word avoidances would place him on a level above borderline. Further details on this placement are given in the sections on diagnosis that follow.

Stuttering Severity Instrument (SSI-3)

Using the 200-syllable or longer samples gathered earlier, you should carefully follow the guidelines in the examiner's manual of the SSI-3 to determine a child's stuttering frequency, duration, and physical concomitants scores. Use of the SSI-3 is described more fully in Chapter 6. Using the definitions of stuttering given by Riley (1994) in the manual, which essentially are what I referred to earlier as "stuttering-like disfluencies," you can use the Total Overall Score to derive a percentile ranking of the child, which compares him to the norms for children who stutter. In addition, rankings that range from Very Mild to Very Severe can also be derived from the Total Overall Score. It is possible, however, that normally disfluent children may be rated as stuttering at the Very Mild level on the SSI-3. Thus, clinical judgment, informed by your analyses of the types and frequencies of disfluencies, must be used to sort out which children are actually stuttering and which are not. The SSI-3 is not a tool for differentiating stuttering from normal disfluency but for assessing a child's severity.

Speech Rate

I assess preschool children's speech rate using the speech sample obtained for the SSI-3. Counting and timing procedures were described in the section on assessment of speech rate in Chapter 6. One sample of speech rates for preschool children is given in Table 6–3. If a child is stuttering and his speech rate is substantially below the range for his age, the extent to which stuttering slows his rate of speech may be a problem for both listeners and the child. Children whose rates are substantially above the norms—or who sound like they are talking too fast—may have the disorder of cluttering, which is described in more detail in Chapter 13.

Feelings and Attitudes

I assess preschoolers' feelings about stuttering by asking about them in the parent interview, by observing parent-child interactions, and by bringing up the topic of stuttering, when appropriate, with the child during our interaction. Feelings and attitudes among preschoolers range from apparent unawareness of difficulty, to mild embarrassment, to extreme hypersensitivity. For example, a child may appear slightly uncomfortable when I ask him why he has come to visit me but may respond that it's because he has trouble talking. At the other extreme, a child may cry at the prospect of talking about his speech and act deeply embarrassed and uncommunicative, even if I gingerly approach the topic of speech or "getting stuck." I am often able to learn a great deal by watching videos of my interactions with a child. I find that being able to devote my undivided attention to observing and replaying key segments of recorded interactions provides a rich payload of information about a child's feelings that may not have been apparent to me in the face-to-face meeting. Parent interviews are also a valuable source for learning whether a child is simply frustrated with his disfluencies or whether his feelings escalate at times into embarrassment and downright fear.

Assessment of the feelings and attitudes of a preschooler leads me to conclude tentatively whether a child (1) is unaware of his disfluencies; (2) is occasionally aware of them and, even then, is seldom and only transiently bothered by them; (3) is aware and frustrated by them; or (4) is highly aware, frustrated, and afraid of them. The levels of awareness and emotion that a child has about his stuttering are an important consideration in planning treatment, as we shall see.

Other Speech and Language Behaviors

When I evaluate a preschool child's speech for stuttering, I also screen for possible articulation, language, and voice problems. In addition, I make sure that his hearing has been checked recently and, if not, arrange to have a hearing screening.

A child's language and articulation problems can usually be detected in the recorded parent-child or clinician-child interactions. When I suspect problems in these areas, I administer formal tests. You may wish to consult Bernthal (1994), Bernthal and Bankson (1998), Hoffman, Schuckers, and Daniloff (1989), or Weiss, Gordon, and Lillywhite (1987) for testing articulatory and phonological disorders, and Paul (1995) for assessing language problems. I will discuss the management of concomitant articulation and language disorders in Chapter 10, which deals with treatment of beginning stuttering.

My view of the relationship between language and stuttering, which I described in Chapter 3, is that one of the pressures on a child who stutters may result from language that is much more advanced than motor development. Thus, in evaluating a child's language and articulation, I explore the possibility that his language exceeds age expectations. In addition, I observe his language usage and motor abilities and question parents about his general motor development and the intelligibility of his speech.

When language development outstrips motor development, there may be a risk that a child will try to produce long sentences at an adult pace with a speech system that is better suited to a slower rate. A child's motivation to speak quickly may come from his own eagerness to express complex thoughts or from his parents' pleasure at his adult-like speech. For a child who stutters and who also has advanced expressive language abilities for his age, rate of speech production may be an important factor to target in treatment. How this is done depends on the child's level of stuttering. If the child is relatively unaware of his stuttering and does not seem to be reacting to it with escape or avoidance behaviors and his frequency of stuttering is relatively low, I am likely to use an indirect treatment approach. I would train parents to use a slower speech rate when speaking to the child as part of the treatment, with the expectation that their model of a slower speaking rate will influence the child to speak more slowly, thereby putting fluency within his reach. In such cases, I also explore ways in which the family may be putting pressure inadvertently on the child's language skills by stimulating language development.

Verbal activities that some parents enjoy most with their children, such as puns, word play, and teaching the child multisyllable words, may convey to a child that the parents place high value on verbal ability. For most children, this would be an incentive to develop their verbal skills. But for children vulnerable to fluency breakdowns, parents' pride in their verbal proficiency may stress their ability to perform, resulting in increased disfluency. For those children who are really struggling with stuttering, parents' focus on verbal performance may create in the children feelings of shame at their verbal ineptitude.

As I review my observations of a child's speech and language, I consider not only the possibility that a child's language is advanced relative to his speech motor abilities, but also the possibility that his motor abilities are markedly delayed. A few children have motor problems that impair their coordination of respiration, phonation, and articulation with language production. Many are aware that speech is difficult for them and have already felt frustration and shame, not just about stuttering, but about the way they speak and how they perform other fine motor tasks. Therefore, I think it is important to help these children improve their feelings about themselves as talkers while the parents and I work on their speech motor skills. These children seem to benefit especially from models of slow speech as well as activities that teach them to speak more slowly.

In addition to exploring the possibility of language and articulation difficulties, I also assess a child's voice. A hoarse voice may be especially significant in a preschool child who stutters because it may be a sign that the child has increased tension in his laryngeal muscles to cope with stuttering. I look closely at how the child is handling his blocks and listen for signs of excess laryngeal tension, such as pitch rises, increases in loudness, and hard glottal attacks. Because many of the techniques I use in treatment of stuttering result in a more relaxed style of speech because of increased fluency, I usually don't treat voice separately from stuttering. However, if a child has voice problems other than hoarseness or if hoarseness does not diminish with stuttering therapy, I refer the child to an otolaryngologist and follow treatment approaches such as those suggested by Boone and McFarlane (1988) and Colton and Casper (1996).

Other Factors

In Chapter 3, I described a number of possible developmental influences on stuttering. In this section, I will review them briefly so that they may be recognized if they are important in a particular preschool child's stuttering. Because much of this information can be obtained from a parent interview, you may wish to consult Chapter 3 for further details on developmental influences before conducting a parent interview.

Physical Development

I like to ascertain whether a child has age-appropriate gross motor skills and whether his oral motor development is typical. Figure 3–2 in Chapter 3 presents information about motor development. Most children learn to walk at about 1 year but usually do not learn to walk and talk at the same time. If a child I am evaluating was delayed in walking but average or advanced in talking, I may explore the possibility that the onset and evolution of his stuttering was associated with his delayed motor development.

Cognitive Development

When I consider a child's cognitive development, I want to learn whether there is cognitive delay, which can be associated with increased disfluency. I also want to know if a child may be going through a period of rapid cognitive growth that might, hypothetically, take a temporary toll on fluency.

Social-Emotional Development

As a child grows, various tensions develop between him, his parents, and his siblings. Between ages 2 to 3 and 4 to 5 years, many children may display negativity in ways that are felt throughout the family. When I ask a child's parents about conditions surrounding the onset or worsening of a child's stuttering, I explore social-emotional factors, as well as environmental and developmental factors.

In Chapter 3, I described various life events that may affect a child's stuttering. In the parent interview, I examine life events surrounding the onset of stuttering to see if upsetting events or ongoing situations may be linked to the child's stuttering. Some events, like the birth of a sibling, may be happy ones, but they can create disturbances in the psychological balance of a family.

Speech and Language Environment

I have referred to the child's communication environment before, but here I will be more explicit. Many children have their hands full trying to compete verbally with fast-talking, articulate adults. Children who stutter may find this particularly hard. I listen to the recording sent by the parents and watch parent-child interactions carefully for indications of a complicated verbal environment, such as rapid speech models without pauses, that may be like rough water to a new swimmer.

Diagnosis

Now let us turn to the task of pulling together the information gathered in an assessment and making a diagnosis of a young client's problems. One of the clinical questions that must be answered is whether the child is truly stuttering. Once you have (tentatively) answered that, you can answer the other clinical questions and describe the child's stuttering, his reactions to it, and an appropriate treatment choice.

Determining Developmental and Treatment Level

In determining what an appropriate treatment may be, I begin by trying to determine if a preschool child is normally disfluent and, if not, his level of stuttering: borderline or beginning stuttering. In the following paragraphs, I briefly review these levels, which were described in detail in Chapter 5.

Normal Disfluency

All of the following characteristics must be met for a child to be considered normally disfluent. The child has fewer than 10 disfluencies per 100 words; the disfluencies consist mostly of multisyllable word and phrase repetitions, revisions, and interjections. When disfluencies are repetitions, they will have two or fewer repeated units per repetition that are slow and regular in tempo. The ratio of stuttering-like disfluencies to total disfluencies will be less than 50%. All disfluencies will be relatively relaxed, and the child will seem to be hardly aware of them and certainly will not be upset when he is aware.

A child may be considered to have borderline or beginning stuttering if he has any of the characteristics described in following paragraphs. Place him at the level—borderline or beginning—that includes the child's most salient characteristics.

Borderline Stuttering

The child I place in this category has more than 10 disfluencies per 100 words, but they are loose and relaxed. They may be part-word repetitions and single-syllable word repetitions, as well as prolongations, and the repetitions may have more than two repeated units per instance. Stuttering-like disfluencies will be above 50% (Yairi, 1997a), and the disfluencies may cluster on adjacent sounds (LaSalle and Conture, 1995).

Beginning Stuttering

The key features at this level are the presence of tension and hurry in the child's stuttering. Disfluencies may take the form of rapid, abrupt repetitions, pitch rises during repetitions and prolongations, difficulty starting airflow or phonation, and signs of facial tension. A beginning stutterer shows that he is aware of his stuttering and may be quite frustrated by it. He may use a variety of escape behaviors, such as head nods or eye blinks in terminating blocks. Occasional avoidance may occur. For example, a child who has developed language to the point of using "I" instead of "me" but begins to stutter on "I" at the beginnings of sentences may begin substituting "Me" for "I" to avoid the frustration of stuttering on "I."

Some children are relatively advanced for beginning stutterers. Except for their age and the way they would be treated in therapy, they might be considered at the intermediate level. The child I place at this level has most of the characteristics of the preceding levels plus noticeable avoidance behaviors. He avoids words and situations, and his behavior and demeanor clearly suggest that he feels both fear and shame about stuttering. For example, he may use a variety of starters to begin sentences and look away or appear embarrassed when he stutters.

Although I use information from all sources to determine a child's developmental and treatment level, I have found that my own observations of parent-child and clinician-child interactions are most useful in making this (tentative) decision. Parents are helpful in describing long-term changes in their child's stuttering, but they frequently miss avoidance behaviors, such as starters, circumlocutions, and postponements, which are critical indicators of this more advanced level of stuttering. Parents' reports do provide, however, as much information about a child's feelings and attitudes as I usually gather in observing interactions in the clinic. Thus, parent reports plus my own observations provide valuable, complementary data. A vital adjunct to direct observations are video recordings of parent-child and clinician-child interactions. I sometimes revise my initial placement of a child in a developmental/treatment level after viewing video of the interactions I have already directly observed.

Risk Factors for Persistent Stuttering

Risk factors are those elements within a child or in his environment that make it more or less likely that he will persist in his stuttering (Guitar and Guitar, 2000). I described much of the evidence for these factors in the chapters on Constitutional Factors in Stuttering (Chapter 2) and Developmental, Environmental, and Learning Factors (Chapter 3). You'll be able to get the information you need to determine a child's risk of persistent stuttering from the case history form, questionnaires, parent interviews, and observations of the child.

Factors Within the Child

The first of these factors is a child's family history. If the child's family history shows that one or more relatives had persistent stuttering and did not recover without treatment, the child is more likely to have persistent stuttering (Ambrose, Cox, and Yairi, 1997). The second factor is that, if the child is a boy, he is more likely to persist in stuttering (Ambrose, Cox, and Yairi, 1997). The third factor is the speech and language skills of a child. If his language, phonological, or nonverbal intelligence skills are poor, he is more likely to persist in stuttering (Yairi et al, 1996). More recent studies, however, have questioned whether or not language skills are predictive of persistence (Watkins, Yairi, and Ambrose, 1999). Another consideration regarding language is the relationship between a child's vocabulary and other measures of expressive language. Conture (2001) suggests that children whose vocabulary scores are 20% or more higher than their expressive language scores are at higher risk for continued stuttering or extended treatment. A fourth risk factor is the child's sensitivity. There is, thus far, only weak evidence supporting this factor (Conture, 2001; Guitar, 2002), but my clinical observations suggest that children who appear to be fearless extroverts are more likely to recover without treatment, but those who appear to be more inhibited are likely to take longer in treatment to recover than other childen. The last within-child risk factor is the child's reaction to his stuttering. This may interact with the previous factor, sensitivity, and make it more likely that more sensitive children will develop escape and avoidance reactions and have more negative emotions in reaction to their stuttering. If persistent stuttering is, as we suspect, a complex of conditioned reactions that are sustained because they are learned under conditions of elevated emotions, then those children who show more of these learned reactions may be more likely to persist in their stuttering.

Factors Within the Child's Environment

These risk factors are typically in the child's relationships or home life (e.g., other's reactions, family communication style, family expectations, events in the child's life, and the family's daily schedule). Support for their importance comes less from well-controlled studies of their effect on a child's stuttering than on clinical observations, both mine and those of other clinicians.

The first of these factors—others' reactions to the child's stuttering—is essentially whether or not the family is supportive or critical of the child's speech. My own clinical observation is that it is helpful if parents acknowledge stuttering in positive, empathetic ways, but it is not helpful if parents (or other listeners) are anxious or negative in reacting to the child's stuttering. Parental anxiety about stuttering interacts with a child's sensitivity; more sensitive children are probably more affected by parents' anxiety than less sensitive children.

The second factor is family communication style. Studies by Kloth et al (1999) and Rommel et al (2000), reviewed in Chapter 3, suggest that when parents' language is quite complex, children who stutter are more likely to persist in stuttering. Thus, an analysis of parent-child interactions may give some indication of whether it might be beneficial, in some cases, to help the family talk with the child using language that is not so far above his level.

The family's expectations for the child's performance can be a third risk factor. A child who stutters may grow up in a family in which high academic, athletic, and social or verbal performance are important family values. If he doesn't naturally excel in the areas that are important to his family, he may feel inadequate, and this may worsen his stuttering. A young man I once worked with came from a family of debaters, and when his high school teachers corrected his speech in their efforts to help him become a "silver-tongued orator," he became self-conscious of his minor disfluencies and developed a long-standing stuttering problem.

A fourth risk factor is events in a child's life that assault his sense of security. As I discussed in the chapter on developmental factors, I have often found that emotional events, such as the birth of a sibling, the death of a relative, or emotional conflict in the home, appear to have triggered stuttering or made it worse. I know of no hard data that link stuttering to such events, but many clinicians have observed them and have spoken and written about them (e.g., Van Riper, 1982). In any case, it is helpful to find out from the case history and the parent interview if the onset or exacerbation of a child's stuttering seems to be tied to such events. Acknowledging to a family that life events may precipitate or worsen stuttering may help them understand their child's stuttering and perhaps feel less like they have caused it. Moreover, sometimes stress in a home is ongoing, and you will be able to help the parents lessen the stress or can refer them to a counselor who may help them.

The last risk factor is a family's daily schedule. As I suggested in the description of parent interviews, it is helpful to ask parents what a typical day in the child's life is like. I have frequently heard parents say that their child stutters more when he is excited or anxious, and very busy schedules can sometimes increase a child's level of emotional arousal. This risk factor may make a difference for some children but not others, and you can explore its relevance in the parent interview. Later, after you have gained a fuller understanding of the child and his family's needs and expectations, you can make an educated guess about whether the family's schedule may be affecting the child's speech. If so, you can then work with the family to determine if they will try to reduce the number of activities the child is involved in.

Drawing the Information Together

After I have completed the assessment tasks, I consolidate the information I have gathered, develop a tentative diagnosis, and meet with the family in a closing interview to discuss my findings and their desires and expectations. If I had been able to get a recording from the parents beforehand, I would have carefully analyzed it before the assessment and would present the results of my analysis in the closing interview. The same is obviously true for the other information I obtained before the assessment, such as the Behavioral Style Questionnaire (McDevitt and Carey, 1995) that was described in Chapter 6. Some data, like my analysis of the recordings of parent-child and clinician-child interactions, may not be immediately available but will be included in my assessment report. Thus, for the closing interview, I rely on a combination of previously acquired quantitative data, some of the quantitative data I acquired as I talked with the child, such as frequency of stuttering, and the qualitative data gleaned from my observations and interview questions.

Prior to the closing interview, I spend a few minutes studying my findings or discussing them with students or colleagues if I have been working with a team. I try to make sure that I have obtained enough information to answer two key questions: What is this child's developmental/treatment level, and what is the appropriate treatment? Working with the family, we can decide where to go from here.

Closing Interview: Recommendations and Follow-Up

I begin with positive comments about the child and the family and then describe to the family characteristics of the child's stuttering that I observed in parent-child and clinician-child interactions and the preassessment recording, if I obtained one. I stay away from jargon and strive to be as clear and straightforward as possible as I briefly describe the child's behaviors, review the more important information that the parents provided in the case history and our interview, and estimate the seriousness of the child's problem. If stuttering is a serious concern, I say so, and if the parents have expressed feelings of guilt about their child's stuttering, I again reassure them that they are not to blame but that they will be crucial in helping to resolve it. At this point, it is important to describe appropriate treatment approaches, such as environmental changes, indirect treatment, and direct treatment, which will differ depending on the developmental/treatment level of the child's problem.

Recommendations for Children with Normal Disfluency

If I believe that a child's speech is normally disfluent, I deal with the family's concerns rather than the child's disfluencies. Most families benefit from knowing how I reached my tentative conclusion, so I provide them with information about normal disfluency, such as the following. During their preschool years, many normal children pass through periods of disfluency. Interjections, revisions, pauses, repetitions, and prolongations are common during these periods, but they usually occur in fewer than 10 of every 100 words. Interjections and revisions are more common than part-word repetitions, and part-word repetitions usually have only 1 or 2 repeated units per disfluency. Children who are normally disfluent are largely unaware of their disfluencies, do not react negatively to them, and gradually outgrow them.

In most cases, I use analogies to help the family understand their child's disfluent speech. For example, I may point out that learning to speak is like learning many other skills, such as riding a bike or learning to skate, and that a learner falls down a lot in the early stages. I look for analogies that will fit the family's experiences to help them understand why their child is disfluent and how valuable an accepting environment can be for a child's self-esteem. Parents who are concerned about their child's normal disfluencies usually feel reassured when they find out that this is normal. In those rare cases, when parents are still not convinced that their child's speech disfluencies are normal, I teach them how to slow their speaking rates, pause frequently, simplify their language, and relieve other pressures that we mutually agree to change. Then, I set up another appointment to discuss their progress and the child's speech. If parents really are concerned and seem likely to continue worrying and perhaps correcting their child's speech, a few sessions focused on the normalcy of their child's speech and the changes they have made in the family's environment may be an ounce of prevention.

I keep the door wide open for all parents of normally disfluent children. I reassure them that I am available to talk with them if they become concerned again, and will be ready to work with them if their child does begin to stutter.

Recommendations for Children with Borderline or Beginning Stuttering

For those children evaluated within 12 months of the onset of stuttering, there are guidelines to help decide which children should begin treatment and which can be followed for a period of time without treatment. Table 7–1 lists some of the characteristics of children who have a high probability of recovering without treatment. Children whose stuttering-like disfluencies (part-word and single-syllable word repetitions, prolongations, or blocks) decrease during the first 12 months after onset are likely to recover. If other factors listed in Table 7–1 also characterize the child, the likelihood of recovery may be increased.

I believe that any preschool child who has borderline or beginning stuttering should be either treated or followed carefully for several months. For those children close to onset whose stuttering is diminishing and whose families are not overly concerned, I stay in contact by telephone or email for several months. However, if families are highly concerned or the child's stuttering is not decreasing, I begin treatment as soon as possible.

My closing interview with these parents is usually the first of many sessions we will spend together. Consequently, I don't need to accomplish everything in this meeting. Because treatment of any preschool child who stutters is often focused on the home environment, we often begin our discussion with things the parents can do at home. The chapters on treating children with borderline and beginning stuttering (Chapters 9 and 10) contain more extensive discussions and guidelines for involving the family in treatment, but I will make some initial suggestions here.

Table 7–1   Factors That May Be Associated With Increased Likelihood of Recovery From Stuttering Without Treatment[a]

Factor	Comment
1. Decrease in stutteringly like disfluencies during the 12 months after onset	This is an important predictor of recovery. It applies to children with borderline, beginning, and intermediate-level stuttering.
2. Female	Evidence suggests females are more likely to recover.
3. No relatives who stutter; or relatives have recovered from stuttering	Preliminary evidence suggests that persistent stuttering may run in families.
4. Good language and articulation skills	Both receptive and expressive language skills should be considered. Evidence of early phonological problems may predict persistent stuttering.
5. Good nonverbal intelligence scores	Children with persistent stuttering had normal, but slightly lower nonverbal skills.
6. Outgoing, carefree temperament	Our clinical experience suggests these children who begin to stutter often outgrow it.

[a]When a young preschool child is assessed within 1 year of stuttering onset.
Factors 1 to 5 are based on evidence cited in Andrews et al (1993) and in studies of Yairi and Ambrose (1992) and Yairi et al (1996).

In my experience, parents who are active in the ongoing assessment process from the beginning feel more hopeful, less guilty, and more motivated to be involved in treatment (see also Zebrowski and Kelly, 2002). Therefore, in the closing interview, I ask parents of children who have borderline or beginning stuttering to begin observing and recording the day-to-day variations in their child's fluency. Having them assess fluency in the home environment also gives me a more valid indication of changes in stuttering than if assessments are done only in the clinic. I teach parents to use the Severity Rating Scale (Fig. 6–2; Onslow, Andrews, and Costa, 1990; Onslow, Packman, and Harrison, 2002), which is a form on which they record, at the end of each day, a number from 1 (no stuttering) to 10 (extremely severe stuttering), which is their estimate of the severity of their child's stuttering. Parents begin by rating the severity of the child's stuttering during the parent-child interaction sample just recorded. The clinician also rates the severity of this sample. If the parents' and clinician's ratings differ by more than 1 point, the parents and clinician discuss the ratings and watch the recording of the interaction to help them come to a consensus. If more than one parent or another family member will be using the Severity Rating Scale, each person should be trained until his or her ratings are within 1 point of the clinician's rating of each sample. More discussion of using this rating scale is provided in the chapters on borderline and beginning stuttering. In addition to rating the child's severity every day, parents can record comments and questions they would like to discuss when we meet at the next session.

If a child with borderline stuttering is being followed but not formally treated, severity ratings are an important part of the monitoring process. Clinicians can obtain information about the child's stuttering via phone calls or email on a regular basis, and parents can report their severity ratings for each day as well as discuss issues of concern and ask questions. In addition to monitoring the severity of a child's stuttering, it is often helpful to brainstorm with the parents about ways in which the environment might be made as facilitating as possible for their child's speech. I'll discuss this in more detail in the following paragraphs.

For the child with borderline stuttering who is being treated (i.e., a child whose parents are very concerned or who has multiple risk factors for persistent stuttering), the closing interview is a time when further appointments may be set up and changes in the family environment can be initiated. Such changes will be determined by the clinician's observations of parent-child interactions, the parent interview, and ideas that parents may have about what they would like to change. In my experience, one of the most powerful ways that parents can facilitate fluency is to set aside 10 to 15 minutes each day, preferably in the morning, for child-directed interactions. This is a one-on-one interaction without other children interrupting. In two-parent homes, parents may need to alternate which one does the one-on-one activity so that the other parent can watch the other children. Or, a parent may conduct the session when the siblings are at school or napping. During these interactions, the parent primarily listens to the child and plays whatever games the child chooses. When the parent speaks, he or she should use a slow rate with frequent pauses, somewhat like television's Mr. Rogers. I have found this works best if the clinician models this interaction style and then watches the parent carry it out. More information about changing the family environment is given in the chapter on treatment of borderline stuttering (Chapter 9).

I also give parents of children with borderline stuttering reading material or a video recording to help them better understand stuttering and what they can do to help their child. The book, *Stuttering and Your Child—Questions and Answers* (Conture, 2002), gives many good suggestions and is available from the Stuttering Foundation of America (www.stutteringhelp.org) for $2. The video, *Stuttering and the Preschool Child-Help for Families* (Guitar and Guitar, 2000, SFA publication #70), is also available from the Foundation for $5. Another video, *Preventing Stuttering in the Preschool Child: A Video Program for Parents* (Skinner and McKeehan, 1996; Communication Skill Builders) is highly instructive.

For preschool children with beginning level stuttering, I begin treatment as soon as possible. For stuttering at this level, I use a direct approach. Options for therapy should be described to the parents, and they, with the clinician's guidance, should make an informed choice. In some cases, the family will be able to make their decision immediately. In other cases, they may need time to consider the possibilities. If they choose to begin treatment soon, one or more family members should be trained immediately in recording daily severity ratings, and the next session should be scheduled. They should be asked to bring in their severity ratings if the session could be scheduled within a week or two. If it has to be delayed, the clinician should be in contact with the family through email or telephone each week to discuss their severity ratings until formal treatment can begin. Once that begins, parents can bring in their severity ratings each week to discuss them with the clinician.

If treatment cannot begin for several weeks, I ask a parent or other family member to conduct one-on-one interactions with their child as was just described for a child with borderline stuttering. If the family is able to begin treatment immediately, the clinician should start the parents on appropriate activities. Clinicians who carry out therapy themselves with the child will probably have a parent watch the first few sessions before beginning direct activities at home. My own preference is to use the Lidcombe Program (Onslow, Packman, and Harrison, 2002), which is a parent-delivered treatment. Consequently, if therapy can begin immediately, I describe the first phase of this treatment program to the parents, which is a daily parent-child session conducted at home. Parents engage the child in an activity at an appropriate linguistic level to elicit fluent speech and reinforce fluent utterances. After explaining this to the parent, I model this type of interaction and then observe the parent as he or she tries it. The Lidcombe Program and other direct and indirect approaches are described in Chapter 10.

The closing interview should end when the family seems to have a good understanding of the clinician's findings, and they and the clinician agree what the next steps should be. Because a family may come up with new questions and concerns in the days following the evaluation, it is important to conclude the interview with information about how they can contact the clinician.

School-Age Child

Preassessment

Clinical Questions

As with preschool-age children, it is important to begin an evaluation with certain questions in mind. What is this child's frequency of stuttering? What types of disfluencies does he display, and what is the percentage of stutter-like disfluencies? What is the child's severity? What is his speech rate? With rare exceptions, the question of whether the youngster is normally disfluent or stuttering is not at issue. By age 6, most children who stutter do so in ways that are quite different from the normal disfluencies typical for their age. Another question is: what emotions and attitudes does the child have about stuttering and about speaking? School children with notable fear and avoidance may need special attention to these feelings and behaviors. Information about risk factors (e.g., gender, family history) are important but not as critical as they are for a preschool child. By the time a child is in school, natural recovery is less likely than in the preschool years; thus, an absence of risk factors doesn't warrant withholding or delaying treatment.

Information from the child's teachers, the clinician's observations of his speech in class and in the treatment room, and information from his family are all required to assign the child a developmental/treatment level. Questions about treatment of children in the public schools can be answered only in the context of federal and state laws, which are considered in the next section. With any school-age child, it is vital to determine the child's school performance and how stuttering interferes with it.

Public School Considerations

The Individuals with Disabilities Education Act (IDEA '97) and individual state laws mandate the procedures that public school clinicians must use for gathering information about a child's disability and deciding on treatment. In most states, a "pre-referral prevention/intervention" process is used when a teacher encounters a child who stutters in the classroom (Moore-Brown and Montgomery, 2001). Speech-language pathologists are usually members of a team that consults with the teacher and parents to determine if a child's difficulty can be resolved by making changes in the educational setting. An example of such modifications might be discussions between the child and teacher about how the teacher can facilitate the child's class participation. If stuttering continues to be a problem in the classroom after the modificatons have been in place for a designated time period, the teacher or parent can refer the child for further evaluation. The next step, evaluation by a multidisciplinary team, is usually taken in response to a referral or as the result of a clinician's identification of a child through screening. As part of this evaluation, the clinician discreetly observes the child in the classroom and confirms (or disconfirms) that the child is stuttering. The clinician then discusses the child's problem with the teacher and the school's special education administrator. Next, the clinician, teacher, or administrator contacts the child's parents to ask permission to do a formal evaluation of the child. If permission is given, the clinician gathers information on as many dimensions of the child's stuttering as possible. Typically, this will include the frequency, severity, and types of stuttering observed in two or more situations; the child's feelings and attitudes about stuttering and speaking; concomitant speech or language problems; and overall communicative performance. The clinician uses standardized tests (such as the SSI-3), observations, and interviews with the child and his family as well as with his teachers and others at school who know him. After this information is gathered, a team composed of the clincian, teacher, special education administrator, and the parents meet to decide two issues. The first is whether the child's stuttering problems meet the state's criteria for eligibililty, and the second is whether the child's stuttering adversely affects his educational performance. These two issues will be discussed in detail later in this chapter, after the sections on the parent, teacher, and child interview.

Initial Contact with Parents

Whether contact is made because the child has been referred to the school clinician or because the parents have made an appointment at a private clinic, the clinician's most important task is to listen and try to understand the parents' point of view. If the school clinician is telephoning the parents for permission to evaluate their child, she should describe the process by which the child was identified and convey her and the school's desire to help the child achieve his potential as an effective communicator. It will be helpful to describe briefly the disfluency that identified the child as stuttering and to find out if the parents have also noticed it. The clinician should calmly convey her interest in the child and his stuttering in an accepting tone of voice, particularly because parents may fear that they are being blamed for the child's stuttering. It may help also to comment that current views suggest that stuttering may be the result of how the child's brain is organized, although its exact cause is unknown. The evaluation process should be described and permission sought. If the parents agree to an evaluation, this is a good time to ask them to fill out a case history form and, if possible, send a video recording of the child's speech. It may be beneficial for the clinician to talk to the child as well and ask his permission to have his parents video record his speech at home. In some cases, the home video is easier to obtain once the clinician has gotten to know the child and has conveyed her acceptance and interest in the child's stuttering.

In cases where parents have made an appointment for an evaluation at a clinic, the clinician should call the parents and let them know what will take place in the evaluation, get some preliminary information about the child and his stuttering, let them know they will receive a case history to complete and return, and request a video from home prior to the evaluation. As with the school clinician's telephone call, it is most important that the parents' point of view about stuttering be understood. Even though they will have a chance to talk over their concerns in person, they may also want to talk and ask questions in this preliminary telephone call.

Case History Form

This form is shown in Figure 7–2 and is the same one used for preschool children. Some of the questions about speech and language development may be difficult for parents to recall. This is not critical for evaluating a school-age child, but it is important to probe for other speech and language problems that may be contributing factors in the school-age child's stuttering. An important section on this form deals with how the problem has changed since it was first noticed, what has been done about it, and how others have reacted to it. In addition, the section on educational history lets us know if the child is having problems in school. This is covered at greater length in the section on academic adjustment.

Audio-Video Recording

Obtaining a recording (preferably a videotape) of the child speaking at home or elsewhere will help clinicians prepare for the evaluation because they can measure the sample ahead of time and plan the assessment more carefully. For example, if a sample from home has little or no stuttering, the clinician may want to obtain another sample in a more difficult speaking situation. Up to a point, more varied samples of a child's speech lead to a more valid assessment. If a pre-evaluation sample has lots of avoidance behaviors on it, clinicians can prepare questions to ask the child about what he does when he expects to stutter.

Assessment

Parent Interview

This description of the parent interview assumes that the parents have brought their child to a clinic for the evaluation. When the evaluation is school-based, the clinician can get much of this information by telephone and follow-up with a face-to-face meeting at school.

Begin a clinic-based interview by making some positive observations about the child and his family and then describe the course of the evaluation. Before obtaining more background information to fill in gaps left by the case history, ask parents to describe their concerns about their child's speech. I use essentially the same questions as those I ask preschool children's parents (see the section on interviewing parents of the preschool child). However, I also ask parents of a school-age child about his school experiences. Does he like school? Does his speech seem to bother him there? Do you think he participates less in school because of his stuttering? Is he teased or bullied about his stuttering? Do you think he stutters more at school than at home? Has he gotten therapy at school? Has that helped? Has he liked it?

As I ask parents questions about the child's stuttering at home and school, I listen for responses that may help me understand why the child's stuttering has persisted into elementary school. Here are some of the questions I think about as I try to assimilate the information I am getting from the parent: Is the child sensitive about his stuttering? Are the family and child comfortable talking about stuttering? Is the family supportive of the child and his ways of coping with his stuttering? Is the family motivated to participate in therapy?

I also keep in mind that the parents are probably doing their best, given the expectations with which *they* grew up. One of the most important things clinicians can do in parent interviews is to convey an acceptance of the parents as they are and to point out the helpful things they have done for their child.

Teacher Interview

The more assistance we can get from a child's teachers, the more we can help the child. We need to approach teachers with respect for their heavy responsibilities and their concern for their students, including the one with whom we are working. But we also should anticipate that they may neither understand nor know what we do to help a child who stutters. As I talk with a teacher, for example, I try to sense what they would like to know about stuttering and my treatment approach. The following questions serve as guidelines for the types of things I want to find out.

1. **Does the child talk in class? Does he stutter? What is his stuttering like? How does he seem to feel about his stuttering and about himself as a communicator?**

   Here, I am trying to determine how much the child stutters in class and whether his stuttering keeps him from talking as much as he might otherwise if he did not stutter. I may also get a flavor of how the teacher feels about the child, his communication abilities, and his stuttering.

2. **Does stuttering interfere with the child's performance in school?**

   This question is obviously related to the previous one about the child's stuttering in class. But it also may give us some information about how much the child may avoid speaking, especially volunteering in class. I ask about disparities between his oral and written performance; a large disparity may indicate that he declines to talk, or says "I don't know," even when he knows the answers.

3. **Do other children tease him about stuttering?**

   Most school-age children who stutter are teased, and I want to get more information about how much he is teased and how it affects him.

4. **How does the teacher feel about stuttering and how does he or she react to it?**

   I am often able to get this information indirectly, from what he or she said before, but, if not, I ask directly. Teachers are also likely to ask how they *should* respond to a child's stuttering, which is an important issue because a teacher's response often influences how the class responds. This and other issues related to the child's speech in the classroom are discussed in the chapter on intermediate stuttering (Chapter 11).

Classroom Observation

In addition to the information obtained from teacher and parent interviews, direct observation can help clinicians understand the severity of a child's stuttering and the degree to which it interferes with his academic adjustment. If a child is to receive services in the school, the clinician must establish that the child's stuttering is interfering with his education. One way to verify this is by first-hand observation of a child in the classroom.

You should arrange with the teacher to come to the classroom at a time when the child will have opportunities to participate in class and observe the class as unobtrusively as you can. By observing the class when many students are participating, not just when the child you are evaluating is talking, you will not call as much attention to him. Most school-age children want to be like their peers and dread being singled out.

Child/Student Interview

After I obtain parents' consent to evaluate a child, I ask the child to come to the treatment room where I talk with him for a while. School-age clients sometimes tell me that it helps just to have someone to talk to about stuttering and other things that are bothering them. This can occur only after a trusting relationship is established, and the first interview is the first step in building that relationship.

In our first encounter, it is important for a child to feel that I am genuinely interested in him as well as his stuttering. I usually begin by asking what he likes to do, who his friends are, and who is in his family. Then I tell him a little about myself and how I work with othe kids who sometimes get stuck on words. As the child talks, I note whether he stutters or not and how he stutters. When a child's body language and behavior tell me he's comfortable in the session, I talk to him about his speech. The following questions are not asked one right after another but over a session or two. Often, it is more effective to make the question a comment, such as phrasing the first question below as: "Sometimes kids have trouble getting words out. Their words just seem to stick a little bit." Then, leave some silence to see if the youngster will talk about his own speech.

1. **Do you ever think that you have any trouble talking?**

   I rarely see school-age stutterers who are unaware of their difficulty. However, if a child regards his problem as minor or seems genuinely unaware of the problem, I avoid giving it undue emphasis or creating an unfavorable attitude about it. Thus, my first talk with a child is usually low key, and if he truly doesn't seem to be bothered by his stuttering, although his parents and teachers are, I respect his perception and try to treat it as a relatively minor problem, but I remain aware that the child may be bothered by his stuttering much more than he wishes to let on at first.

2. **What happens when you get stuck on a word? When does it happen? Is it different at different times?**

   I am looking for several things here. One is to learn the words the child uses to describe his stuttering so that I can use them when talking with him about it. I also want to find out if the child is unaware of some of his stuttering behaviors, if they seem to be too painful for him to face, or if he just doesn't like talking about them. Even more important, these questions let a child know that the clinician really wants to understand his problem.

3. **Have you learned to use any helpers or "tricks" to get words out? Do you sometimes avoid certain words?**

With this question, I can convey that I understand what some people do when they stutter. I can also let a child know that I am nonjudgmental about the "tricks" he uses, by conveying my acceptance and interest in his descriptions. In addition, I am also exploring which level the child's stuttering has reached by determining if he is using escape and avoidance behaviors.

4. **Are certain speaking situations more difficult? Do you avoid them?**

This is another question that helps me understand what a child is experiencing, while conveying my understanding.

5. **Most kids who stutter get teased or picked on about their speech. Does it ever happen to you? What do you do when that happens? How does it affect you?**

Many children who stutter are teased but are not willing to talk about it straightaway with someone they don't know well. So this question is a "feeler," and if the child denies being teased, the clinician should not dwell on it now.

6. **How do you feel about your speech?**

To help a child express feelings about stuttering, I can suggest some possibilities by asking, "Does it make you mad sometimes?" or "Do you wish you didn't get stuck?" Don't be surprised, however, if a child says it doesn't bother him because his feelings may have been rejected, perhaps unintentionally, by adults. Adults may say, for instance, "You shouldn't feel that way," or "Why do you let it bother you?" An effective clinician will show the child that whatever feelings he has are okay and that the clinician is really trying to understand. Real discussions of feelings probably won't begin until a child has learned to trust the clinician deeply. But, in this first interview, I may be able to infer what some of the child's feelings are and, from that, understand how far his stuttering has advanced.

Another avenue to elicit feelings is through drawing pictures. For some children, drawing makes it easier to talk about feelings. The child doesn't have to look directly at the clinician, and his self-consciousness may be decreased by his focus on drawing. I usually suggest to a child that both of us draw whatever we would like, and as we are drawing, I talk about feelings. If this goes well, I bridge the gap between the drawing and talking by suggesting that the child might want to draw a picture of what stuttering is like or what he feels like when he stutters. I have found that this technique can make extensive discussion of feelings much easier for some children. In some cases, children have used their drawings when they talked about stuttering with their class, once therapy has helped them feel more comfortable with themselves and their speech.

Some of the activities in the workbook, *The School-Age Child Who Stutters: Working Effectively with Attitudes and Emotions* (Chmela and Reardon, 2001), are helpful in exploring a child's emotions in both the evaluation and treatment. I will discuss some of these a little later.

7. **How do your parents feel about his speech? Do they ever say anything or give you advice?**

   This helps me determine what sorts of experiences the child may have been going through at home. One parent may be much less accepting of a child's stuttering than the other. Whatever I find out may help me enlist the parents' participation in treatment.

8. **Can you think of anything else important for me to know about you or about the trouble you sometimes have when you talk?"**

   This lets the child know that I am interested in him and that his ideas are important to me.

Speech Samples

Preliminaries

With a school-age child, I video record him talking for 10 minutes about school and other activities in the therapy room. I prefer not to turn on the recorder the moment the child walks into the room. Instead, after talking for a few minutes, I ask the child if he would mind my recording our conversation as we talk. If it's ok with the child, I record a sample that includes, optimally, 300-400 syllables of his speech. For those few children who are reluctant at first, I explain that I need a recording of their speech to understand their stuttering better. In rare cases, I might need to postpone recording until the child is more comfortable with me. After recording the speech sample, I ask the child to read approximately 200 syllables of age-appropriate material. I often use the SSI-3 examiner's manual, which has 200-syllable reading passages at the 3rd, 5th, and 7th grade levels.

If possible, I also obtain a video recording from home for a second sample. In some instances, you may not be able to get a second recorded sample from home or elsewhere. It is important, however, to observe the child's speech in several settings, even if you are not able to record it. For these other samples, write down your impressions of the child's stuttering, including the amount of stuttering and the core and secondary behaviors you observed.

Pattern of Disfluencies

During interviews with teachers, parents, and the child himself, as well as from speech samples, I gather information about when and how a child stutters. A school-age child is likely to show beginning or intermediate stuttering, so I want to know as much as possible about the amount of tension in the child's stuttering, the escape behaviors he uses, and the extent to which he avoids words and situations. As with adults or adolescents who stutter, I use this information not only to decide at which developmental/treatment level to place the child, but I also use it, when appropriate, to plan the process of unlearning conditioned responses, which, once created, now maintain the child's pattern of stuttering.

Stuttering Severity Instrument (SSI-3)

I need samples of conversational speech and reading from which to calculate scores on the SSI-3. Administration and scoring of the SSI-3 were described in Chapter 6.

Speech Rate

The samples you collect for rating severity with the SSI-3 can also be used to assess the child's speaking rate. The purpose of assessing speech rate is to get some idea of how much the child's stuttering interferes with the rate of speech he normally uses. As I help the child manage his stuttering, I expect a steady increase in his speech rate toward normal levels.

Normal speech rates for school children in Vermont between the ages of 6 and 12 years, measured in syllables per minute, are given in Table 6–3. These rates were obtained from children's conversations with a clinician about Christmas, hobbies, school, and home activities. They were calculated by including normal pauses in their conversation but excluding pauses longer than 2 seconds for thought. It is reasonable to expect that children's speech rates in other states will be similar.

Trial Therapy

Trial therapy with a school-age child will help me understand what approach might work with this particular child as well as what may be difficult for him. If the child is able to make significant, although temporary, changes in his stuttering in this brief treatment, he will gain hope and motivation for our work together.

I usually begin by asking the child to identify moments of voluntary stuttering in my own speech. I explain that I will be putting stutters in my speech and want to see if he can catch me. It's more fun if I can use a small reward for his successes. I then tell him about my favorite recent movie or television show (something he can later do himself) and put in a variety of stutters in my speech. As I talk and encourage him to catch my stutters, I let him know how good he is when he catches one of my stutters without my help and hand him a piece of candy. After a few successful catches, I reverse our roles and have him put in some stutters—pretend or real—as he talks about a movie, tv show, or any other handy topic, and I try to "catch him." Each time, I make a positive comment about his stutter and give him a reward. Rewarding stutters of school-age children causes no harm; in fact, it reduces negative emotion.

A next step is to see if he can hold on to a stutter. As always, I first demonstrate what I'm asking the child to do. I have the child signal me by pointing to me when he wants me to stutter and make me hold on to the stutter for several seconds by continuing to keep his finger pointing at me. Then, I reverse roles and coach him to hold on to either voluntary or real stutters. In so doing, I also coach him, while he's holding on to the stutter, to let it go slowly and loosely when he's ready to move on. Typically, my models, my enthusiasm, and the reinforcements I use enable most children to be able to carry out these activities. It is important to note if the child cannot do these activities, which suggests a higher level of fear or an inability to focus on the task. These possibilities usually mean that a child needs a slower approach, and I will consider teaching him fluency skills before attempting stuttering modification.

Trial therapy using fluency skills simply involves teaching the child one or two of the fluency skills described in Chapter 11 on intermediate stuttering. I use a word list and give the child an example by producing each word myself before he tries it, using a slow rate and gentle onset of voicing. The severity of the child's stuttering will determine how slowly I begin the word; my aim is to use modeling of slow rate and easy onset to produce fluency in the child. Once he can say words after me in that slow fashion, I then ask him to say each of several words again, but without my model. If he can do this, I create sentences beginning with those words said slowly and with an easy onset (but with the remainder of the sentence produced at a near-normal rate) and again assess whether he can repeat them fluently with my model and then without.

These exercises help me determine how well the child can make changes in his speech and his stutters. By using a large amount of modeling and appropriate reinforcement, I can often take the child quite far along in the time I have.

Feelings and Attitudes

A fair measure of a child's feelings and attitudes is the clinician's judgment, which usually improves as she gets to know the child better. Nevertheless, the clinician should be able to get a pretty good indication of a child's feelings and attitudes from the first interview. Some indications will emerge from your discussion with the child about his feelings, and some will emerge from observations of his behavior. Watch how the child responds when asked about his stuttering, and note how much he avoids stuttering. When the child does stutter, observe how calm he is and how good his eye contact is.

After the clinician has gotten to know the child a bit, she may want to administer a paper and pencil assessment of attitude. Figure 6–4 in the previous chapter depicts the A-19 scale (Guitar and Grims, 1977), which is a measure developed to assess children's communication attitudes. This scale consists of questions that were found to distinguish children who stutter from those who do not. Hence, if treatment is effective, a child's attitude about communication may change, although this has not been established by research.

In addition to the A-19, the Communication Attitude Test (CAT) (Fig. 6–5), which was developed by Brutten, has been tested on nonstutering children (Brutten and Dunham, 1989) and shown to differentiate them from stuttering children (De Nil and Brutten, 1991).

Many informal methods of assessing feelings and attitudes are given in the workbook, *The School-Age Child Who Stutters: Working Effectively with Attitudes and Emotions* (Chmela and Reardon, 2001). These include such activities as a "Worry Ladder," in which a child lists his worries in a hierarchy, and "Hands Down," which elicits things the child likes and does not like about himself. Although the reliability and validity of these tools have not been determined, they provide useful starting points for communication about feelings and attitudes.

With some children, both formal and informal methods of assessing feelings will be productive during the evaluation. But others will hold back until they have developed a trusting relationship with the clinician. Thus, clinicians should be mindful that information about a child's feelings and attitudes obtained in a first meeting may not be complete or accurate.

Other Speech and Language Disorders

In my discussion of the preschool child, I described the importance of screening language, articulation, and voice. The same abilities should be screened in the school-age child. Conture (2001) suggests using the "Sounds in Words" subtest of the Goldman-Fistoe Test of Articulation (Goldman and Fristoe, 1986) for phonology; the Clinical Evaluaton of Language Fundamentals-3, Screening Test (Semel, Wiig, and Secord, 1996) for language; and the Peabody Picture Vocabulary Test (Dunn and Dunn, 1997) and Expressive Vocabulary Test (Williams, 1997) for vocabulary. The child may have a previously diagnosed language or articulation (or, to a lesser extent, voice) problem and may be in therapy. If so, the clinician should seek out details of any current or previous therapy. If a child is receiving or has received articulation or language therapy in the past, the clinician should find out details about the type of treatment the child received and how the child responded. Did his articulation or language difficulties improve? Did his stuttering first appear or worsen during treatment? If so, the clinician should pay particular attention to indications that the child may think of himself as a poor speaker and may believe that speaking is difficult. The interviews and questionnaires I suggested in the previous section on feelings and attitudes will help you explore this possibility, and the therapy approaches described in the chapters on beginning- and intermediate-level stuttering are designed to help a child regain confidence in his ability to speak easily and well.

Other Factors

Other factors can influence the outcome of treatment. We recommend evaluating all factors that may have precipitated or are maintaining a child's stuttering, so that they may be included in the child's overall treatment plan.

Physical Development

My main concern in this area is that motor development may be lagging behind language development. A child with speech-motor delays may benefit from therapy that helps him coordinate respiration, phonation, and articulation, thereby reducing stuttering. He may also benefit from procedures that help him learn to stutter easily and openly, rather than becoming tense and frustrated, if his fluency breaks down under stress. Such children's treatment should also focus on building their self-esteem, which may be low in children who are not well coordinated.

Cognitive Development

I try to find out whether or not cognitive stresses of school may be increasing the general demands experienced by the child, which I'll discuss further in a following section on academic adjustment. If a child has academic difficulty or a learning disability, we may need to adjust our approach to treatment to make sure that he understands our explanations and examples.

Social-Emotional Development

I am interested in how well a child fits in with his classmates, how comfortable he feels about talking and relating to others, and how often he feels a need to hide his stuttering. Some children are friendly and outgoing, even though they stutter, and are supported by their classmates. These social skills are a positive factor in their prognoses for recovery from stuttering. Other children have not outgrown their self-centeredness, and stuttering compounds their self-concern and keeps them from relating easily to others. Such children need help in relating more easily to their classmates. Evaluation of this component can be accomplished through teacher, parent, and child interviews; classroom observation may be helpful, too.

I am also concerned with the extent to which a child's home environment provides support and security. This information comes primarily from parent and child interviews. Parents often provide insight into conditions surrounding the onset of stuttering and conditions under which it gets better or worse. I sift through this information, and with the parents' help, determine whether something can be done to improve the child's self-esteem. For some children, school psychologists have been helpful in building self-esteem and helping them improve their social adjustment.

Academic Adjustment

Parent, child, and teacher interviews allow me to find out how well the child is doing in school and how much he likes it. Stuttering may appear for the first time or worsen when a child is under the stress of learning many new things. For example, reading aloud in class when just learning to read is likely to put substantial demands on a child's resources for language formulation and speech production. The child must make "second-order mappings of meanings and lexical units from speech" (Gibson, 1972), while simultaneously translating the written representation into units appropriate for speech production. Thus, some academic challenges may be more demanding for a child who stutters, and his stuttering in school should be understood in relation to this. In practical terms, clinicians can determine if a child needs extra help in certain academic areas through discussions with his teachers about which speaking situations in school are most difficult for him. If the child has more difficulty in certain academic situations, these should be given extra attention in treatment when planning generalization of more fluent speech.

Diagnosis

At this point, in a clinic-based evaluation, the clinician pulls together the information collected from the case history; parent, teacher, and child interviews; speech samples; and classroom observations. This information helps the clinician determine the developmental/treatment level of the child's stuttering, which will give direction for treatment.

Most school children are at beginning or intermediate levels of stuttering. Beginning-level stuttering is characterized by physical tension, hurry, escape behaviors, awareness of difficulty, and feelings of frustration. The intermediate level also involves tension, hurry, escape behaviors, and frustration, as well as avoidance behaviors as a result of fear and anticipation of stuttering. In addition to a child's stuttering behaviors and feelings, current developmental and environmental pressures must be considered in planning treatment. Such pressures can be uncovered from parent, teacher, and child interviews and the speech sample. Some pressures may result from other speech and language disorders, motor problems, or pressures in the child's home. Goals can formulated, with the parents' input, for alleviating those pressures that can be changed and helping the child cope with those that can't be changed. Some pressures can be dealt with in treatment, but others may require parent counseling or referral to other professionals.

Closing Interview

The closing interview provides an opportunity to summarize my immediate impressions for the parents and make recommendations about treatment. It also provides an opportunity to discuss the crucial role parents can play in reducing environmental pressures. I point out the many beneficial things they have done about their child's speech and assure them that stuttering was not caused by anything they have done. Although some parents may have created conditions in which a child's predisposition to stutter has been transformed into a serious problem, it does not help to make an issue of this. Rather, we want to convince them that they are in a key position to help.

After describing clearly and simply what I observed about the child's stuttering, I summarize my thinking about appropriate treatment. I do this in only general terms because parents' main concerns at this time are not the details of treatment but the prospects for their child's future. Therefore, I rely on my experience to describe likely outcomes. For example, I might say that a combination of many factors will determine the child's outcome. These include the natural increases in fluency that occur as a child matures, feelings of self-acceptance that a child develops when he finds that people accept him whether or not he has trouble with his speech, and his learning ways to speak more fluently. When I talk about the child's prognosis, I always include some aspect of the parents' role, such as their acceptance of the child's speech or their participation in treatment, as part of the formula for recovery.

After summarizing my impressions and describing some of the ingredients for recovery, I discuss some of the things the parents can do to promote recovery. Specific suggestions depend on findings from our interviews, but the sections on parent counseling in the chapters on treatment of beginning and intermediate levels of stuttering present general ideas for parents' involvement. Discussion of the family's involvement in therapy is the most important part of the closing interview and, in fact, may continue for several more meetings. If I treat the child directly and in a clinic rather than in a school setting, I meet with parents weekly as part of treatment. In these meetings, I continue to help them explore how various changes in the home environment can facilitate their child's fluency.

Public School Setting

The sequence dictated by IDEA (1997), after a referral for stuttering is made, is for the multidisciplinary team to develop an assessment plan and carry it out. After the clinician gathers information using tests, observations, and interviews, she writes a report describing the affective, behavioral, and cognitive aspects of the child's stuttering and his current performance in academic, nonacademic, and extracurricular activities. The assessment report should be brief (e.g., two pages) and understandable by lay readers, such as the child's parents.

Then, an Individualized Education Program (IEP) team is appointed to consider the report and other information. The IEP team must decide the two issues mentioned earlier: does the child meet the state's eligibility standards, and does the child's stuttering have an adverse effect on his education? The first of these issues is resolved by the data the clinician gathered, particularly the information about the frequency and severity of the child's stuttering and his feelings and attitudes. The second issue is usually more complex because it is necessary to show that the child does not perform as well he might in school because of his stuttering. For example, the team can conclude that his stuttering prevents him from participating as much as he might in class or in extracurricular activities with his peers. Evidence of this can be obtained from measures of communicative functioning in school, such as the *Teacher's Assessment of Student Communication*

Competency (Smith, McCauley, and Guitar, 2000), observations of the child in the school, and interviews with teachers and parents. Lisa Scott Trautman (personal communication, July 30, 2003) noted that adverse effects can be shown by demonstrating that the child cannot meet the school district's curriculum objectives because of his stuttering. Examples of such objectives might be that students will be active in class discussions or that students must be able to speak effectively in front of a group.

If the evaluation determines that the student is eligible for services, an IEP team develops measurable goals and short-term objectives (also called "benchmarks") as well as services to be provided that will help the student improve his performance in all aspects of the educational setting. These goals and objectives are considered in detail in the chapters on treatment of beginning and intermediate stuttering.

Adolescents and Adults

Preassessment

Clinic Versus School Assessment

This section is written as though the evalution is being carried out in a clinic rather than a school. When the setting is a public school, the evaluation process is determined by the Individuals with Disabilities Education Act (IDEA '97) and the laws of each state. The guidelines for this process were described in the previous section on evaluating a school-age child. For the adolescent, an additional consideration is his participation in the IEP process and his transition beyond high school. When a student reaches age 14, his input is sought by the IEP team, and he gradually becomes an active member of the team, not only with regard to his present situation, but also in terms of his aspirations beyond secondary school. When a student reaches age 16, transition plans are a mandated part of the IEP. At age 18, students take over responsibility from their parents for signing off on documentation.

Case History Form

A case history form is sent to adult clients (those over age 18 years and beyond high school) several weeks before their appointment. A copy of this form is shown in Figure 7–3. Because adolescents are often seen in schools, the clinician encourages them to fill out the form, with help from their parents for parts of it.

This form requests information that would be appropriate for most speech-language disorders and can be used with all adult clients referred for speech or language problems. It also allows the clinician to learn ahead of time whether the client referred for stuttering may have a different or an additional disorder. The form also gives the clinician information about the extent to which stuttering, if that is the problem, affects a client's life.

Attitude Questionnaires

I assess clients' communication attitudes through observations, interview questions, and questionnaires. Because I want to be able to analyze completed questionnaires before the diagnostic interview, I prefer to send them to clients and ask them to complete and return

Note: Please complete and return this form before your appointment. Thank you.

Speech Clinic
Stuttering Case History Form Adult & Adolescent

Date: _____

Name: _____

Address: _____ Tel: _____

_____

Date of Birth: _____ Place of Birth: _____

Social Security: _____ Referring Physician: _____

Sex: _____ Marital Status: _____

Educational level: _____ Occupation: _____

Employed by: _____

Referred to this Center by: _____

Name of spouse/nearest relative: _____

Address: _____ Tel: _____

_____

History of Stuttering

Are there other individuals in your family background or immediate family who stutter?
_____

Give approximte age at which your stuttering was first noticed _____
Who first noticed or mentioned your stuttering? _____
In what situation did this occur? _____
_____

Describe any situations or conditions that you associate with the onset of stuttering
_____

What were the first signs of your stuttering? (if you don't remember, you might ask parents or siblings) _____
_____

Was the stuttering always the same or did it occur in several different ways? _____
_____

If the stuttering occurred by different ways, how were they different from one another? _____
_____

Did the first blocks soon to be located in the tongue? Lips? Chest? Diaphragm? Tiroat? (Circle your answer.)
Approximately how long did each block (on one word) seem to last? _____
Was the stutterling easy or was there force at the time when the stuttering was first noticed? _____

Figure 7–3 *Case history form for adults and adolescents.*

Were the words that were stuttered at the beginning of sentences, or were they scattered throughout the sentence being said?_____
_____

When stuttering first began, was there any avoidance of speaking because of it?
Give examples, if any,_____
_____

At the time when stuttering was first noticed, what was your reaction?
(Check all that apply)
Awareness that speech was different? ____ Indifference to it?   ____ Other? ____
Surprise?   ____ Anger or frustration?____
Fear of stuttering again?   ____ Shame?   ____
What attempts have been made to treat the stuttering problem? _____
_____
_____

Development of Stuttering

Since the onset, have there been any changes in stuttering symptoms?
(Check all that apply.)
Increase in number of repetitions per word. _____
Change in amount of force used (Increased?) _____(Decreased?)_____
Increase in amount of stuttering _____
Increase in length of block _____
Periods of no stuttering _____
More precise in speech attempts _____
Lowered voice loudness _____
Slower rate of speech _____
Change in location of force when stuttering (if force is present) _____
Looking a way from listener _____
Describe any that apply _____
_____

Were there any periods (weeks/months) when the stuttering disappeared? ____
_____

Were there any periods (weeks/months)when stuttering increased? _____
_____

Can you give an explanation for these 'worse' periods? _____
_____

Current Stuttering

Are there any situations that are particularly difficult? If so, please describe,_____
_____
_____

List any situations that never cause difficulty. _____
_____

Figure 7–3   (Continued)

Answer the following 'yes' or 'no' as they apply to your stuttering.
Do you stutter when you

Talk to young children?	___	Recite memorized material?	___
Say your name	___	Ask questions?	___
Answer direct questions?	___	Talk to strangers?	___
Talk to adults, superiors at work, teachers?	___	Speak when tired?	___
Use new words that are unfamiliar?	___	Speak when excited?	___
Use the telephone?	___	Talk to family members?	___
Read aloud?	___	Talk to friends?	___

Do you feel that stuttering interferes with your career? ___Social relationships? ___
Success in school? _____ Success on the job? _____ Daily use? _____

Do you know any stutterers? _____Describe your relationship with them_____
_____.
_____

Describe what your stuttering currently looks and sounds like._____
_____
_____
_____

Medical Development and Family History

If possible, describe your mother's health during pregnancy and/or your birth
history (ie, complications). _____
_____
_____

Describe any development problems during infancy or early childhood (i.e., late
in walking, feeding problems, food allergies, late in talking)_____
_____
_____

Are you: Rightly handed? _____Leftly handed? _____Both? _____Is therte evidence of visual, artistic abilities in your family?_____
_____

Were you sensitive as a child? _____Would you describe yourself as sensitive
now?_____

List any significant illnesses, injuries, and operations:

Name	Date	Fever	Complications	Treatment	Physician's Name

Figure 7–3   *(Continued)*

List of present physical disabilities. _____
_____

Any chronic illnesses, allergies, or physical conditions? _____
_____

Is your vision normal? _____ Hearing normal?_____
List any medications you take regularly or are taking currently. _____
_____

Describe any learning or reading problems you experienced as a child or are currently experiencing._____
_____

Do any members of your family have speech or language problems or learning disabilities? If so, describe_____
_____

Social History

Hobbies _____
Leisure time activities _____
Describe any previous therapy you have participated in to aid your fluency. When? Where? With whom? For how long? Outcome_____
_____
_____
_____

Add anything else you would like to include and think might be important._____
_____
_____
_____

If, in order to help you, it is appropriate to send reports to other agencies or professional persons, or to contact other agencies or professional persons for additional information, please indicate your permission by signing below.
I authorize and request (fill in name of clinician or clinic) to obtain and/or exchange pertinent medical/educational information. I understand that all information will be kept confidential.
Signed: _____
Date: _____
If signed by person other than client, please state name and capacity of that persons _____
_____

Please return this completed form at least 2 weeks before your evaluation.

Figure 7–3 (Continued)

the questionnaires before the interview. If this is not possible, clients can complete them when they arrive for an evaluation before the initial interview or, as a less desireable alternative, after the initial interview. Prior to the interview, follow-up questions based on information from the case history and questionnaires, which are described in the section on feelings and attitudes, can be prepared to further explore a client's attitudes.

Audio-Video Recording

It is important to sample a client's speech in several situations to get an adequate picture of his stuttering. I ask clients to video- or audiotape themselves talking in one or two different situations outside the clinic and get the tape to me prior to the evaluation. It is usually easy for clients to record themselves talking to someone on the phone, recording only their own voices and not the person on the other end of the line. Some clients can also record themselves talking face-to-face with a friend or family member. If I view the recording(s) before an evaluation, I am better prepared to understand the client's stuttering and to plan various trial-therapy strategies.

Assessment

Interview

I begin by welcoming the client and reviewing the procedures I will use to evaluate his problem, such as interviewing him about his stuttering and his feelings and attitudes, videotaping his speaking and reading, examining what he does when he stutters, and trying to determine if he can change it. I let him know that, after the initial part of his evaluation, I will ask him to wait while I analyze the information I've obtained before meeting with him to share my findings and recommendations. If there are any forms or questionnaires I haven't already obtained from him, I'll have him complete those while I analyze the other data.

I begin our interview with an open-ended question such as, "Tell me the problem that brings you here today" or "Why don't you tell me about your stuttering." The first might be used if I don't know what is motivating the client to come for an evaluation at this time; the second question I use when I already know, from prior information, why the client has come right now.

Once a client has had a chance to describe his speech problem, I ask further questions to try to get a deeper understanding. The following questions are typical questions that I ask, with a brief commentary about each. Sometimes, I group several questions together (e.g., a question to start the client talking about a particular topic and follow-up questions that I ask if the first question doesn't elicit the desired information).

1. **When did you begin to stutter? How has the way you stutter changed over the years?**

   I realize that, in answering the first part of this question, a client may just be reporting what parents told him about his stuttering. The accuracy of his response may be questionable, but at least I'll learn his perception of the onset. The second part of the question—about changes over the years—may reveal what kinds of things affect the way a client stutters. Does he stutter more severely because of a recent job change or a threat to his self-esteem, such as a divorce or loss of employment? Less frequently, I may find out that a client began to stutter in late adolescence or as an adult. If so, I would want to consider the possibility of neurogenic or psychogenic stuttering, which is discussed briefly in the section on diagnosis and more fully in Chapter 13, on other fluency disorders.

2. **What do you believe caused you to stutter?**

This may give some insights about a client's motivation. For example, a woman reported that her mother and several brothers stuttered and that her stuttering was, therefore, a genetic problem that could not be helped. This led us to confront the issue of whether or not she was likely to change.

In addition, I sometimes find that clients have misinformation about possible causes of their stuttering. If I can give them more appropriate information, their attitudes about the problem may change, and their motivation may increase. I have met individuals who come to the evaluation believing that their problem is entirely psychological. After I discuss current views of stuttering, they are relieved to know that they can modify their speech without long-term psychotherapy.

3. **Does anyone else in your family stutter?**

I might find that a parent stutters, which can be significant, because a parent's attitudes about his or her own stuttering may have had a profound effect on the client. Moreover, knowing about other family members who stutter and how they have responded to it may provide a better understanding of the factors related to this client's stuttering, which may be useful in treatment. For example, someone I am interviewing may have had a parent who stuttered but who never talked about it. I might then want to explore whether the individual I am working with feels especially ashamed of his stuttering or feels it gives him an important bond with the parent.

4. **Have you ever had therapy for your stuttering? What did the therapy consist of? How effective do you think it was?**

This information is important in planning therapy. For example, if a client had received a type of therapy that he felt did not help, it would be unwise to use that type of therapy with this client. But if a client has had success with therapy but has regressed slightly or moved away before treatment was finished, using this type of therapy again may be most appropriate. It is important that clinicians be familiar with various types of therapy that clients may have undergone. Most current therapies emphasize either modifying stuttering behaviors or learning to talk in ways that eliminate stuttering.

5. **Has your stuttering changed or caused you more problems recently? Why did you come in for help at the present time?**

Responses to these questions allow clinicians to see the current problems faced by the client and also obtain some inkling of the client's motivation. For example, a client may have been offered a promotion if he can improve his speech or may have recently learned of the clinic's treatment program and is hoping for some relief from a long-standing problem. The following four questions about the client's pattern of stuttering are closely related to one another.

6. **Are there times or situations when you stutter more? Less? What are they?**

7. **Do you avoid certain speaking situations in which you expect to stutter? If so, which ones?**

8. **Do you avoid certain words that you expect to stutter on? Do you substitute one word for another if you expect to stutter? Do you talk around words or topics so you won't stutter?**

9. **Do you use any "tricks" to get words out? Escape behaviors?**

These four questions will provide information that is useful in planning therapy because they tell us something about the client's most difficult situations, how he feels about them, and how he deals with them. This information may also corroborate what has been learned from the questionnaires that the client completed and will also reveal how aware he is of his stuttering behaviors.

10. **Have your academic or vocational choices or performance been affected because you stutter? How?**

The client's answers can be used to help plan later stages of treatment in which new behaviors and new challenges are attempted. They may also prompt the clinician to refer clients in later stages of treatment to an academic or vocational counselor to help them make more appropriate choices for themselves.

11. **Have your relationships with people been affected because you stutter? How?**

As with question 10, I can use this information to plan a client's hierarchy of generalization, moving from easy to difficult social situations gradually if the client finds social interactions difficult. I also need to know how much a client blames his stuttering for any of the difficulties he has in social interactions. A client may be socially inhibited because he is sensitive and vulnerable to expected listener reactions. Such sensitivity can be assessed by observing his facial affect and body movements while stuttering. If he appears to be relatively unaffected emotionally by his stuttering but professes to have difficulty relating to people, he may benefit from counseling or psychotherapy that focuses on resolving this interpersonal difficulty.

The decision to refer an individual for psychotherapy as an adjunct to stuttering therapy can seldom be made in the evaluation session. Some time and a few therapy sessions are needed to learn more about a person and to develop the client's trust before a successful referral can be made. If psychotherapy is recommended too hastily, a client may feel that I think his stuttering is too great a problem for me to handle, perhaps an insurmountable problem. But if I work with him and he starts making some progress before I refer, he will likely feel supported and may be more likely to benefit from psychotherapy.

12. **What are your feelings or attitudes toward your stuttering? What do you think other people think about your stuttering?**

A client's responses will be used to help determine some of the foci of treatment, such as desensitization procedures to decrease his shame and guilt about stuttering. Perceptions about others' views of his stuttering may need to be confronted with various "reality-testing" tasks to find out what people really think.

13. **What are your family's (parents', spouse's, children's) feelings, attitudes, and reactions toward your stuttering and toward the prospect of your being in therapy?**

This information can identify sources that may positively or negatively affect a client's motivation and may be an important consideration in planning therapy.

14. **Is there anything else that you think we ought to know about your stuttering?**

This gives the client a chance to get anything off his chest that he may be holding back or an opportunity to discuss issues that occurred to him only after other questions were asked.

15. **Do you have any questions you'd like to ask me?**

Sometimes an adolescent or adult has questions about stuttering that he has been reluctant to ask, and this may give the clinician an opportunity to answer them. On the other hand, a client may want to ask about the length and type of treatment or other issues that are best dealt with after his assessment is completed. In this case, the clinician explains why she needs to delay responding but will keep the questions in mind to answer during the closing interview.

Speech Sample

In this part of the evaluation, the client's overt stuttering behaviors are assessed. Although I always videotape the entire evaluation, if the client has given permission, I pay particular attention to the taping of this section because I will need to analyze it carefully afterward. Clinicians use a variety of procedures for assessing overt stuttering. Next, I'll describe in detail the tool I currently use and then note other available options.

Stuttering Severity

As indicated in the previous chapter, the Stuttering Severity Instrument (SSI-3) is a moderately reliable tool that is commonly used to assess the severity of stuttering. To obtain appropriate samples, I have the client talk about a familiar topic, such as his work, school, hobbies, vacations, sports, or entertainment. It is important to get about at least 300 syllables of the client's talking, so 5 or 10 minutes are usually enough, depending on the client's fluency. Then, I provide the client material at an appropriate reading level, such as the passages in the SSI-3 examiner's manual, and ask him to read aloud for about 3 minutes to get 200 or more syllables of reading;

As I noted earlier, we often gather more than one sample of spontaneous speech from adults and adolescents. A sample of speech during a telephone conversation in the clinic can be video recorded and scored using the SSI-3. In addition, I use samples the client has brought or sent in. If the sample from another environment is audio recorded rather than video recorded, I score it for both frequency of stuttering and speech rate.

Other Measures of Stuttering

If I am assessing stuttering frequently or assessing samples that I cannot analyze visually, such as those audio recorded by a client in his natural environment, I use a combination of frequency of stuttering (percentage of syllables stuttered) and speech rate (syllables spoken per minute). These measures, which were first described in Andrews and Ingham (1971), together require much less time than the SSI.

Starkweather (1991) has presented a case for capturing the amount of time that stuttering takes. This is done by totaling the duration of all disfluencies and pauses in a sample and dividing this total by the overall time spent in speaking, thereby giving the clinician a measure of how much an individual's stuttering interferes with the rate he can communicate information.

As part of a determined effort to improve the reliability of stuttering measures, Ingham and his co-workers (Ingham, Cordes, and Gow, 1993; Ingham, Cordes, and Finn, 1993) developed a time-interval system of assessment. They have shown that, when judges determine whether or not 4-second intervals of continuous speech contain one or more stutters, interjudge reliability is higher than when moments of stuttering are counted; however, the clinical usefulness of this procedure has not been determined.

Speech Rate

In addition to measuring stuttering severity using the SSI, I also assess a client's speech rate. I believe, as many other clinicians do, that speaking rate often reflects the severity of stuttering, as well as its effect on communication. If a client's speech rate is markedly slower than normal, communication may be difficult for him. A description of the procedure for measuring speech rate was given in Chapter 6, "Preliminaries to Assessment."

Normal speaking rates of adults range from around 115 to 165 words per minute, or about 162 to 230 syllables per minute, with a mean of 196 syllables per minute (Andrews and Ingham, 1971). Adults' normal rates for reading aloud are faster, ranging from about 150 to 190 words per minute (Darley and Spriestersbach, 1978), or about 210 to 265 syllables per minute (Andrews and Ingham, 1971).

Pattern of Disfluencies

Throughout my evaluation of adult or adolescent stutterers, I observe the client's patterns of stutters. For example, I try to determine roughly the proportions of core behaviors that are repetitions, prolongations, or blocks and ask myself a number of questions about the client's stuttering. During blocks, where and how does he shut off airflow or voicing? What are his escape and avoidance behaviors? Is he able to tolerate being in blocks, or does he speak in unusual or vague ways to avoid stuttering? More details on various escape and avoidance patterns can be found in Chapter 5 on the development of stuttering.

As I explore the behaviors that constitute a client's stuttering, I comment on them, question him about how typical this sample of his stuttering is, and ask about the escape and avoidance behaviors we've observed. If a client doesn't seem too uncomfortable confronting his stuttering, I ask him to teach me how to stutter like he does, and we work together, with both the client and myself emulating his various types of stuttering. This need not be an exhaustive exploration, because I will do much more in treatment. Here, I am trying to accomplish three tasks: (1) model an "approach" rather than "avoidance" attitude toward stuttering, showing calmness and objectivity about behaviors that the client may feel are shameful and perhaps even terrifying; (2) study the client's emotional reaction when he comes face-to-face with his stuttering and perhaps reduce some of his fear; and (3) teach both of us about what the client does when he stutters so that he can begin to learn how to change it.

Trial Therapy

I try therapy techniques with clients during their assessment sessions for several reasons. First, I try to get an idea of how a client responds to different therapy approaches, which provides me with information I may use in talking with him about possible treatments. Second, trial therapy can help me to make differential diagnosis between developmental stuttering and stuttering with a neurological or psychological etiology. Third, it gives clients a preview of things to come and provides them with hope and motivation to follow through on treatment.

I begin by asking a client to modify his stuttering, which can be done easily in the context of studying his patterns of disfluency, as described in the preceding section. In fact, this exploration of stuttering with a client is a condensed version of the first stage of treatment that aims to change stuttering to an easier pattern. Once a client is able to emulate his stuttering to a small degree, I carry out trial therapy by coaching him through the following sequence: (1) having him "freeze" during a moment of stuttering and maintain the level of physical tension and posture of his stuttering as I encourage him to stay in the moment of stuttering; (2) having him become aware of what he is doing in terms of physically tensing muscles, holding his breath, and pushing against jammed postures; and (3) having him change elements that are maintaining stutters by (a) releasing their excess physical tension wherever he can feel it, (b) moving rigidly held structures, (c) getting voicing or airflow going, and/or (d) allowing himself to breathe. I may stop a client's trial therapy here if he is unable to release physical tension or does it only with obvious difficulty.

If clients seem able to make these changes easily, I go one step further. I ask them to hold on to the stutter, which has become voluntary by now, prolong the airflow or voicing for several seconds, and then produce the remainder of the word slowly. If a client is able to do this with coaching, I ask him to do it while reading without my coaching. This is enough. No matter how much or how little our client is able to do, I want to stop when he is feeling successful.

Another approach to trial therapy is to change the client's habitual way of talking so that stuttering is decreased substantially or prevented. I begin by reducing my own speech rate as I describe the aim of this exercise to the client, which is to produce words very, very slowly. I use a written sentence that begins with a vowel or a glide, going over it word by word, teaching the client to use gradual and gentle onsets of voicing and to stretch each sound, whether vowel or consonant. The clinician needs to provide a good model for each word and to give feedback frequently. When words are produced slowly enough, with each part of the speech production system (respiration, phonation, and articulation) moving in slow motion and without excess tension, fluency results. After a client is able to produce each word of the sentence in this way, he is then coached to produce the entire sentence, linking each word to the next. Breath supply should be monitored closely, so that pauses for breath are taken whenever the client would take a breath naturally. Again, accurate modeling and frequent feedback are vitally important.

As an example, the sentence, "Apples are a red fruit," should take from 15 to 20 seconds to produce, with a pause for a new breath after the word "a." The /p/ in "Apples," the /d/ in "red," and the /t/ in "fruit," each should be produced without stopping airflow, making these plosives sound like fricatives. If clients are particularly adept at this, they can be taken all the way to saying short sentences in conversational speech that are produced in this slow, fluent manner. However, clients who have difficulty should be coached only through the production of the short, written sentence, and care should be taken to stop this activity before they experience notable failure.

Feelings and Attitudes

A variety of questionnaires can be used to assess various aspects of a stutterer's feelings and attitudes about communication and stuttering. In Chapter 6, I described those questionnaires that I use regularly. These include the Modified Erickson Scale of Communication Attitudes (S-24) (Andrews and Cutler, 1974), the Stutterer's Self-Rating of Reactions to Speech Situations (Johnson, Darley, and Spriestersbach, 1952), the Perceptions of Stuttering Inventory (PSI) (Woolf, 1967), and the Locus of Control of Behavior Scale (Craig, Franklin, and Andrews, 1984).

Other Speech and Language Behaviors

As I interact with a client during the interview, I informally assess his comprehension and production of language, his articulation, and his voice. I also screen his hearing. If I suspect that there may be an articulation, language, or voice problem, I follow up with further evaluations. Adolescent language assessment procedures can be found in McLoughlin and Lewis (1990), and procedures for assessment of articulation can be found in Hoffman, Schuckers, and Daniloff (1989). I let a client's concern about other disorders guide us in treatment. If, as I have found occasionally, a stuttering client also lisps, I discuss it with him. If he is not concerned, I don't feel it is necessary to treat that problem. However, if I feel that an articulation, language, or other problem handicaps a client communicatively, I advise treatment for that problem also. Sometimes I deal with voice problems differently. I have found that some stutterers may be hoarse, but I suspect this may be the result of laryngeal tension related to stuttering. If stuttering treatment is successful, hoarseness may disappear. Again, I take my cue from the client. If the problem bothers him and isn't remediated by treatment, I address it. If hoarseness is of recent origin and not associated with a cold, I may refer him for an otolaryngological examination to rule out serious laryngeal pathology.

Other Factors

In this section, I discuss the evaluation of the following factors: intelligence, academic adjustment, psychological adjustment, and vocational adjustment. Each of these factors can affect the treatment of an adult or adolescent stutterer and, therefore, must be considered in planning therapy. The factors are considered briefly here, but some are covered in depth in the chapter on other fluency disorders (Chapter 13).

If a client has below-normal intelligence, he may have difficulty following the regimen of a typical therapy program. Usually, clinicians know beforehand if a client scheduled for an evaluation has Down Syndrome or some other condition characterized by below-normal intelligence. Adolescent stutterers in schools are usually identified as developmentally delayed, if they are, and are also likely to be in a special class. Adults, too, are usually identified as mentally handicapped if this is the case, because either the referral source will report this or a guardian will have filled out the case history form.

Problems of academic adjustment in an adolescent who stutters usually become apparent from either the original referral or interviews with the child's teachers as part of the evaluation process. These interviews are described in more detail in the section on the school-age child. An example of poor academic adjustment relevant to stuttering could be a student's conflict with a teacher who insists on oral presentations that the student is unwilling to do. The IDEA '97 process mandates a team approach to solving such problems. This process will be described in the chapters on treatment.

The research reviewed in Chapter 2 suggests that there are no group differences in the psychological health of stutterers and nonstutterers. However, we sometimes see individuals who stutter who do not function well in their environment. They may be unable to achieve a satisfying marriage, unable to hold a job, or socially withdrawn. Clinicians need to be alert to the effects that adjustment problems may have on treatment. If psychological problems are suspected of interfering with treatment progress, the clinician may wish to refer the client for a psychological evaluation. In such cases, the clinician should take care to ask professional colleagues for recommendations of the most effective psychotherapists in the area.

Psychological problems that are relevant to stuttering also may become apparent during the interview when the onset of stuttering is explored. Sudden onset after a psychological trauma, particularly if onset is in late adolescence or adulthood, may indicate psychogenic stuttering. I have found that, if the psychological effects of the trauma have subsided, an adolescent or adult client may respond well to the integrated approach to treatment described in Chapter 12. If it is clear that psychological factors are still affecting the client's speech and behavior or if there is doubt, I refer the client for a psychological evaluation. Unless the disorder is a psychosis, in which case stuttering therapy may not be recommended, clients with psychological problems may respond well to a combination of psychotherapy and stuttering therapy.

Interview with Parents of Adolescent

When I evaluate an adolescent who stutters, I also talk with his parents separately from the adolescent to obtain more background information about the student, to give them an opportunity to express their concerns and feelings privately, and to tell them about the evaluation process and the options for treatment.

I begin the interview by asking the parents to describe the problem as they see it and encourage them to express their fears, concerns, and frustrations, as I listen carefully. I try to get an understanding of how their child functions within the family and usually ask such questions as: "What is his stuttering like at home?" "How does he seem to feel about it—is he embarrassed or does he show fear of talking or anger?" "How do you feel about it?" "What are your and other family members' reactions to it; what do you do when he stutters?" "Has he been seen anywhere else for therapy?" "If so, what were the results?" Although parents may ask what can be done to help their child and what they should do, I prefer to wait until after I have seen the youngster before answering these questions.

Adolescents strive to become more and more independent of their parents, and I have found that therapy works best if an adolescent is treated as an adult. I begin fostering independence by talking first to teenage clients separately from their parents so that they can give me their own views of the situation and how they view the prospect of treatment. After this and after our meeting with the parents, I meet with the parents and teenage clients together to seek mutual agreement about their respective roles in treatment. This is often an important time. It serves to let teens know that I respect their ability to work independently from the parents, and it serves to let the parents know that they can be most helpful by being supportive but not directive.

Diagnosis

After I gather the information just described, I need to determine whether the client stutters and, if so, what treatment level is appropriate. Typically, teenage clients are advanced stutterers; however, some are still in the intermediate stage. But first, let us consider the possibility that a teenager turns out *not* to be a stutterer.

In rare cases, teens who are normally but highly disfluent may be referred by teachers, employers, or friends. Most have phrase repetitions, circumlocutions, revisions, and hesitations, which are the types of disfluencies described in Chapter 5 as normal. Such disfluencies are observed relatively infrequently after children's elementary school years; however, some adolescents and adults may simply be at the disfluent end of the continuum of normal fluency. In addition to the differences in type and number of disfluencies, secondary behaviors and negative feelings and attitudes will be absent. Our role in such cases is to explain to the individual and to the referring person, if there is one, that this kind of speech is not abnormal and need not be of concern. It may also be emphasized to the referring source that excessive attention to these disfluencies may be more harmful than helpful. If the client or referring person feels strongly that the disfluent speech interferes with communication, a fluency-oriented treatment described in the chapters on treating intermediate and advanced stuttering may be offered to the client.

Another need for differential diagnosis, in addition to identifying cases of normal disfluency, is ensuring that cluttering, neurogenic disfluency, and psychogenic disfluency are distinguished from stuttering. Moreover, it is also necessary to rule out disfluencies caused by word-finding difficulties that we might find in persons with a learning disability.

Some of the salient features of cluttering in adults and adolescents are rapid, sometimes unintelligible speech, frequent repetitions of syllables, words, or phrases, lack of awareness or concern about their speech, disorganized thought processes, and language problems. Cluttering often coexists with stuttering, and both disorders may respond to a highly structured, fluency-shaping approach for treatment. Evaluation and treatment procedures for cluttering are described in Chapter 13.

Neurogenic disfluency in adolescents or adults is usually the result of stroke, head trauma, or neurological disease. Symptoms are likely to be repetitive disfluencies but may include blockages as well. Because stuttering commonly begins in childhood, if a client reports onset of stuttering after age 12, a neurogenic-based disorder is a possibility. In almost all such cases, onsets of neurogenic-based fluency problems are clearly linked to a well-defined episode of acquired neurological damage. A section of Chapter 13 is devoted to evaluation and treatment of neurogenic stuttering.

Disfluency that begins in adolescence or adulthood can also result from psychological trauma. When late-onset disfluencies are seen that are associated with psychological stress and conflict or the onset of a psychiatric condition, psychogenic disfluency should be suspected. Traditional treatments, such as those described in the chapters on treatment of intermediate and advanced stuttering, may or may not be helpful. The patient should be referred for both psychological and neurological assessments, so that treatment needed in these areas will be identified and provided. See Chapter 13 for more information.

When a clinician determines that stuttering treatment would be appropriate for a client, whether the stuttering had a typical onset during early childhood or has another etiology, the focus turns to a consideration of what level of treatment to select for the client. As I indicated earlier, adult and adolescent stutterers are most likely to be at advanced developmental and treatment levels. Signs of this level include the core behaviors of repetitions, prolongations, and blocks, all with tension; the secondary behaviors of escape and avoidance; and negative feelings and attitudes about communication in general and stuttering in particular.

Determining Developmental and Treatment Level

The determination of a developmental/treatment level for an adolescent or adult stutterer is based largely on the client's age. Intermediate and advanced treatment approaches are well suited for clients whose core behaviors are blocks, who have escape and avoidance behaviors as secondary symptoms, and whose attitudes about speech are relatively negative. A client suited to the advanced-level treatment will usually have more entrenched negative attitudes about speech and himself as a speaker simply because he has been stuttering longer. The major difference between intermediate and advanced treatment levels is that more independence and responsibility are required of clients at the advanced level. Consequently, clinicians ordinarily place adult clients at the advanced level but determine an adolescent's placement based on how much responsibility he can take for self-therapy.

Intermediate Stuttering

A client whose stuttering is at the intermediate level will probably be younger than 14 years old. His stuttering pattern will be characterized by escape and avoidance behaviors and considerable tension on blocks, prolongations, and repetitions. He will also be avoiding some speaking situations. Moreover, his feelings and attitudes, as revealed in interviews with him and with his parents and teachers and in questionnaires, will suggest many negative speech attitudes.

Advanced Stuttering

Individuals who fit into the advanced developmental/treatment level are 14 years or older and sufficiently mature to handle the assignments used in advanced treatment. Their stuttering pattern is similar to the intermediate stutterer's, but their patterns of avoidance and escape may be more habituated (i.e., patterns appear to be highly automatized and rapidly performed). They will probably avoid difficult speaking situations whenever possible, and I often find strong negative self-concepts and negative anticipations of listener reactions, as well. An advanced stutterer may feel, for example, "I must be awfully incompetent to talk like this" or "People think I'm dumb because I stutter."

Closing Interview

I will assume here that the client is a stutterer. By this point in the evaluation, I have a pretty good picture of his stuttering and how I will start therapy. I begin by summarizing my impression of his stuttering pattern (i.e., core and secondary behaviors) and his attitudes and feelings. One of my aims is to let him know I have some understanding of his stuttering and why he does what he does when he stutters. I feel it is important to let him know that, given his level of stuttering, it is no surprise that he would use the various secondary behaviors and avoidance tactics that he does. I accept these behaviors rather than criticize them and let him know that I feel we can work with him and help him discover other ways to respond. I try to ensure that he feels he will not be alone, that I will be working alongside him, and that I will gradually give him more and more responsibility to work on his own.

Then, I briefly describe some therapy options and discuss the possibilities with him. With my guidance, the client and I decide on a treatment approach. Afterward, I give him an assignment to begin the process of his taking responsibility for part of his treatment. This will also take advantage of the fact that many adult clients are highly motivated to change at the time they come for an evaluation. I generally don't do this with adolescents, but there are exceptions. Some adolescent clients are reluctant to participate in therapy, rather than being highly motivated, because of their desire to close ranks with their peers and distance themselves from adults. With adolescents, I often end our evaluation session by striking a bargain to try at least four sessions of therapy before they make a decision about treatment. I may also give them the booklet, *Do You Stutter: A Guide for Teens* (Fraser and Perkins, 1987), and the video, *Do You Stutter: Straight Talk for Teens* (Guitar and Guitar, 2003), so that they can learn about therapy on their own and develop realistic and motivating expectations about its potential outcome.

At the end of the closing interview, I ask a client if he has any questions about the evaluation. I also try to answer the questions asked in the initial interview that I postponed for response until after the evaluation. Adults and adolescents sometimes ask how long treatment will take. This is a reasonable question, given that they need to budget time and money to undertake treatment, but I have no easy answer for this difficult question. With appropriate cautions about individual differences and unexpected issues, I reply that, with hard work and a willingness to tackle difficult situations and to confront fears with my help, I believe that considerable progress can be made with a year of treatment.

Summary

- In evaluating a client who may stutter, your task is to decide (1) if his disfluencies warrant treatment; (2) if so, what are the important characteristics of his history, current environment, speech behaviors, and reactions; and (3) what treatment do these characteristics indicate?

- In assessing a preschool child, the important questions to answer are whether the child is stuttering or is normally disfluent, what are the probabilities that he will recover without treatment, and if treatment is needed, should it be indirect (for borderline stuttering) or direct (for beginning stuttering).

- It is important to obtain some information prior to the formal assessment. This includes a recording of the child's speech at home and a completed case history.

- Key elements of the assessment for a preschool child are (1) observation of parent-child interaction, (2) parent interview, (3) clinician-child interaction, (4) analysis of child's speech, (5) screening of language, articulation, and voice, (6) determining risk factors,

(7) deciding on the child's need for treatment, and (8) making follow-up recommendations to family.

■ In assessing a school-age child, the important questions are how supportive the parents are of the child's problem, how the stuttering is affecting the child's performance in school, how the child feels about his stuttering and how motivated he is to work on it, and how supportive the child's teachers are.

■ The assessment of the school-age child may proceed differently if he is been seen in a clinic or at school. If seen at school, the IDEA affects the process and mandates how assessment is carried out. If seen in a clinic, the clinician will have more contact with the family but needs to reach out to the school setting.

■ Key elements of the assessment for a school-age child are (1) initial contact and formal interview with the child's parents, (2) interview with the child's teachers, (3) interview with the child, (4) analysis of speech, (5) trial therapy, (6) assessment of other factors, including academic adjustment, and (7) determination of appropriate treatment.

■ In assessing an adolescent or adult, the important questions are the client's level of motivation and ability to carry out assignments independently, the severity of stuttering and degree of avoidance, the client's feelings and attitudes about his stuttering, whether the problem is typical "developmental" stuttering or is cluttering or psychogenic or neurogenic stuttering, and the appropriate type of treatment.

■ Key elements of the assessment of an adolescent or adult are (1) obtaining preliminary case history, attitude questionnaires, and recordings made outside of the clinic, (2) interview with client, (3) analysis of speech, (4) trial therapy, (5) parent interview if adolescent, (6) determination of appropriate treatment, and (7) summary and recommendations in closing interview with client.

■ Whether the person is to be treated as a normally disfluent speaker or as someone who stutters depends on your interpretation rather than a score. You must weigh what you see and hear to determine whether they indicate stuttering, normal disfluency, or even another disorder. From the flood of information you have gathered, you must extract the essential characteristics that support your choice of treatment.

■ To hone your judgment, make evaluations a continuing process. The procedures I have suggested for assessment and diagnosis in this chapter will give you a good start, but stuttering is highly variable, and no individual can be understood in just an hour or two. Consequently, you will overlook an important element at times, and sometimes a vital clue will not be present in the samples of behavior you see during an evaluation. With good follow-up evaluation of a client, you will be able to change decisions and redirect therapy as additional information and understanding become available. You will also be able to evaluate the effectiveness of your treatment and improve it, when needed.

Study Questions

1. How do you determine whether a preschool child is stuttering or is normally disfluent?

2. Why is it useful to obtain audio-video recordings of a preschool child's stuttering before the evaluation?

3. What are some indications that a parent of a preschool child who stutters feels she or he is to blame? How can you help them deal with those feelings?

4. What do you tell the parent of a preschool or school-age child who asks you what causes stuttering?

5. What are the variables assessed in the speech of a preschooler to determine his developmental/treatment level.

6. What are the advantages and disadvantages of talking to a child about his stuttering.

7. Compare the involvement of the parent and the teacher in the evaluation of a school-age child.

8. In what various ways do we assess the impact of the school environment on the school-age child who stutters?

9. What are the benefits of obtaining both a reading and a conversation sample with school children and adults?

10. In the section on evaluation of the adult and adolescent, what different pieces of information that you may gather from the interview questions help you to assess the client's motivation?

11. What are two reasons we suggest for continuing evaluation after the initial assessment of clients who stutter?

12. Compare the assessment of the feelings and attitudes of a school-age child with their assessment in an adult.

13. What is the role of the IEP team in the management of a school-age child who stutters?

14. What are the goals of trial therapy?

15. What are the major questions to be answered in the evaluation of an adult?

SUGGESTED PROJECTS

1. Role play the part of a clinician in a parent interview, having a friend or classmate play the part of a parent. Practice your listening skills by only listening and asking no questions as the "parent" describes in detail his or her child's stuttering problem. Switch roles, and then compare your impressions of the experience both as the parent and as the clinician.

2. Pair up with a friend or classmate who could pretend to stutter or with a person who stutters and practice trial therapy that is appropriate for a school–age child and then appropriate for an adult. Try both approaches, modifying stutters to make them less severe and modifying speech to produce fluency.

3. Pair up with a friend or classmate who doesn't stutter and have them talk rapidly about a complex topic so he or she produces normal disfluencies. See if they are able to "catch" their normal disfluencies and hold onto them (for example, turn

single repetitions into multiple repetitions or make prolongations longer). Can this be done with normal disfluencies? With only certain types of normal disfluencies?

(4.) Find websites on the internet that contain helpful information for (1) parents of children who stutter, (2) school-age children who stutter, and (3) adults who stutter.

(5.) One of the challenges for clinicians is to get a good speech sample from a child who may be somewhat shy or reluctant to talk to someone they don't know well. Experiment with different ways of interacting with a child until you find a "best" method. For example, try asking lots of questions, try just playing quietly alongside a child, and try playing with a child and making comments about things you are playing together with.

Suggested Readings

Conture, E. (2001). Assessment and Evaluation. In *Stuttering: Its Nature, Diagnosis, and Treatment.* **Boston: Allyn & Bacon.**

In this chapter, Conture covers many details of the assessment not dealt with in this chapter that you have just read. Among these are finer points of audio and video recording, general interview procedures, and analysis of the speech sample. Conture also discusses concomitant problems like attention deficit hyperactivity disorder, Tourette's syndrome, neuromotor problems, and word finding problems.

Guitar, B. (2005). Stuttering. In Parker and Zuckerman (Eds), *Behavioral and Developmental Pediatrics–A Handbook for Primary Care.* **Baltimore: Lippincott, Williams & Wilkins.**

This brief chapter for pediatricians summarizes key questions and important information for parents, criteria for referral, and initial treatment strategies.

Shafir, R.Z. (2000). *The Zen of Listening: Mindful Communication in the Age of Distraction.* **Wheaton, IL: The Theosophical Publishing House.**

This is an excellent introduction to the practice of careful listening. Shafir is a speech-language pathologist who has developed her ability to listen to clients and writes eloquently about the healing powers of mindful listening.

Yairi, E., and Ambrose, N. (2005). Assessment of early stuttering. In *Early Childhood Stuttering.* **Austin, TX: Pro-Ed.**

This chapter gives a thorough description, based on assessment experience with hundreds of children, of how to obtain samples and analyze speech of preschool children who stutter. Information regarding prognosis is given by the experts.

Yairi, E., and Ambrose, N. (2005). Parent involvement and counseling. In *Early Childhood Stuttering.* **Austin, TX: Pro-Ed.**

The authors critically review the literature on ways in which parents can be involved in treatment of early childhood stuttering and conclude that there is little evidence to support any of the approaches.

Yaruss, S. (2003). Facing the challenge of treating stuttering in the schools: Part 1. Selecting goals and strategies for success. *Seminars in Speech and Language,* **23:August 2002.**

This volume of "Seminars" is a rich source of information for school clinicians. Experienced clinicians, many of whom work in the schools, have written chapters on a wide variety of topics, including interpreting IDEA '97, doing an evaluation in a school setting, and planning therapy for school-age children.

Chapter 8

Preliminaries to Treatment

Before presenting the details of treatment, I want to provide some background for the procedures you use, as well as how and why you use them. In this chapter, I will present some ideas about the clinicians who work with people who stutter and how their beliefs about the nature of stuttering influence treatment decisions. I will also describe in some detail commonly held goals for stuttering therapy and the procedures used to achieve them. Let's begin with you, the clinician.

Clinicians' Attributes

The clinician is probably the most important ingredient in stuttering therapy, other than the client. Whether therapy's major focus is behavioral, cognitive, or affective, a clinician's knowledge, skills, and personality have a major influence on outcome. In this section, I will discuss some of the attributes that I think make a clinician effective, and I will suggest how these attributes can be developed. Unfortunately, there are no data that I'm aware of to support the importance, for stuttering therapy, of these attributes, although Rogers (e.g., 1961) and others have spent a considerable amount of time and effort measuring the effects of some of these clinician attributes on treatment success in psychotherapy.

Much of my thinking about the treatment process has been influenced by my experiences as a client and a student of Charles Van Riper. Let us begin, then, with Van Riper's (1975a) description of three clinician characteristics: empathy, warmth, and genuineness.

Empathy

Empathy, in this context, is the ability to understand the feelings, thoughts, and behaviors of someone who stutters. This is, of course, a little easier for clinicians who stutter. However, Van Riper's own clinician, Bryng Bryngleson, was a fluent speaker who showed an impressive understanding of individuals who stutter. Once, when Van Riper was frustrated at his own inability to stutter purposefully to strangers and exhausted from trying again and again, he sought out Bryngleson in his office. Bryng, as he was called, jumped up from his chair and headed for the door, saying "It's okay, Van, just follow me and watch." Bryng then went into a tobacco store, walked up to the clerk, and pretended to stutter with the longest, loudest stutter that Van Riper had ever witnessed. That single gesture had a huge impact on Van Riper because he felt deeply supported by Bryngleson's acceptance of his failure and willingness to risk ridicule to help him.

You may wonder how you can become a truly empathetic clinician. You can increase your empathy with all your clients by working on your ability to listen deeply and acceptingly. It will also help to observe clients' body language, their posture, and the words they use. Van Riper said that he could improve his understanding of a client's feelings if he assumed the same body posture that the client had. You can also get some idea of what clients experience by going out in public, like Bryngelson did, and stuttering voluntarily, although you don't have to stutter as long or as loud. Reading stories written by people who stutter and parents of children who stutter will also help you better understand the experiences that have shaped their feelings. Good examples of such writings are *Living with Stuttering: Stories, Basics, Resources, and Hope.* (St. Louis, 2001) and *Forty Years After Therapy: One Man's Story* (Helliesen, 2002). I'll describe these books and others in the suggested readings at the end of this chapter.

Warmth

This attribute has also been referred to as "unconditional positive regard" (Rogers, 1957). Much of it is conveyed in the tone of voice, facial expression, and body language of the clinician. Clients whose clinician has this warmth feel accepted, liked, and nurtured.

This creates an environment that supports learning and unlearning, and helps clients make difficult changes. Warmth also is expressed in the comments the clinician makes when a client has done something well. It often surprises me, when I watch a videotape of one of my therapy sessions, how many opportunities I miss reinforcing the client with a "Good!" or "Well done!" Clinicians should become aware of how much or how little they show enthusiasm and give encouragement to their clients. These are important tools of therapy.

Genuineness

A third clinician characteristic that Van Riper (1975) described is "genuineness," which he equated with Rogers' (1961) "congruence." Both terms refer to a clinician's honesty and self-acceptance; the clinician just tries to be who she is, "roughness, pimples, warts, and everything" as Oliver Cromwell said on having his portrait painted. Genuineness allows clinicians to be honest with their clients, without sugar coating the hard lumps of reality that must be digested if real progress is to be made. For example, Van Riper said to one of his clients, with his characteristic bluntness, "Why do you have to have all that junk in your speech? Can't you just go ahead and say the word, starting with the first sound and working your way through it slowly, syllable by syllable?" (Van Riper, 1975b). When a client senses the clinician's genuineness, he gains trust and begins to believe that his clinician means it when she asks about his thoughts and feelings, that he can let go and honestly express his frustration, fear, hate, and anger, convinced that the clinician will understand and accept him and his feelings, and be strong enough to be unhurt by them. Clinicians can cultivate their genuineness and strength by being open about their limitations and learning self-acceptance through psychotherapy, spiritual practice, or other experiences that help us accept both our weaknesses and our strengths.

An effective tool for fostering improvement in clinical skills and attributes is videotaping oneself during treatment and watching it after the session. This can be painful initially because it's easy to focus on our flaws rather than our finesse. But we can overcome this tendency and begin to see our effective behaviors as well as our mistakes. If you try this, you will find that, after watching several sessions, your uncomfortable feelings will gradually decrease, and you will be able to study each tape and take pride in your improvements while noting things to work on. Videotape or audiotape replay is a powerful way to improve your clinical practice.

A Preference for Evidence-Based Practice

There are more traits than those three traits just listed that characterize good clinicians. One is a clinician's desire and ability to base her clinical practice on evidence. In choosing tools and approaches for evaluating and treating someone who stutters, a good clinician knows how to find evidence of the reliability and validity of diagnostic measures and data supporting the effectiveness of various treatment approaches. She works together with the client or family in the diagnostic evaluation and thereafter to determine which treatment approach is likely to meet the client's or family's goals most effectively. She frequently measures the client's progress during treatment to assess the effectiveness of the approach she is using and is flexible, creative, and insightful enough to find ways of altering treatment if it is not working as well as it should. Many treatments, including those described in this text, have relatively little data that support their effectiveness. This does not preclude their being used, but a clinician should be careful to assess how well they work for her clients with measures made before, during, and after treatment. Ideas and information on evidence-based practice can be found in Bothe (2004), Frattali (1998), Guitar (2004), Pietranton (2003), and Sackett et al (2000). In the treatment chapters that follow, I will suggest how to measure changes in behaviors that are targeted for treatment.

A Commitment to Continuing Education

Another important attribute for clinicians is the habit of continually updating knowledge gained in graduate school. New methods of evaluation and treatment are developed every year, and new data on treatment effectiveness become available. It is vital for the clinician to keep up to date with the latest and best practices. Journals are the best source of this information, but recent editions of books that review diagnostic and treatment methods for stuttering can also be helpful. For the very latest publications, Internet search engines can scan the literature on stuttering, and the American Speech-Language-Hearing Association (ASHA) has recently made a search engine called "The Dome" available to members at a low monthly cost. New approaches to treatment often require training, and short courses at the annual ASHA convention and workshops offered through schools, hospitals, state associations, and other institutions are excellent sources of such training. However, before adopting a new approach, a clinician should critically analyze the quality of evidence that supports its claim to effectiveness, as described in the next section.

Critical Thinking and Creativity

Clinicians should become discriminating consumers and ask, "Which new diagnostic tools and treatment approaches are effective and which clients are they appropriate for?" Some new approaches are not all they are cracked up to be. For example, many years ago, a well-known psychologist and his colleagues (Azrin and Nunn, 1974) suggested that teaching clients to take a breath and relax before speaking was an effective treatment for stuttering. Researchers at another clinic tested the approach and found it to be far less effective than its developers had claimed (Andrews and Tanner, 1982). Nevertheless, there may be some aspects of relaxation and breathing that are useful for some clients in the hands of a clinician who becomes skilled at integrating these tools into a broader approach.

Another critical question is, "Will this approach work for my clients in my environment?" Often a treatment that works under laboratory conditions with carefully selected subjects does not work as well in the real world of a public school, for example. But a clinician may be able to adapt an approach to suit her situation. For instance, an approach developed for young children in tightly controlled clinical studies with total fluency as its goal may need to be altered so that some degree of easy and open stuttering is an acceptable outcome when this approach is used with older children.

Clinicians' Beliefs

It is important for clinicians to weigh their beliefs about the nature of stuttering against the available data and then develop clinical procedures compatible with those beliefs supported by the data. My own beliefs about the etiology and development of stuttering that were presented in the first few chapters are reviewed here only in enough detail to illustrate how a clinician's theoretical view affects her clinical decisions.

I believe that predisposing physiological factors interact with developmental and environmental influences to produce or exacerbate core behaviors that often (but not always) begin as repetitions. When a child responds to these early disfluencies with increased tension and hurried speech, various secondary or coping behaviors and negative feelings and attitudes are acquired. Escape behaviors are learned through instrumental conditioning, speech fears are learned through classical conditioning, and word and situation avoidances are learned through avoidance conditioning. All of these factors and how they contribute to stuttering are reflected in the developmental/treatment levels I described in Chapter 5.

So, how does this point of view about the etiology and development of stuttering affect treatment? Let's use the management of school-age children who stutter to illustrate this point. In my view, a child's treatment plan is determined by his level of stuttering, and each advance in level requires new components in treatment. A second-grader with beginning stuttering who is not embarrassed or afraid to talk and who doesn't avoid talking should be treated differently than a fifth-grader with intermediate-level stuttering who is beginning to develop fears and avoidances in response to his stuttering. The second-grader may be treated with an approach that doesn't deal with negative feelings and avoidance behaviors, but this fifth-grader needs to have help with these aspects of his stuttering. In contrast, a clinician with other beliefs about the nature and development of stuttering or the effects of treatment on negative emotions and avoidances might treat both children with the same approach.

Another way in which a clinician's beliefs can affect management is in the assessment procedures she uses. Assessment tools should provide clinicians with information that is essential for planning treatment and measuring progress. In evaluating the second-grader and fifth-grader just described, I would evaluate each child's feelings and attitudes about his speech, as well as his use of word and situation avoidances, to accurately determine each child's developmental/treatment level and decide which aspects of the problem to focus on first. Another clinician, for example, one who has no theory of the etiology and development of stuttering, might simply want to measure each child's frequency and severity of stuttering.

A third way in which a clinician's beliefs about the nature, development, and treatment of stuttering can affect clinical behavior is in counseling the parents of her clients. In counseling the parents of these two school-age children, my beliefs would guide me to describe the etiology of stuttering as being unknown at present but as probably related to the way a child's brain processes speech and language. Using terminology appropriate to the parents, I would talk about brain processing that may predispose a child to stutter, and I would emphasize that this suggests that things that parents do don't cause stuttering. I would also explain that the child's way of processing speech and language can be changed; consequently, parents can be vital in helping a child overcome or manage it. I would also discuss with parents the importance of factors in the environment that might be contributing to the child's stuttering problem and discuss ways of modifying these factors. Last, I would use my understanding of the development and nature of stuttering to give parents a general idea of the course of therapy and possible outcome. Clinicians with other beliefs might not go into the nature of stuttering because they feel it is not well understood and, instead, would just counsel the parents about their role in the child's treatment.

Treatment Goals

Treatment goals will vary with a clinician's beliefs and a client's developmental/treatment level. It is still possible, however, to describe most of the goals that clinicians have for clients who stutter and to suggest which goals are likely to be paramount for which level. Individuals differ in their strengths and weaknesses at the outset of treatment, and these change as treatment proceeds. Thus, a clinician needs to ask herself, "What does this client need? What does he need from me? What does he need from me right now? And why?" (Van Riper, 1975, p. 477).

The clinician is not the only one who determines the goals of treatment. Clients and their families have an important role to play in choosing goals that are important for them. Ongoing discussions between clinicians and clients about treatment goals will strengthen clients' motivation to achieve them and enhance the relationship between the clients and clinicians. The following statement by Donald Baer, an eminent behavioral psychologist, expresses this philosophy.

> It seems only reasonable to learn that when stutterers are given control of the therapeutic consequences that presumably can change their output, some of them choose different targets than would their therapists or, probably, other stutterers, and some of them target not so much their speech output as they do a private response that they describe as sense of "imminent loss of control." (Baer, 1990, p. 35)

The selection of goals presented in this section owes much to the *Guidelines for Practice in Stuttering Treatment* (American Speech-Language-Hearing Association, 1995).

Reduce the Frequency of Stuttering

This can be achieved in a variety of ways, but it is important to reduce the frequency of stuttering without creating other behaviors, such as taking deep breaths before speaking, that are distracting to the listener (and speaker) and may, therefore, hamper communication. This goal is appropriate for all developmental/treatment levels of stuttering; note that for children at the borderline and beginning levels, the goal should be to reduce frequency of stuttering to zero.

Reduce the Abnormality of Stuttering

Much of the abnormality of stuttering comes from the conditioned tension and struggle behaviors that occur during moments of stuttering, and reducing this tension and struggle is an important goal for clients who are at intermediate or advanced developmental/treatment levels. In addition, such escape behaviors as eye blinks and head nods are also appropriate targets for treatment. It may not be possible to eliminate all clients' stuttering, but it can be changed so that it is easy and comfortable both for the speaker and the listener and doesn't interfere with communication. Van Riper and other experienced stuttering clinicians have suggested that a stutterer may not always have a choice about whether he stutters or not but he does have a choice about how he stutters. This choice includes stuttering in a way that is easier and briefer than his old habitual pattern.

Reduce Negative Feelings About Stuttering and About Speaking

Clients who have more sensitive temperaments may be more vulnerable to feelings of embarrassment, fear, shame, and other negative feelings. These can quickly become part of a cycle in which stuttering gives rise to negative feelings, which, in turn, increase tension and other struggle behaviors that generate more negative feelings. Classical conditioning plays a major role in this cycle, so that deconditioning and counter-conditioning, which will be discussed in the treatment chapters, are useful. Reducing negative feelings is an important goal for clients with intermediate and advanced stuttering. These feelings need to be attacked directly in clients who have strong negative feelings but may be dealt with indirectly if a client is able to substantially reduce the frequency and abnormality of his stuttering. A major difference among treatment approaches is in how they deal with clients' negative feelings.

Reduce Negative Thoughts and Attitudes About Stuttering and About Speaking

In Chapter 5, I described how people who stutter might develop negative self-concepts through repeated experiences of stuttering and perceiving, correctly or incorrectly, that listeners are impatient or disapproving. As these perceptions become more and more deeply ingrained, they begin to affect a stutterer's expectations in speaking situations, which increases the likelihood that he will begin speaking with fixed, tense articulatory postures that trigger stuttering. Treatment of intermediate and especially advanced levels of stuttering may include working directly on negative thoughts and attitudes, or a clinician may assume that they will be improved by repeated experiences of improved fluency.

Reduce Avoidance

Avoidance behaviors, as you will remember, are evasive maneuvers taken by individuals to keep from stuttering. Sometimes they may occur very close in time to the expected stutter, such as saying "um" or "well" just before attempting to say a feared word. Other times, they may be quite separated from the expected stuttering, such as not volunteering to be in a school play or driving some distance to talk to someone rather than telephoning her. Some stutterers may have an innate predisposition to avoid because of their temperaments, as suggested in Chapters 2 and 3. Avoidances keep stuttering "hot," because they prevent an individual from learning that it is possible to stutter in an easy fashion and communicate well. Reducing avoidance is usually not the first treatment goal on the list, although it may be the most important goal for more advanced levels of stuttering. Usually, before helping a client reduce avoidances, clinicians need to help him reduce negative emotions about stuttering and teach him to stutter more easily. Reducing avoidances is a major goal for intermediate- and advanced-level stuttering, although some approaches work indirectly.

Increase Overall Communication Abilities

The ability to communicate easily and well varies a great deal from client to client. It may be affected by severity of stuttering, temperament, avoidances, and communication models in the family. For many of us who work with individuals who stutter, effective communication is a major goal of treatment. Some clients will become effective communicators once the frequency and severity of their stuttering, along with their negative feelings and attitudes about speaking and stuttering, have been reduced. For other clients, guided practice and structured experiences in effective communication are essential. Once clients feel they can communicate effectively, they often begin to seek out talking experiences, their avoidances drop away, and they become comfortable and open about any remaining stuttering that occurs. The goal of effective communication is most needed for clients with intermediate and advanced stuttering, who have developed avoidances. Many of these clients, especially clients with more severe stuttering, have been preoccupied with their stuttering and have not spent much time learning to communicate effectively (Curlee, personal communication, March 3, 2004).

Create an Environment That Facilitates Fluency

This goal is paramount for working with borderline stuttering, which can often be treated by helping the family reduce pressures on the child's speech and increase positive aspects of the child's speaking environment. For example, family members can spend one-on-one time with the child, using a slow speech rate and careful listening skills, thereby increasing the child's daily opportunities to experience fluency. This goal may also be important for beginning and intermediate stuttering, but if such children are in school, teachers and aides, as well as family members, need to be enlisted in facilitating the child's fluency. Clients with advanced stuttering can make their environments facilitating to both fluency and easy stuttering by being open about their stuttering and sharing with others how listeners can be most helpful to them.

Therapy Procedures

The aim of this section is to outline the tools and strategies that clinicians can use to work on each of the treatment goals that I have just described. By understanding which procedures are most likely to be useful in achieving each goal, clinicians can select those procedures that best suit each client and that are in accord with their own beliefs. The procedures outlined here are fully described in the therapy sections on each developmental/treatment level.

Procedures to Reduce the Frequency of Stuttering

Operant conditioning procedures are often part of treatment approaches for achieving this goal and typically involve reinforcement for fluency and mild punishment for stuttering. Note that the word "punishment" is used in a technical sense, referring to any stimulus that reduces the frequency of a behavior, rather than anything hurtful.

Rewards may be verbal, such as the clinician's praise or approval, or tangible, such as tokens that can be redeemed for snacks, prizes, or an opportunity to take a turn in a game. Mild punishment may simply be calling attention to a stutter or requesting the individual to try the word again. Rewards for fluency and mild punishment for stuttering are most often the primary tools used for beginning stuttering and are often coupled with a hierarchy based on the complexity and length of utterances. In this case, clients move from producing one or two words fluently, to saying longer phrases, and then to spontaneous speech. Reward and punishment may also be used as "shaping" tools for intermediate- or advanced-level stuttering, in which clients begin by speaking in a way that produces instant fluency (such as speaking very slowly) and then progress to more and more normal-sounding speech in more and more difficult situations. The general name for treatments that focus on increasing fluency rather than decreasing the abnormality of stuttering is fluency shaping.

Procedures to Reduce the Abnormality of Stuttering

Many approaches do not target the abnormality of stuttering because they depend on reducing the frequency of stuttering to near zero. Therapies that specifically target the abnormality of stuttering most often use reward and mild punishment to change long and tense stutters into increasingly briefer and more relaxed ones and to diminish clients' use of escape and avoidance behaviors. To meet this goal, reward and punishment are used most often in the context of a systematic program for reducing negative emotions (see next goal). Such programs are founded on the belief that negative emotions elicit increased tension, escape, and avoidance behaviors and that such behaviors are maintained by negative reinforcement (i.e., reduction/elimination of the eliciting negative emotion). These approaches are often referred to as "stuttering modification." A classic stuttering modification approach is that of Van Riper (1973, 1975b), which uses a progression of having the client (1) learn to correct a stutter immediately after it occurs by saying it again but in an easier fashion, then (2) learn to change a stutter into an easier production of the sound while it's still going on, and then (3) learn to start a word the client expects to stutter on in an easy, slow, relaxed fashion that makes the stutter very mild. Interestingly, both stuttering modification and fluency shaping, despite the fact that they start out so differently, often end up with a similar result: a modified style of speaking that contains brief disfluencies that are produced in a slightly slower than normal way of talking.

Procedures to Reduce Negative Feelings About Stuttering and Speaking

This goal is directly addressed by clinicians who believe that negative emotions are a crucial part of intermediate and advanced stuttering but are unlikely to diminish as a by-product of reducing the frequency of stuttering. Instead, these clinicians use deconditioning or counter-conditioning to deal with such feelings because many of these emotions have been classically conditioned to be associated with stuttering. This approach entails associating stuttering with neutral or positive experiences. Clinicians can do this in many ways, as you will see later in the descriptions of various treatments. One example is having clients stay in the moment of stuttering (i.e., continue stuttering rather than finishing the word), while the clinician comments approvingly; another example is having school-age children compete with each other to see who can produce the longest or loudest or funniest stutter. Voluntary stuttering is also a powerful way to reduce negative emotions. By deliberately producing the kinds of stuttering that previously elicited embarrassment and fear, clients begin to feel in control of themselves and the situation, and their negative emotions begin to subside. Clinicians' models of voluntary stuttering while remaining calm are also a potent tool for desensitizing clients to the negative emotions associated with stuttering.

Negative emotions associated with speaking are often the products of repeated experiences of embarrassment, fear, and shame while stuttering in certain situations. One example of a situation that can elicit these emotions for someone who stutters is having to say his name when a teacher or group leader says, "Let's go around the circle and introduce ourselves." Such emotions are often reduced when clients learn to use techniques that reduce the frequency and abnormality of their stuttering and then re-experience the situation repeatedly without embarrassment, fear, and shame. In addition, the negative emotions of many clients are reduced when they are open about their stuttering and put their listeners at ease by commenting on it. Because negative emotions are often the products of negative thoughts and expectations, the procedures described for the next goal are also appropriate for dealing with a client's negative emotions about speaking.

A final procedure for dealing with negative emotion is counseling. This is one of the most important ways of helping parents of children who stutter, and it is also a crucial element in working with the emotions associated with intermediate and advanced stuttering. Principles of counseling are described in each treatment chapter, but it is worth noting here that *listening* is one of the most critical aspects of counseling. Empathetic listening and other aspects of counseling are discussed in *Counseling Persons with Communication Disorders and Their Families* (Luterman, 2001) and illustrated in the videotape *Counseling* (Zebrowski, Guitar, and Guitar, 2002). An excellent guide to improving listening skills is *The Zen of Listening* (Shafir, 2000).

Procedures to Reduce Negative Thoughts and Attitudes About Stuttering and Speaking

There are a number of therapy procedures that can help clients become more realistic about how listeners perceive them and what this may mean to them. Cognitive therapy, for example, can be an excellent technique for helping clients think and feel more positively about their speech, listeners, and the situations that have elicited negative emotions in the past. Clients can learn to examine their thought processes and to understand how what they *think* influences what they *feel* and how they *act*, particularly in regard to such maladaptive behavior as muscular tensing that leads to more stuttering. Some clinicians use cognitive therapy as their sole treatment; others use cognitive therapy as a supplement to techniques for learning to speak fluently or to stutter in an easier way. The book, *Cognitive Therapy: Basics and Beyond* (Beck, 1995), is a good source for learning this approach, and I will discuss cognitive therapy in the chapter on advanced stuttering.

Procedures to Reduce Avoidance

Some clients have very little avoidance, and once they learn to speak fluently, they enter speaking situations freely, without expectation of difficulty. Others, however, because of temperament, learning, or both, have a strong tendency for avoidance. Minor avoidances may appear in beginning stuttering, but avoidance is a problem that must be addressed at the intermediate and advanced levels. Treatment to reduce avoidance should begin by reducing negative emotions, particularly fears of stuttering and of listeners' reactions. Fear of stuttering can be tackled by rewarding clients with praise, support, or tangible reinforcement for "catching" a stutter and holding on to it. Fear of listeners' reactions can be lessened by clients voluntarily stuttering to acquaintances and strangers. When a stutterer can deliberately imitate his typical stuttering pattern and pretend to stutter, he finally feels in control during a stutter; in addition, the feeling of "stuttering" while also feeling in control is highly rewarding. Reducing fear is not enough, however. Studies of animal behavior have shown that, even when avoidance symptoms disappear after fear is reduced, fear eventually returns and so do its symptoms, like conditioned avoidance behaviors (Ayres, 1998). Thus, new responses to the old stimuli must be taught. In stuttering therapy, an example of learning a new response to an old stimulus is for a stutterer to slow his speech rate as he says a word he expects to stutter on. This is an aspect of the "preparatory set" used in many stuttering modification approaches, as well as the "downshifting" to a slower rate before attempting a difficult word, which may be taught in fluency-shaping programs.

Avoidances are not confined to the moment just before a difficult word. Individuals who stutter may also avoid opportunities to speak by pretending to be busy when the telephone rings or by waiting for someone else to make introductions of new acquaintances. These avoidances can be treated by helping a client construct a hierarchy of easy to difficult speaking situations in which he can use newly learned stuttering modification or fluency-shaping techniques. Clinicians can also motivate clients to continue seeking out new situations in which they can be open about their stuttering and can use their new strategies to manage stuttering. At meetings of the SpeakEasy Associations of Australia and the U.S. and conventions of the National Stuttering Association, there are always impressive testimonials by clients who have sought out public speaking opportunities, joined Toastmasters, or found other ways of increasing their approach behaviors and decreasing their tendency to avoid stuttering and speaking.

Procedures to Increase Overall Communication Abilities

For many children, adolescents, and adults, communication blossoms when fears of stuttering and listeners' reactions are reduced and ease of speaking is increased. For others, long-standing habits of avoiding speaking situations and the accompanying lack of social experience have stunted the growth of their communication skills. For still others, concomitant problems, such as attention deficit or extreme shyness, may have prevented them from learning how to communicate well. Communication skills should be addressed in treatment whenever it appears that they are not appropriately developed. Observations of a client's communication and reports from a school-age child's teachers will indicate the areas that may need to be addressed. Specific skills that can be worked on include eye contact, turn-taking, maintaining a topic, making relevant contributions to conversation, speaking intelligibly, clarifying and repairing what was said, and developing a willingness to initiate and maintain communicative interactions with others (Kent, 1993; Smith, McCauley, and Guitar, 2000). Although these skills can be worked on individually, group therapy provides excellent opportunities for clients to practice the skills. Direct instruction, modeling, role-playing, and videotaped feedback with discussion can be used to teach and refine communication skills.

Procedures to Create an Environment That Facilitates Fluency

Preschool-age children, especially those on the borderline between normal disfluency and stuttering, may need only a little change in their environment for their stuttering to disappear permanently (Starkweather, Gottwald, and Halfond, 1990; Gottwald and Starkweather, 1999). Treatment focuses on parents (e.g., counseling the parents to reduce their anxieties, modeling for them, and continuing to support the changes they make). Parent-child interactions are usually the key element of the environment that can be changed to facilitate fluency. Video recordings and playback of these interactions in the clinic or observations at home, coupled with parent counseling, can help parents improve how they communicate with their child (Guitar et al, 1992). Parents usually work on creating a facilitating environment during brief, one-on-one daily sessions with the child. In some families, other aspects of the environment may need to be changed, such as the home's hurried pace of life, stressful life events, and the communication styles of other family members. Preschoolers with beginning-level stuttering may also benefit from a direct approach, involving contingencies for fluent speech and stuttering.

For school-age children, the creation of facilitating environments may include working with the child's family, but the school setting may be equally important, if not more so. Clinicians often work in partnership with a child or adolescent to make school a "fluency-friendly" environment. The clinician may arrange meetings with the child and his teachers to improve the teachers' understanding of his stuttering and to open lines of communication between the child and his teachers. A child's peers can be invited to treatment so that they may improve their understanding of the child's stuttering, while the process of the child's openness about his stuttering with other children is begun.

Freely discussing his stuttering with other students is one of the most effective ways for a school-age child to make his environment more fluency friendly. For some children, a powerful boost can be given to therapy's progress if they are able, with the clinician's help and support, to make a presentation to their class about the nature of stuttering, in general, and their stuttering, in particular. Not all children are willing to take this risk.

Openness about stuttering is also a major way in which adults can create a supportive environment. By commenting on their stuttering, by showing a sense of humor about it, and by sharing what techniques they're working on, adults who stutter can create environments in which their listeners are quite comfortable with the adults' stuttering. This helps them feel free to use various fluency-enhancing techniques.

My own treatment for each level and the treatments of several other clinicians are presented in the next four chapters. Both my own approaches and those of other clinicians have been developed and refined, usually over several years' of trial and error. When possible, supporting data are provided for each treatment, but in many cases, where such data are not available, I suggest what data would be appropriate.

Summary

- The clinician's attributes are a vital ingredient in treatment success.

- Empathy, genuineness, and warmth are three clinician attributes that have been suggested to be important by Van Riper (1975a).

- A vital component of best clinical practice is choosing evaluation procedures and tools that have been shown to be valid and reliable.

- Best clinical practice dictates (1) choosing treatment procedures that have reliable and valid evidence of effectiveness, (2) adapting treatment procedures to fit clients' needs, and (3) continuing to assess improvement in attributes that have been chosen as goals for treatment.

- Continuing education is vital to keep abreast of new approaches and new evidence of effectiveness of diagnostic and treatment procedures.

- It is important for clinicians to develop an informed set of beliefs about the nature of stuttering and to fit assessment and treatment procedures to those beliefs.

- Goals for treatment and for continuing assessment should come from not only the clinician's beliefs but also from the client's (or his family's) informed choices.

- Treatment procedures for meeting these goals can include methods of reducing frequency and severity of stuttering and secondary behaviors, reducing emotions and thoughts that interfere with fluency, increasing communication abilities, and developing environments that facilitate fluency.

Study Questions

1. What are the three important characteristics of a clinician described by Van Riper?

2. How might each of these characteristics facilitate progress in treatment?

3. What are the characteristics of evidence-based practice?

4. How might two clinicians' beliefs about the nature of stuttering result in two very different treatment approaches? How might these beliefs result in two similar treatment approaches?

5. Which of the treatment goals described in this chapter are appropriate for borderline stuttering?

6. Which treatment goals are appropriate for beginning stuttering?

7. Which treatment goals are appropriate for intermediate stuttering?

8. Which treatment goals are appropriate for advanced stuttering?

9. Describe the differences between the "fluency shaping" and "stuttering modification" approaches to treatment.

10. How might reducing negative emotion reduce stuttering frequency?

11. How might reducing stuttering frequency reduce negative emotion?

12. Describe, for each developmental/treatment level, which goal (reducing negative emotion or reducing stuttering frequency) you would start with and why.

SUGGESTED PROJECTS

(1) Videotape yourself and a client during an evaluation or a treatment session. The first time you watch it, note only the things you think you do well. The second time you watch it, note two things you would like to improve. Meet with a colleague or supervisor and discuss how to improve the things you would like to and then work on those aspects in another session, and videotape yourself again. Watch this new tape for improvements in the behavior(s) you have chosen to work on.

(2) Choose a test you use (or would like to use) in your evaluation procedures, and try to find evidence of its validity and reliability.

(3) Choose a treatment procedure you use (or would like to use), and search the literature to see if you can locate any information about its effectiveness.

(4) Find a stuttering treatment approach that is described in detail and determine what the goals of treatment are, what the procedures to reach these goals are, and whether there is a description of how to measure progress of these goals. Examples of such approaches are: *Systematic Fluency Training for Young Children* by Richard Shine (Pro-Ed, Austin, TX), *Fun with Fluency–Direct Therapy with the Young Child* by Patty Walton and Mary Wallace (Imaginart International, Inc, Bisbee, AZ), *Cooper Personalized Fluency Control Therapy for Children* by Eugene and Crystal Cooper (Pro-Ed, Austin, TX), and *A Primer for Stuttering Therapy* by Howard Schwartz (Allyn and Bacon, Boston).

(5) Describe in detail your own beliefs about the nature of stuttering applied to children with intermediate stuttering. Given these beliefs, what therapy goals do you have for a child with intermediate stuttering?

Suggested Readings

Bothe, A. (Ed) (2004). *Evidence-Based Treatment of Stuttering: Empirical Bases and Clinical Applications.* **Mahwah, NJ: Lawrence Earlbaum.**

This text, available in hardcopy or electronic format, contains chapters dealing with data on stuttering treatments and the scientific basis of treatment approaches.

Cordes, A., and Ingham, R. (Eds) (1998). *Treatment Efficacy for Stuttering: A Search for Empirical Bases.* **San Diego: Singular.**

This is an excellent volume of papers by clinician-researchers who are searching for a scientific foundation for the treatment of stuttering. As the introduction makes clear, this book is the outcome of a continuing series of conferences on this topic.

Guitar, B., and Peters, T. (2003). *Stuttering: An Integration of Contemporary Therapies.* **Memphis, TN: Stuttering Foundation of America. www.stutteringhelp.org.**

This book describes in detail the two approaches mentioned in this chapter: fluency shaping and stuttering modification.

Manning, W. (2001). *Clinical Decision Making in Fluency Disorders* **(ed 2). San Diego: Singular.**

The first chapter describes many aspects of the clinician as well as of the clinical interaction in stuttering therapy. Also relevant to the material discussed earlier is Chapter 6, "Facilitating the Change Process." Manning describes goals for treatment and subtleties of how and when to work toward them.

Proceedings of the NINCD Workshop on Treatment Efficacy Research in Stuttering, September 21-22, 1992. *Journal of Fluency Disorders*, **18 (2&3), September, 1993.**

This issue of the journal contains chapters by more than a dozen specialists in stuttering treatment and research. Each chapter deals with an area related to treatment efficacy. Although they are somewhat out of date, these chapters are good examples of the kind of literature reviews that need to be redone every 2 or 3 years.

Shapiro, D. (1999). The Clinician: A Paragon of Change. Unit IV. In *Stuttering Intervention: A Collaborative Journey to Fluency Freedom.* **Austin, TX: Pro-Ed.**

This section of this textbook contains two chapters on clinician characteristics. Chapter 11 deals with the "magic" of the client-clinician relationship and touches on many of the attributes needed by effective clinicians. Chapter 12 discusses the processes of students becoming qualified clinicians. The author discusses the many aspects of supervision and analysis of clinical interactions.

Van Riper, C. (1975a). The Stutterer's Clinician. In J. Eisenson (Ed), *Stuttering: A Second Symposium.* **New York: Harper & Row.**

This ancient chapter is still a useful description of the attributes that may be important in clinicians who treat stutterers. It also contains excellent sections on clinicians' roles in motivating clients and discusses the subject of whether clinicians who themselves stutter should treat clients who stutter.

Chapter 9

Treatment of Borderline Stuttering

An Integrated Approach

Treatment of borderline stuttering combines two principles, working with the environment to decrease stress and working with the child to increase fluency. The initial focus is on the family and on decreasing their concern, trying to understand their feelings, and helping them change selected aspects of the family-child interactions. If a child's family can discover ways to facilitate the child's fluency, they become confident in their ability to effect change and are able to assume long-term responsibility for the child's fluency. If this is not effective or is slow to take effect, direct work on the child's speech by both the clinician and family is appropriate.

Author's Beliefs

Nature of Stuttering

As I described in Chapters 4 and 5, borderline stuttering occurs as a result of the interplay between the a child's constitutional predispositions and the stresses resulting from developmental demands and the environment. Treatment for a borderline stutterer is based on the assumption that stresses on the child and his speech can be decreased, his stuttering will taper off, and he will become normally fluent. I believe that the plasticity of normal neural maturation allows most of these children to compensate for constitutional predispositions toward stuttering. For such flexibility in development to blossom into normal fluency, however, the clinician and family must provide an environment that fosters fluency and diminishes negative experiences with speaking. And this must be done promptly. If too much time passes, the child may become negatively aware of his stuttering and become frustrated by it. If this happens, frustration combined with the child's concern about negative listener reactions may push his stuttering beyond the borderline level into beginning and even intermediate stuttering. These more advanced levels of stuttering are usually more resistant to treatment.

With borderline stuttering, I seldom treat the child directly, at least not at first. Instead, I work with the child's family to help them reduce environmental stresses. Stress is normal in the life of every child, but the child with borderline stuttering may simply be more vulnerable to fluency breakdown under normal stresses. As you will see in my description of clinical procedures, I usually begin by informing and educating family members about ways they can reduce stresses and foster fluency. I demonstrate a facilitating style of communicative interaction as a model for the family and meet with them once a week to support and guide their efforts in finding ways to help their child.

If indirect therapy is not effective in reducing stuttering after 6 weeks or if the child's stuttering proves to be more advanced than initially thought, I add more direct procedures. My direct approach for borderline stuttering, which assumes that the child is aware of stuttering, consists of a hierarchy of activities that focus on playing with stuttering and changing it to a milder form.

Speech Behaviors Targeted For Therapy

Because I don't treat the child's speech directly, none of the child's speech behaviors are specifically targeted for direct change. Instead, the family's interaction styles, including both speech and nonspeech behaviors, are the focus of treatment. For example, I help family members learn to speak in a slow and relaxed manner, and I support their efforts to make other aspects of their interactions with the child who stutters as unstressful as possible. In those rare instances when this approach doesn't soon decrease stuttering, the child's repetitions and prolongations are targeted for change.

Fluency Goals

I believe that all children who stutter at the borderline level can achieve spontaneous fluency. With effective early intervention, this goal is readily achievable because the child's maturing nervous system gradually increases his capacity for fluent speech.

Feelings and Attitudes

The main focus of treatment is on the behaviors of family members and others who interact frequently with the child. Consequently, the child's feelings and attitudes are not directly dealt with. However, as the family and I monitor the child's fluency, we try to ensure that he is not developing negative attitudes about speaking or about his disfluencies. If the child's borderline stuttering persists and shows periodic worsening, he may become more frustrated by it when it is at its worst and may soon acquire the escape behaviors seen in beginning stuttering. In these cases, the addition of more direct intervention is used to deal with such feelings.

Maintenance Procedures

Many children with borderline stuttering achieve fluent speech soon after their families have made some environmental modifications, and most maintain fluency without further treatment. However, it is important to keep in contact with the family even after formal treatment has stopped to prevent their reverting to old, more stressful interaction patterns. This contact, through telephone calls or email, is gradually faded.

Clinical Methods

Working with borderline stuttering involves a variety of therapy procedures. I educate families by providing them with videotapes and reading material to help them understand the nature of stuttering and the ways in which they can help their child become more fluent. I counsel families by listening to their concerns and trying to understand their hopes, desires, fears, and frustrations. I brainstorm and problem solve with families when I help them choose aspects of their interaction patterns to modify. I collect data on the child's speech and on the family's perceptions of his stuttering and fluency. And finally, I provide support as the child's stuttering decreases and the family strives to maintain their new styles of interaction.

Clinical Procedures: Indirect Treatment

Indirect treatment begins during the evaluation. As I described in the preschool section of Chapter 6, part of the evaluation involves studying family interactions, listening to descriptions of the home environment, and asking about factors that may be associated with fluctuations in the child's fluency. When the stuttering is diagnosed as being at the borderline or beginning level, families are provided with materials to help them understand what their role in treatment may be. I often ask families to watch the video, *Stuttering and the Preschool Child: Help for Families* (Guitar, Guitar, and Fraser, 2001; Stuttering Foundation video #70; www.stutteringhelp.org), and then discuss it with them at the first treatment session. Other material for family education is described in the Suggested Readings section at the end of this chapter.

If you followed the procedures in Chapter 6 for evaluating a preschool child, you will have done a preliminary analysis of factors in the environment that may make a vulnerable child more disfluent. In the following section, I provide more details on this analysis.

Studying Family Interaction Patterns

The family's interaction patterns, which can be assessed from videotapes or observed directly, often give clues about aspects of how the family talks or interacts with the child that may stress the child's fluency. Remember, these stresses are usually not from abnormal or negative family interactions. They are often typical patterns of talking among family members. However, the vulnerable child may benefit from some modification of them. One of the first things I do in treating the borderline stutterer is to help the family decide which aspects of their interactions should be considered for change. Here are some aspects of conversational interactions that are "normal" in busy homes but that may put pressure on a borderline stutterer:

1. High rates of speech
2. Rapid-fire conversational pace (lack of pauses between speakers)
3. Interruptions
4. Frequent open-ended questions
5. Many critical or corrective comments
6. Inadequate or inconsistent listening to what the child says
7. Vocabulary far above the child's level
8. Advanced levels of syntax

After observing 10 or 15 minutes of family-child interaction, an experienced clinician usually has some hypotheses about which variables might be important to help the family change. For example, family members' speech rates may be unusually fast, or they may interrupt each other frequently when conversing, or they may convey high expectations of the child through critical or corrective comments.

Less experienced clinicians may want to follow the suggestions in Table 9–1 for developing their skills for assessing family interaction variables. As was described in Chapter 7, it is helpful to have a recording of a family interaction before the evaluation, and I ask the family to record 10 minutes of a typical conversational interaction with the child when he is likely to stutter. This might be, for example, at a time when one or more family members are playing together with the child.

In some cases, it will not be possible for the family to make a recording before the evaluation; or, it may be that a noisy recording prevents assessment of key variables. In these instances, the family interaction recorded in the clinic can be used. Family members

---

Table 9–1 Suggestions for Quantifying Family-Child Interaction Patterns

1. **High rates of speech.** Count the number of syllables spoken by each family member interacting with the child. Next, using a stopwatch, measure the amount of time each individual speaks. Be sure to stop timing whenever they stop speaking or pause for more than 2 seconds. Resume timing as soon as the speaking continues. Then, calculate the time in minutes to hundredths of a minute (e.g., 1 minute and 13 seconds would be 1.22 minutes). Divide the total number of syllables spoken by the time in minutes to obtain the number of syllables per minute (SPM). For example, if a family member speaks 366 syllables in 1.22 minutes, their rate of speech is 300 SPM. Normal adult speaking rates are 180 to 220 SPM. Thus, this is a fast rate of speech.

2. **Rapid-fire conversational pace (lack of pauses between speakers).** Using a stopwatch, measure intervals from when the child stops speaking and when another family member begins. If these intervals average less than 1 second, the pace of conversation is rapid.

3. **Interruptions.** Count the number of sentences or sentence-like utterances the child speaks during the sample and the number of times a family member interrupts the child. Divide the number of interruptions by the total number of sentences. If more than 10% of the interruptions, the child may feel pressure to speak quickly.

4. **Frequent questions.** Count the number of sentences spoken by family members to the child and the number of sentences that are questions. Divide the number of questions by the total number of sentences. If more than 25% of the utterances are questions, the child may feel pressure from having to answer questions.

5. **Many critical or directive comments.** Each sentence of family members should be characterized as being either "critical/directive" or "accepting/nondirective." Sentences characterized as critical/directive would be (1) those that convey that the speaker does not unconditionally accept the child, his actions, or his words; (2) those that pressure the child to speak or direct the child's activity; and (3) those spoken with a tone of voice that is stern or incredulous. The number of sentences that are critical should be divided by the total number of sentences. If the percentage of critical/directive comments is higher than 50%, the child may feel stress from high standards in the family.

6. **Inadequate or inconsistent listening to what the child says.** Assess the content of family members' sentences during each speaking turn. Note whether family members are responding to the content of the child's utterances. If more than 50% of family members' utterances ignore the topic the child has been speaking about, the child may feel he is not being heard.

7. **Vocabulary far above child's level.** Compare the vocabulary level of family members' speech with that of the child. If more than only a small amount of the family members' vocabulary exceeds the child's receptive level, the child may feel pressure when trying to understand family members' vocabulary.

8. **Advanced levels of syntax.** Assess the syntax used by family members when speaking to the child. If more than only a small amount is considerably above the child's current receptive level, the child may feel pressure not only to understand family members, but also to use syntax that he has yet to master.

---

are asked to interact with the child in a room outfitted with an array of quiet materials (paper, crayons, dolls, and games) to ensure an audible recording. Once a good recording is in hand, the clinician can make a transcript of a 10- or 15-minute interaction and quantify the eight variables listed in Table 9–1. Some clinicians will not be able to record the family interaction pattern but will make notes as they directly observe it.

Involving the Family in Change

During the diagnostic evaluation (see Chapter 7 for details), I also gather information about other important aspects of the child's environment. These include such things as the busyness of the family's daily schedule, the amount of individual attention the child receives, and how the family reacts to the child's stuttering. Using this information, I develop some tentative hypotheses about which factors may be important in influencing this child's stuttering. I keep these hypotheses to myself for the moment, first because they may be wrong and second because it is more effective for the family to lead the way in choosing what and how to change. Toward the end of a diagnostic session, I summarize my findings about the child's speech, concluding with a description of his borderline level of stuttering, and then help the family decide how to facilitate the child's fluency.

I begin by telling the family, using appropriate vocabulary, that research suggests that stuttering first arises from an innate predisposition toward disfluency. Therefore, the child's stuttering wasn't caused by something they did or did not do. I point out that a child who has a predisposition to stutter may be especially sensitive to certain speech pressures that are typical of a normal home environment. Such pressures may trigger the appearance of stuttering in the first place or may make it harder for the child to outgrow it. I note that other children have improved when their families have been able to create an environment that is especially helpful to fluent speech. I make it clear that, although they did not cause the child's stuttering, there is much they can do to help him overcome it.

I ask the family to observe and make notes about the child's stuttering and fluency for 1 week, and then I schedule a second session. I also suggest specific areas for the family to observe based on my experience with other families, such as their speech rate and conversational pace. I also suggest areas that I hypothesize may be important to their child. I try to be nondirective and guide them with suggestions, such as those in Table 9–2, and with materials for parents of children who stutter, such as the video *If Your Child Stutters: Help for Families,* which is available from the Stuttering Foundation.

The First Treatment Session

In the first session after a diagnostic evaluation, I help the family begin to change the child's environment. I discuss their observations and readings with them, establishing a supportive, nonjudgmental relationship and remaining alert to comments that suggest they feel they may have caused their child's stuttering. Such feelings are not unusual and need to be acknowledged as natural; however, I always suggest reasons why it is unlikely that they caused their child's stuttering. For example, I may point out that their other children, who grew up in the same environment, don't stutter. I have found that reducing family members' guilt and anxiety makes it easier for them to focus on the changes in family interactions and household routines that we will be discussing. In the sharing of ideas to facilitate a child's fluency, I usually talk about changes in both family-child interactions and the household routine. Changes in interaction patterns are often more subtle and may be difficult to make. Therefore, I offer to role-play the interactions that I and the family mutually consider important to try to change.

Modeling Interaction

I ask the family to observe me playing with the child as I model one or two changes, such as a slower rate of speech and increased pausing. If I have a room with a one-way mirror, the family can observe from another room. If another clinician or a student is available,

---

Table 9–2   Things Families Can Do to Help the Borderline Stutterer

1. **Listening time.** All children benefit from feeling that what they have to say is important. This is especially true for the child who is beginning to stutter. Set aside some time each day as "listening time" with your child. Make it 15 to 20 minutes at about the same time each day, so your child can depend on it. During that time, refrain from making suggestions or giving instructions. Merely "be there" for the child, listening attentively to what he or she says or quietly playing alongside the child, if he or she chooses not to talk.

2. **Slow rate.** Family members may reduce their conversational rate of speech to a slow, soothing style. Speech should sound relaxed and calm, with comfortable pauses throughout. Fred Rogers on the television show "Mr. Rogers' Neighborhood" is a good model.

3. **Pauses.** The pace of conversation can be kept appropriately slow if the speaker pauses 1 to 2 seconds before starting to talk. This also helps to keep the speaker from interrupting another speaker.

4. **Positive comments.** Make many positive and accepting comments about what your child is saying and doing. Limit corrections or criticisms to important issues. Changes for the better usually happen more quickly when someone feels they are okay as they are. The child who feels good about himself will be better able to use "listening time," "slow rate," and "pauses" to gain more fluency.

5. **Fewer questions.** It is natural to ask a child many questions in order to encourage him to learn new things and to display that knowledge. However, this makes some children feel "under the gun." So, it may be a good idea to decrease demanding questions and instructions. If you are worried that your child won't learn enough if you are too laid back, keep in mind that learning comes naturally to children. They learn best from your interest in things, especially from your interest and positive comments about the things they do and say.

I have this person observe with the family and point out good examples of the interaction style I am modeling and also ask the other clinician or student to point out not-so-good examples in my interaction. A family trying to change is rarely helped by a perfect model. Sometimes, I model interactions without a one-way mirror or someone to help me by playing with the child while the family sits nearby and observes (Fig. 9–1). After the interaction, we discuss the things I have been trying to model for them.

After 5 or 10 minutes of letting the family observe, I invite them to participate. Sometimes, I have only one family member participate at a time. At other times, both parents or other family members participate. Who participates depends on what we are working on as well as which family members have attended the session. When a family member participates in the play session, I pull back and let him or her be the primary player. I observe family members and note whether or not they are demonstrating the desired behaviors. If they are, I continue to observe and let them practice. If not, I usually rejoin the interaction and provide further models of the desired behavior.

After another 5 or 10 minutes of observing a parent or other family member play with the child, I arrange to talk briefly with the family in private toward the end of the session. Knowing how difficult such changes can be, I give as much positive feedback as I can about the interaction, even if I can praise only their efforts to change. Gordon Blood (personal communication, 1994), an accomplished stuttering clinician, says that he tries to use a 5:1 ratio of positive to corrective comments. Even if a family member has shown little change, I search for ways of making the experience of trying to change as positive as possible.

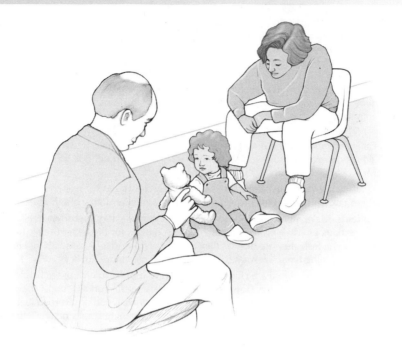

Figure 9–1   *Clinician models interaction patterns while the mother observes.*

Discussing Changes in Family Routine

In addition to changing conversational interaction patterns, a family may identify other stresses on the child that need to be changed, such as the amount of individual attention the child receives and the "busyness" of the family's schedule. My main function in helping families work on such stresses is to give them information about areas of changes that others have found helpful and to be a sounding board for their plans for changing. I encourage them to assess, informally, the effects of these changes on the child's fluency and his overall adjustment. Although my praise and appreciation may help, a significant change in the child's stuttering is the real motivator.

One factor in parent-child interaction is of particular importance: the attention that a child receives from his parents contributes immensely to his self-esteem, which, in turn, affects fluency. When a child senses that his mother or father understands him and genuinely cares about him (cares about what he likes to do, what he thinks about things, and how he feels), the child feels more comfortable with himself, is less anxious, and is better able to speak easily. For many children with borderline stuttering, a little more one-on-one time spent with a parent each day, preferably in the morning, can boost fluency tremendously. Although the morning can be the most difficult time for parents who work outside the home, work on fluency in the morning can have a positive effect on the child's speech for the rest of the day. The time does not need to be long, just 15 to 20 minutes, but the parent needs to be with the child in a place where they won't be interrupted.

The child should choose what to play or talk about, and the parent should follow the child's lead, participating as the child directs. As a parent becomes more and more comfortable with this nondirective play, he or she may want to explore ways of helping the child feel really understood. One of the parents we worked with, for example, would "mirror" her child's momentary emotions as they built a tower of blocks together. When the child placed a block on the tower and it fell off, she would quietly murmur a word of disappointment, echoing the child's facial expression. This child made impressive gains in fluency in only a few weeks, and I believe that this parent's deep attention to the child may have contributed significantly to this change. Although not every parent could be expected to achieve the level of empathetic response that this mother did, increased caring attention is probably a realistic goal for most families.

Attentive play can become child-directed conversations as a child grows older, and such conversations can continue the process of helping the child develop a sense of being loved, understood, and appreciated. An excellent description of one-on-one time between parents and school-age children can be found in the article, "Making Time for Your Child" by Stanley Greenspan, M.D., in *Parents* (August, 1993). With borderline stutterers, we often work with families in changing the family-child interaction style as well as setting aside a one-on-one time each day. This combination gives family members a specific time to practice fluency-facilitating verbal interactions. If it is done in the morning, the child may be calmer and more receptive to the relaxed interaction style and may carry over the fluency achieved to the remainder of the day.

At the end of the first therapy session, I help families to formulate plans for implementing changes and for continuing to note conditions associated with the child's fluency and stuttering. I encourage them not to take on too much but to concentrate on just one or two changes, and I arrange to meet with them again within 1 or 2 weeks to continue assessing, guiding, and supporting their attempts to help the child.

Subsequent Sessions

In sessions that follow, I am eager to find out if family members have tried to change aspects of the child's environment. However, I avoid asking them directly when I first greet them. Even "How's it going?" asked routinely at the beginning of every session may make our expectations weigh heavily on them. Instead, I endeavor to maintain a positive, low-pressure interaction style as a model of what we want them to use with their child and this also allows them to decide how they'd like to begin. As family members describe what they have been observing and doing since the last session, I carefully look for things to praise. As I said before, families often feel that they are to blame for their child's stuttering; therefore, it is vital to give them sincere, positive feedback about what they are *doing well.* It is also the best way to help anyone learn new skills.

Sometimes families report that their attempts to make changes have been fairly successful. For example, they may have been able to slow their speaking rates and to simplify their language and may have seen improvement in their child. I let them know that their changes have been key factors in the child's improvement and stress the importance of continuing them. It is easy to resume old patterns after some improvement occurs, whether it's the challenge of losing weight or helping a child become more fluent.

Each child and family are unique in how they respond to treatment, but it is possible to note some common trends. For example, some children become much more fluent soon after the family makes one or two changes in their environment. Occasionally, a child may become fluent immediately after an initial session, possibly because the family is much less anxious about his disfluencies after sharing their concerns with a professional. Whatever the cause, early and immediate fluency gains should be viewed with cautious optimism. I share the family's pleasure at such dramatic change but suggest that their child's fluency may be fragile and will need to be nurtured by our continued efforts to create a facilitative environment.

Sometimes the path toward fluency is rough and irregular. The child may make a little or no progress or may improve for a while and then return to his old pattern of disfluency. When this happens and the family or clinician feels frustrated by slow progress, further exploration of the family's feelings about the child's stuttering is called for. Many times family members worry about the child's future, afraid that stuttering will be a serious handicap for him. Sometimes there is lingering guilt about having caused his stuttering. Often it is hard for parents to accept the blemish they feel that stuttering is on the family image.

Whatever the source of a family's anxieties, their concern about stuttering may easily radiate to the child in their reactions to his stutters. Unwittingly, family members may show their anxiety or disappointment through facial expressions or body language, which may make the child "hesitate to hesitate" and, thus, stutter more severely. Open and frank discussions with the family about their feelings and concerns are likely to be more helpful at this point than trying to change their reactions. In such discussions, the clinician's role is to make it easier for the family to talk about their concerns; so I listen carefully, try my best to understand them, and convey my understanding with acceptance and respect. When family members feel understood and accepted, it is easier for them to share their feelings and accept them. When this occurs, some feelings may change, and in turn, the child's stuttering may decrease, possibly because his stuttering no longer seems so terrible.

Another barrier to changing a family's interaction patterns is the fact that some styles of interaction reflect important cultural values. For example, in the urban eastern United States, family members frequently finish each others' sentences, conveying a closeness and solidarity within the family that is highly valued. If they are asked to speak more slowly and pause between speakers' turn takings, such changes would conflict with one of the family's implicit cultural values. Another example might be parents who frequently teach, correct, and criticize their children's behavior. This "instructional" mode of interaction may reflect the importance that the family's culture places on education.

I believe it is important to explore how the family feels about changes they are considering. In some cases, they can find ways to change other variables that will be as effective, thereby leaving unchanged those interactions that are of value to the family. Several years ago, I worked with a parent who spoke very rapidly to her child who was showing some borderline stuttering. She resisted changing her speech rate because "it isn't the way we talk." In addition, she was frequently critical of her child's behavior. Consequently, I trained her to use positive reinforcement for fluency, as described in the treatment of beginnng stuttering, which I adapted from Onslow, Andrews, and Lincoln (1994), and asked her to let her child know, with upbeat statements of praise, that she liked his smooth fluency. The child's stuttering diminished almost immediately, and she was delighted with her ability to help her child.

Sometimes a family may resist change and doesn't fully participate in treatment. There may be psychological issues that need to be resolved through referral to a family counselor, or the family may have other, more serious problems to cope with. In such cases, I talk with the family directly about my concerns. This usually leads to an open discussion of their situation, a referral to a family counselor, or, in rare cases, their decision to withdraw the child from stuttering therapy for the time being. If this happens, I let the family know that I remain available to them, and I try to stay in contact by occasional phone calls or emails to make it easier for them to resume the child's therapy if they wish to.

Maintenance

Indirect treatment of a borderline stutterer is often effective within five or six sessions, over a period of 1 or 2 months. The child's speech becomes markedly less disfluent. Part-word repetitions become whole-word or phrase repetitions, and the family's concerns about the child's speech diminish. When this happens, I review the changes the family has made with them and the changes in their child's stuttering that reflect his improvement. Using this information, I help the family develop a plan to deal with periods of increased stress that may prompt stuttering to reappear. Most families feel that they have a handle on how to reduce stress on their child at this stage of therapy, and their experiences in observing and changing their behaviors have given them confidence. If their child's stuttering suddenly increases, they know how to examine their speech rates or attentiveness when talking to the child and how to examine other aspects of their interactions and implement needed changes.

Effective maintenance for borderline stuttering is the result of two things: (1) helping the family to view the child's stuttering more objectively, with less anxiety, guilt, or panic, and (2) building the family's confidence in their own ability to implement problem-solving skills they've learned to use when the child's disfluencies increase. Sometimes, however, despite a family's best efforts to respond constructively, stuttering returns. This may occur after an increase in stress from some trauma or from normal life events, such as moving to a new house, or it may accompany a growth spurt in the child's language. On the other hand, it may be unexplainable. Whatever the cause, the family should feel comfortable getting back in contact with the clinician. I let each family know at the end of therapy that relapse is possible and is not abnormal and that I would look forward to seeing the child again if help is needed.

Supporting Data

Several years ago, my colleagues and I published a study that evaluated the effect of changing parent-child interactions with a 5-year-old child who stuttered (Guitar et al, 1992). Although this child's level of stuttering was at the beginning level rather than borderline, the principles of working with the family on their interaction style were similar to those described for borderline stuttering. Our approach to treatment was to videotape parent-child interactions over five treatment sessions and view them with each parent. When viewing the videotapes, we let the parent decide what to work on in the intervening week and then videotaped a new parent-child interaction after a week of work on changing the behavior they had selected. After six sessions, the child's stuttering had diminished to the level of normal disfluency; we followed the child for 10 years and the stuttering never reappeared.

Further supporting data on this approach will be presented in the outcome measures of the Michael Palin Centre's treatment of preschool children in Chapter 10. Moreover, a new report by Franken, Kielstra-van der Schalk, and Boelens (in press) provides evidence of the effectiveness of parent-child interaction therapy.

Clinical Procedures: Direct Treatment

My approaches to therapy change as I learn more about children who stutter and treatment options. Recently my choice of a direct treatment approach for those borderline stutterers who have not responded to indirect treatment has been the Lidcombe program, which described in detail in Chapter 10. The material in this section on direct treatment has been helpful in the past, and I would recommend it to those clinicians who do not choose to use the Lidcombe program or who have not yet been trained in it.

I don't use direct treatment with every child who is a borderline stutterer, but it is a powerful alternative when indirect treatment does not decrease the child's stuttering after 6 weeks or if the family's anxiety about the child's speech is abnormally high. The causes of failure with an indirect approach are often unknown. Sometimes, a family seems unable to modify the child's environment as planned, or they do, but the child's stuttering persists unchanged or increases. In these few cases, if the child's disfluency remains at the borderline (rather than beginning) level, I try a slightly more direct approach, as described in the next section.

Direct Treatment for Mild Borderline Stuttering

Most children with borderline stuttering are only slightly aware of their disfluencies. Their repetitions appear relaxed, and they show no signs of extra effort or attempts to "fight" their stutters. They also are normally fluent a great deal of the time and have, I think, the capacity to develop entirely normal fluency. Consequently, when I use direct treatment for mild borderline stuttering, I focus on the child's fluency, assuming that they will easily be able to increase the amount of fluency they have and "outgrow" their stuttering with our help. I follow much of the behavioral management strategies used by the Lidcombe Program, which is described in Chapter 10. I train parents to respond to fluency with praise, and unlike the Lidcombe Program, I ask them to ignore stuttering unless the child is momentarily distressed by a stutter, in which case, I suggest the parents comment acceptingly on it. Thus, it is not, strictly speaking, a Lidcombe approach.

I usually begin by training one of the child's parents to use praise for fluency during the daily one-on-one time with the child. The parent might say, "Gee that was really smooth talking," or "I like the way you said that." The clinician and parent should decide how frequently to use positive reinforcement, but most children are annoyed by praise if the parent gives it too often. A good ratio to begin with is one praise for about every fifth fluent utterance. These fluent utterances do not need to be consecutive.

As in parent-child interaction therapy, parents keep daily logs of the child's overall fluency for each day, using the 1 to 10 severity ratings described earlier. When the child has made substantial progress in decreasing severity, the clinician guides the parent in gradually replacing praise for fluency in the daily one-on-one sessions with praise used occasionally during other activities during the day. While the parent is carrying out this direct therapy, it is critical for him or her to attend weekly meetings with the clinician to demonstrate using the procedure, to share severity ratings, and to discuss progress and problems. It is also important for the family to continue one-on-one sessions with the child and to continue the changes made in their interactions and family lifestyle.

Direct Treatment for More Severe Borderline Stuttering

Some children with borderline stuttering are beginning to have negative feelings about their disfluencies but are not showing the full-blown signs of physical tension or escape behaviors that characterize beginning stutterers. Still, they may occasionally express real frustration with their stuttering. Others may evidence signs of both borderline and beginning stuttering, as predominantly easy repetitions become physically tense and abrupt under stress, leading the child to begin showing signs of alarm. These are children whom we feel are vulnerable to stress and who need to be inoculated against the negative emotions that they are beginning to attach to stuttering and that will get stronger unless we address these emotions without delay.

Typically, I work with children having more severe borderline stuttering for about 45 minutes each week. I also continue to provide encouragement and support to the family in helping them make the child's environment as facilitating to fluency as possible. Our direct treatment activities are presented in a hierarchy that the clinician and child ascend as far as is necessary to bring the child's disfluencies into the range of normal. Progressive steps are taken when the clinician senses that a child is feeling competent at the current step. Thus, progress may be rapid or slow or sudden or gradual, depending on the child's feeling of comfort and mastery with the tasks at hand. There is no need to hurry this process. It should take place within the context of games and activities that make the focus on stuttering casual. The clinician needs to remain alert to the child's immediate sense of confidence and self-esteem in selecting the moment to move the child to the next step in the treatment hierarchy.

Modeling Easy Stutters

I begin direct treatment rather indirectly by providing models of easy stuttering in my speech. If the child's repetitions are fast and abrupt, my models are slow with gradual endings. If the child has many repetitions or long prolongations, I repeat only a few times or prolong sounds briefly. These models are done casually during play with the child. I don't produce them immediately after the child stutters but insert them randomly, about once every two or three sentences, as if I were stuttering as I talked.

Once the child has become acclimated to the models of easy stuttering after 10 or 15 minutes of play, I begin to make accepting comments about them. I might say, for example, "Hmmmm, I bounced a bit on that word, didn't I?" or "That word stuck a little, but that's okay." Most children appear to be shyly interested in what I am talking about, and direct therapy can continue to develop. A few, however, may react negatively and say such things as, "Don't do that!" or "I don't like it when you do that." For them, direct therapy needs to proceed slowly to allow my acceptance and support during play activities to gradually counteract the child's anxiety.

If the child has begun to experience the first pangs of frustration from stuttering, which can be inferred from his questions or complaints about getting stuck on words, I will try to help the child express this. Even though I am making comments that show acceptance of my own stuttering, I occasionally may produce a longer than usual stutter and say, "Sometimes they go on for a long time. That feels weird." I continue to try to sense what the child is feeling and to empathize as naturally as possible. I use this emphatic focus not only when I am modeling easy stutters, but throughout direct treatment.

For children who evidence periods of acute frustration with their stuttering, parents should be coached on how to make emphatic statements in a calm, soothing, slow style when the child is going through a difficult time. As I do direct therapy, I try to involve the parents in appropriate activities both at home and in the clinic. If their indirect treatment has not been effective, I need to be sure they do not feel pushed aside by my direct therapy.

The Child Begins Active Participation—"Catch Me"

When I sense that a child is comfortable with my easy stuttering models, I see if the child will take part. I may say, for example, "Can you help me? Sometimes when I get stuck on a word, it goes on and on. Then I try to make my stuck words real slow and loose, and it helps me get unstuck. But sometimes I forget. If you hear me go on and on like thi-thi-thi-thi-thi-this, just say, 'There's one,' and I'll try to make it slow and loose." When the child catches me, I will change a fast, tight repetition to a slow, loose one. As I model stuck words, I choose a style of stuttering similar to the child's.

Praise should flow liberally when the child catches one of my modeled stutters. This provides the child with an initial sense of competence that is associated with something he previously felt to be out of control. For many children, tangible rewards, such as small snacks or turns at a game, are important motivators and should be used along with praise to establish the child's ability to catch the clinician's stutters.

The Child Begins Active Participation—Play

This stage can either follow or precede "Catch Me." It depends on the clinician's judgment about which activity would be more comfortable for the child. Sometimes you may start one of these two stages but find the child is not ready and switch to the other. The "Play" stage engages a child in following the clinician's lead in playfully imitating disfluencies that are similar to his own, such as repeated or prolonged sounds. The purpose is to desensitize the child to the frustration that sometimes arises in borderline stuttering. It is a process that may take place because play can give a child a sense of mastery without the risk of failure. The concept of play is quite interesting. Many scientists speculate that children's play is an opportunity for them to practice and master skills that are needed in adulthood. Playing with stuttering may take advantage of children's natural tendency to play and provide them with the pleasure of mastery and control over something that has been frustrating and, sometimes, even frightening.

Take, for example, the child who stutters primarily in a repetitive fashion. The clinician might say, "Let's play a game of saying some sounds over and over and see how many times we can say them. I bet I can say a sound five times! Watch this. Ba-ba-ba-ba-ba! Can you do it five times?" Or, it can begin by making sounds for animals, puppets, or other toys: "Hey, this is a zebragella! It goes 'lllllla! llllla!' (using prolongations). Then it jumps around like this ('jump-jump-jump') and eats carpet ('eat-eat-eat')."

The clinician and child can keep incorporating such play into their routine as long as the child finds it fun. From playing with repeated or prolonged sounds, the clinician can build a bridge to playing with repeated or prolonged sounds in conversation and, in time, to the child's actual stutters.

The Child Produces Intentional Stutters

After the child is able to catch the clinician's stutters and appears comfortable doing it, the clinician should begin looking for opportunities to ask the child to produce a stutter intentionally. This can be done most easily by pretending to have trouble producing slow, loose stutters. For instance, the clinician might say, "I can't seem to make this one slow and loose. Can you show me how to do it?" Again, this should be done intermittently and casually mixed in with other activities.

Praise and, if needed, tangible rewards are used to help the child build confidence. When the child is able to produce slow and loose stutters, the clinician can let the parents know, in the child's presence, about this accomplishment, focusing on the child's ability to teach the clinician. If the child seems proud of this accomplishment, the clinician can take advantage of this opportunity and have the child show intentional stutters to the parents. This not only desensitizes the child to stuttering with the parent, but it also desensitizes parents to the child's stuttering and models acceptance of the child's stuttering for them.

The Child Changes His Own Real Stutters

For many children whose stuttering fluctuates between borderline and beginning levels, these direct therapy activities, combined with a facilitating environment provided by parents, may be enough to advance their fluency into the normal range within a few months. For those whose stuttering persists, still another stage of direct therapy may be necessary. In such cases, I look for opportunities when the child seems ready to modify his own stutters.

I begin by responding to a few of the child's real stutters with accepting comments to help the child feel comfortable with his stutters. I might say, with an accepting voice, "Oh, that one was a little bumpy on 'my-my-my car...,'" and then return to the business of playing. After further play, when the child stutters again, the clinician can model an easier and slower style of stuttering on the same word and comment positively about it. I then ask the child to imitate my easier stutter and praise him for doing so, using reinforements and guidance to shape his stuttering to a slow, relaxed style.

I look for slightly slower and easier stutters in the child's speech and reward them. Even if the child intentionally stutters, but in an easier way than he stuttered previously, I reward him. From this point on, the clinician uses a combination of modeling and reinforcement to shape the child's stuttering. It is the deliberate slowness and "easiness" with which the child produces repetitions or prolongations, along with the sense of playing with stuttering, that make it possible for the child to begin feeling a sense of control. This, in turn, should reduce his frustration and fear, further diminish tension, and enable him to move through stutters with minimal effort.

After the child is able to make his stutters slower and easier in the clinic, generalization may occur away from the clinic without the need for formal transfer activities. Such "spontaneous" generalization may be a result of the child's increased self-esteem from gaining mastery over behavior he previously felt uncomfortable about and felt was out of his control. Consequently, emphasis should be placed on the stutters that a child handles successfully, rather than when he loses control.

If generalization is not occurring automatically, I work with family members to make the child's ability to play with and modify stutters a point of pride at home. Initially, the child can teach parents and siblings to stutter in the clinic under the clinician's guidance. Then the clinician can work with the child at home and involve family members when appropriate, so that the parents learn to use positive reinforcement selectively to increase the child's slow and easy stutters and let him know that he is appreciated. Even though the emphasis here is on slow and easy stutters, the effects of speech and language maturation and the increasing confidence that the child feels in his speech as a result of reduced frustration should result in normal fluency.

Other Clinicians

The approaches of several other clinicians are described here. Many of these approaches are used not only for borderline stuttering, but for beginning stuttering as well. I have selected them because they all involve the child's family, which I consider of major importance when working with borderline stuttering. The degree of intervention ranges from monitoring the child's stuttering to helping parents change their interaction patterns to direct work on the child's way of speaking, if needed.

With the exception of Conture's approach, the effectiveness of these treatments has not been formally assessed. Clinicians using them should be aware of this fact and, as with any approach, should carefully assess their own effectiveness when using any of them, even when using those that have supporting data. As suggested in Chapter 8, baseline measures of the child's stuttering at the beginning of treatment should be made in a valid and reliable way. Because preschool children are highly variable, recordings of the child's speech should be made at home as well as in a clinical setting. The Stuttering Severity Instrument-3 should be used to assess frequency and severity. When treatment begins, weekly measures of progress should be made; percentage of syllables stuttered in the clinic and daily severity ratings of speech at home made by a parent are effective and efficient. When the child has achieved fluent speech (severity ratings at home of 1 [normal fluency] and less than 1% syllables stuttered in the clinic), a maintenace program should be started, involving continued measurement at home and during gradually faded clinic visits. Children with borderline stuttering can be expected to achieve stable, normally fluent speech within 6 months.

Richard Curlee

Curlee (1993, 1999) believes that most young preschool-age children who begin to stutter will recover within 2 years of onset without treatment, which is supported by findings from several longitudinal studies (Andrews and Harris, 1964; Yairi and Ambrose, 1999; Mansson, 2000). Consequently, his approach to borderline stuttering focuses on identifying which children should receive treatment without delay and which are likely to stop stuttering if treatment is deferred while their disfluencies are monitored systematically.

His diagnostic and evaluation procedures begin by obtaining a thorough case history from the parents several days before their child is seen in the clinic. The parents are asked how long they have been concerned about the child's fluency, what kinds of disfluencies are causing concern, how the child's disfluencies changed since they first became concerned, if the child reacts emotionally to his disfluency or expresses concern about it, and if there is a family history of stuttering. At the conclusion of the interview, the parents are given a Stuttering Foundation of America booklet to read and are asked to videotape the child talking with them or other family members and to bring the recording to the clinic when they return for the child's evaluation.

The clinical evaluation begins with observation and videotaping of the child and parents interacting together with a game or book brought from home. He, or another clinician, then enters the room and joins the parents' and child's interaction. From time to time, speech-language screening procedures are mixed in with games and play to determine if the child's speech and language skills are age-appropriate. After detailed analyses of the child's stuttering-like disfluencies from the videotapes of parent-child interactions at home and at the clinic and with the clinician are completed, another meeting with the parents is scheduled to discuss evaluation findings and to consider the child's management alternatives.

When evaluating a child's stuttering on the initial visit and subsequent recordings, Curlee makes careful observations of the child's stuttering pattern. Taking into account research of Yairi (1997a) and others, Curlee suggests that a child's stuttering is more likely to become chronic if the following disfluency types are increasing: multiple-unit repetitions (li-li-li-li-like this), prolongations, and tense pauses with fixed articulatory postures (blocks). In addition, he notes that muscle tension associated with stuttering, escape, and avoidance behaviors and a child's negative emotional reactions to stuttering are signs that stuttering may be worsening. If recordings show that these signs are more consistent or increasing as the child is monitored over a period of 6 months, he recommends that treatment begin without further delay.

On the other hand, there are certain indications that suggest to Curlee that treatment may be deferred for a year or more without harming the child or adversely affecting later treatment. These indications are: (1) if a child has been stuttering for less than a year, (2) stuttering has not become more frequent, consistent, or severe during this period, (3) no other speech or language problems are present, and (4) neither the family nor the child is distressed by the child's stuttering. In these cases, Curlee asks the parents to decide if they want treatment to begin as soon as possible or prefer to defer treatment while active monitoring of the child's speech is initiated to determine whether stuttering will stop without the child receiving treatment or it appears to be persisting and is, therefore, in need of treatment.

Monitoring consists of having the family audiotape or videotape the child's speech during various interactions, which are analyzed monthly by the clinician. Clinic visits by the child and parent are scheduled every 2 or 3 months. However, if analyses of the recordings and reports from parents indicate that the child's stuttering is decreasing, clinic visits may be delayed as long as 6 months.

For some children, however, Curlee does not use systematic monitoring, but he initiates treatment immediately after the initial evaluation. These are children for whom a number of critical factors suggest that stuttering is likely to persist unless treatment is initiated. These factors include the presence of frequent stuttering-like disfluencies together with one or more other speech-language problems, a family history of persistent stuttering, and the presence of consistent stuttering-like disfluencies that are not diminishing over a period of a year. Curlee also initiates treatment if the family requests treatment instead of systematic monitoring but states that most parents decide to initiate monitoring procedures for a while. With some families, Curlee may begin therapy by working with family-child interaction patterns if his analysis of their speech rate, length and complexity of utterances, and turn-switching pauses appear to place stress on the child. In other cases, he may use a home-based direct treatment, such as the Lidcombe approach described in Chapter 10, or he may opt for a two or three session per week treatment regimen in the clinic.

Curlee does not provide outcome data on his approach, but it should be noted that the emphasis of his writings are on the process of choosing which young children to treat and which to monitor for a period before deciding whether or not to treat. Substantial data on the Lidcombe approach are available in the next chapter.

Edward Conture

Conture's therapy for preschool children (Conture, 2001; Conture and Melnick, 1999) is carried out in separate parent and child groups that meet concurrently, one time per week. The two groups meet for 12-week blocks, although most children need more than one block of treatment to reach the dismissal phase. The group of mothers and fathers are provided information, suggestions, and opportunities to help them facilitate their child's fluency. They also discuss child-rearing issues that directly affect their child's ability to receive maximal benefit from treatment. Such issues include behavior management and fostering an appropriate degree of independence in their child. The children's group helps the children learn the skills of effective communication and gives them tools to use when they have trouble talking. It is conducted with each child sitting on a small rug on the floor, except when the parents join the group in the last 15 minutes when they all sit at tables and chairs.

Communicative Interactions

Activities in the children's group begin with rules that foster good communication, which include listening when someone else is talking, taking turns in conversations, and not interrupting. These rules are described to the child verbally and augmented by brightly colored pictures depicting each of the three rules. Much of the parent group activities are focused on improved communicative interactions that dovetail with these rules, so that parent-child conversations at home increasingly facilitate the child's development of fluency, related speech and language behaviors, and ease of communication. The following strategies are learned by the parents over the course of the 12 weeks:

- Not interrupting the child
- Speaking more slowly to the child
- Appropriately adjusting the length and complexity of utterances to meet requirements of the communicative situation

- Decreasing the number of corrections of the child's speech, language, and related communicative behaviors
- Not talking for the child

Parents in the group are asked first to observe their speaking behaviors with their child, as well as the child's speaking behaviors, and then encouraged to discuss their observations with the group. Subsequently, parents learn how to make changes in these behaviors and practice them in a single setting, once a day for 10 to 20 minutes. This helps them experience and learn these changes in a relatively controlled setting, such as nightly bedtime rituals, before trying them in more spontaneous situations, such as during conversations at the dinner table. The first new behavior parents are asked to practice is to pause for one second after the child finishes speaking before they start speaking. This change will reduce how often parents are interrupting their child and creates a more relaxed speaking environment for the child, one in which he is more likely to feel that he doesn't have to hurry to speak. The pause will also reduce the extent to which parental communicative behavior may encroach on the time during which the child may be planning and producing spoken language.

Subsequently, parents discuss and practice other new behaviors on the list and are encouraged to use the group to support each other in planning situations in which they can try out these changes and then share the results of their efforts. Parents are most successful when they don't try to change all of their behaviors in all situations but work on only one or two at a time in such specific situations as talking with their child at a meal or reading a bedtime story.

Direct Therapy

For most of the children, one or two blocks of group treatment (12 or 24 sessions) will be adequate to make them fluent enough to be gradually weaned from therapy. For those children who don't recover during this period and who may have more advanced symptoms or concomitant problems, a more direct approach is used. This involves both individual therapy and group treatment in which the child is taught to stutter more easily. Stuttering is discussed in terms of "hard" and "easy" ways to say words. Repetitions, prolongations, and blocks are identified by terms such as "bumping," "skidding," and "getting stuck" so that the clinician and child can discuss them easily in terms that are appropriate for the child. The child tries out, both individually and with other children in the group, ways of modifying stuttering as he speaks. Parents learn about the techniques that their child is learning so that they can facilitate these changes both in the clinic and at home. For example, a child may be working on a technique called "change out" in which he reduces the tension on a stuttered word and then completes it slowly. When he is familiar with this technique, parents can acknowledge when the child uses it.

Throughout treatment, parents are provided with graphic descriptions of how their child is doing. These "therapy graphs" depict three pieces of information: (1) total disfluencies per 100 words, (2) stuttered disfluencies per 100 words, and (3) total nonstuttered disfluencies per 100 words. These graphs are used during therapy sessions as well as during scheduled parent-clinician counseling sessions to help parents understand their child's progress as well as help the clinician plan short-term and long-term goals for each child.

Supporting Data

Treatment continues until the child is ready to be dismissed. The criterion for dismissal is "an average of 3% or less stutterings per 100 words across an 8-week period" (Conture, 2001, p. 40). Based on evidence collected in the clinic, 70% of the children in this program are ready for dismissal within 12 to 36 weeks. Another 10% take longer but still reach readiness for dismissal. Some of the remaining 20% develop "reasonably fluent" speech but not as a result of the parent-child groups. Some of the factors that appear to predict failure of this parent-child group treatment for stuttering are poor attendance, nonparticipation of parents in the group, a child's sensitive temperament, concomitant speech and language problems, pervasive anxiety, and attention deficit disorder.

Conture stresses the importance of the fact that once a child is ready for dismissal, treatment is not abruptly terminated but gradually faded. First, the child's treatment changes from once a week to once every other week, then to once a month, once every 3 months, and finally, every 6 months for a year. If stuttering reappears at any time during this period, the child can be brought back into treatment until he regains fluency. Although this schedule of fading is the best approach, the time of a child's dismissal is sometimes negotiated with the parents. Some parents want to continue with regular treatment longer than may be necessary, which is only allowed if it is believed to be in the child's best long-term interest. Other parents want to discontinue treatment after the child has become fluent but before gradual fading of treatment has been completed. In these cases, parents' wishes are acceded to, but the door is left open for them to return if necessary. Based on his experience, Conture rejects a one-size-fits-all approach to determining the length of treatment and criterion for termination. Instead, he considers the individual needs of each child, the nature of his problem, his learning history, the parents' concerns, and the extent of their involvement in therapy in determining each child's pace in moving from skill acquisition to maintenance to dismissal.

Lois Nelson

Lois Nelson's intervention approach to a child with borderline stuttering focuses on the verbal interaction patterns that adults use when talking with the child (Nelson, 1985; personal communication, April 29, 2004). She models for parents a speaking style that incorporates the following guidelines for conversation with the child.

1. Adults should slow their speech rate around the child and should also convey to him, both verbally and nonverbally, that there is no reason to hurry when he talks, that adults have time to listen.

2. Adults should reduce the number of questions they ask the child by commenting instead of questioning. Comments should be brief statements about what the child may be thinking, doing, or feeling. For example, "You seem to like that red truck. It goes really fast on the carpet."

3. Let the child decide when he wants to talk in a social situation. Avoid putting him on the spot by asking him to recite or tell an adult about an event that happened.

4. Stay in the "here and now" when talking with the child. Talk about what is right in front of the child, rather than about things or events that are far removed in time or space.

5. Help the child feel that he is being heard and understood by echoing part of what he has just said. This will also make talking fun for the child because he will feel that he can determine the topic.

6. As much as possible, adults should try to convey nonverbally that they are listening by keeping good eye contact when the child is talking.

7. Reduce language pressure on the child. Refrain from teaching him and just enjoy being in his presence. Use short, simple sentences, pause frequently so he can talk, and allow time for silences.

After interacting with the child, Nelson consults with the parents, and together they choose only one change in their interaction pattern based on these guidelines for parents to practice. She may suggest a particular style of interaction change for the parents to begin with by assessing which one has been most effective in reducing the child's stuttering. To help parents understand the potential effectiveness of the changes she's asking them to make, Nelson prepares a transcript of the child's speech in his interaction with her and uses it to illustrate to the parents how much reduction in stuttering took place in response to her change in interaction style.

Parents vary greatly in their need for support in changing their verbal interaction patterns. Some elect to try it immediately on their own, with Nelson providing guidance over the telephone. Others prefer to work jointly with Nelson for several sessions before trying it on their own with her intermittent guidance. After parents appear to be able to use the new style of interacting about 75% of the time, Nelson teaches them a second change in interaction style and coaches them in mastering it. All the while, parents are reporting on changes in the child's stuttering that are taking place, possibly as a response to the new interaction style. To the extent possible, parents encourage grandparents and significant others to adopt the new styles of interacting. In some cases, a child's preschool teachers can incorporate these interaction styles into their programs with the child.

Nelson reports (personal communication, April 29, 2004) that more than half the children with borderline stuttering she works with have signs of word retrieval and language formulation problems. These may be children who are advanced in some aspects of language but normal and delayed in others. They, Nelson believes, need time to develop language at their own pace. This can be accomplished by using various strategies, such as having parents slow their speech rates as well as reducing any indirect demands they may be placing on the child to produce advanced language.

Stuttering Foundation of America (SFA)

The Stuttering Foundation's online store on their website (www.stutteringhelp.org) currently has available two booklets and a video designed for parents of preschool-age children who are beginning to stutter. Ainsworth and Fraser's booklet, *If Your Child Stutters: A Guide for Parents,* 6th edition (2005), helps families to differentiate between normal disfluency and stuttering and provides guidelines to help them create fluency-facilitating environments.

Conture's *Stuttering and Your Child: Questions and Answers,* 3rd edition (2002), provides families, teachers, and others with information about stuttering and how children who stutter can be helped. It covers a wide range of issues, including stuttering versus normal disfluency, the possible causes of stuttering, changing the home environment, dealing with others' responses to the child's stuttering, and treatment. Although formal aspects of treatment are left to professionals, specific advice on how parents, babysitters, day care centers, and teachers can help children who stutter is given in highlighted pages. Parents are instructed how to be good listeners, how to increase the times when their child feels he is being heard, and how to reduce both conversational and lifestyle pressures on the child. Babysitters and day care centers are advised to react as normally as possible to the child and to treat him like other children, while ensuring that he has plenty of time to say what he wants to say without feeling rushed. Teachers are encouraged to give the child support for oral recitations, allow him the same speaking opportunities as other children, and help the entire class to develop good speaking and listening practices.

The Stuttering Foundation's most recent publication on the treatment of borderline stuttering is the videotape and DVD, *Stuttering and the Preschool Child: Help for Families* (Guitar, Guitar, and Fraser, 2001). This video, in both English and Spanish, was designed to be used by families working alone, as a preliminary tool, as well as by those who are in treatment with a speech-language pathologist. The video teaches families to make changes in the child's environment primarily in two areas: communicative interaction and family lifestyle. It also describes when to get help from a speech-language pathologist and what to expect in an evaluation and from treatment.

All of the Stuttering Foundation's publications emphasize that families are not the cause of stuttering but that families can create an environment that facilitates the growth of fluency. The following suggestions for changes in families' conversational interactions are described in detail in both publications, and parents demonstrate them in the video.

- Talk more slowly
- Use plenty of pauses in your speech, after the child finishes talking
- Ask the child fewer questions
- Spend time physically close to the child, such as having him in your lap when you read to him
- Allow silent time in conversations so that the child doesn't feel compelled to talk and isn't interrupted
- Help the child learn to take turns talking

The following suggestions are for families wishing to change some aspects of their lifestyle to facilitate their child's fluency:

- Try to find an opportunity each day, preferably in the morning, when special attention can be given to the child so that he is getting one-on-one time with a parent or another caregiver. During this time, the focus should be on listening to the child and letting him direct the play. The best interactions at these times are those when the parent is talking little and is primarily there for the child as he talks and plays.
- Slow the pace of life, when possible. Give the family more time to do fewer things.
- Develop regular, consistent times for meals, naps, and bedtimes.
- Use reasonable and consistent discipline.
- Make sure the child gets plenty of rest.

- Provide plenty of time for the child to transition from one thing to another. For example, getting ready to go to a birthday party after playing quietly at home may require an extra 10 or 20 minutes because the two activities are so different.

In addition to these ideas for changing a child's environment, the Stuttering Foundation's publications suggest that families become aware of what events or situations are associated with the ups and downs of their child's fluency. Some children who stutter are more sensitive to common, everyday life stresses; things that may not bother most children may cause a child who stutters to become more disfluent. Some examples might be visits by strangers, holidays, a parent coming home from work, or an argument between parents. If it can be predicted when more stressful events might occur, extra support can be provided to the child during such situations.

Families who are working with their child on their own are advised that if their child's stuttering does not show a gradual decrease after these changes have been in place for over a month, they should seek help from a speech-language pathologist who specializes in treating childhood stuttering.

In addition to an extensive online bookstore with many low-cost publications and video material, the SFA website also has a page with guidelines from the American Speech Language Hearing Association for seeking insurance coverage for stuttering evaluation and treatment (www.stutteringhelp.org/insuranc.htm).

Susan Meyers Fosnot and Lee Woodford

Fosnot and Woodford's (1992) approach has three major components: differential assessment, treatment of the child, and parent counseling. Differential assessment begins with the clinician obtaining background information through a telephone interview with the parents and a case history form. Then, she arranges to observe the child interacting with each parent and screens the child's language, articulation, voice, and hearing. The parent-child interactions are videotape or audiotaped and subjected to a "microanalysis." Fosnot and Woodford detail how to transcribe and score the bidirectional interactions between the parents and child. Assessment results in one of the following decisions about treatment. Normally disfluent children without other speech, language, or hearing disorders are followed-up for several years to ensure that fluency is stabilized. Normally disfluent children with other speech-language disorders are given appropriate treatment that incorporates fluency monitoring. Children who stutter are enrolled in fluency therapy, and their parents are counseled to help them change the child's environment.

Fosnot and Woodford's child treatment component uses cognitive and behavioral principles to teach children three rules for facilitating fluency. The first rule is to use slow speech, which is taught using stories, activities, and puppets to help young children grasp the concept of slow versus fast talking and to practice speaking slowly with normal intonation and stress. The second rule is to talk smoothly, so that part-word repetitions and sound prolongations are transformed into an effortless, easy style of speech. The concept of smooth versus bumpy is taught with foods such as peanut butter, finger paints, and picture books. The third rule is to take turns when talking, which is an outgrowth of research suggesting that young children are more disfluent when they interrupt someone (Davis, 1940). The clinician teaches turn-taking with a story book, a

"Mr. Turn-Taker" animal, and games that incorporate turn-taking with speaking slowly and beginning speech smoothly.

After a child has learned the three rules for fluency and is able to remain fluent in spontaneous conversation with the clinician, she introduces the concept of "pressure" that can disrupt fluent speech. Games and activities using a "Mr. Pressure" mask are used to help the child understand and resist pressure on fluency from fast talkers and interruptions. After the child has learned to remain fluent in the face of pressures used during these games, the clinician introduces the child's parents into the therapy setting. Using data from the child's initial assessment, the clinician selects parents' behaviors that are most in need of change and coaches them on how to make their interactions more facilitating to their child's fluency. Parents then take what they have learned in therapy sessions and apply it in their interactions with the child at home, with feedback and reinforcement from the clinician.

Fosnot and Woodford's approach also has a data collection component, which is used to assess the success of treatment and determine when to move from one stage of therapy to the next. The authors provide instructions for assessing and charting fluency at each stage, preparing the child for "graduation" from therapy, and planning follow-up procedures. While the child is in direct therapy, the parents receive group counseling to help them better understand their child and his problem and how to make their home a fluency-facilitating environment. The authors carefully structure the activities and topics they use in parent counseling.

Beatrice Stocker and Robert Goldfarb

The Stocker Probe (1995) is an assessment tool and a treatment approach. It is based on evidence that children's stuttering varies with the level of communicative demand. For example, children stutter less when asked, "Is this hot or cold?" than they do when they're asked to make up a story. The assessment phase measures how much stuttering occurs at each of five different levels of communicative demand: (1) descriptions of objects with alternatives offered, such as, "Is it round or square?"; (2) simple "wh-" questions, such as, "What is it?"; (3) more complex "Wh-" questions, such as, "What do you do with it?"; (4) open-ended descriptions, such as. "Tell me everything you know about this"; and finally, (5) a request to make up a story about an object. The clinician records how much stuttering occurs at each level of demand.

Treatment begins at a level of demand in which the child showed no disfluency. The clinician rewards the child for successively longer periods of fluent speech, which are timed by a stopwatch, at this level until the child is fluent for "three consecutive sixty-second periods of fluency." Then the child moves to the next higher level of demand, and the clinician continues rewarding him for fluency at that level. If the child is disfluent, the clinician resets the stopwatch to zero and has the child respond to another question or probe. Gradually, using successive approximations, the child learns to be fluent for longer and longer periods of time at higher and higher levels of communicative demand.

Clinicians are given substantial leeway in using materials, beyond those provided, to keep therapy interesting for the child. In addition to direct treatment of the child, the clinician councils the parents to lower demands on the child's speech at home until the child has moved far enough up the demand hierarchy in therapy to remain fluent at the highest levels of demand in all situations.

Summary

- Borderline stuttering is characterized by an excess of normal disfluencies, particularly part-word repetitions and single-syllable whole-word repetitions. Although the child may have a high frequency of disfluencies and may repeat sounds many times, he typically is not frustrated or embarrassed by the disfluencies. If these emotional reactions do occur, they are usually transitory. Onset of stuttering is relatively recent (less than a year).

- The occurrence of borderline stuttering is thought to be the result of an interaction between a child's predisposition and typical developmental and environmental stresses. The family is not to blame for the stuttering but can be vital in creating a facilitating environment that increases fluency.

- Treatment is usually focused on helping families make changes in their conversational interactions and in family routines.

- Changes in the family's interaction patterns include helping family members: (1) slow their speech rates, (2) pause for 2 or 3 seconds after the child finishes talking before they begin to speak, (3) listen attentively to what the child is saying, (4) ensure appropriate turn-taking by all members of the family, including the child, (5) ask fewer questions that lead to long answers, and (6) use vocabulary and sentence complexity that are close to the child's level when speaking to him.

- Changes in the family routine should include the following. Arrange a time, preferably in the morning, when one parent or caregiver can have 10 to 15 minutes of uninterrupted time with the child. During this time, the parent should be primarily there for the child, listening and paying attention to what the child is saying and doing, and appropriately reflecting the child's feelings. This can be a time in which a parent or caregiver practices the interaction patterns suggested earlier.

- The family should be encouraged to carry out the following changes in their lifestyle: (1) create structures and predictable routines to increase the child's sense of security, (2) slow the pace of family life, so that there are calm transitions from one activity to another, (3) ensure that the child's life is not too busy or rushed, and (4) use consistent, reasonable discipline with the child to ensure that he feels his family is in control.

- If a child's stuttering does not decline within a month or 6 weeks, more direct treatment should be undertaken. For mild borderline stuttering, parents are taught to use occasional praise for fluency during one-on-one sessions with the child. For more severe borderline stuttering, the child is taught to change harder stutters into easier ones, using modeling, playing with stuttering, voluntary stuttering, and reinforcing slow, easy stutters in his spontaneous speech.

- Other clinicians' indirect approaches to borderline stuttering include parent counseling coupled with monitoring of children with few risk factors, group therapy, and work with families on changing communicative interaction patterns and family lifestyles.

- One other clinician's direct approach teaches children to use slow and smooth speech and to take turns in conversation. Another approach assesses the linguistic level at which a child is fluent, then moves the child through a hierarchy of longer and more complex responses while keeping him fluent for longer periods of time.

Study Questions

1. What are some aspects of family conversational interactions that may put pressure on the child with borderline stuttering?

2. What changes can a family make in their home to relieve speech and language pressures?

3. Discuss how the clinician can facilitate changes in family routines that may help the child's fluency.

4. What are some of the barriers to change that are found in some families? How can the clinician help the family overcome these barriers?

5. Compare my direct approach to a mild borderline stutterer with an approach for a severe borderline stutterer.

6. Compare one of the other clinician's more indirect therapies with one of the more direct therapies.

SUGGESTED PROJECTS

(**1**) Conduct an informal ABAB study of the effect of slowing your speech rate on a conversational partner who is not aware of the purpose of your study. You will need to record your conversation so that you can analyze the data afterwords. In the first A condition, conduct several minutes of conversation at a normal rate; in the first B condition, conduct the same amount of conversation at a slower rate. Then repeat the two rates in two subsequent A and B conditions. Was your speaking partner affected by your speaking rate, by slowing down when you slowed down and by speaking at a normal rate when you did?

(**2**) Pretend that you are the parent of a child who is beginning to stutter. Search the library and the internet for advice about how to help your child and determine whether there is consistency in the advice or whether conflicting information is given.

(**3**) Examine the materials presented in this chapter from other clincians and determine whether the approaches are designed just for borderline stuttering or whether the authors intend them for beginning-level stuttering as well.

Suggested Readings

Ainsworth, S., and Fraser, J. (2005). *If Your Child Stutters: A Guide for Parents* (ed 6). Memphis: Stuttering Foundation of America.
This inexpensive booklet gives advice to parents who think their child is beginning to stutter.

Chmela, K. (2004). *Working With Preschoolers Who Stutter: Successful Intervention Strategies.* **Videotape or DVD format. Memphis: Stuttering Foundation of America.**

This is a video of a convention presentation designed to teach clinicians how to work with preschool children who stutter, using modeling of easy, relaxed speech when talking to children and counseling parents to develop a fluency-friendly environment.

Conture, E. (Ed) (2002). *Stuttering and Your Child: Questions and Answers.* **Memphis: Stuttering Foundation of America.**

This booklet provides answers for parents to commonly asked questions about stuttering in young children.

Curlee, R.F. (1993). Identification and management of beginning stuttering. In R.F. Curlee (Ed), *Stuttering and Related Disorders of Fluency.* **New York: Thieme Medical Publishers.**

This chapter describes procedures to evaluate children who may be stuttering, to select those who need therapy, and to follow-up when appropriate.

Curlee, R.F. (1999). Identification and case selection guidelines for early childhood stuttering. In R.F. Curlee (Ed), *Stuttering and Related Disorders of Fluency* **(ed 2). New York: Thieme Medical Publishers.**

This chapter updates Curlee's procedures for evaluation and case selection but does not provide the specifics on therapy given in the 1993 version.

Fosnot, S.M., and Woodford, L.L. (1992). *The Fluency Development System for Young Children.* **Buffalo: United Educational Services, Inc.**

This kit supplies all the props and materials needed to evaluate stuttering in young children, provide therapy, and counsel their parents.

Gottwald, S., and Starkweather, C.W. (1995). Fluency intervention for preschoolers and their families in the public schools. *Language, Speech, and Hearing Services in Schools,* **26:115–126.**

This article describes assessment and treatment procedures used by a variety of clinicians for young children who stutter.

Guitar, B., et al. (1992). Parent verbal interaction and speech rate. *Journal of Speech and Hearing Research,* **35:742–754.**

This article describes therapy with parents of a young child who stutters and the analysis of parent-child interactions.

Roseman, B., and Johnson, K. (1998). *Easy Does It® for Fluency: Preschool/Primary.* **East Moline, IL: LinguiSystems.**

This manual and materials book provides instruction and materials for stuttering therapy for children, from ages 2 to 6 years. The focus is on teaching fluency through the establishment of "easy speech" through modeling and then progressing up a linguistic and situational hierarchy. Desensitization to fluency disruptors is included, as well as maintenance of fluency. Some suggestions for combining phonological and fluency therapy are provided.

Nelson, L. (1985). Language formulation related to dysfluency and stuttering. In *Stuttering Therapy: Prevention and Intervention With Children.* **Memphis: Stuttering Foundation of America.**

This chapter delineates Lois Nelson's treatment strategies for preschoolers who stutter. It is a distillation of many years of experience with stuttering children.

Reville, J. (1988). *The Many Voices of Paws.* **Princeton Junction, NJ: Speech Bin.**

This is a manual for speech-language pathologists and parents to help them work with preschool children who stutter. A slow, easy style of speaking is taught with the help of a poem about a cat named "Paws."

Starkweather, C.W., Gottwald, S.R., and Halfond, M.H. (1990). *Stuttering Prevention: A Clinical Method.* **Englewood Cliffs, NJ: Prentice-Hall.**

This book details a program of assessment and treatment for children who stutter and for their parents.

Stocker, B., and Goldfarb, R. (1995). *The Stocker Probe for Fluency and Language.* Vero Beach, FL: The Speech Bin.

Walton, P., and Wallace, M. (1998). *Fun With Fluency. Bisbee,* AZ: Imaginart International, Inc.
This manual provides extensive information about working with both borderline and beginning stuttering. Both indirect and direct treatment are covered, information and materials for working with parents and teachers is provided, and many activities for children ages 2 to 7 are suggested.

Chapter **10**

Treatment of Beginning Stuttering

An Integrated Approach

Children with beginning stuttering are usually between 3 and 6 years of age, but some children may be 7 or 8 years old. They have probably been stuttering for at least several months, and now their parents may well be concerned that it is not a transient problem that will disappear on its own. What follows are some details on core and secondary behaviors of stuttering, as well as feelings and attitudes. These children's most common core stuttering behaviors are part-word repetitions that are produced rapidly, usually with irregular rhythm. Some prolongations may also be present. Both the repetitions and prolongations may contain excessive tension, which can be heard as abrupt endings to the repetitions and increases in vocal pitch in repetitions and prolongations. Blocks may be present but will probably not be the predominant core behavior. Secondary behaviors are typically escape devices, such as eye blinks, head nods, and increases in pitch. A few avoidance maneuvers, such as starting sentences with extra sounds like "uh," may be observed. Children with beginning stuttering usually feel frustrated with their difficulty in talking but have not yet developed a fear of stuttering or learned to be ashamed of their speech. In rare cases, if the frequency of stuttering becomes extremely high, these children may put their hands to their mouth to push words out or may momentarily avoid talking.

Author's Beliefs

Nature of Stuttering

I believe that beginning stuttering arises when children's basic sensory-motor difficulty interacts with their temperament and other developmental and environmental influences to produce or exacerbate repetitions, prolongations, and blocks. This is essentially the position taken by Wendell Johnson (1959), who suggested that the problem of stuttering arises as a result of interactions among (1) the amount of the child's disfluency, (2) the reaction of his listeners to the disfluency, and (3) the child's sensitivity to his own disfluency and to listeners' reactions. I would add to Johnson's list of interacting factors any pressures that a child may feel internally (for example, to speak quickly and in long, complex sentences) and any anxieties the child may experience as the result of moving, the birth of a sibling, or other life events.

In some children, beginning stuttering emerges gradually, after they have gone through a period of borderline stuttering and have begun to respond to negative experiences of repetitive disfluencies with increased tension. In other children, beginning stuttering appears quickly, close to the onset of stuttering. Their increased tension may be a rapid response to their distress when their attempts to talk are frustrated by runaway repetitions. As children attempt to cope with these core behaviors, they develop a variety of escape behaviors that are instrumentally reinforced. Their eye blinks, head nods, and pitch increases are rewarded when they are associated with the release of the child's stutters. Gradually, classical conditioning influences when and where the child's stuttering occurs. Negative emotional experiences that are associated with stuttering are etched into memory and associated with various contexts, such as the telephone, impatient listeners, or particular words. As stuttering spreads and becomes more pervasive and more consistently present, these children become aware of their stuttering, although they have little shame of it and do not dread speaking situations. Because of the plasticity of the brain at this age, some beginning stutterers develop better sensory-motor control of speech, and their stuttering goes out the door it entered. Their stutters diminish in frequency and severity and disappear or become a minor nuisance. Other children, perhaps those with more widespread sensory-motor deficits, more sensitive temperament, or larger doses of other developmental and environmental stresses, continue to stutter and may develop more advanced symptoms.

Like Oliver Bloodstein (1975), I believe that if we can provide a beginning stutterer with a sufficient number of positive, fluent speaking experiences during treatment, fluency will replace stuttering. Perhaps the daily, structured practice of fluency in the approach I use reinforces the neural pathways for fluent speech so that they become more robust, more automatic, and more resistant to stress. This may happen best when treatment takes place at home, where stuttering is most common. It also appears effective if natural fluency is elicited in highly structured situations, systematically reinforced, and then carefully transferred to more and more real-life situations in which stuttering is occurring.

The increased fluency gained through treatment reduces the opportunities a child has to respond to any remaining disfluencies with tension, frustration, or escape and starting behaviors. It also allows time for the child's physiological system to mature and for normal fluency patterns to become stabilized.

Speech Behaviors Targeted For Therapy

Which speech behaviors are targeted for the beginning stutterer? In the major approach I advocate in this section, the Lidcombe Program, the clinician teaches the parent first to reinforce the child's fluent speech, and then respond to stutters. The parent uses appropriate and varied verbal contingencies immediately after fluent utterances but comments neutrally on stutters much less frequently or gently asks the child to try the word again immediately after she stutters.

Fluency Goals

Almost all children who are treated with effective therapy for beginning stuttering will gain or regain spontaneous, normal fluency. Typically, a year or two after treatment ends, the children will have little or no recollection of having stuttered and will not have to monitor their speech or work at being fluent.

Feelings and Attitudes

As noted earlier, a child with beginning stuttering has only occasional frustration and intermittent concern about talking. She has not yet developed conditioned fears or avoidances of stuttering. Thus, it is unnecessary to focus directly on feelings and attitudes in therapy with a beginning stutterer.

The feelings and attitudes of these children are, however, influenced by the family. The clinician teaches the family member providing the at home treatment to be matter-of-fact about the child's "smooth" and "bumpy" speech. The clinician and family member openly discuss the child's stuttering during their weekly meetings when the child is also present. These aspects of treatment reduce any embarassment or shame that was associated with stuttering and foster the child's acceptance of stuttering as just a little mistake, like bumping into a table or falling off a tricycle. This is a far cry from the "conspirancy of silence" that formerly characterized the treatment of children who stutter.

Maintenance Procedures

Systematically fading contact with the child and her family is vital for maintenance of fluency. In my experience, if families leave treatment after fluency is achieved without having participated in a maintenace program, stuttering is very likely to return. Thus, it is important for clinicians to stress the imporance of maintenance procedures at the outset of treatment. Moreover, the clinician and family should continue with careful data collection as contact is faded, so that the family can return to regular weekly meetings and discuss appropriate contingencies for fluency and stuttering if any relapse occurs.

Clinical Methods

For the last 5 years, I have been using the Lidcombe Program (Onslow, Costa, and Rue, 1990; Onslow, Packman, and Harrison, 2003) to treat preschool children with beginning stuttering. I was initially trained in using this program in a workshop led by Rosalee Shenker. Subsequently, I developed more expertise through consultation and mentoring from Rosalee and my colleagues, Julie Reville and Melissa Bruce. Follow-up training with Elisabeth Harrison further sharpened my skills. For readers interested in using this approach, I urge you to obtain formal training at one of the many workshops offered around the world by the Lidcombe Consortium. In Canada and the U.S., contact Rosalee Shenker (rosalee.shenker@mcgill.ca); in the United Kingdom, contact Mary Kingston (kingstonamee@talk21.com) or Rosemary Hayhow (rosemarie@speech-therapy.org.uk); in Australia, contact asrc.su.cpe@fhs.usyd.edu.au. More information on the Lidcombe Program is available at www3.fhs.usyd.edu.au/asrcwww/treatment/lidcombe.htm.

Overview

The Lidcombe Program uses operant conditioning procedures, which are delivered by a parent in the home during conversations each day and guided by weekly meetings with the clinician. Treatment begins in structured conversations designed to elicit a maximum of fluent speech by the child, so that the child receives mostly positive reinforcement. Approximately every fifth fluent utterance is followed by *praise* (e.g., "That was really good smooth talking!"), *acknowledgement of fluency* (e.g., a very low-key "That was smooth."), or *request for self-evaluation* (e.g., "Was that smooth?"). When the child stutters, the parent provides an occasional *acknowledgement of the stutter* ("That was a little bumpy.") or *a gentle request for self-correction* (e.g., "Can you say 'truck' again without the bump?"). The ratio of verbal contingencies for fluency to verbal contingencies for stuttering is kept very high (about 5:1) to make the program a positive experience for the child. As the child's stuttering decreases, treatment is delivered in unstructured conversations each day. Once the child is fluent in all situations, treatment is gradually faded in a systematic fashion. Throughout the program, the clinician and parent regularly assess the child's stuttering and use those measures to make treatment decisions.

Stage 1: First Clinic Visit

In the first clinic visit, the clinician meets with the parent (or other caregiver) and child to accomplish three goals: (1) to assess the child's stuttering, (2) to explain severity ratings to the parent, and (3) to teach the parent to conduct daily treatment conversations. Stage 1 clinic visits are typically 1 hour in duration.

The clinician assesses the child's stuttering using a measure of syllables stuttered during conversation between the child, her parent, and the clinician during an activity that the child enjoys. For a valid sample, approximately 300 syllables of the child's speech should be assessed, which usually takes about 10 minutes. Measuring percent syllables stuttered is best done online as the child is talking, rather than from a videotape, using either a stopwatch and calculator (as described in Chapter 6) or a True Talk® hand-held counting device (www.truetalk.com.au). I make no attempt to hide the fact that I am assessing the child's speech; if the child asks about it, I usually say something like, "I'm just counting how many smooth words you say." Once I assess the sample, I let the parent know the child's score, and we discuss how it compares to the child's speech in other situations.

Each day the parent uses the Severity Rating Scale (see Chapter 6) to assess the child's stuttering at home. It is a 10-point scale that the parent completes at the end of every day, reflecting his or her judgment of the child's stuttering severity that day. A 1 on the scale represents no stuttering, a 2 represents extremely mild stuttering, and a 10 represents extremely severe stuttering. After discussing the scale with the parent, I ask her to tell me what rating she would give the child's speech in the clinic that day, which I compare with my own rating. It is usually possible, with only a little discussion, to ensure that the parent is using the scale appropriately. On the rare occasion that the parent's rating differs from mine by more than 1 point, I explain how I came up with my rating and then try to determine if the parent seems to understand my rationale and is likely to be accurate in her future ratings. If I have doubts, I use video clips of the child's speech to help teach the parent how to use the scale. I typically ask the parents to make videotapes of the child's speech at home during the first few weeks of treatment so that I can continue to "calibrate" the parent's ratings. Once I'm sure the parent understands the scale, I ask him or her to rate the child's speech at the end of every day and to bring the ratings to our weekly meetings. The standard Lidcombe procedure has the parent bring in a chart that displays each day's severity ratings of the child. I encourage the parents to add comments to the chart if the child has gone through a period of increased stuttering, sickness, or other event that the parent feels may have an impact on severity or the child's response to treatment.

The final thing I accomplish in the first clinic visit is to show the parent how to conduct the daily structured treatment conversations. It is most important to create situations that are not only fun, but that also stimulate a lot of fluent speech in the child. This enables the parent to begin treatment using a great deal of positive verbal contingencies for fluency. To demonstrate for the parent, I begin by using a picture book or picture cards with the child to elicit short, fluent utterances. To keep the child's interest, I talk with a lot of enthusiasm and move through the pictures quickly. With children who have more severe stuttering, I may need to elicit single words or even single-syllable words. Children who have milder stuttering can usually remain mostly fluent saying short phrases of three or four words. I usually name a picture or two myself, as a model for the

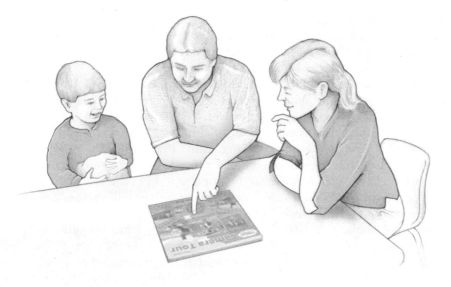

Figure 10–1 *Clinician teaching father to conduct treatment in structured conversation.*

child, and then ask her to name some pictures. After the fifth fluent utterance, I praise her fluency immediately by saying something specifically about her speech, such as, "That was really smooth talking!" or "You said that really smoothly!" It is important to make the praise directly relevant to the child's fluency, rather than general praise. After modeling for the parent, I ask her or him to work with the child, and I coach the parent if necessary (Fig. 10–1).

One of the mistakes parents often make when they first begin is to use positive verbal contingencies for fluent speech that are too general. They might say, for example, "That's good" or "You're doing well." In this case, I simply restate the need for specific praise and observe the parents doing it. Another common error is for parents to let the child make longer responses than are appropriate, thereby allowing more stuttered than fluent utterances to occur. Fortunately, a little discussion and lots of modeling will usually clear this up. For those children who need to start at the one- or two-word utterance stage, specifically praising their use of one or two words will help keep them at this level until it is appropriate for them to move to longer utterances.

As I mentioned earlier, it is crucial that the parent make the treatment conversations fun for the child. It may be helpful to suggest games and activities for the sessions. Table 10–1 lists some of the activities that parents can use with the child in these structured conversations.

At the end of the first clinic visit, I review the activities and tasks the parent will be doing over the coming week and respond to any questions she has. Some parents benefit from taking notes or being given a written description of things they will be doing; others like to have a follow-up email. In all cases, I encourage them to call or email me if they have any questions or concerns during the week.

Table 10–1   Suggested Games and Activities for Structured Treatment Conversations

- Grab-bag. The parent puts interesting items into a large cloth bag or pillowcase, and the child guesses what each is by reaching into the bag and feeling the item.
- Picture naming. Using picture books or picture cards, the child names each picture. At the one-word level, the child only names the pictured object. As longer utterances are permitted, the child can use a carrier phrase such as "That's a _____," or she can name the item and its color, such as "Red rabbit."
- Reading a story. Parent and child look at a familiar book while the parent reads or tells the story. To elicit a word or phrase, the parent asks the child to complete a sentence, such as "Then Goldilocks said, 'Somebody's been sleeping in my _____.'"
- Rhyme closing. Parent makes up a rhyme and leaves the last word blank, like "There was a boy who lived in Kalamazoo. He liked to climb mountains so he could get a good _____."

Stage 1: Subsequent Clinic Visits

Most subsequent clinic visits have three goals: (1) to assess the child's stuttering, (2) to discuss the current progress, and (3) to introduce new procedures when appropriate. Each session begins with the clinician's assessment of the child's stuttering, as described earlier. In the first few clinic visits, it is often helpful to ask the parent to rate the child's severity on the 1-10 scale during the 5- or 10-minute assessment period. This enables the clinician to determine if the parent's ratings are still similar to her own. Accurate parent severity ratings are essential to the integrity of the treatment program. These ratings, along with the clinician's assessment of percent syllables stuttered (%SS), determine whether treatment is progressing successfully and signal when to fade structured treatment conversations and transition to treatment in unstructured conversations. They also indicate when to move from Stage 1 to Stage 2 of the Lidcombe Program.

After the clinician's assessment of %SS, the clinician and parent discuss the week's severity ratings and home treatment conversations. As they talk, the child usually plays by herself, with some interaction and encouragement from the parent and the clinician. The openness with which discussions of the week's progress take place is a hallmark of the Lidcombe Program. There is no attempt to keep the child from overhearing the parent and clinician talk about the child's stuttering. The matter-of-fact manner in which the clinician and parent discuss the child's speech seems to me to make it more likely that both the parent and child will feel less anxious about the child's stuttering and may reduce any shame the child might feel about her difficulty. During the parent's and clinician's discussion, some children often make noise to call attention to themselves. In my experience, this is not because the child objects to the discussion of her stuttering but is only an attempt to get the focus back on herself. At such times, it may be helpful if the clinician simply asks the child, "Can I talk to your mommy for just a minute and then we'll play again?"

As the clinician looks over the parent's severity ratings, she may ask about the days in which ratings are higher or lower than average. Or, the clinician and parent may brainstorm solutions to problems that may be indicated by lack of change in the ratings. This is often a time when videotapes of the treatment conversations from home are useful, so that the clinician can assess how they are being conducted. It is also helpful to have the parent demonstrate during each clinic visit how he or she is using verbal contingencies during the sessions at home.

When adequate progress is being made and home severity ratings and clinic assessments indicate that the child is becoming more fluent, new treatment procedures can be introduced.

Once a parent is appropriately reinforcing fluency, she or he may be taught to use verbal contingencies for stuttering. The mildest is verbally acknowledging the occurrence of an unambiguous stutter. Only unambiguous stutters should be acknowledged because normal disfluencies should not be treated as stutters. The descriptions of normal disfluencies and stuttered disfluencies in Chapter 5 clarify this difference. I typically model an acknowledgment of stuttering for the parent, which is given after about five instances of contingencies for fluent utterances. It is important that the parent learn to use contingencies for fluency several times before using a verbal contingency on stuttered speech. When I demonstrate acknowledgment of stuttering, I use comments like "a little bumpy one there" or "that one was a little bumpy." I make the statement quietly, immediately after the stutter, and without any negative inflection in my voice. After I have modeled acknowledging stutters, I ask the parent to try it but only after she or he has praised several of the child's fluent utterances. Most children hardly seem to notice the acknowledgment, although some may stop momentarily and look at the parent when it is given. Typically, I ask parents to continue using contingencies for fluency and begin using acknowledgment of stuttering for a week before introducing further verbal contingencies for stuttering.

In the following weekly meeting, I introduce requests for self-correction of unambiguous stuttering. This verbal contingency asks the child to say the stuttered word again with a phrase like, "Can you say 'I' again?" or "Can you say that word again?" Such requests are made in a positive, supportive manner, and it is important that the parent practice this contingency after the clinician demonstrates it. Some parents may be hesitant to request a self-correction and may convey their concern to the child. Others may inadvertently use a slightly negative or impatient tone when asking for a correction. However, a patient clinician's modeling and subsequent coaching can do wonders to shape parents' responses into helpful, supportive requests.

After the child has repeated the word fluently, the parent should praise the self-correction with comments like, "Nice job of making that word smooth." If a child ignores a parent's request for self-correction or refuses to self-correct, the parent just moves on. If the child says the word again but stutters again, the parent may say something supportive like, "That's okay; sometimes those words are hard."

In the subsequent weeks, the clinician monitors the child's progress and ensures that the parent is delivering verbal contingencies effectively. The clinician also checks to see that the child is enjoying the structured treatment conversations and is responding well to the contingencies for both fluency and stuttering. Every child and every family are different, so the program must be individualized in each case. For example, some children may indicate they are uncomfortable with such praise as, "That was really smooth talking." In this case, the parent can ask the child what she would like the parent to say when she is talking smoothly. Alternatively, the parent can use one of the other verbal contingencies for fluency. Some children who don't react well to praise will happily respond to requests to self-evaluate their fluency. One child I worked with preferred that the parent put a penny in a jar, which made a nice "plink" sound, rather than verbally praise her fluency.

Stage 1: Introducing Unstructured Treatment Conversations

When treatment has progressed well for 2 or 3 weeks and severity ratings and %SS indicate improvement, a gradual transition can be made from structured to unstructured treatment conversations. Thus, verbal contingencies of praise, acknowledgment of stutters, and requests for correction can now be given in typical daily conversations, such as during meals, riding in the car, shopping, and playing. When treatment is first introduced in unstructured conversations, structured treatment usually continues for a time to make the transition easy. When unstructured treatment has been going well for a week or two and stuttering continues to decrease, structured sessions can be faded gradually. For example, each week one or two structured conversations may be dropped until they have all been discontinued and replaced with unstructured treatment.

There are several reasons why structured treatment may subsequently be reinstated. One is if stuttering increases for a day or more; in this situation, structured treatment may be conducted until the child's fluency has returned to earlier levels. Another reason for continuing or reinstating structured treatment is if the child asks to have these conversations. Most children enjoy one-on-one time with a parent, and many ask for a structured conversation occasionally after the conversations have been discontinued. A third reason for continuing structured conversations for a period of time as the transition to unstructured sessions is made is if the parent requests it. Sometimes parents feel that things are going so well in structured sessions that they believe the transition to unstructured sessions should be made slowly.

Several issues may warrant consideration when unstructured treatment is just getting underway. Parents may wish to begin with just praise for fluent utterances and then add acknowledgment for fluency and for stuttering, requests for self-evaluation, and finally, requests for self-correction of stuttering. If problems appear in response to any of these verbal contingencies, they can be solved immediately. It is also important that verbal contingencies not be given relentlessly throughout each day but are used selectively at first, so that the parent can judge how the child is responding. If the child reacts well, which is usually the case, the parent can begin using verbal contingencies in more and more conversations but, at the same time, the parent should make sure that the child is not overwhelmed by too frequent attention to her speech. The child needs to experience the normal flow of conversation for its own sake, rather than feel that everything she says is being evaluated.

Another issue that may arise relative to unstructured treatment is who is giving the verbal contingencies. Although only one parent may have been conducting the structured treatment, both parents, and even other family members, may be involved in the unstructured treatment. However, this must be done very carefully and be individualized for each family. Other adults in the home or older siblings may be appropriate in some cases, whereas a sibling close to the child's age may not be. If a child is responsive to the contingencies given by one parent in unstructured conversations, I usually try adding another family member and evaluate the child's response. It is recommended for the clinician to meet with any family members who are giving verbal contingencies to ensure that they understand how crucial it is that five times as much praise for fluency be given as requests for self-correction of stuttering and that requests for self-correction be done in a supportive manner.

Unstructured treatment at home and weekly meetings in the clinic continue until the child is essentially fluent. This point is reached when two criteria are met for 3 weeks in a row: (1) the parent's severity ratings of the child's stuttering are all 1 and 2, with at least four of the ratings being 1, and (2) the percentage of syllables stuttered by the child at the clinic is below 1%. If the clinician has any doubts about the reliability and validity of the parent's severity ratings, she should request that the parent bring an audio or video recording of the child's speech at home to confirm that the criteria are met.

Stage 2: Maintenance

One of the most important components of the Lidcombe Program is its maintenance procedure. Because relapse is common in stuttering treatment, parents are cautioned when they begin Stage 1 of the Lidcombe Program that it is essential that they continue to work with the clinician through the end of Stage 2. They are reminded of this throughout Stage 1 so that the procedures of the second stage are expected. Stage 2 consists of 30-minute clinic visits that are scheduled at gradually greater intervals. Typically, there are two visits at 2-week intervals, then two visits at 4-week intervals, then two visits at 8-week intervals, and finally, one visit 16 weeks later. During this period, parents continue to provide verbal contingencies for fluency and stuttering just as they did during Stage 1, but the clinician guides the parents in gradually decreasing their child's verbal contingencies until they are completely discontinued.

To progress through this schedule of visits, the child must maintain the same level of fluency achieved to begin Stage 2 (less than 1%SS in the clinic and severity ratings of 1 and 2, with at least four ratings of 1). When the parent and child come in for a scheduled clinic visit, the usual assessment of the child's %SS takes place followed by a discussion of how the child's speech has been since the previous visit. This discussion, as always, is facilitated by the parent's severity ratings and reports of how the child is responding to verbal contingencies. At each visit, the clinician and parent decide whether to continue decreasing the frequency of clinic visits or to make some changes, such as keeping to the current decreasing frequency of visits, resuming unstructured treatment conversations, or reinstating both structured and unstructured treatment. It is also possible that some aspect of the verbal contingencies may need to be adjusted. For example, sometimes a child becomes so fluent that, when stutters do occur, parents or other family members apply contingencies to stuttering without concurrently giving the appropriate number of contingencies for fluency. Sometimes making this adjustment will solve a problem of returning stuttering. In other cases, stuttering reappears because of momentary stress. In this case, reinstating weekly visits may help the parent and clinician get the child back on track.

Stage 2 takes about a year to complete for most children who stutter. Although minor relapses may occur, parents are usually able to accurately assess what changes need to be made to bring the child back to essentially fluent speech.

Problem Solving

Generally, the Lidcombe Program runs smoothly, without much difficulty, if clinicians follow the program carefully. However, it is common for minor problems to arise during

Stages 1 and 2. This section describes some common problems that may occur and their possible solutions. For more detailed descriptions of troubleshooting and special cases, see *The Lidcombe Program of Early Stuttering Intervention—A Clinician's Guide* (Onslow, Packman, and Harrison, 2003).

Sometimes, progress toward fluent speech is stalled for several weeks, or previous gains are momentarily lost. If so, I usually begin by talking to the parent about what he or she thinks might be occurring. Parents are often able to pinpoint something they have changed about the way they are doing treatment. Or, it may be that a parent misunderstands some aspect of treatment. Thus, it helps to have parents demonstrate how they conduct treatment during each clinic visit, and it may be even more helpful to have them bring in a videotape of treatment at home. Examples of things that may go wrong include: (1) parents are less attentive to praising fluent speech regularly, so that fewer positive reinforcements are made than requests for corrections, (2) parents become lax about the consistency of structured treatment conversations, so that many days are missed, (3) other family members, while trying to be helpful, make mistakes in providing verbal contingencies because they have not been trained, (4) structured treatment conversations are so ponderous that the child doesn't enjoy them, and (5) the child is not generating enough fluency in structured treatment.

The problems that arise from misunderstanding the parameters of treatment can usually be resolved by supportive feedback and guidance of the parent and modeling of appropriate behavior. Other issues, such as conducting treatment inconsistently, may require brainstorming with the parent about how treatment can be conducted more regularly. If a child isn't enjoying conversations, progress will be stalled. But it is not difficult to coach parents in delivering treatment in ways that are enjoyable, effective, and fun for both parent and child. Clinicians who have worked with preschool-age children have usually learned how to keep a child interested and achieve therapy goals at the same time. It may be appropriate for other family members to become involved in unstructured treatment conversations, but they should be trained by the clinician to deliver contingencies effectively. Structured treatment may be shared by both parents or other caregivers, but the clinician should ensure that whoever is delivering treatment is doing so accurately, and direct training is the best way to achieve this.

With children who have moderate or severe stuttering, it is critical to structure their treatment conversations so that the child is largely fluent and only stutters occasionally. This can be done by creating a linguistic hierarchy in which the child begins using short utterances and then moves to longer ones when the child is consistently fluent; ascending this hierarchy may take several days. Some parents need specific instructions on how to achieve this. The clinician can model conversations for the parent using pictures for single word naming, differentially reinforcing briefer utterances, and requesting the child to say just one word. In treatment conversations at home, the parent can then model for the child what is expected and continue to use differential reinforcement to control the child's output.

The Lidcombe Program is an effective treatment approach but should but used only after attending a training workshop conducted by the Lidcombe Program Trainers Consortium. Information about workshops, research articles on treatment outcome, and a treatment manual are available on the Australian Stuttering Research Centre website (www.fhs.usyd.edu.au/ASRC).

Outcome Data

A number of studies have reported that the Lidcombe Program is effective in eliminating stuttering in preschoolers. A long-term outcome study of 42 children treated with the program showed that their stuttering was at near-zero levels 4 to 7 years after treatment (Lincoln and Onslow, 1997). The results of a 12-week randomized control trial involving 10 preschoolers in a Lidcombe treatment group and 13 preschoolers in a no-treatment group indicated that the treated children had significantly less stuttering than the untreated children. Other research reported that the median number of clinic visits needed to complete Stage 1 treatment, in a sample of 316 children, was 11 clinic visits (Kingston et al, 2002). In response to concerns expressed by critics that the Lidcombe Program might produce negative psychological effects, Woods et al (2002) compared pre- and post-treatment measures of the *Child Behavior Checklist* (Achenbach, 1988) and the *Attachment Q-Set* (Waters, 1995) and found no ill effects of treatment on the children's psychological health. In fact, the *Child Behavior Checklist* showed improvement in the children's behavior. A randomized control trial has shown significantly ($p = 0.003$) greater improvement in Lidcombe treatment ($n = 29$) versus control ($n = 25$). Effect size was 2.3% SS (Jones et al, in press).

Other Clinicians

Frances Cook and Willie Botterill

At the Michael Palin Centre for Stammering Children, Frances Cook and Willie Botterill have developed a treatment for beginning stuttering based on the parent-child interaction therapy of Lena Rustin (1991). This approach rests on the assumption that changing the way parents communicate with their child will change how the child talks, and the child will gradually become more and more fluent. Several research studies support the hypothesis that the parents' communication style is associated with the child's fluency (Guitar, 1978; Guitar et al, 1992; Kasprisin-Burelli, Egolf, and Shames, 1972; Meyers and Freeman, 1985a,b; Stephanson-Opsal and Bernstein Ratner, 1988).

The Michael Palin Centre approach begins with a thorough evaluation of a child's strengths and needs. The child's receptive and expressive language, articulation, speech rate, and sensitivity are assessed. Particular attention is given to analyzing, with the parents' help, social situations and linguistic contexts that are associated with increases and decreases in the child's stuttering. The clinician also stresses to the parents that nothing they have done has *caused* their child's stuttering but that their participation in treatment is vital in helping the child. Part of the assessment is videotaped so that interactions of the parents and child in a play situation can be analyzed later. The parents' language, speech rate, amount of questioning, pausing, and other aspects of communication in the interaction are evaluated. Chapter 7 gives further details about analyzing parent-child interactions.

Once the assessment, including the clinician's analysis of the videotape, is completed, the parents and clinician meet to discuss the findings. The results of the assessment are described in terms of the child's strengths and needs, and the parents' ideas are sought about what facilitates the child's fluency. The parents may have observed, for example, that the child is more fluent when she has had plenty of rest but less fluent when she is competing for speaking time, such as at the dinner table. The parents' ideas are valued and incorporated into treatment. The clinician then views the videotape with the parents and emphasizes what helpful things the parents are already doing, such as commenting rather than questioning or pausing for a few seconds when the child finishes a speaking turn rather than talking immediately. If the parents observe that they are talking too fast, the clinician finds examples on the video of when they are talking slower, at a more facilitating rate. The overarching principle behind changing parents' interaction behaviors is to find ways of giving the child more time to plan and execute speech.

In this first session, the parents and clinician begin a routine that will continue for 6 weeks. Together, they develop a plan for changing parent-child interactions based on one new target each week, such as increasing the parents' pause time after the child speaks. The parents work on the new target daily, in 5-minute sessions with the child. In addition, they assess the child's fluency intermittently on a 1- to 9-point scale. They also complete two other self-assessment scales that reflect their own anxiety and their confidence in managing the child's stuttering. Using these scales, the clinician can monitor both the parents' and the child's progress outside the clinic.

In subsequent sessions during the initial 6 weeks of treatment, the clinician reviews the parents' homework and then videotapes each parent interacting separately with the child. The clinician then reviews the two videotapes with both parents together. While watching his or her own videotape, each parent picks out several interactions that he or she is pleased with and one behavior that needs to be changed. In consultation with the clinician, improving these interactions becomes the parents' homework the next week, which they work on during their daily 5-minute interaction sessions with the child. Although much of the emphasis is on their communication interactions, the parents also learn to use praise of other skills to build up the child's confidence. The book *How to Talk So Kids Will Listen and How to Listen So Kids Will Talk* by Faver and Mazlish (1999) is used for teaching parents to praise their child once each day for something specific the child did.

After 6 weeks of meeting with the clinician, the parents work on their own at home for a second 6-week period of "consolidation" of their new behaviors. Parents send homework record sheets and assessment scales to the clinician each week and continue to work on behavioral changes during the daily 5-minute interaction times that each parent has with the child. The clinician responds via email, phone, or regular mail. At the end of this 6-week consolidation period, the family meets with the clinician for a review of progress. If the child's fluency is significantly better and continuing to improve, the parents are asked to continue working on the changes they are making, and another review is scheduled 6 weeks later. If the child's fluency is not improving, more direct treatment is introduced, such as the Lidcombe Program described earlier in this chapter or the approach of Fosnot and Woodford (1992) described in Chapter 9.

Clinician-researchers at the Michael Palin Centre (Cook, Millard, and Nicholas, 2004) reported outcome data on six children between the ages of 3-0 and 4-11 whose lengths of time since onset were all greater than 12 months (mean time since onset = 20.3 months). Children were assessed 1-year after treatment and were found to have reduced stuttering from a mean pre-therapy level of 8.4% syllables stuttered to a mean of 2.7%. Four of the six children significantly reduced stuttering with both parents; the other two children significantly reduced stuttering with one of their two parents. Outcome was not related to stuttering severity at pre-treatment.

Diane Hill and Hugo Gregory

Diane Hill and Hugo Gregory (Gregory, 2003) believe that stuttering develops as the result of an interaction between the child's predisposing factors and the communicative and interpersonal stress of her environment. Their treatment approach, therefore, focuses on both the parents and the child. A complete description of this approach is available in a chapter by Hill in Gregory's book (Hill, 2003). For the child with beginning stuttering, treatment consists of six stages, which are worked on sequentially, although some continue throughout treatment.

1. Provide Feedback to Help Parents Develop an Understanding of the Stuttering Problem

In this first stage, the clinician educates the parents about the nature of stuttering and its development. She also engages the parents in treatment by explaining the importance of their participation and the benefit of early intervention. The clinician then trains the parents to identify various types of disfluencies and the circumstances in which they occur. They learn to chart the disfluencies that the child displays in her daily life, what and to whom she was communicating, the child's awareness of her disfluencies, and other aspects of the situation that may have been an influence. The exploration and discussion of these aspects of the child's stuttering and her environment continue throughout treatment, which are supported by group meetings with the parents.

2. Facilitate Development of Fluency Skills

Treatment sessions usually begin with some free play, which is essential for younger children. During this time, the clinician models slow, easy, relaxed speech that is characterized by easy initiations of speech, a slightly slower than normal rate, and smooth transitions between units of speech. The clinician also moves slowly and in a relaxed way. This relatively unstructured aspect of the session is then changed to more structured games in which the child is asked to emulate the clinician's slow, relaxed speech and is reinforced for following the clinician's speech model more and more accurately. The clinician ensures that the child's speech sounds as natural as possible, so that as the child learns to use easy, relaxed speech in more and more situations, it is essentially normal sounding and fluent.

3. Support Generalization and Transfer of Fluency Skills by Systematically Progressing through Hierarchies of Response

This stage of treatment is designed to help a child progress from producing single words easily and fluently in games to speaking with natural, fluent speech in all situations. Hill (2003) provides a detailed set of hierarchies to use with children, which begins with two- to three-word phrases and then progresses to multi-sentence responses and then to narratives. She includes hierarchies for propositionality, topic importance, stimuli, location, physical activity, and people present, as well as descriptions of how clinicians can facilitate the child's progress through the hierarchies (Fig. 10-2).

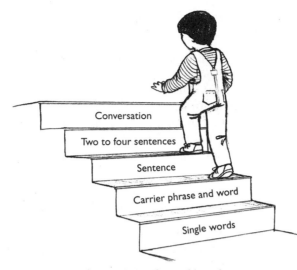

Figure 10–2 *Fluency hierarchy.*

As the child progresses up the hierarchy, the clinician introduces various pressures and potential fluency disruptors to prepare the child for generalizing fluency to the real world. Parents' charts of the child's disfluencies outside the clinic are valuable in identifying those stressors to which the child is vulnerable. Just as a weakened form of smallpox is used to inoculate a person against the real thing, stressors are introduced in treatment in mild forms at first to ensure success. The fluency disruptors are then increased in magnitude but always in a manner that strengthens the child's tolerance, as described in Van Riper (1973).

A further procedure used by Hill to increase generalization is to place a child in a children's therapy group, which allows the child to learn from other children who are practicing fluent, easy, relaxed speech. It also provides a realistic context in which the clinician can facilitate the child's fluency during such activities as competitive speaking, talking in a group, and meeting new people, which are situations that may be stressful.

4. Identify and Modify Child Factors with the Potential to Interfere with the Development of Fluency

Some children have difficulties in addition to stuttering that may interfere with their learning to become fluent using easy, relaxed speech. For example, many children who stutter have other concomitant speech-language disorders, such as phonological errors, language delay, or word-finding difficulties. A section at the end of this chapter suggests how treatment of these other communication problems may be integrated with stuttering therapy. Problems other than communication difficulties may also interfere with learning to become fluent, such as shyness and aggression. Some of these problems, in milder form, may be handled by the clinician as stuttering treatment is progressing, but more severe forms of the problems may require referral to other professionals trained to deal with these specific issues.

5. Integrating Cognitive, Affective, and Behavioral Aspects of Therapy

The clinician needs to be aware of normal cognitive, affective, and behavioral development in order to determine whether or not a child has difficulty in one or more of these domains. Generally, as with the mild problems discussed earlier, work on these areas can be incorporated into stuttering treatment. Children with cognitive delays, for example, may need more concrete activities to help them understand and use slow and easy, relaxed speech. Children who are fearful of making mistakes and trying new things can be helped by a clinician who works with them on new tasks and models making and accepting her own mistakes.

6. Gradually Phase Out Treatment and Implement a Follow-Up Plan

Hill recommends a formal plan for gradually decreasing the frequency of contact with a child and her family. When a child has sustained normal fluency or borderline level of stuttering or has had 2% or less stuttering-like disfluencies for 2 months, phasing out of treatment contacts begins. Contact with the clinician decreases initially from twice a week to once a week for 2 and a half months, then once a month for 2 months. Parents are encouraged to take the lead in monitoring and solving problems concerning the child's fluency but are urged to stay in contact with the clinician by telephone. After 6 months, a formal re-check at the clinic is undertaken.

Hill reports that "successful intervention may take 8 to 12 months, but approximately 5 percent of these children have persisting problems that require referral for family counseling or psychoeducational consultation and/or longer-term speech-language therapy" (Hill, 2003, pp. 183-184). This suggests that 95% of the clients treated with this therapy may be successful long-term, but specific follow-up data are not presented.

Tim Mackesey

Using an approach to stuttering he calls "F.A.S.T. Fluency," an acronym for Family and SLP Treatment, Mackesey works directly with children 2 to 6 years old and involves parents at all stages of therapy. For those children who are relatively mild stutterers, Mackesey uses a structure that is similar to the Lidcombe program. To begin, Mackesey models therapy for the parents in the clinic. The parents then demonstrate the therapy for him and then work in a similar way at home. Parents are taught to play "fluency" games with their children twice each day at home. They reinforce fluency in increasingly natural situations, so that reinforcement for fluency becomes a normal part of the child's day. Verbal contingencies are not used with stuttering, unlike the Lidcombe program. As treatment goes on in the clinic as well as at home, Mackesey introduces various distractors, such as putting time pressure on the child and creating excitement, while continuing to reinforce fluency.

For preschool children with more severe stuttering, Mackesey teaches the equivalent of a "pull-out." The child holds on to a stutter while it's occurring and gradually relaxes the tension and finishes the word. He demonstrates this to children using such activities as trying to pull a stuck sock out of a mostly closed bureau drawer. As children (and their parents) learn the skill of using a pull-out when a stutter occurs, they are taught the accompanying concept that patience achieves more than force. Once they have the idea of using a pull-out, he asks them to "catch bumpy words" and ease out of them. Mackesey notes that both he and parents observe that children rapidly adopt the relaxed release of stutters in place of forcing words out.

Once these more severely stuttering preschool children have practiced the pull-outs and have learned the concept, Mackesey begins cueing the children, during moments of stuttering, to use pull-outs. He interrupts a child who is stuck in a moment of stuttering by using a tactile and auditory cue, such as a gentle touch accompanied by a verbal prompt, like "Oops, say _____ (whatever the word is)." He then praises the child with a comment like, "Wow! You fixed that bumpy word!" Once a child has mastered these pull-outs in response to cueing (and sometimes without it), Mackesey teaches parents to use it. He is very careful to ensure that parents are using it properly and only in situations where the child would feel comfortable (i.e., at home and not in public). Both praise for fixing stutters and intermittent praise for fluent utterances are given.

The children's skill at being able to fix their own stuttered words is transferred to the home environment with the help of reinforcers such as poster boards in the kitchen on which children can attach stickers to columns labeled "I can talk smooth" and "I can fix my words."

Mackesey measures stuttering in percent syllables stuttered at the beginning of treatment and intermittently throughout treatment as well as in follow-ups after treatment has ended. Mackesey's criteria for success is less than 1% syllables stuttered, measured at least 3 months after treatment via clinic visits or taped conversational samples submitted by mail. In 5 years, he has treated 63 children, and 59 of them have been treated successfully. Eighty percent of these children were between 8 months and 5 years after treatment. Average treatment time was nine clinic visits. Two children dropped out of the program, and two children were not able to be contacted for follow-up because they moved out of state.

Woodruff Starkweather, Sheryl Gottwald, and Murray Halfond

Starkweather, Gottwald, and Halfond use three treatment strategies to help the child with beginning stuttering: individual parent counseling, group parent counseling, and modification of the child's speech (Gottwald and Starkweather, 1999; Starkweather, Gottwald, and Halfond, 1990).

The initial component of individual parent counseling provides parents with information about the nature of stuttering. For example, the clinician informs them that stuttering is highly variable and that many factors may influence its ups and downs, including factors that they may be able to change. The family is also introduced to an etiological model of stuttering, which explains it as emerging from interactions between the child's capacities and the demands placed on the child. The clinician also helps the family to find ways of talking about stuttering with their child. They learn to support the child by commenting sensitively when she has difficulty getting a word out. Open acknowledgment of stuttering is intended to reduce the child's and the family's negative feelings about stuttering.

During individual counseling (Fig. 10–3), families are also taught to change other aspects of their behavior that may be affecting their child's fluency. For example, family members may learn to respond to the child's stuttering without interrupting, looking

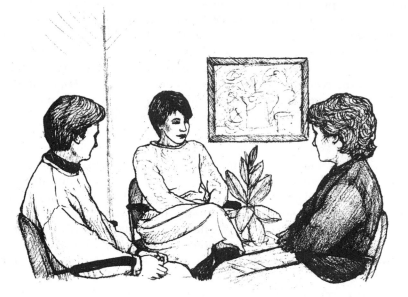

Figure 10–3 *Counseling with a family.*

away, or otherwise conveying impatience. To decrease pressure from the family's speech and language environment on the child, family members may be taught to slow their speech rates, pause more frequently, and simplify their language when talking with the child. To increase the child's self-esteem, families may be urged to create times each day when the child has a parent's full attention. Sometimes, family members may be bombarding the child with questions or otherwise pressing him to speak. As a remedy, they are shown how to talk about what they are thinking and doing as they play with the child, thereby modeling the behavior they want to encourage.

In addition to changing behavior directly related to speech, families are also counseled about other stresses in the home. For example, Starkweather and his colleagues note that a hectic family lifestyle can exacerbate a child's stuttering. Once parents understand that a too-busy family schedule may be a factor in their child's stuttering, they are often able to reduce the hustle and bustle in the home and are gratified when their child's stuttering subsequently diminishes. In addition, a slower pace and lifestyle can often provide increased satisfaction for all family members.

Starkweather, Gottwald, and Halfond's approach uses group parent counseling to supplement individual family counseling. As members of a group, parents receive support from one another and can share ideas for helping their children. The clinician's role is to help the group members develop a sense of mutual trust by modeling concern, acceptance, and respect for all group members and their ideas and feelings. Generally, the group talks about topics they select, although the clinician also may suggest topics that are often concerns of most members, such as regression during treatment and at termination of treatment.

The third component of this therapy, which is modification of the child's speech, incorporates both parent and clinician modeling and reinforcement, as well as the clinician's direct instruction, when needed. Direct instruction in changing stuttering with older preschool-age children is a natural outgrowth of the parents and clinician talking openly about stuttering with the child. The procedures that the authors use to modify a child's speech are as follows.

First, when an evaluation indicates that a child is talking faster than usual for her age or is using more complex language, the clinician and parent model speech rates and language that are more appropriate for the child. The aim is to encourage the child to talk in ways that do not stress her ability.

Second, the clinician uses modeling, instruction, and reinforcement to help the child stutter more simply and loosely, thereby making it more like stuttering often is when it first appears. Their approach attempts to move the child backwards on what they consider to be the developmental sequence of stuttering. They hypothesize that most children who stutter begin with relaxed, slow, whole-word repetitions, then develop part-word repetitions or prolongations, and progress to increasingly tense and rapid repetitions and tense prolongations, until finally reaching the stage of tense blockages of speech. Consequently, if a child stutters with considerable tension and struggle, she's taught to stutter with easy prolongations of sounds and then easy, slow repetitions. Individual and group parent counseling and modification of the child's speech continue until the family environment and the child's speech have met the following two criteria. First, the environment has changed enough so that major stresses have diminished and the family seems to understand the dynamics that may exist between environmental stresses and the child's stuttering. Second, the child's stuttering has decreased to the point at which she is normally disfluent, with an occasional mild instance of stuttering.

Starkweather and his colleagues report that most of the children they have treated have regained normal fluency. Of 39 children who they treated using this approach, seven dropped out, and of the remaining 32 children, 29 recovered completely, and three were still in treatment at the time of the report. The average child requires about 12 sessions of therapy using this approach, although some children require much more before therapy can be terminated.

Janis Costello Ingham

Janis Ingham is a leading advocate of operant conditioning and programmed instruction procedures in the treatment of a beginning stutterer. She refers to her treatment procedures as the extended length of utterance (ELU) program. A detailed description of her ELU program is provided in a chapter titled, "Behavioral Treatment of Young Children Who Stutter: An Extended Length of Utterance Method" (Ingham, J.C., 1999).

Ingham's ELU program is a clinician-delivered therapy that uses feedback to the child via positive and negative reinforcement of the child's speech. Therapy moves the child from short, fluent utterances to longer fluent utterances in the treatment room and then to spontaneous fluent conversation in all environments. The program begins by using picture cards to elicit brief utterances by the child. When the child is fluent during sessions, which should be most of the time, the clinician delivers positive reinforcers, either praise or, if needed, a token that can be redeemed for a tangible prize. When the child stutters, the clinician says "stop" in a gentle voice, and the child stops speaking for a few seconds.

Criteria for each step must be passed before the child moves to the next step, requiring her to produce longer fluent utterances. For example, the criterion for the first step using picture cards is 10 consecutive fluent utterances. There are also criteria for failing to pass a step, such as seven consecutive stuttered trials or 100 trials without passing the criterion. If a child fails a step, the clinician creates a "branching" step, which is designed to help the child pass the failed step. Sometimes a branching step will consist of adjusting the clinician's feedback to the child to increase her motivation, sometimes it will be an easier, intermediate step between the successful step that preceded the failed step, and sometimes it will just be an opportunity for the child to refocus her attention on the task.

The progression of the child's fluent responses begins with single-syllable words and gradually advances to longer and longer conversational speech. After 20 successful steps, the program reaches a criterion requiring the child to converse fluently for 5 minutes in the therapy setting. Most children, especially younger children, will be fluent in all situations by the time they have completed the program's last step in the treatment room. However, for those children who have not generalized fluency to all situations, Ingham provides advice about encouraging self-management, parent training, and inclusion of a peer or sibling in treatment to enhance a child's generalization.

Self-management is developed through having the child involved more and more in choosing treatment tasks and contingencies. The children may, for example, bring pictures and books from home to use for stimuli, choose conversational topics, and pick their own reinforcers, including what they receive in exchange for tokens earned, as well as the words the clinician uses for praise and acknowledging stutters. Children may also be encouraged to record their own responses and share their data sheets with their family. The older the child, the better able they may be to employ self-management. Some children are able to monitor their own levels of fluency, and if accurate, they can be encouraged to use self-reinforcement for fluent utterances and self-corrections for stuttering.

Parent training in this treatment program can be similar to that used in the Lidcombe Program, with the clinician demonstrating treatment procedures and the parent trying them out in the clinic and then providing treatment at home. Training must ensure that the parent learns to distinguish between stuttering and normal speech, including normal disfluencies. In some cases, instead of providing treatment at home, parents will only be asked to positively reinforce fluent speech in the home and other environments. Peers, siblings, and teachers may also be involved in such treatment activities to enhance generalization of the child's stutter-free speech to all environments.

Ingham reported data in "Behavioral Treatment of Young Children Who Stutter: An Extended Length of Utterance Method" (Ingham, 1999) for a small number of children who were 3 to 5 years of age, indicating that their stuttering was eliminated.

Treatment of Concomitant Speech and Language Problems

One of the clinical issues that should be considered, especially with beginning stuttering, is the management of concomitant speech and language problems. Research has indicated that some of these children are delayed in their speech and language development, especially in their articulation or phonological development. When using the Lidcombe

Program, it is imperative that only stuttering be treated during Stage 1, when the parent and child are highly involved in working on fluency. Typically, the Lidcombe Program up to Stage 1 is conducted first and then any other speech or language problem would be treated. In some cases, however, when another problem is particularly severe, treatment can be focused on that problem first until appropriate improvement is made. Then Stage 1 of Lidcombe can be implemented, and treatment of the other problem(s) can be resumed when Stage 1 is finished. During treatment on the Lidcombe program, it is crucial that parents understand that the focus is only on fluency so that their severity ratings are not affected by the other disorder(s).

A number of clinicians not using the Lidcombe Program have recommended a variety of ways of responding to other, concomitant speech and language problems in beginning stutterers. We will discuss the contributions of Conture, Louko, and Edwards, Gregory and Hill, Ratner, Wall and Myers, and Riley and Riley to this issue.

In discussing the contributions of these clinicians, I will limit my remarks primarily to their views on the clinical management of concomitant speech and language problems as they interface with the treatment of the stuttering and not discuss their overall treatment approach to stuttering.

Edward Conture, Linda Louko, and Mary Louise Edwards

Conture, Louko, and Edwards (1993) developed a treatment approach for children with fluency and phonological problems that tempers the demands of articulation therapy while providing support for increased fluency. These researchers work on both problems at the same time but use an indirect approach for the articulation problems. This avoids the demands of traditional "corrective" articulation therapy. Their approach provides the child with plenty of models of target phonemes through extensive auditory stimulation and opportunities for improved production. This is done in an accepting environment rather than correcting the child when he is wrong and asking him to try again with more attention and effort. Thus, this approach does not stress the child's production capacities as much as a traditional approach to articulation therapy. Conture, Louko, and Edwards also incorporate a variety of fluency facilitating techniques, such as slow speaking rate, relaxed manner of speaking, reduced interruptions, and increased interspeaker pause time. This is done while they work on articulation to enhance the child's overall fluency when under the stress of attempting to produce new phonological structures. This approach is contrasted with other approaches in the section on Ratner's overview of these therapies.

Diane Hill

Diane Hill (Hill, 2003) believes that it is best for 3- to 4-year-old children having concomitant phonological, language, or word-finding problems to begin treatment with work on fluency. In working on fluency, she systematically increases the length and complexity of a child's utterances from single-word responses, to phrases, to sentences, and, finally, to conversation. Hill suggests that this strategy readily lends itself to working on language or phonological delays. Once fluency is established at the sentence level, some work on phonology or language may be introduced. As work on fluency continues, one activity per session can be focused on a concomitant problem, such as phonology for example.

Hill believes that clinicians should use a low-key approach in treatment that does not place too much demand on a child's fluency. When the child's phonology is delayed, the clinician can begin with receptive training and then follow with a sequence of working on phonemic change, sound play, sound approximation, and rehearsal of correct sound production in a few target sounds. If language is an issue, the clinician again begins with receptive training, followed by integrating practice with proper syntactic forms into the fluency hierarchy of more and more complex language. For example, the clinician provides appropriate instructions and materials and has the child practice a specific syntactic structure while using easy, relaxed speech.

Gregory and Hill (1980) reported that a significant percentage of the young stutterers they see have word-finding problems. Hill believes that the first goal is to help these children feel comfortable with pauses in their speech. Therefore, she models delays in responding to naming tasks and then says something like, "I can't think of what that is called, but everybody has problems like this sometimes." Of course, she also gives the child ample time to recall words. Her second goal is to provide these children with a strategy for retrieving words by helping the child learn to build associations between objects and their semantic attributes, such as function, size, shape, color, and other characteristics. Then, she creates situations for the child to practice using this strategy to retrieve words during naming tasks.

Hill (2003) also works with parents to improve the speech and language models to which their child is exposed at home. For example, if parents speak too rapidly, ask too many questions too quickly, or do not listen to the child, she instructs and models more appropriate speech and language behaviors for them to use around the child.

Nan Ratner

Ratner discussed several models for working with children who stutter and have other concomitant speech or language disorders (Ratner, 1995). The sequential model typically treats the language or articulation problem first, with the hope that once this problem is resolved, stuttering will no longer be a problem for the child. If it is not improved, the child's stuttering may become more severe, more chronic, and more resistant to treatment, either because of the demands of the language or articulation therapy she received or simply because her stuttering remained untreated for an extended period of time.

The concurrent model avoids this problem by beginning treatment of fluency simultaneously with treatment of the other disorder(s). When this approach is used effectively, two principles are followed. First, the child practices fluency only with language and phonological structures that have already been mastered. Second, phonological or language therapy procedures avoid demands that may make the child excessively self-conscious of his errors. This can prevent him from using excessive physical or mental efforts in the production of the forms targeted for therapy (Conture, Louko, and Edwards, 1993).

A third model, the blended model, also works on both fluency and the other disorder(s) at the same time, which provides extra support of fluency. The clinician and child speak with slow rates, gentle onsets, relaxed movements, ample pauses within and between utterances, and careful turn taking. Training and modeling of this style of speaking are crucial for success. As new phonological and linguistic structures are mastered, they are practiced with more normal speech characteristics (e.g., normal rate, and so on). A particular advantage of the blended approach is that it gives the child an opportunity to tackle difficult utterances with complex language and challenging phonology while having the support of fluency facilitators. Thus, the child learns to maintain fluency in the face of high demands (see the section on the approach of Conture, Louko, and Edwards).

The fourth and final model, the cyclic model, alternates fluency treatment with language or phonology therapy over the course of the year. Ratner points out that this provides children with initial periods of concentrated learning of new skills, followed by opportunities for spontaneous generalization of these skills to other settings.

Glyndon and Jeanna Riley

Glyndon and Jeanna Riley (1984) advocate a "component model" of treatment for children at "Intervention Level II: Chronic Stuttering." By treating underlying components of stuttering, they report that children regain normal fluency in most cases. At this intervention level, they do not attempt to modify a child's moments of stuttering or reinforce his fluent responses. They treat only what they see as underlying and maintaining components of stuttering.

There are nine components in the Rileys' model. Four are "neurogenic" components, and five are "traditional" components. The neurogenic components are attending disorders, auditory processing disorders, sentence formulation disorders, and oral motor disorders. The five traditional components are disruptive communicative environment, unrealistic parental expectations, abnormal parental need for the child to stutter, high self-expectations by the child, and manipulative stuttering. In my view, three of these components (auditory processing disorders, sentence formulation disorders, and disruptive communicative environment) may best be viewed as concomitant speech and language problems.

Riley and Riley (1984) report that approximately 27% of their young stutterers have auditory processing disorders. By auditory processing disorders, they mean that the child has problems receiving and manipulating auditory information. Such children may have any of the following problems: retaining auditory images, making figure-ground distinctions, or selecting meaningful from nonmeaningful auditory signals. Treatment goals depend on a child's particular auditory processing problem but often include increasing the child's auditory memory or his ability to follow verbal directions. Riley and Riley recommend a number of commercially available programs for improving children's receptive language abilities.

Sentence formulation disorders may include the following types of problems: word retrieval problems, word order problems involving reversals and transpositions, and formulation problems involving incomplete and fragmented sentences. They report that approximately 30% of their young stutterers have such problems. Treatment goals depend on a child's particular problems. A number of commercially available materials based on generative grammar, and not those based simply on utterance length, are recommended for treating these types of expressive language difficulties. Riley and Riley (1984) also stress the importance of a careful analysis of a child's syntax so that treatment is targeted at the child's level of language abilities.

Riley and Riley (1984) report that 53% of their young stutterers come from disruptive communicative environments that are fluency disrupters in a child's environment, such as the child having difficulty getting the parents' attention, being interrupted while talking, or being rushed while speaking. In such cases, the Rileys counsel parents regarding the importance of reducing such fluency disrupters.

Meryl Wall and Florence Myers

Meryl Wall and Florence Myers (1984) note that some clinicians are reluctant to work on a young stutterer's concomitant speech or language problems because they fear that calling attention to the child's speech and language will exacerbate stuttering. They believe, however, that such fear is largely unjustified. Their basic approach to therapy (Wall and Myers, 1995) for all children who stutter has a "language-based orientation," in which they control the length and semantic-syntactic complexity of the child's utterances. Therapy typically goes through the following sequence: two- and three-word phrases, simple sentences, complex sentences, picture descriptions, storytelling, and conversation.

Wall and Myers indicate that this method of sequencing linguistic tasks ensures that the length and semantic-syntactic complexity of therapy activities are kept within the child's capacity. In the early stages of therapy, vocabulary should consist of words already in the child's repertoire.

In the later stages, new words can be added to the child's lexicon. In a similar manner, syntactic structures already in the child's repertoire are used in early stages of treatment. Later on, new grammatical structures can be gradually introduced in their normal developmental sequence. Wall and Myers recommend that clinicians move a child through this sequence of linguistic tasks, with easy speech or pull-outs being incorporated with the work on new vocabulary or new syntactic structures.

What about a child with a phonological or articulation disorder? Wall and Myers (1995) recommend that such problems be treated after fluency has been stabilized if the child's disability is mild and not interfering with speech intelligibility. However, if the disability is interfering with intelligibility, the problem should be dealt with immediately because it may be adding considerable stress to the child's communicative attempts. If treatment of a phonological or articulation disorder is begun, Wall and Myers recommend that the phoneme or phoneme group selected for treatment be one that is the easiest for the child to produce. Words and syntactic structures selected for practice material should be ones with which the child can easily cope. Work on speech sound production can be integrated with work on fluency. For example, practice of a new sound in a word can be integrated with practice of easy speech.

Wall and Myers (1995) also have suggestions for parents of a child with both stuttering and delayed speech and language. If the parents talk fast, they are asked to talk more slowly around the child. If they use language that clearly exceeds the child's semantic-syntactic skill, they are asked to simplify their language when talking to the child. To help parents make these changes and become better fluency models for their child, Wall and Myers encourage parents to watch the clinician working with their child and observe how she modifies her speech rate and language to enhance the child's fluency.

In addition to improving the fluency models that parents present to their child, Wall and Myers (1995) also discuss with parents other ways to use language at home to enhance their child's fluency. They point out that questions that require short responses usually elicit more fluency than open-ended questions that require longer, more complex answers. For example, "Did you have fun at Ted's birthday party?" usually elicits a shorter and more fluent response than "What did you do at Ted's birthday party?" In using these and other strategies, Wall and Myers help parents provide their child with a linguistic environment that is more conducive to fluency.

Summary

- The author believes that beginning stuttering arises from an interaction between children's constitutional predispositions interacting with developmental and environmental influences to produce primarily repetitive disfluencies with increased tension. Escape behaviors are also an important component of the disorder, as children experience increasing frustration with their inability to complete a word.

- Children with beginning stuttering usually have a large amount of fluency that can be reinforced and generalized to situations that previously elicited stuttering.

- The Lidcombe Program is a parent-delivered, operant conditioning program for preschoolers in which the parent is guided to conduct daily treatment conversations and apply verbal contingencies to fluency and stuttering. Treatment begins in structured conversations and quickly moves to unstructured conversations throughout the day, so that treatment is conducted in the children's natural speaking environment, necessitating little work on generalization. Once the child is fluent in all situations, the clinician manages a phased withdrawal of clinic contact with careful monitoring of progress so that the family can respond to any relapses by reinstating needed features of treatment and then return to the fading process.

- Other treatments for stuttering include: (1) Cook and Botterill's parent-child interaction therapy; (2) Hill and Gregory's combination of parent counseling and teaching the child fluency skills, generalizing them, and developing a resistance to fluency disruptors; (3) Starkweather, Gottwald, and Murray's parent counseling and speech modification approach; and (4) Ingham's operant conditioning and programmed instruction for children, which replaces stuttering with fluency and engages parents to become clincians at home.

- In the Lidcombe Program, work on other communication disorders precedes or, more typically, follows Stage 1 of treatment. In other treatment approaches, clinicians often integrate work on fluency with other concomitant speech or language problems.

Study Questions

1. Describe Stage 1 and Stage 2 of the Lidcombe Program for the beginning stutterer. What is the goal of each phase?
2. Describe structured and unstructured treatment conversations in the Lidcombe program.

3. Describe the two major ways of collecting data on the child's progress in the Lidcombe Program.

4. Describe how the two different types of data are used to guide the child's progress in the Lidcombe Program.

5. Compare the Lidcombe Program with (1) Cook and Botterill's approach and (2) Hill and Gregory's approach. In what ways are they similar, and in what ways are the different?

6. Basing your answer on Conture, Louko, and Edwards', Gregory and Hill's, and Wall and Myers' approaches, describe how the treatment of beginning stuttering and other speech and language disorders can be integrated.

7. What are the four approaches to treating concomitant problems described by Ratner?

SUGGESTED PROJECTS

(1) Develop a hierarchy, based on length and complexity of utterances that could be used by a clinician who is working with beginning stuttering and wants to move from single words to conversational speech.

(2) Develop a hierarchy, based on increasing social complexity, for a child with beginning stuttering. Design it for use by a typical, two-parent family with older and younger siblings and grandparents who visit frequently.

(3) Interview the family of a child with beginning stuttering who was treated successfully. Find out what they perceived to be the most helpful aspects of treatment and what advice they would give to other families just beginning treatment.

Suggested Readings

Bernstein Ratner, N. (1995). Treating the child who stutters with concomitant language and phonological impairment. *Language, Speech, and Hearing Services in Schools,* 26:180–186.
  In this insightful overview of the treatment of children with concomitant disorders, Bernstein Ratner identifies several models that have evolved.

Conture, E. (2001). *Stuttering: Its Nature, Diagnosis, and Treatment.* **Boston: Allyn & Bacon.**
  Chapter 3 of Conture's text (Remediation: Children Who Stutter) describes treatment of beginning stuttering with excellent analogies that will appeal to children and make sense to clinicians. Sections of this chapter on working with children who stutter and who also have other communcation problems are also excellent.

Conture, E., Louko, L., and Edwards, M.L. (1993). Simultaneously treating stuttering and disordered phonology in children: Experimental therapy, preliminary findings. *American Journal of Speech-Language Pathology,* 2:72–81.
  This article details how to use indirect articulation therapy with children at both beginning and intermediate levels of stuttering.

Gregory, H.H. (2003). *Stuttering Therapy: Rationale and Procedures.* **Boston: Allyn & Bacon.**

The chapter on treating stuttering in the early stages of development is quite relevant to beginning stuttering, particularly the "Comprehensive Fluency Development Program." Diane Hill's description of relaxation and modeling, as well as generalization of fluency skills, may be helpful for many clinicians not using the Lidcombe Program.

Onslow, M., Packman, A., and Harrison, E. (2003). *The Lidcombe Program of Early Stuttering Intervention: A Clinician's Guide.* **Austin, TX: Pro-Ed.**

This is a complete guide for both new and experienced clinicians who have been trained to use the Lidcombe Program. It is very clear and filled with clinical wisdom.

Ramig, P., and Dodge, D. (2005). *The Child and Adolescent Stuttering Therapy and Activity Resource Guide.* **Clifton Park, NY: Thompson Delmar Learning.**

There are a vast array of activities and techniques in this book for use by clinicians using almost any approach to treatment. The book also covers evaluation, treatment planning, and report writing.

Riley, G.D., and Riley, J. (1984). A component model for treating stuttering in children. In M. Peins (Ed), *Contemporary Approaches in Stuttering Therapy.* **Boston: Little, Brown, & Company.**

This chapter describes treatment for oral motor, language, and other problems that may be components of stuttering in children.

Shapiro, D. (1999). *Stuttering Intervention: A Collaborative Journey to Fluency Freedom.* **Austin, TX: Pro-Ed.**

The section on direct intervention in the chapter on intervention with preschool children has many excellent suggestions for treatment, including ideas for building up resistance to fluency disruptors and encouraging expression of emotion.

Wall, M.J., and Myers, F.L. (1995). *Clinical Management of Childhood Stuttering* **(ed 2). Austin, TX: Pro-Ed.**

This edition includes a complete treatment approach for beginning and intermediate stutterers. It appears to be available from Amazon.com.

Zebrowski, P.M., and Kelly, E. (2002). *Manual of Stuttering Intervention.* **Clifton Park, NY: Singular.**

The chapter on treatment of the preschool child, particularly treatment of those children who are likely to persist in stuttering, contains many excellent ideas for direct work on stuttering. Many case examples are given.

Chapter 11

Treatment of Intermediate Stuttering

An Integrated Approach .

The child with intermediate stuttering is usually an elementary or junior high school student between 6 and 13 years of age who has been stuttering for several years. I use the word "child" to refer to a client, but I am aware that when a youngster is 10 years or older, he is more like an adolescent in many ways than like a child. The typical intermediate stutterer exhibits tense part-word and monosyllabic whole-word repetitions, as well as tense prolongations; however, blocks with tension and struggle are the most evident sign of stuttering. This child may use escape devices, such as body movements or brief verbalizations (e.g., "uh"), to break free of stutters. He may also use various avoidance strategies such as starters, word substitutions, circumlocutions, and evasion of difficult speaking situations. He experiences more frustration and embarrassment than beginning stutterers do and has distinct anticipation of stuttering on specific sounds, words, and many speaking situations. His major fear is the moment of stuttering itself, and he has a definite concept of himself as a stutterer.

My approach to intermediate stuttering is markedly different from the fluency shaping I use with beginning stuttering. I typically begin treatment with a stuttering modification approach, which focuses on decreasing the child's fear and increasing his understanding of stuttering. After that, treatment progresses to teaching the child to use "superfluency," which is a style of speaking that incorporates fluency-shaping components such as slow speech rate and gentle onset of phonation. In the later stages of treatment, I help the child replace anticipated or actual stutters by "turning on" superfluency.

Author's Beliefs

Nature of Stuttering

I believe that, in intermediate levels of stuttering, neurophysiological factors combined with a vulnerable temperament interact with developmental and environmental factors to prevent natural recovery and produce or exacerbate the core behaviors of repetitions, prolongations, and mild blocks. Children respond to these disfluencies with increased tension that, in turn, increases the frequency and duration of repetitions, prolongations, and blocks. As young stutterers experience more and more of these increasingly severe core behaviors, their emotions flare up, and a host of secondary behaviors arise.

To the frustrations and embarrassments of beginning stuttering are added anticipatory fears. These fears spread through classical conditioning to many sounds, words, and speaking situations and soon beget avoidance behaviors. Children with intermediate stuttering begin to avoid feared words and situations by using starters, postponements, substitutions, circumlocutions, and just saying, "I don't know" when asked a question. Avoidance behaviors are reinforced when children are intermittantly successful in preventing stuttering. Because longer and more abnormal moments of stuttering lead to more negative listener reactions and, in turn, to more avoidances, children with intermediate stuttering develop the belief that stuttering is bad and, therefore, that they are bad when they stutter. Shame about their speech then becomes a feature of their daily life.

Because the tension response, escape and avoidance behaviors, and negative feelings and attitudes are all learned, I believe they can be modified by new learning. The context for this change must be an accepting, supportive environment that focuses on the child as a person, rather than just on his stuttering. Many intermediate stutterers feel that they have failed in previous therapy and thus have disappointed their parents and teachers because they did not become fluent. Thus, I must help these children feel accepted with their current level of stuttering, as well as help them experience mastery and success with their speech.

If treatment can provide an intermediate stutterer with a sufficient number of emotionally positive speaking experiences in therapy, such as experiences in which he feels "in control" of his speech, the increased fluency and positive feelings associated with speaking will generalize to other environments. The clinician can use operant and classical conditioning principles to achieve this. Furthermore, because predisposing neurophysiological factors may contribute to the core behaviors in the speech of many intermediate stutterers, it is also important to help children at this age cope effectively with any remaining disruptions in their speech. These twin goals of positive speaking experiences and coping with the remaining stuttering can be achieved using a combination of stuttering modification and fluency shaping. In implementing these goals with an intermediate stutterer, I need to keep in mind the child's age and maturity because these will influence the selection of clinical procedures.

Finally, it is important to reduce developmental and environmental influences that may be contributing to the child's stuttering. I can do this by working with the child's parents and classroom teachers, helping them create an environment that accepts the child, regardless of his progress with speech, and thus that helps him feel free to work on his speech, thereby facilitating change. In addition, I help the child communicate directly with his parents and teachers about how they can best help him deal with his stuttering.

Speech Behaviors Targeted for Therapy

The speech behaviors targeted for intermediate stuttering therapy are both stuttered and fluent speech. Unlike treatment of beginning stuttering, this therapy begins with a focus on stuttering behaviors that are first explored and then changed. Subsequently, fluent speech becomes the target for therapy and is shaped using various tools, such as easy onsets and light contacts.

Fluency Goals

Which fluency goals are realistic for intermediate stutterers? Some intermediate stutterers may become normal or spontaneously fluent speakers, which is more likely for younger than for older intermediate stutterers. Typically, an intermediate stutterer will need to use controlled fluency to sound normal. This is often a difficult task for a youngster (or indeed any speaker) to do on a consistent basis. Although he may use controlled fluency in some situations, a child this age often may not have the motivation or self-discipline to control fluency throughout his daily talking. Thus, I believe that a realistic fluency goal for many intermediate stutterers is acceptable stuttering; that is, fluency mixed with mild or very mild stuttering.

Feelings and Attitudes

How much attention should be given to an intermediate stutterer's feelings and attitudes about his speech? Whenever a child is experiencing frustration and embarrassment and is beginning to experience some fear related to speech, as is usually the case for intermediate stutterers, I believe it is important to reduce these negative feelings. Furthermore, because these children are beginning to avoid certain words and speaking situations, it is important to eliminate or reduce these avoidances.

Maintenance Procedures

The typical intermediate stutterer needs more hours of treatment than a beginning stutterer. And after formal treatment has ended, it is likely that he will need continued contact to maintain improvements in his fluency. A systematic, planned program of gradual fading of treatment contact and continuing assessment of improvements is recommended. In addition, if he can become a mentor to younger children who stutter, it will help him maintain fluency, as well as bolster his self-esteem.

Clinical Methods

My approach to intermediate stuttering is to use a combination of stuttering modification and fluency-shaping strategies for the child. Soon after I begin therapy with the child, I also work with the child's parents and the teachers to create "stuttering friendly" environments that increase the child's comfort using the techniques we learn together in treatment. The measures I use to assess progress are described in the section titled "Progress and Outcome Measures."

Clinical Procedures: Working with a Child

My clinical methods for intermediate stuttering have been influenced by many people, but Charles Van Riper has been my prime inspiration. Many of the techniques and much of the philosophy in my approach come straight from a chapter in Van Riper's treatment book entitled, "The Young Confirmed Stutterer" (Van Riper, 1973). I am also indebted to Richard Boemhler for my understanding of how to replace stuttering with controlled normal fluency and to Julie Reville, who shared her intuitive clinical approaches with this age group. Many activities that she and I developed for treating children with intermediate stuttering are presented in our workbook, *Easy Talker* (Guitar and Reville, 1997).

Key Concepts

Van Riper (1973) cited fear, avoidance, struggle, and shame as four major characteristics of the intermediate stutterer. I will begin with a brief snapshot of these factors and how they can be dealt with in treatment.

1. *Fear and avoidance are major factors in intermediate stuttering.* Fear produces tension, making it difficult for youngsters to change their old, struggled patterns to more relaxed, forward-moving ways of saying words. Treatment, then, must reduce fear either directly or indirectly. The focus of this fear is getting stuck in a stutter. These children have had numerous experiences of their mouth and tongue and throat being jammed up and unable to move, and they don't want it to happen again. Because of this, they have learned to avoid words and situations and to employ starters and postponements. Avoidance is a very natural response to something unpleasant, especially for more sensitive children. To counteract it, therapy must tip the balance toward an "approach" attitude by helping children explore their stuttering, learn about it, and learn new responses to old cues.

2. *Struggle must be reduced to approximate normal speech.* Struggle arises when a child desperately wants to get a word out and to finish the communication but has contracted his muscles so tightly that the word can't come out. You can better understand a stutterer's experience if you imagine yourself stuck and in a hurry to get unstuck, for example, being stuck in traffic when you are late for an important meeting or trying to open a stuck door when a taxi's waiting. The child, when a sound is stuck, feels helpless, out of control, and frustrated; he pushes harder and harder; tension spills out to muscles throughout his face; and finally, the sound spurts out. Relief! The word is finished, communication is completed, and struggle is rewarded. Therapy to deal with this cycle of struggle and reward must use a two-pronged approach: (1) reducing the negative emotions and rewarding the easier speech that results, and (2) teaching the child to use controlled fluency (which I call "superfluency") instead of stuttering.

3. *Reduce shame by openness.* Bill Murphy has spoken and written in some detail about the shame associated with stuttering. His video, *The School-Age Child Who Stutters: Dealing Effectively with Guilt and Shame* (Stuttering Foundation publication #86, 1999) is an excellent resource for clinicians. Murphy notes that, whereas guilt is associated with something you have done, shame is related to the way you are. Thus, the intermediate stutterer has begun to feel that stuttering is a part of him;

he calls himself a stutterer, and it is the way he is. Shame can often be reduced by being more open about shaming experiences. For example, individuals who were sexually abused as children are sometimes ashamed because of it; however, they discover that, when they talk about their experiences to counselors or very close friends, they feel relief from the shame. This occurs with stuttering as well. When a child can talk to an accepting clinician about his stuttering experiences, especially negative listener reactions, his shame decreases. When he can talk to his parents about his stuttering and they can listen and accept his feelings, his shame decreases more. When he can talk to his peers, maybe even his whole class, his shame may almost disappear.

There are two more key concepts to keep in mind when working with intermediate stuttering. I have learned them through my own experience and by watching colleagues work with children who stutter.

4. *Therapy must be fun.* Most school-age children are ashamed and anxious about their stuttering. Rewards and games take the sting out of stuttering and reduce the anxiety associated with having to work on something shameful and difficult. Children in school settings are often reluctant to come to therapy, as so vividly portrayed by David Sedaris in *Me Talk Pretty One Day* (Sedaris, 2000). To draw them in, clinicians need to make therapy exciting, interesting, and above all, emotionally safe. When I worked in a junior high school in Washington D.C., kids thought it was cool to go to the "speech room," where there were always interesting games on tap, including poker. After we started the poker, even the principal wanted to come for a visit.

Many times, when a school-age child is reluctant to come to therapy or work on his speech, all that may be needed is an effective reward system. I have had success with Jolly Rancher Hard Candies, Skittles, and Gummy Worms. Every child will have his own favorites, and parents can be consulted about what is ok with them. With youngsters who are transferring new skills to outside situations, I have used a point system so they can earn food at a nearby shopping mall. In the session before a child and I go to the mall, we plan what we will do and how many points each assignment will bring. When I am working in the treatment room, I stock up with children's favorite rewards and let them earn candies, or sips of soda, or time playing a game after they achieve each objective. Snack reinforcers are highly effective for children in a therapy group, too. In our school kids' group, I use M&Ms to reward new behaviors, such as easy voluntary stutters. The competitive spirit usually ensures that every child in the group has filled his paper cup with M&Ms by the end of the session.

5. *Clinicians should first perform any tasks they ask children to perform.* Van Riper (1973) uses the term "identification" in a variety of ways. It is not only a term for getting to know one's stuttering, but it also describes the bond between the clinician and client. For the youngster with intermediate stuttering, a major factor in treatment is that the child identifies with the clinician and, therefore, wishes to please and emulate her. On the clinician's part, this means that she must be accepting of the child, be interested in him as a person, and must also model the behaviors that she wants the child to learn. Whether she's teaching easy stuttering or gentle onsets, the clinician must show the child what the new skill looks and sounds like. When she wants him to use easy stuttering on the phone, she should make the first phone call.

Beginning Therapy

In this first phase of treatment, I have a number of objectives. First, I help a child explore his stuttering; in part, this means that we talk about the moments of stuttering when they happen. As the child explores his stuttering, I try to help him understand what is happening when he stutters. Also, I help him identify easy stutters in his speech and suggest that those forms of easy talking are one of our goals for therapy. When he learns how to use easy stutters whenever he wants, to replace hard stuttering, we'll call it his "superfluency." This intensifying of the goal takes us into the realm of children's dreams and sets the stage for future accomplishments. Exploring, understanding, and setting our target for therapy are three objectives that are all interwoven into the fabric of our first phase of therapy.

When I meet a child for the first time, I let him know that I'm here to help him with his stuttering, but first I want to know more about him. I ask about what he likes to do after school and on the weekends, as well as about his family, his likes, and his dislikes. I want him to see that I'm a good listener and hope this emerges naturally out of my real interest in his world. His daily life, his favorite activities, and his experiences provide the metaphors and analogies that we will use as we work together on his stuttering. As we talk, I convey my comfort with his stuttering by my relaxed attention during his moments of stuttering. At first, I just watch and listen carefully to learn what he does when he stutters; eventually, when he seems to be ready, I help him explore his stutters, as described in the following paragraphs.

Exploring

Exploring is the opposite of avoiding; it is an "approach" behavior that reduces negative emotions. When I proposed a theoretical background for persistent stuttering in Chapter 4, I speculated that the temperament of many children who have developed intermediate-level stuttering may be biased toward avoidance and withdrawal from threatening stimuli. This idea is put into practice by engaging such youngsters in activities that counteract their natural tendency to avoid.

Exploring the Goals of Therapy

It is important for a child to know where he's going in therapy and to know that the clinician has a map to guide him on his trip through sometimes difficult territory. Depending on his age, I will ask him about past therapy, what he learned, and what he'd like to get out of therapy. Most school-age children will probably answer that they would like their stuttering to be totally gone. I might say, in response, that we can work toward that goal, but then I would ask him if it would be ok if he had a little stuttering sometimes when he's excited or in a hurry. I let him know that, at first, he and I will be working to get to know his stuttering and what makes it happen, and then we'll work on helping him change his talking so that it will be easier. I might tell him this at the very beginning of therapy or after several sessions. It's often helpful to draw some pictures or diagrams to make the activities and sequence of therapy easier to grasp.

Exploring Beliefs About Stuttering

I think it is important for an intermediate stutterer to be given some explanation for his stuttering. He knows he stutters and has been stuttering probably for a number of years, and he needs to have an explanation for why he talks differently than his friends. So, what do I say to this child?

Choosing words that are appropriate for the child's age and comprehension level, I let him know that stuttering is not his fault and that much of it is learned and can be unlearned. I let him know that he must already be a good learner to have learned all the things he does when he stutters. This means he will be good at learning some new, easier ways of handling his stutters. To help him realize that stuttering is not his fault, I may say that just like some kids have trouble drawing pictures of things or other kids find it hard to play a musical instrument, he has a little more trouble getting words out smoothly if he is talking fast and has lots of ideas to get out. I let him know about famous people who also have the same problem, like the movie actors Bruce Willis, James Earl Jones (Darth Vader in "Star Wars"), and Nicholas Brendon (star of the TV show "Buffy the Vampire Slayer"). Lots of famous people stutter, but they have learned to change their stuttering so it is hardly noticeable and so can he.

I go on to explain that any inborn tendency to stutter accounts only for the fact that, sometimes when he talks fast or is excited or tired, he finds that he stumbles over words. This is the part I call natural stuttering. Other parts, the most bothersome parts, like getting really tight when he stutters or putting in extra sounds or eye blinks, are learned. If they are learned, he can change them. One tool I sometimes use to help teach intermediate stutterers about stuttering is the videotape, *Stuttering: Straight Talk for Teens,* which is available from the Stuttering Foundation of America (Guitar and Guitar, 2003). The Stuttering Foundation videos *Stuttering: Straight Talk for Teachers* and *Stuttering: For Kids by Kids* also have great examples of kids who stutter talking about the difficulties they face and how they have worked on their speech.

In helping a child to better understand his stuttering, I think it is beneficial for him to know that a lot of children stutter and that he is not the only person in the world who stutters. Often a child may not know any other child who stutters and may believe that he is one of only a very few who have this problem. So, I tell him that about 1 in 100 children stutter and that there are over 2 million people in the United States and millions more around the world who stutter. I believe this sort of information helps a child to feel less alone because of his stuttering.

Exploring the Core Behaviors of Stuttering

I guide a child to approach and explore the core behaviors of his stuttering using three principles taken from research on phobias in animals and humans (Mineka, 1985). These principles, adapted for stuttering, are: (1) the clinician must be unafraid of stuttering; (2) the child must explore his stuttering; and (3) the longer the child is able to remain in contact with moments of stuttering, the more his fear will be reduced.

The clinician can demonstrate her lack of fear of stuttering by her curiosity about the child's stuttering, by having the child teach her to imitate his stuttering, and by taking the lead in practicing in many situations. The clinician should cultivate and renew her own lack of fear of stuttering. She should be able to pseudo-stutter comfortably when talking with the child alone, as well as in public, to acquaintances and strangers.

The second principle, that the child must explore his stuttering, is the basis of much of the activity in this first phase of treatment. After I get to know a child and he feels at ease with me, I bring up the topic of stuttering with him. My aim is to help him become interested in his stuttering, rather than denying it and hoping it will go away. Because talking about stuttering is often uncomfortable for a child, I begin our discussions when we are drawing pictures, playing a game, or doing something else the child enjoys. Thus, I can alternate between helping the child explore his stuttering and moving back to an activity that is fun. To begin, I simply comment on the child's stuttering in an accepting manner. For instance, I may say something like "Hey, you really eased out of that one pretty well," or "That was a tough one, huh?" I take note of how he responds and whether he appears uncomfortable or whether he acknowledges his stuttering, even subtly and nonverbally, when I comment on it. This first approach to stuttering may go quite easily if I have won the child's trust and he is not excessively embarrassed by his stuttering. However, many children at the intermediate level feel helpless, frustrated, and ashamed about their stuttering. Fortunately, most can be helped to face their stuttering if I proceed slowly.

For a particularly sensitive child, I begin by providing him with a feeling of mastery over something else, such as a board game, drawing, or "shooting hoops" in the therapy room. I then alternate between exploring his stuttering and giving him relief through other activities of his choice. As I explore a child's stuttering with him, I not only comment on it but also ask him to describe what he's doing when he stutters. For example, I might say, "Okay, there was an interesting one. What did you do when you stuttered on that word?" Then, I help him feel and identify what he actually does when he stutters. For many children, this focus on stuttering behavior is an openness that can change their emotions from shame and helpless confusion to a more hopeful and objective outlook.

At some point during early exploration of a child's stuttering, I teach him about "speech helpers," which are the lungs, larynx, and articulators, and their involvement in speech production. A cardboard or plywood cutout of a head, neck, and chest with speech helpers drawn in may help (see Exercise 1-1 in *Easy Talker*, our workbook that is listed in Suggested Readings at the end of the chapter). For a more sensitive child, I start with instructions about how speech helpers work during fluent speech and later explore what the child does with his speech helpers when he stutters. For children who are less emotional about their stuttering, I incorporate instruction about speech helpers into our exploration of what they are doing when they stutter.

Once a child is able to tolerate discussing his stuttering for a few minutes, I move on to activities that focus more consistently on stuttering. I begin by having the child try to "catch me" stuttering. I throw in a few easy stutters and ask him to let me know by signaling whenever he notices a stutter in my speech. Easy stutters can be repetitions, prolongations, or blocks, but they are produced slowly and without much tension. I reward him when he successfully catches my easy stutters, and I sometimes talk about what I did when I got stuck. This lets him know that I am not afraid of stuttering and, in turn, provides a model of talking objectively about stuttering. Most clinicians can do this legitimately even though they don't stutter. Most children know that the clinician's stutters are voluntary and are ok with it. After several minutes of putting easy stutters in my speech, I might ask the child to signal me when *he* stutters. If he misses many of them, I comment on a few that he has missed. I am careful to find some easier stutters in his speech and compare them with harder ones. I discuss with the child, as I have earlier, that this is one of our goals for therapy: to replace his hard stuttering with easier talking that I call "superfluency."

An important aim at this stage is to continue making stuttering something that we can talk about. This openness decreases some of the fear, frustration, and shame associated with stuttering. I can judge progress on this goal by noticing how a child reacts when I put stuttering in my speech and when I ask him to explore his stuttering. I continue to question the child about his stutters, while I maintain an interested, enthusiastic, accepting style of inquiry. What did he do when he stuttered? Where was it tight? Could he show me again what it sounded like? Again, I continually assess how much confrontation a child can tolerate and intersperse it with activities the child enjoys. An important focus of this phase of therapy is easy stuttering. Therefore, as the youngster and I explore his stuttering together, I help him identify relatively easy and relaxed stutters in his current speech. Because I have filled my own speech with models of these, the child is usually familiar with these targets. It will help, however, if I audio or video record his speech and play back those segments in which there are only good examples of easy stuttering. With an initial emphasis on these mild stutters, we can then move to longer and tenser stutters that the child can readily identify in his own speech.

The third principle taken from the phobia literature suggests that extended amounts of time in contact with stuttering will help reduce fear of it. The idea of being "in contact" with stuttering behavior may have an important meaning in the context of speech motor control. A child who has been stuttering persistently for several years may have lost proprioceptive awareness of his speech or may never have had it to an appropriate degree. This may make it difficult for him to use proprioceptive information to coordinate speech movements. Therefore, as a child explores his stuttering, I help him increase his awareness of what he's doing when he stutters, particularly for more severe moments of stuttering. If I can guide him to stay in the moment of stuttering beyond the time when he can release the block, he can feel what he's doing and then will realize that he can control the tension and movement of his speech structures. The shift that he will feel as he holds on to stutters for an extended period of time will seem like a change from being out of control to being in control. It may, indeed, result from a change in the activity of brain areas that control speech movements, such as a shift from a motor area of the brain that is not well supplied with sensory feedback to a motor area with better sensory information (Guitar et al, 1988).

Exploring Secondary Behaviors

The aim of the exploration phase of therapy is not to identify every aspect of a child's stuttering in great detail but to develop an "approach" attitude, to decrease fear, and to learn the rudiments of easier stuttering and easier talking. However, most children with intermediate stuttering have some avoidance behaviors, and if we can help these children become aware of them, avoidances are likely to diminish. I usually begin by mentioning some examples of starters, postponements, and other avoidance behaviors that I have seen in other children. For instance, I may tell the child about other kids I know who use "well" or "um" before difficult words, who don't talk in class because they're afraid they might stutter, or who substitute easy words for hard ones. I make it clear that these avoidances are very understandable and nothing to be ashamed of, but they also get in the way of being able to talk easily. By sharing such examples with the child and asking him if he has tried any of them, I make it easier for him to be open about the secondary behaviors he uses or at least those he is aware of using. If a child has difficulty identifying or discussing secondary behaviors, I put it aside for the moment. He may be better able to explore these behaviors after he has learned some coping skills.

Exploring Feelings

In addition to identifying the strategies that a child uses to hide or avoid his stuttering, I also explore the feelings underlying his need to use them. Many children are unwilling or perhaps unable to discuss in much detail their feelings of embarrassment or fear associated with stuttering. I do not push a child on this point, but let him know that these sorts of feelings are understandable and natural. I encourage his expression of such feelings, reinforce any of his comments about them, and continue to show my acceptance. I use several approaches to help a child express, and thereby diminish, feelings about stuttering. I often comment on the experiences and feelings that other children have when they stutter, such as the angry and sad feelings that result from being teased, being told by adults to slow down, having words finished for them, and being interrupted. Kristin Chmela and Nina Reardon have produced an excellent workbook to help children express and manage their feelings about their stuttering and about themselves (Chmela and Reardon, 2001).

I find that some children express their feelings more freely through drawings. Thus, I often ask them to draw pictures of what stuttering is like. I begin by telling the child that some stutters are like a stuck door (or whatever is most relevant to his type of stutters), and I draw something that represents the feeling. I usually make jaggedly lines to represent frustration and talk to the child about how stutters like that might feel. Then, I ask the child to draw a picture showing how it feels when he gets stuck on a word. In explaining his drawing, the child is often able to express how he feels. Therefore, I use drawing throughout therapy to help the child deal with old feelings of hurt and new feelings that are encountered during various stages of therapy. My experience has been that children's feelings often affect their fluency. The more practice they get in expressing their feelings, the less those feelings interfere with talking.

By now, the child has shared with me his moments of stuttering and the strategies he uses to hide them. Moreover, he has found me to be an understanding and accepting listener. Some deconditioning of speech fears has already occurred, and the child has also learned some of the terms I will be using in the remaining phases of therapy. Thus, some basic groundwork has been laid for the following phases of treatment.

Teaching Fluency Skills

In *Treatment of the Young Confirmed Stutterer*, Van Riper advocates building up the child's fluency: "We always try to increase the amount of fluency in these children and we want them to feel it and recognize it when it does occur rather than to focus their attention only on the stuttering" (Van Riper, 1973, p. 434). Following Van Riper's lead, I teach these children to create fluent speech by using a variety of skills. Once a child has learned these skills, he can use them to replace stuttering with controlled fluency. The preceding phase of exploration has set the stage for this work by reducing the child's fear of stuttering. He will then be calm enough in difficult speaking situations to perceive upcoming stuttering, plan a response, and be able to use his fluency skills to move through the feared word(s) slowly, carefully, and smoothly.

There are some intermediate-level stutterers who are more like beginning stutterers in their relative lack of fear toward stuttering. These youngsters may begin therapy by learning fluency skills to replace stuttering. In some cases, intermediate stutterers may have fear of stuttering but be unable to make progress in confronting their fears until they have increased their fluency and, thus, may benefit from starting with fluency skills training.

Specific Fluency Skills

The skills described in this section are also described in the workbook, *Easy Talker* (Guitar and Reville, 1997), which includes reproducible worksheets for each skill. There is no magic to the order in which these skills should be taught. In this section, I begin by describing what skills I think are the easiest before going on to those that are a little harder or more abstract. They may be taught in any order or all at once; with the latter option, the clinician models fluency with flexible rate, easy onsets, light contacts, and proprioception and then shapes the child's responses.

Flexible Rate

Flexible rate is simply slowing down the production of a word, especially the first syllable (Boehmler, personal communication, 2003). Slowing is thought to be effective in reducing stuttering by allowing more time for language planning and motor execution (see "Fluency-Inducing Conditions" in Chapter 1). This skill is called "flexible rate" rather than "slow rate" to emphasize that only those syllables on which stuttering is expected are slowed, not the surrounding speech. I also think that "flexible rate" is more acceptable to school-age children who may be tired of hearing people tell them to "slow down."

Flexible rate is taught first by having the clinician model production of words in which the first syllable and the transition to the second syllable are said in a way that slows all of the sounds equally. Vowels, fricatives, nasals, sibilants, and glides are lengthened, and plosives and affricates are produced to sound more like fricatives, without stopping the sound or airflow. After the clinician's model, the child produces the word with flexible rate, and successive approximations of the target (i.e., improvements) are reinforced. Practice should include all the sounds of the language; a good resource for words to use for this is *40,000 Selected Words* (Blockcolsk, Frazer, and Frazer, 1987). Younger children may be helped to learn flexible rate by running an obstacle course of chairs and tables, in which they have to slow down as they move around obstacles but can speed up in parts of the course without obstacles. As you and the child run the obstacle course, you can tell a joke or a story and slow down both your speech and your movements as you negotiate the obstacles. Older children can get the idea by using analogies from their areas of interest. For example, some video games have race cars that can be slowed down on curves and sped up on straight aways.

Easy Onsets

These are labeled as "Ee-Oo's" in our *Easy Talker* workbook (Guitar and Reville, 1997); they refer to an easy or gentle onset of voicing. My perception of my own stuttering is that if I begin a "feared" sound with a rapid onset of voicing (i.e., a hard glottal attack), I get myself into a "stuck" posture that feels like I can't move it. But if I start my vocal folds vibrating gently at first, I can usually get voicing going without stuttering. For me and probably for many others who stutter (but not all), vowels in word-initial positions are easier to use with an easy onset than are consonants. Vowels following a word-initial voiceless consonant, however, are fairly difficult for me. For example, I might prolong the /s/ in "sun" and may block on the /u/ unless I consciously employ a gentle onset on the /u/.

Again, teaching easy onsets is like teaching flexible rate. You model the target behavior on lots of different sounds and then have the child imitate your models and reinforce his successive approximations. Some children, particular younger ones, may be helped to get the concept by performing an action, such as bringing their hands together slowly, as they produce an easy onset.

Light Contacts

Just as a hard glottal attack can trigger stuttering, so too can hard articulatory contacts. When someone who stutters anticipates difficulty with a sound, he'll often "preset" his articulators into a stuck position before starting a word or he may even rehearse the stuttering behavior (Van Riper, 1936). Producing consonants with light contacts prevents the stoppage of airflow and/or voicing that can trigger stuttering. Light contacts are taught by modeling a style of producing consonants with relaxed articulators and continuous flow of air or voice, depending on the consonant. Plosives and affricates should be slightly distorted so that they sound like fricatives but are still intelligible. For example, when I produce the /b/ in "Barry" using a light contact, I slow down the movement into and out of the lip "closure." Instead of stopping the airflow and voicing by closing my lips, I let my lips loosely vibrate and allow the /b/ sound semi-closure continue for a little longer than normal. For a /p/, my lips barely touch and air flows out of my not-quite-closed lips, creating a slight turbulence so that it sounds a little like an /f/.

Teaching a child to use light contacts is accomplished by modeling a variety of words with initial consonants and reinforcing the child's successive approximations of the target. To make the concept more interesting and perhaps clearer, you can use a variety of games to demonstrate light contact. For example, you might try catching soap bubbles or throwing and catching water balloons or raw eggs. Some games that build towers or require you to gently pick-up an object (like jackstraws, also called pick-up sticks) may depict a light, gentle touch in a vivid way. Once a child gets the basic idea of using light contacts in speech, you can combine flexible rate, easy onsets, and light contacts together in practice on multisyllable words, while using these skills on the first syllable and transition to the second syllable and finishing the word at a normal rate.

Proprioception

In the present context, proprioception refers to sensory feedback from mechanoreceptors in muscles of the lips, jaw, and tongue (Abbs, 1996). This feedback may be crucial in controlling speech movements, and its use as a concept in stuttering therapy may have originated from Van Riper, who suggested that, "...some of the stutterer's difficulties seem to originate in the auditory processing system. [Therefore,] if we can get him to concentrate upon proprioceptive feedback rather than auditory feedback we can bypass these difficulties" (Van Riper, 1973, p. 211). Recent brain imaging studies reviewed in Chapter 2 support Van Riper's contention that the auditory systems of people who stutter may be dysfunctional (e.g. Ingham, 2003; Stager et al, 2003), but there is also evidence that other sensory systems may not be functioning normally either (e.g., DeNil and Abbs, 1991). The effectiveness of teaching proprioception may be that it promotes conscious attention to sensory information from the articulators, perhaps bypassing inefficient automatic sensory monitoring systems and thereby normalizing sensory-motor control.

Children can be taught to use proprioception in a number of ways. One of my former students, David Stuller, has taught proprioception by having a child first hold a raisin in his mouth and report on its taste, shape, size, and other attributes. This activity tunes the child into sensations from his mouth before introducing speech, which may have negative associations for more severe or more sensitive intermediate stutterers. Children can also learn proprioception by picking a word from a list and then closing their eyes and silently moving their articulators for this word and being rewarded when the clinician guesses the word. During this game, children can be coached to feel the movements of their lips, tongue, and jaw as they say a word. Proprioceptive awareness can also be enhanced by using masking noise or delayed auditory feedback to interfere with self-hearing. Although it is not always easy to judge accurately whether or not a child is using proprioception, I look for slightly exaggerated, slow movements to verify that a child is trying to feel the movements of his articulators.

Once a child seems to have acquired proprioception skills, they can be combined with flexible rate, easy onsets, and light contacts as described in the next section. I call using the combination of all these skills "superfluency."

Replacing Stuttering with Superfluency

The use of superfluency to replace stuttering begins with practice on fluent speech. I start with three-word sentences like, "I am great!" and have the child practice putting superfluency on the first syllable and the transition to the second. Using multiple letters to represent superfluency, I would depict its production like this: "IIIIaam great." By first modeling the production and then listening and watching the child imitate it, the clinician shapes the child's superfluency skills. Clear and enthusiastic feedback to the child will help him learn; a reward system will make learning fun.

At first, it is important to ensure that all the elements (flexible rate, easy onset, light contacts, and proprioception) are present. Later on, when a child has learned to use superfluency successfully, he may develop his own version that may use only those elements necessary for him to be fluent. Some children become quite fluent and may need to use superfluency only rarely because, for them, having a tool that replaces stuttering with fluency gives them confidence and replaces anticipation of stuttering with anticipation of fluency. Thus, they appear to no longer put their articulators in anticipatory postures or have anticipatory tension that triggers stuttering.

After starting with a simple three-word sentence, the clinician continues drilling the child on superfluency using both long and short sentences, with a variety of initial sounds and with superfluency used in a variety of positions. At first, she has the child imitate her model but then fades the strength of that cue. The more successful the child is in learning good quality superfluency, the less the clinician needs to model the sentences. For those sentences not imitated after the clinician's model, the child can read the sentence from a list using superfluency on words that are circled. Here are a few sentences to use: "Just do it!" "Show me the money," "Yes, we have no bananas," and "Get away from the car." Video or audiotape playback of the child's successful utterances can be helpful in creating an auditory target in the child's mind to guide him.

After a youngster has mastered the use of superfluency on fluent utterances at the one-word level, the focus should be on conversation. At first, the clinician should model superfluency on many of her utterances, both on sentence-initial words and on initial sounds of other words in sentences. The child should be rewarded for superfluency during the time he is working to master it in conversation, but systematic fading of his rewards should be used to make the skill independent of the clinician's feedback. In any case, the activity must be fun for the child, especially if he is taken out of class for therapy. I often use rewards that release frustration toward past stuttering, such as shooting a ping-pong ball gun or throwing a stuffed rat at cans and bottles that have pictures of "stutters" taped to them. A ball-shooting burp gun is available from www.HammacherSchlemmer.com.

Some children respond well to concrete representations of new skills they are trying to learn. To help them get the idea of shifting into superfluency from normal speech as they attempt a difficult word, I use the idea of "downshifting" a car or truck. In Vermont, it's easy to have kids imagine they are driving a 4-wheel drive truck and need to downshift when they see deep snow ahead. In other areas, downshifting may be needed before driving through deep mud or up a steep hill. Downshifting can be acted out by the clinician and child by talking and changing into superfluency as they talk when encountering pretend snow, mud, or a hill while walking around the therapy room. Some children may have trouble perceiving when they might stutter on an upcoming word. These children can often be helped in two ways. First, they may be given a little training on the side, using reinforcement for stopping after a stutter, then during a stutter, and finally before a potential stutter. Second, they may benefit from massed practice of superfluency on fluent words, letting the shift into superfluency before an anticipated stutter become automatic.

During the conversation, because superfluency on fluent utterances is being rewarded, the child will probably get into a mind set that will make it easy for him to use superfluency with words on which he expects difficulty. Sometimes you can tell when a child uses superfluency on an expected stutter, rather than an expected fluent word, and sometimes you can't. However, the child can often tell you when he is actually using it on an expected stutter, and you should give him an extra reward for these times. There is no harm done when the child uses superfluency on an "expected" stutter that was really just a fluent word. The more practice the better. When the child has replaced stutters with superfluency in the therapy room and superfluency is comfortable for him to use, he can begin using it in structured situations.

Transferring Superfluency to Structured Situations

This section describes not only the specifics of transferring fluency skills, but also additional elements, such as being open about stuttering, which will help make transfer successful and aid in maintenance.

Transfer of superfluency to replace stuttering with other listeners and in other situations begins by setting up a hierarchy with the child of easy-to-difficult situations, in which the child and I can use voluntary downshifts to superfluency together. I use the word "voluntary" here to mean that superfluency is used on nonfeared words, that is, words that the child doesn't expect to stutter on. In the context of using voluntary superfluency, anticipated stutters will eventually occur, and the child will be primed to replace them with superfluency. We begin each session by working together to plan a hierarchy and determine the number of reward points for each accomplishment. At this time, I am getting information from the parents about the child's progress at home.

At an appropriate level of difficulty in the hierarchy, I bring the parents into therapy and have the child teach them about downshifting into superfluency and then develop a plan to have the child use both voluntary and real (when stuttering is expected) downshifts at home. One or both parents, depending on the child's preference, should help him keep a log of the number of downshifts he makes each day. However, involving parents as therapy helpers is not effective for some children. They prefer not to have their parents function in this way but merely want their parents to be supportive listeners. In such cases, I telephone the child at home and have him tape-record himself when transferring superfluency into speech at home.

By now, the child may be speaking with little difficulty in many situations, but some situations are probably still giving him problems. As I continue the transfer process, I turn more attention to those situations in which the child is having trouble using superfluency successfully to replace his stuttering.

Desensitizing the Child to Fluency Disrupters

Most children at intermediate levels of stuttering have an "Achilles heel," and sometimes, they seem to have one on each foot. For example, some find it hard to maintain fluency when they are talking in a group where children are interrupting each other. Others have more difficulty when telling a story or joke to a friend or when talking in a noisy environment like an industrial arts (shop) class. When a child is vulnerable to particular situations, I begin by role-playing the situations in the safety of the treatment room, and then I gradually move the child into more life-like approximations of the situations. If the child has difficulty using superfluency when he's being interrupted, we plan some role-plays. I let the child interrupt me so that I can model using superfluency, with all its bells and whistles, to retain a calm, smooth utterance despite the interruptions. We then switch roles, and I interrupt him. When we have done that and he seems to be confident in using superfluency to deal with interruptions when talking to me, we enlist other children or adults to help out in the role-playing. By doing this many times over many sessions, the child usually learns to handle this type of difficult situation.

Scaffolding

I have found it useful with some children to "scaffold" their use of superfluency by letting the listener(s) know that we are working on our speech and sometimes by coaching the child in that fluency-friendly environment. I am always careful to plan this beforehand with the child and ensure that he is comfortable with it. For example, I may tell a stranger in a mall that the child and I are working on our speech and we'd like to ask him some questions. Depending on the child's readiness, I may ask the first question or the child may. If the situation has been difficult in the past, I may coach the child in his use of superfluency as he speaks by giving him subtle signals that we have worked out beforehand.

Transfer on the telephone lends itself to a great deal of scaffolding, which can be faded as the child is more and more successful. For example, the clinician and child may plan a variety of gestures or signs that can provide support as the child makes telephone calls to practice superfluency. If we are practicing voluntary superfluency, which is always a good thing to do, I'll make the first phone call and have the child signal me to put in superfluency whenever he wants. Then we will reverse roles. Sometimes, physical contact helps focus a child on his speech even in the face of some fear. If you and the child are comfortable with it, you could place your hand on the child's arm and squeeze it to let him know you notice that he has shifted to superfluency or to remind him to do so.

Reducing Fear and Avoidance

Some children take a little longer than others to transfer their superfluency skills. They may have learned fears and avoidances that will require a concerted effort to overcome. It helps many children in this situation to deal with their fears if the right analogies or comparisons can be found. I get them to think about other fears they have overcome or about people they know, such as family members, who are afraid of such things as the dark, bugs, snakes, or swimming in deep water, and I enlist the child's help in listing ways they might overcome their fears. I also look for examples in pop culture, like Harry Potter or Spiderman. By analyzing how people get over their fears and describing the rewards of facing fears and conquering them, I am often able to motivate children to tackle their fears of difficult words and situations.

In preparing to help a child plan a hierarchy to overcome fear and avoidance, I make up a hypothetical situation. For example, I might talk about overcoming fear of jumping off the high diving board at the local swimming pool (Fig. 11–1) and suggest, if the child wanted to overcome his fear of the high board, it would be best for him to start by jumping

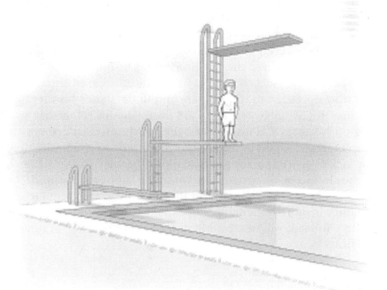

Figure 11–1   *Using an easy to hard hierarchy to overcome fear and avoidance.*

off the side of the pool. When he could imagine being comfortable with this, he could imagine jumping off the low board. After becoming comfortable with diving off the low board, he would be ready to take on the medium-high board. Eventually, he would reach the high diving board. After jumping off the high diving board a number of times, he would find himself no longer afraid of it. Therefore, there would be no reason for him to avoid the high diving board any more. I then explain to the child that I will use this same easy-to-hard strategy, or hierarchies, to help him overcome his speech fears and avoidances.

It is usually easier to help a child overcome his fear and avoidance of particular words than of particular situations. This is because I can provide the child with more support in confronting word fears in the therapy room than I can provide when he confronts his situational fears in daily life. I can also use feared words over and over again within the therapy situation. For example, I worked with a young intermediate stutterer who consistently substituted "me" for "I." This was not because of a language disorder, and his parents reported that he had used "I" appropriately for a number of years before he began using this substitution. With this child, I began to practice saying "I" in unison with him, while we both used superfluency saying the word, and strongly reinforced his efforts. Next, we used "I" many, many times in carrier phrases while playing games, with both of us using superfluency when saying "I." Gradually, the child regained his confidence in saying "I." Within a week or two, his avoidance of "I" was eliminated in therapy, and his parents reported that he was again using this pronoun appropriately at home.

Now, let's consider the situation of a child being afraid to speak aloud in the classroom. In this case, I would invite, with the child's consent, one or two of his classmates into therapy. I would play the role of the classroom teacher and have this small group of two or three children ask and answer questions. When the child began to feel comfortable doing this, I would expand the group to three or four classmates. Next, it might be helpful for the child, and the rest of us, to go to his classroom during the noon hour or at recess. After explaining our goal and therapy procedures to the classroom teacher, I would have the child sit at his desk and have the teacher ask questions about his lessons. These activities are about as far as I can go in simulating a child's fear of this situation. The child needs to take the last step of these therapy procedures by himself. He has been successful in a series of situations that successively approximate his feared situation, and his classroom teacher is now sensitized to his problem and understands his therapy. The chances are that, after some initial ambivalence, he will overcome his reluctance to talk in class.

In working on his fears and avoidances, the child must understand that he doesn't have to be completely successful in using superfluency in all situations all of the time. In fact, as he first tackles feared words and situations, he may stutter in his old way many times. Even so, he should be rewarded for trying. The "approach attitude," which I sometimes refer to as "Seeking Out" (Guitar and Reville, 1997), may reduce fear and tension so that superfluency is more obtainable. Repeated exposure to the feared objects, when supported by the clinician, will make a big difference in transfer of new skills to feared words and situations.

Coping with Teasing

It is important to minimize any teasing that a child is receiving because of his stuttering. The clinician can deal with it at any time, but it may be helpful to address teasing after the child has mastered some fluency skills and is transferring them. I address this issue in more detail when I discuss counseling parents and classroom teachers. Regardless of how hard parents, teachers, clinicians, and friends may try to eliminate teasing, I doubt that it is possible to eliminate all of it. Thus, I try to give a child some defenses against the teasing that he is likely to receive.

I agree with Van Riper (1973) that the best defense against teasing is acceptance, if a child is emotionally mature enough to feel and express acceptance. For example, if a child can say, "I know I stutter, but I'm working on it," or some similar statement, this will disarm most teasers. Nobody likes to tease someone who does not appear to be bothered. Running away, on the other hand, just reinforces teasing. Nevertheless, I have found that it is difficult for a school-age child to calmly accept and admit his stuttering to tormentors. When I have been successful, I have done the following things.

First, I discuss the importance of calmly and openly admitting stuttering to teasers, rather than saying nothing. I explain how this type of response usually discourages teasers. I then explore with the child the sorts of statements he can imagine himself making. The words he uses must be words with which he feels comfortable. Next, I initiate role-playing with the child. As I play the role of the teaser, the child's task is to respond calmly to my heckling. He practices saying the types of statements he has chosen to use to counteract the teasing. I role-play this many times until the child feels comfortable with his response and can see himself doing this in a real-life situation. Finally, the day comes when he tries out this new behavior. I hope it works, but if it does not, I am there to give the child support and encouragement.

I have also found that, if I have two or more children who stutter or if I can form a group of several children who have speech or language problems, we can write and perform a play together about a child who stutters who triumphs over teasing.

Some children are especially sensitive to teasing and need patience and understanding as they work to develop effective responses. These children may have more inhibited temperaments, and their first reaction to a threatening situation is to withdraw or avoid. Hence, these children need practice in asserting themselves. In our role-playing, I experiment with a variety of ways in which the child can feel that he confronted the teaser. For some children, it might be teasing back; for others, it might be reporting the teaser to a teacher or the principal. A tactic taught by Bill Murphy, an experienced speech pathologist who also stutters, is to have children say "So?" back to the teaser after every taunt. Because it's a short utterance, children who stutter can often say it fluently and with gusto. Other excellent advice is contained in a recent publication by Murphy and others titled, *Bullying and Teasing: Helping Children Who Stutter* (Yaruss et al, 2004).

Being Open About Stuttering

One of the best ways to combat fear, embarrassment, and the physical tension that these emotions often elicit is to be open about stuttering, to talk about it casually with friends, to refer to it in humorous ways when it happens, and to educate people about it. Children differ widely in their readiness to be open about their stuttering. However, once most of them feel some sense of mastery over what has made them feel helpless in the past, they are much more able to let people know about it. If a child stutters in class, I rehearse casual comments that he can make about his stuttering when he is giving an oral report or answering a question in class. He might say, for example, "My report is about how maple syrup is produced. Before I begin, I just want to say that I'll probably stutter sometime while I'm talking, but don't let it bother you. I'm learning to deal with it." Or, he might say, "It makes it easier for me if you can keep pretty good eye contact with me when I get stuttery." Basically, it is not so much the content that is important as the fact that the child acknowledges his stuttering and that he's working on it. He feels good that he has acknowledged it, and his audience is more comfortable than if he stutters and tries to hide it.

A child may also benefit from developing a repertoire of casual comments to make about his stuttering if he gets particularly hung up on a word while talking to friends, relatives, or strangers. He might learn to say, "Wow! I really got hung up there," or, "I'm really running into a lot of blocks; I'd better slow down a bit." In my experience, the most effective comments are those that the child comes up with spontaneously, when he feels comfortable with his stuttering. These are unforced, often funny remarks that put the child and his listeners at ease.

Teaching other children and his teachers about stuttering can be a powerful tool in combating the shame and embarrassment that often accompany a school-age child's stuttering. Although this can be done with small groups of students brought into the therapy room or in meetings with the child and his teachers, our experience has been that, eventually, sharing information about stuttering in front of the entire class is extremely effective for many children. When and if a child is ready to do this, we work together to prepare, rehearse, and then give a presentation that informs the class about stuttering in general and the child's own stuttering in particular. A question-and-answer period is a crucial part of the presentation because it gives the child's classmates a chance to express their curiosity about stuttering. It also gives the child an opportunity to become an expert in the very behavior that previously made him feel so helpless.

Here is an example of how this can work. A second grader who was very sensitive about his stuttering was also rather proud of a brief segment on a local television station that showed him working on his stuttering. He was willing to show a videotape of this segment in class and answer questions about his stuttering. The following year, I accompanied him to class for a full-scale presentation about stuttering. This presentation included posters he had made, demonstrations of therapy techniques, and a question-and-answer segment. A year after this program, the child had a particularly rocky beginning to the school year because his stuttering had returned full-force after his family moved to a new house in a new neighborhood. However, he was still willing to do another presentation with me. This time he used more videotaped clips of himself talking, because he was more reluctant to talk at length, and talked to the class about some of the "ups and downs" in his progress with stuttering.

Maintaining Improvement

By this point in therapy, a child is usually speaking well in most situations. He is having a great deal of natural fluency in many situations and either superfluency or acceptable stuttering in others. His speech fears and avoidances have been eliminated or significantly reduced. I do not dismiss the child from therapy at this point but gradually phase him out of therapy. I see him for therapy on a weekly basis for a month or so, then on a twice-monthly basis for another month or so. If all continues to go well, I see him for a series of "check-ups" over the next 2 years, first monthly, then bimonthly, and, finally, once a semester.

During these check-ups, I obtain samples of the child's speech and oral reading and discuss with him how he has been talking in everyday speaking situations. I also interview his parents and classroom teacher about his speech at home and school. If I find that the child's fluency has regressed or that he has begun to use avoidance behaviors again, I re-enroll him in therapy. My experience is that a number of children may have one or two mild regressions before their fluency stabilizes. Such regressions are often associated with the beginning of a school year or with transfers from one school to another or with other disrupting factors.

When I return a child to therapy, it is usually for only a month or two. During these "booster" sessions, he may need to have his fluency-enhancing or stuttering modification skills "tuned up." He may need a brief refresher course on the importance of not avoiding, or he may just need an opportunity to talk to an understanding listener about his stuttering. In time, these regressions and our re-evaluations become farther apart until, finally, the day arrives when the child, his family, and I decide to dismiss him from treatment.

Clinical Procedures: Working with Parents

I have five goals in mind when counseling parents of an intermediate stutterer: (1) explaining the treatment program and the parents' role in it, (2) discussing the possible causes of stuttering, (3) identifying and reducing fluency disrupters, (4) identifying and increasing fluency-enhancing situations, and (5) eliminating teasing. I will discuss each of these goals in turn.

Explaining the Treatment Program and the Parents' Role in It

First, I discuss the stages of our therapy program with the child's parents, letting them know how I hope to take the mystery out of stuttering for the child by exploring with him what he does when he stutters. I also tell them about our goal of teaching the child to use superfluency to replace stuttering and how it is a gradual process. At times, it may even sound like their child is stuttering in slow motion when he uses superfluency. Second, I tell them that therapy may take time, perhaps 1 to 3 years and, in some cases, even longer. Third, I inform them that communicating with their child about his stuttering is important and that they should express their acceptance of his stuttering and acknowledge their understanding that it is often difficult for him to work on it.

Explaining the Possible Causes of Stuttering

I believe it is important for the parents of an intermediate stutterer to be given an explanation of the possible causes of stuttering. I explain current thinking about the nature of stuttering. In some cases, parents have no information about the causes of stuttering. Since I want them to participate in their child's treatment, they need to understand the rationale for our treatment program. Many parents feel guilty about their child's stuttering because of some outdated or inaccurate information they may have. They may have been exposed to an explanation that is no longer valid, or they may have been given some erroneous information by a well-meaning but misinformed friend or relative. Such parents then blame themselves for some supposed misdeed on their part. They need good, current information about the nature of stuttering. Often, just supplying this information relieves them of their guilt. The following materials have been helpful supplements to parent counseling:

1. On the "Stuttering Home Page" website (http://www.mnsu.edu/comdis/kuster/), there is a link titled "Information about Stuttering" which leads to another link for parents of children who stutter. Articles, essays, books, and other materials for parents are provided directly there or are described so that parents can find them elsewhere.

2. On the National Stuttering Association website (http://www.nsastutter.org/), there is a link titled "Information for Parents/Family," which provides useful advice for parents of teens who stutter.

3. On the Stuttering Foundation website (http://www.stuttersfa.org/), a link titled "If You Think Your Child is Stuttering: 7 Ways to Help" provides useful information to parents. The Foundation also has two videos, *Stuttering: Straight Talk for Teens* and *Stuttering: Straight Talk for Teachers,* that are also helpful for parents.

Using language that is appropriate to the parents' level of understanding, I provide the type of information that I presented in the early chapters of this book. I describe how developmental and environmental influences may interact with predisposing physiological and constitutional factors to produce or exacerbate a child's initial repetitions and prolongations. The child responds to these disfluencies with increased tension in his effort to inhibit them. In time, the child also learns a variety of escape and, possibly, starting behaviors to cope with his repetitions and prolongations. I go on to suggest that predisposing physiological factors are most likely neurological in nature and are related to a child's deficits in speech production. I suggest that the child may have problems in timing the fine motor movements required for fluent speech. I add that children who stutter may also have a more sensitive temperament and that could compound the stuttering by making the child more likely to have learned emotional reactions to his speech difficulties. I also note that, in many cases, the predisposing physiological factors may be genetic in origin. Thus, there are many possible sources for his speech difficulty. I also suggest that, because of the way the brain may be organized, their child may have special talents in the areas of drawing, music, and engineering.

I explore, with the parents' assistance, the developmental and environmental influences that may be interacting with the child's predisposing factors to affect his stuttering. These are reviewed in Chapter 3. In some cases, I may not identify any developmental or environmental factors that seem to be contributing to the problem; however, when I do identify one or more possible factors, I attempt to lessen their influence. My experience suggests that, in most cases, the solution to reducing the impact of developmental and environmental influences is fairly straightforward. In a few cases, when it may be more difficult, I have suggested that counseling by a family therapist may be helpful.

I also talk with parents of an intermediate stutterer about avoidance behaviors. I describe these behaviors to them and explain how the child's word and situation avoidances are behaviors he has learned to use in coping with the embarrassment and fear of talking. I also explain how, in therapy, I will be helping the child eliminate his use of these avoidance behaviors.

Some parents feel responsible for their child's stuttering and may feel they need to find a cure for it. While I'm discussing the possible causes of stuttering and after I've mentioned the possible neurological differences in children who stutter, I often bring up the possibility that their child will always stutter but that it needn't interfere with his life. Because this can be such an important issue for parents, I try to judge whether this moment is the right time to discuss it. For example, if this is an initial phone conversation, I might not bring it up at that time. But if this is a face-to-face meeting and we have some time to talk about their concerns, I find it helpful to let parents know that a child who is still stuttering after age 9 or 10 years will probably continue to have at least a little stuttering throughout his life. In saying this, I am sure to indicate that most individuals who stutter into adulthood don't let their stuttering get in the way of their goals, and I will cite some examples of famous people who have achieved success even though they stuttered. At this point, I am careful to let them respond to this information. Parents sometimes envision difficulties in academic, social, and occupation areas for their child who stutters, and it is important for them to express these concerns and for me to listen deeply to them.

Identifying and Reducing Fluency Disrupters

As I explain in later chapters, environmental influences are often critical factors for managing beginning and borderline levels of stuttering. Intermediate-level stuttering is more complex and requires direct treatment of a child's behaviors and attitudes, but environmental factors are important for this level of stuttering as well. An intermediate stutterer's home environment may involve stresses that can be substantially alleviated if the clinician can join forces with an interested, motivated family. I begin by asking family members to observe when the child stutters most and when he stutters least. With this information, I brainstorm with them various ways to reduce potential stresses and to observe the effects on the child's stuttering. For example, some children stutter a lot when there is competition for attention at the dinner table or when several children arrive home from school at the same time, all wanting to talk to their parents. In other cases, changes in a family routine may spark an increase in a child's stuttering. Whatever the sources of stress, I encourage the parents and other family members to take the lead in identifying them and in planning ways of reducing such stress. Even in cases when stress may result from relatively abstract sources, such as a family's attitude that stuttering is shameful, the family is unlikely to change unless they feel that they and their points of view are respected and understood by the clinician. In an accepting environment, a trusting relationship can be developed, and a family may be open to seeing the child and his stuttering in new ways.

Increasing Fluency-Enhancing Situations

During the process of identifying the times when a child stutters more frequently, families also discover there are times when a child is extremely fluent. These may be specific situations or just days or weeks when the child is particularly fluent. Whatever the case, families can find ways of increasing factors that promote fluency and giving a child plenty of opportunities to talk when he is fluent. For example, a child may be especially fluent when he is talking to a parent at bedtime, when he is sleepy and relaxed. This provides a parent an opportunity to comment on the child's "smooth speech" and to let the child know that they can imagine how good it must feel to talk easily. I am also interested in helping parents find ways of increasing fluency-enhancing situations and of reinforcing their child's fluency without implying that the times when he stutters are bad. I can accomplish this by having the family empathize with the child that fluency is great but that stuttering just can't be helped sometimes.

For those children who are willing to work on their fluency with members of their family, a program of home therapy can be developed cooperatively by the child, parent(s), and clinician. Regular contact between the clinician and family members is important to facilitate and guide this component of treatment. Face-to-face meetings are ideal, but phone calls, journals, or email will also suffice. A typical home program would include severity ratings made by both parents of the child's speech at home and by the child of his speech at home and at school. The specific behaviors to be rated and an effective reward system are negotiated by the child, parents, and clinician.

Eliminating Teasing at Home

If any of an intermediate stutterer's siblings are teasing him about his stuttering, his parents need to stop it. I have found the best way to do this is to have parents have a serious talk with the teaser. They need to explain that teasing makes stuttering worse and must be discontinued. Usually, this is sufficient. If it is not, I have found it effective for us to talk to the sibling about the importance of not teasing a young stutterer. Having an adult other than a parent talk seriously about this matter often carries more weight with teasers.

Another important issue for parents is their reactions to teasing by other children at school. Although this is a serious matter, parents may do more harm than good if they are overly upset by teasing. The child who is teased will take his cue from his parents. If parents are anxious or distraught about their child's being teased, the child will be more deeply affected by it. If parents let the school take care of the incident and convey to the child that they have faith in his ability to handle it but are also empathetic to his concerns, they will help the child maintain a good perspective on it.

Clinical Procedures: Working with Classroom Teachers

I believe it is very important to have an intermediate stutterer's classroom teacher involved in the child's treatment program (Fig. 11–2). After all, the child spends as much, if not more, time with the teacher than any other adult. I have four goals in mind when I am working with a classroom teacher: (1) to explain the treatment program and the teacher's role in it, (2) to facilitate the teacher talking with the child about his stuttering, (3) to help the child and teacher work out the child's class participation, and (4) to help the teacher eliminate teasing.

Explaining the Treatment Program and the Teacher's Role in It

Involving the child's classroom teacher(s) in treatment works best if the child gives his permission for this to take place. Even the most reluctant children usually agree to let me make a contact with the teacher. Sometimes, a meeting with several teachers at once is efficient. When I worked as a speech-language pathologist in junior high and elementary schools, I gave in-services about stuttering to teachers at the beginning of the school year. If such in-services can be arranged, the Stuttering Foundation video *Stuttering: Straight*

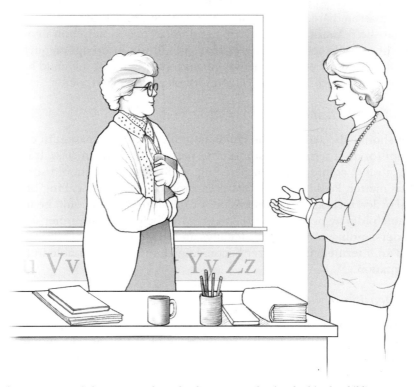

Figure 11–2 *It is important to have the classroom teacher involved in the child's treatment.*

Talk for Teachers makes a powerful addition to a presentation on the problems faced by school children who stutter and how teachers can help them.

It is beneficial for classroom teachers to have an overview of the child's treatment program, so I discuss how I am helping the child increase his fluency, eliminate his avoidance behaviors, and improve his overall communication ability. I want the teacher to understand the rationale behind these procedures. Therefore, I am careful to answer any questions the teacher may have, believing that helping the teacher understand our goals will have at least two benefits: (1) the teacher will have a better understanding of how to interact with the child; and (2) the teacher will be better able to give me feedback regarding the child's fluency in the classroom. I use the Teacher's Assessment of Students' Communicative Competence (TASCC), described in Chapter 6, to measure the child's baseline levels and progress. I also explain the teacher's role in the child's therapy and discuss why and how I would like the teacher to implement the three goals of how to talk with the child about his stuttering, how to help him cope with oral participation, and how to eliminate any teasing he may be receiving. I discuss each of these in the following paragraphs.

Talking with the Child About His Stuttering

A friend of mine recalled going all the way through school, from kindergarten through high school, without any teacher ever mentioning his stuttering. He stuttered severely year after year, and everyone knew he stuttered, but nobody ever acknowledged it. This silence, he said, was very painful. I believe that it is better for a classroom teacher to sit down with an intermediate stutterer and talk calmly with him about his stuttering, letting him know that she is aware of his stuttering and would like to help him in any way possible. The teacher should tell the stutterer that she will not interrupt or hurry him when he is talking. Just this sort of acknowledgment and acceptance of the child's stuttering by a teacher will make the child feel more comfortable in the classroom.

Coping with Oral Participation

The teacher should also talk with the child about his oral participation in class. I believe it is important for an intermediate stutterer to participate orally in class. It is also important for him to feel comfortable participating, and the teacher should seek the child's input on this matter. Possibly some classroom procedure, such as calling on students in alphabetical order, is creating apprehension for the stutterer and could be modified. For example, the child may prefer to be called on early, before his apprehension builds up. With an understanding of the child's feelings and flexibility in procedures, most teachers can help an intermediate stutterer become much more comfortable in his oral classroom participation.

Eliminating Teasing

It is not unusual for stutterers in elementary or junior high school to be teased about stuttering at school. If a classroom teacher becomes aware of teasing, she should attempt to stop it. As I indicated during my previous discussion of teasing in the home, I believe the best way to do this is to have a serious talk with the teaser. The teacher needs to explain that the child's teasing is making the stutterer's speech worse and that he needs to discontinue it immediately. The teacher should make it clear that this behavior will not be tolerated. Some teasers are themselves troubled children and will need help from the school counselor to change their behaviors.

Progress and Outcome Measures

Measures of progress and outcome, as described in Chapter 6, need to be taken to assess the effectiveness of this approach. Data on stuttering and fluency (%SS, SSI-3), measures of attitudes (CAT and A-19), and assessment of communicative competence (Teacher's Assessment of Student's Communicative Competence) can be used to measure progress during treatment and outcome after maintenance.

This concludes the description of my approach to treatment of a child with intermediate stuttering. I now describe the clinical procedures of some other clinicians.

Other Clinicians

Carl Dell: Changing Attitudes and Modifying Stutters

As he says in the book, *Treating the School Age Stutterer: A Guide for Clinicians,* Dell (2000) believes that most stuttering results from a delay in speech motor coordination and suggests that it is similar to such problems as taking longer to develop the gross motor coordinations needed for jumping rope or riding a bike. He believes that many children who begin to stutter are not bothered by their disfluencies and soon outgrow them, but that others become self-conscious about their difficulty, which leads them to speak with tension and effort. They may be responding to their own discomfort with repetitions and prolongations or to the concerns of parents, relatives, or others. Such children are experiencing stuttering as a handicap and need immediate help.

The targets of Dell's therapy include a child's moments of stuttering (repetitions, prolongations, and blocks), but the child's emotional responses to stuttering are equally important. Consequently, Dell begins therapy slowly, because children with intermediate stuttering are likely to be embarrassed and ashamed of their stuttering. Too much confrontation before a trusting relationship is established may cause these children to be turned off by therapy.

Dell indicates that most of the youngsters he works with at the intermediate level of stuttering will have controlled fluency, as well as some mild residual stuttering when they finish therapy. He believes in dismissing intermediate stutterers from treatment when they are confident that they can control their remaining stuttering and before they are completely fluent. This, he believes, gives them a better chance to become their own therapist in the final stage of therapy, when they become more fluent. Dell keeps his door open, however, for the children to return for "booster" sessions of therapy if needed.

Dell believes that a child's feelings and attitudes are of major importance. If a child's frustrations and fears are not dealt with, he will react to stuttering with more and more struggle and avoidance, making it more difficult to treat. Dell enables the child to change his feelings and attitudes by helping him to confront his stuttering and discover ways of changing it. This is done in a communicative atmosphere in which the clinician shows acceptance of stuttering by voluntarily stuttering herself. This allows the child to feel an equal partnership in his therapy and to enjoy it. When working with the child who has intermediate stuttering, Dell also achieves many changes in feelings through direct work on stuttering. The success that the child experiences in making stuttering easier goes a long way toward reducing his frustration and fear of stuttering.

Dell's therapy is conducted in a teaching/counseling style in which the clinician teaches and models a new behavior for the child, then informally reinforces the child for using it. The clinician responds spontaneously to the child's responses and reactions within the framework of working on goals but does not follow steps in a formal program. Data are not systematically collected, but the clinician judges the child's progress informally on the basis of his observations and reports by parents, the teacher, and the child himself.

Direct Treatment of the Child

Dell begins treatment slowly, testing the readiness of a child to confront his stuttering by putting a few voluntary stutters into his own speech, then commenting on them. If the child does not seem uncomfortable, Dell comments on some of the child's stutters and explores them with him. After the child has developed a trusting relationship with the clinician and appears to feel comfortable with his explorations of stuttering, Dell proceeds with direct therapy, which is divided into eight phases: (1) saying words in three ways, (2) locating tension, (3) canceling, (4) changing stuttering to a milder form,

(5) inserting easy stuttering into real speech, (6) changing hard stutters with pull-outs during real speech, (7) building fluency, and (8) building independence.

Three Ways of Saying Words

Dell describes and demonstrates for the child three ways of saying words: the regular or fluent way, the hard stuttering way, and the easy stuttering way. The hard way is characterized by typical stuttering, and the easy way is characterized by effortless prolongations or repetitions. Dell's first step is to have a child identify these three ways of saying words in the clinician's speech as a game in which the child has to identify whether the clinician said a word in a "regular," "hard," or "easy" way. As the game proceeds, the clinician occasionally asks the child to imitate her hard and easy stutters, allowing her to assess the child's readiness to put voluntary stutters into his own speech. When the child seems ready, the clinician changes the game so that they alternate, giving each other words to say with instructions to say them hard or easy.

Because a major goal of this phase is to help a child learn how to produce easy stuttering, the clinician should develop a variety of ways that vividly portray easy stuttering, such as moving two fingers together slowly (Fig. 11–3) or drawing a gentle curve on a piece of paper.

Throughout this and later phases, the clinician stays alert to the child's spontaneous use of easy stutters when he's talking and praises him. If the therapy sessions that focus on the three ways of saying words are enjoyable and successful for the child, he will complete

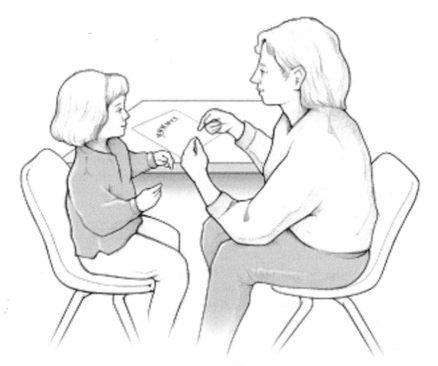

Figure 11–3 *Showing a child how to stutter easily by moving two fingers together slowly.*

this phase with feelings of confidence that he can change his speech and will have less fear of stuttering.

Locating Tension

The next phase, locating tension in speech, is designed to help the child confront and explore stuttering as it is happening. Dell begins by doing some voluntary stuttering and asking the child to help him figure out where he is tensing or what he is doing when he stutters. He encourages the child to stutter voluntarily in the same way as they explore what is going on, thereby laying the groundwork for the child's exploration of his own stuttering. The clinician and child experiment with different types of stutters, which cover those that the child shows in his own speech (repetitions and prolongations) as well as labial, lingual, and laryngeal blocks, when appropriate. When the child can identify the types of stutters and places of tension in the clinician's voluntary stutters, he is encouraged to do the same with his own stutters that the clinician gently points out in the child's spontaneous speech. Before stopping a child after stutters, the clinician should explain that such interruptions are needed to work on stuttering and then help the child confront and briefly explore his stutters during conversations.

Cancellations

After a child has learned to produce easy stutters and to confront his stutters immediately after they have occurred, he is ready to stop after hard stutters and redo them as easy ones. This activity is often frustrating, so it is best to use a structured situation for only a few minutes at a time. Dell recommends that a clinician begin this activity by having the child become the teacher and interrupt the clinician when she produces a hard stutter, then teach her how to say the word, not fluently, but with an easier, more relaxed stutter. These cancellations, unlike other ways of modifying stutters, are not used outside the therapy room because they are too likely to be interrupted in the fast give-and-take of normal conversation. They are a means of helping the child begin to change stutters as they are happening.

Changing Stuttering to a Milder Form

This phase of transforming hard stuttering to easy stuttering begins after the child has mastered cancellations in the previous phase and can redo his hard stuttering as truly loose and relaxed easy stutters. Now, he is ready to change a stutter *as it is happening,* using what Van Riper called "pull-outs." This is begun with the clinician modeling how to make this change during voluntary stutters, then asking the child to imitate her. Basically, this change is simply shifting from a hard to an easy stutter during moments of stuttering and finishing the word without rushing.

Inserting Easy Stuttering into Real Speech

After the child can use pull-outs during voluntary stuttering, the next step is to have him put voluntary, easy stutters in his speech on words that he doesn't expect to stutter on. These easy stutters are like using a voluntary pull-out at the beginning of a nonfeared word. This gives the child a feel for working on stuttering as he is communicating and is also a great desensitization activity.

Changing Hard Stutters with Pull-Outs During Real Speech

Now Dell is ready to teach the child to change hard stutters into easy stutters while he is talking. Dell notes that this is often a difficult task for a child to learn, but once learned, the child is well on the way to recovery. One helpful technique is to touch the child gently when he is caught in a real stutter. The child is to hold on to the block voluntarily until Dell lets go and then to release the block using an easy stutter. Because some children are sensitive about being touched, Dell suggests that clinicians talk with the child before using a touch to signal.

As before, Dell advises the clinician to begin this phase by putting some voluntary stutters in her speech and having the child touch her arm for several seconds while she does this. She continues to stutter until the child releases his touch and then finishes the word slowly and easily. Roles are then reversed, and the clinician gives the child an easy, nonemotional speaking task, such as describing a neutral picture. She explains to the child that, when he stutters, she will touch him and that he is to keep stuttering on the same sound in the same way until she releases her touch and then to finish the word slowly and easily. For example, if the child is stuttering on the /l/ in "like," he is to keep repeating or prolonging the /l/ sound until the clinician removes her hand; if he is having a silent block on the /b/ in "boy," he should continue the block at first and then slowly change the silent /b/ to a voiced /b/, even though this may distort the sound. Then, when the clinician's touch is released, the child slowly finishes the word.

After the child can change hard stutters into easy ones in conversational speech using the clinician's touch, he is asked to do so on his own. As he learns to do this successfully, he can begin to set goals, with the clinician's help, for using these techniques in more difficult situations, such as when talking about a complex topic or with a parent. Before transferring this skill to talking with a parent, the child should teach the parent about easy stuttering with the clinician's help. While the parent learns about easy stuttering in the therapy room, the clinician can also teach the parent how to help the child practice at home and especially how to be supportive of these changes in the child's speech without being intrusive.

Building Fluency

In the building fluency phase, Dell makes sure that the child has plenty of experiences every day in which he is fluent. At the same time, he helps the child work on his stuttering by desensitizing him to fluency disrupters and helping him to transfer his more fluent speech into many different everyday situations. Transfer can begin as soon as the child can change hard stutters into easy ones in conversational speech without the clinician's cue. In the context of a game or in role-playing, the child talks and tries to use easy stutters instead of hard ones, while the clinician gradually increases stress on the child by interrupting the child or looking away while he's talking. If the child begins to have hard stutters instead of easy ones, they stop and discuss what happened and how it might be handled differently. A hierarchy of more and more stressful therapy or real-life situations are devised by the child and clinician together, and the child enters these situations and, as best as he can, uses easy stutters when he stutters. At the same time, the child is open about his stuttering and comments about it when appropriate.

Building Independence

Finally, in the building independence phase, which begins when both the frequency and severity of the child's stuttering are notably diminished and he is confident that he can control his stuttering, Dell gradually fades the child from therapy. He does not believe that the child needs to be totally "cured" before he is dropped from therapy. Rather, when the child is doing well, Dell discontinues therapy for a period of time, allowing him to continue on his own and develop the conviction that he, rather than the clinician, is responsible for the change. If a child regresses a bit, Dell brings him in for one or more booster sessions; often there will be a number of these cycles before the child is finally dismissed.

Working with Parents and Teachers

Parents

Dell begins to work with parents during initial interviews when he seeks information about the child and gives parents information about the nature of stuttering. During his initial conversations with parents, some of Dell's other objectives are to create an open, nonjudgmental atmosphere. This is done so that parents can speak freely about their concerns and vent their feelings of frustration about their child's stuttering, and Dell can help them put some of their unspoken feelings into words. These discussions and informing parents about the nature of stuttering can also go a long way toward relieving parents of any guilt they may feel about their child's stuttering.

After he has begun treating the child, Dell invites parents to observe some of their sessions. When the child is changing hard stutters into easy ones, for example, parents may be invited to participate by letting the child teach them how to stutter easily, a situation in which the child is in a position of mastery, compared with the parents, and which is usually very rewarding for both child and parents.

At this time, the child needs to be consulted about including a further role for the parents in his treatment at home. Some children may allow parents to remind them to use easy stuttering; others may be more comfortable if their parents know what they are working on but are just good listeners. Parents are encouraged to spend a few minutes every day in quiet times with the child; these are times when the parents put aside their own agendas and let the child talk about whatever is on his mind.

In addition, Dell asks parents to keep a diary of the times when their child is most disfluent as well as when he is most fluent. In discussions of events surrounding very disfluent times, Dell helps parents identify and decrease pressures that worsen the child's stuttering. Similarly, he encourages them to find activities and situations that promote the child's fluency and to increase these activities. By establishing a continuing partnership with the parents, in which respect and understanding are paramount, Dell is able to help the child while giving the parents an important role in establishing and maintaining the child's fluency.

Teachers

Dell's counseling of classroom teachers involves providing them with information about stuttering, helping them respond more objectively to the child's stuttering in the classroom, and helping them deal more effectively with the difficult issue of the child's oral participation in the class.

Dell believes that an initial meeting with a teacher in a quiet place is very important. In this setting, the teacher can ask questions about the nature of stuttering, in general, and the nature of this child's stuttering, in particular. By comparing stuttering with other problems that children have, such as making an obvious mistake on a math problem that results in other children laughing, the teacher is better able to see that her response will guide the class and that she needs to ensure that the child who stutters feels confident even though he may have difficulty speaking. In such discussions, clinicians can help the teacher discover how she may be most helpful to the child.

When dealing with the issue of how much verbal participation to expect of a child who stutters, Dell believes this is a topic that the child and teacher can discuss privately and frankly and work out effective strategies for each situation. For example, if the child has to give an oral report, he may prefer to be called on first, so that his fears don't build up. When being called on in class, the child may wish to wait until he feels he is ready and then raise his hand.

In general, Dell finds that helping teachers to understand stuttering is a key to helping children manage their speech in the classroom. With this understanding, teachers can communicate more effectively with a child who stutters and, with the help of the clinician, can work out any difficult situations that arise.

Bruce Ryan: Delayed Auditory Feedback Program

Clinical Methods

Ryan's therapy is based heavily on operant conditioning and programmed instruction principles. This involves a great deal of structure and an emphasis on data collection.

Clinical Procedures: Direct Treatment of the Child

In his 1984 chapter, "Treatment of Stuttering in School Children," Ryan discussed his treatment procedures for intermediate stutterers, whom he refers to as a child who exhibits "severe stuttering." This is our primary reference for this section. The reader may wish to refer to Ryan's more recent book, *Programmed Therapy for Stuttering in Children and Adults–2nd Edition* (Ryan, 2000), for additional information. I will begin by discussing Ryan's direct treatment of the child during establishment, transfer, and maintenance phases. Then I will describe his procedures for counseling the child's parents and classroom teacher.

Establishment

Ryan uses a delayed auditory feedback (DAF) establishment program for intermediate stutterers (Fig. 11–4). This is also the program he typically uses with advanced stutterers. The goal is to have the child speaking fluently with the clinician for 5 minutes in the clinical setting. However, before beginning the program, Ryan ensures that the child understands what is expected of him by providing him an overview of the program. He defines stuttering for the child as any word that contains a repetition, prolongation, or other struggle behavior and explains that he will be reinforced for fluent speech and punished for stuttering. Reinforcement involves verbal praise and sometimes tokens; punishment is a verbal correction. Ryan also administers a pretreatment criterion test, consisting of 5 minutes of reading, monologue, and conversation, which he uses later to assess improvements.

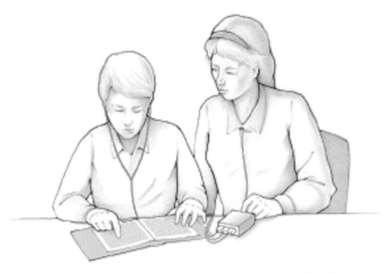

Figure 11–4 *Use of delayed auditory feedback (DAF) to establish fluency.*

The DAF establishment program is a 26-step program that begins by teaching the child to use a "slow, prolonged, fluent pattern of speech." Training starts with Ryan reading sentences aloud with the child and ends with the child reading aloud in a slow, prolonged, fluent pattern for 5 consecutive minutes. Table 11–1 presents an outline of Ryan's DAF program.

The DAF device is introduced using a 250-msec delay, and the child is told to use his slow, prolonged, fluent speech pattern while reading aloud. When he does, his speech pattern is socially reinforced. If the child stutters or speeds up, he is reminded to use slow, prolonged, fluent speech. The child needs to have 5 consecutive minutes of fluent, oral reading at this delay, which means that he needs to meet a criterion of 0 stuttered words per minute (0 SW/M) for 5 consecutive minutes. When he does, DAF is reduced by 50 msec; the child must now complete another 5 consecutive minutes of fluent, oral reading at the new 200-msec delay. In this manner, DAF is systematically reduced in 50-msec steps until the child is reading without the aid of the device. During this process, the child is required to have 5 consecutive minutes of fluent, oral reading at each of six delay times (250, 200, 150, 100, 50, and 0 msec) and 5 consecutive minutes of fluent, oral reading without DAF. As delay time is reduced, the child's speaking rate gradually increases. Eventually, the child is reading aloud fluently without the aid of the DAF device at an oral reading rate that is slightly slower than normal.

After the child completes the reading component of the DAF establishment program, he begins the monologue and conversation stages of the program. These components replicate the steps used for reading, except that the child now engages in either a monologue or a conversation with the clinician. Everything else (i.e., the reinforcement, punishment, 0 SW/M criterion, and so on) remain the same. Ryan reports that most children complete the establishment program speaking fluently at a slightly below-normal speaking rate. After completing the DAF establishment program, the child takes a

Table 11–1   Outline of Ryan's Delayed Auditory Feedback (DAF)
Establishment Program

Antecedent Events	Response	Consequent Event	Criterion
Pattern Training in Reading:			
Instructions to read in a slow, prolonged pattern	Slow, prolonged, fluent reading	"Good"	0 SW/M
Reading:			
Instructions to read. DAF: 250 msec	Slow, prolonged, fluent reading	"Good"	0 SW/M
	Stuttering	"Stop, use your slow, prolonged, fluent pattern"	
Instructions to read. DAF: 200 msec	"	"	"
Instructions to read. DAF: 150 msec	"	"	"
Instructions to read. DAF: 100 msec	"	"	"
Instructions to read. DAF: 50 msec	"	"	"
Instructions to read. DAF: 0 msec	"	"	"
Instructions to read	Fluent reading	"	"
Monologue:			
Repeat the above sequence			
Conversation:			
Repeat the above sequence			

post-establishment criterion test that consists of 5 minutes of reading, monologue, and conversation. If a child has 0.5 SW/M or less, he goes on to the transfer phase. Otherwise, he recycles through portions of the establishment program.

Transfer

The goal of this phase of treatment is to transfer a child's fluency from the therapy room to a variety of other settings and other people. Ryan uses a number of hierarchies, or sequences of speaking situations, arranged from easy to difficult, in which the child practices fluent reading and fluent conversation. During these activities, Ryan instructs the child to speak fluently and continues to reinforce the child's fluency with verbal praise and reminds him to speak fluently if he stutters. The child must continue meeting the 0 SW/M criterion for specified periods of time to pass each step. The transfer program that Ryan uses with intermediate stutterers involves physical setting, audience size, home, school, telephone, stranger, and all-day hierarchies, which are outlined in Table 11–2.

The first step in the transfer program, the "physical setting" hierarchy, involves having the child read and converse with Ryan in five different physical settings, arranged in an easy-to-difficult progression, away from the therapy room. The first step is just outside the therapy room door, and the last step is just outside the young stutterer's classroom.

Table 11–2   Outline of Transfer Program

Antecedent Events	Response	Consequent Event	Criterion
Physical Setting:			
5 steps with clinicial in different physical settings	One minute of fluent reading	"Good"	0 SW/M
	3 minutes of fluent conversation	"Good"	
	Stuttering	"Stop, speak fluently."	
Audience Size:			
3 steps with 3 classmates in therapy room	"	"	"
Home:			
5 steps with parent in therapy room and at home	"	"	"
School:			
4 steps with clinician in school	"	"	"
Telephone:			
11 steps on the telephone	3 minutes of fluent conversation	"	"
Strangers:			
4 steps with strangers	"	"	"
All Day:			
Up to 16 steps (optional)	Up to 16 hours of fluency	"	"

The next hierarchy targets "audience size" and begins with one of the stutterer's classmates joining him and Ryan in the therapy room. The stutterer reads and converses with his classmate, and when he meets the criteria, this procedure is repeated with two and then three of his classmates.

The "home" hierarchy is third, and its first step involves a parent joining Ryan and the child in therapy and being trained to carry out the transfer procedures. The parents have been informed previously that they would be involved in these and other treatment activities (Ryan's parent counseling procedures are discussed in a later section). The first step of the hierarchy is now repeated by the parent and child at home. The remaining steps involve gradual increases in audience size in the home environment by having other family members, and possibly neighbors, join the parent and child as he reads and converses. After successfully completing the home hierarchy, the child is instructed to speak fluently at all times at home, and the parents are instructed to reinforce his fluency.

The fourth hierarchy focuses on the school. Its first step consists of the child reading and conversing with Ryan in the classroom. The last and most difficult step is a speech that the child gives to the entire class. After completing this hierarchy, the young stutterer is instructed to speak fluently at all times in the classroom, and the teacher is asked to reinforce his fluency.

The "telephone" hierarchy is an 11-step program, which begins with the child saying "hello" and "goodbye" into an unplugged telephone. It ends with the child engaging in 3 consecutive minutes of fluent conversation on the telephone with a friend or stranger.

The "stranger" hierarchy begins with the child conversing with people at school, such as the school secretary or principal, and ends with him talking with strangers in local businesses. At each of the four steps in this hierarchy, the child needs to maintain 3 consecutive minutes of fluent conversation.

The final, all-day hierarchy goes as follows. The child is instructed to speak fluently for increasingly longer periods of time each succeeding day. On the first day, he is to speak fluently for 1 hour. On each subsequent day, 1 hour is added until the child is speaking fluently his entire waking day. The parents and teacher have to monitor and record the child's consecutive hours of fluency.

Ryan reports that the child is usually speaking fluently in all speaking situations by the end of the transfer phase and has increased his speaking rate to normal. Ryan gives the child a post-transfer criterion test, and if he passes (0.5 SW/M or less), he goes on to the maintenance phase. If not, the child recycles through portions of the transfer phase.

Maintenance

The goal of Ryan's maintenance phase is for the child to maintain fluent speech in all situations over a 22-month period after completion of the transfer phase. Ryan sees the child and his parents on five separate occasions during this period, which are scheduled in such a manner as to gradually fade the child from therapy. (See Table 11–3 for an outline of this maintenance program.) During each recheck, Ryan administers the criterion test to the child and questions him and his parents about his fluency at home and at school. If the child has 0.5 SW/M or less on the criterion test and is reported to be doing well in all other situations as well, Ryan schedules the next recheck. If a child's speech has regressed, he recycles through portions of the treatment program, depending on the severity of the regression. After a child demonstrates and the parents have reported fluent speech for 2 years, Ryan dismisses the child from treatment.

Table 11–3 Outline of Maintenance Program

Antecedent Events	Response	Consequent Event	Criterion
2 weeks	5 minutes of reading, monologue, and conversation	–	0.5 SW/M or less
1 month	"	"	"
3 months	"	"	"
6 months	"	"	"
12 months	"	"	"

Clinical Procedures: Parent Counseling

Ryan begins working with the parents before beginning the DAF program with a child and explains the program and the overall treatment plan to them. He wants the parents to understand what their child will be doing in therapy and what they can expect in terms of improvement in his speech. Ryan also tries to enlist the parents' cooperation for the "home practice" program and the home and all-day hierarchies of the transfer phase. The home practice program involves the parents helping the child practice being fluent while engaging in reading, monologue, and conversation at home. After the child completes the reading portion of the program, he is ready to begin practice reading at home. At this point, Ryan brings the parents into therapy to teach them how to identify stuttered words and how to carry out treatment procedures at home. They then help the child practice reading 5 minutes daily. After the child completes the monologue portion, home practice is modified to include 2 minutes of reading and 5 minutes of conversation. Later, when the child has completed the conversation mode, home practice is again modified to include 2 minutes of reading, 2 minutes of monologue, and 5 minutes of conversation. This routine continues daily until the child begins the home hierarchy of the transfer program, which we discussed in the home portion section of the transfer program.

Clinical Procedures: Classroom Teacher Counseling

Before beginning the child's treatment, Ryan explains the overall treatment plan to the classroom teacher and enlists her aid in the "school" hierarchy of the transfer phase. He also explains that she may observe improvements in the child's speech at any time during the treatment program.

Outcome Measures

Ryan describes many outcome studies of his therapy in his recent book (Ryan, 2000), but perhaps the most relevant study for the treatment described in this section is a report of the outcome of two treatment programs (Ryan and Ryan, 1995). In that study, five school-age children (mean age = 11 years) who were treated on the DAF program had a mean pre-treatment score of 10.3 stuttered words per minute. After a mean of 18 treatment hours in establishment, transfer, and maintenance components of the program, these five children had a mean of 1.1 stuttered words per minute, measured 14 months after the maintenance phase ended.

June Campbell and Hugo Gregory

June Campbell (Campbell, 2003) and Hugo Gregory (Gregory and Campbell, 1988) have developed a treatment approach for elementary school children who I believe are at an intermediate level of stuttering. Treatment consists of working on a more fluent style of producing speech, on attitudes if necessary, and on modifying school and home environments to enhance fluency.

In the beginning of treatment, Campbell and Gregory teach the child to use a fluency-enhancing skill they describe as an "easy, relaxed approach with smooth movements" (ERA-SM). ERA-SM involves a slower rate of speech and smooth transitions from sound to sound and word to word. These changes occur at the beginning of a word or phrase but not during the entire sentence. The child also learns to "chunk" speech into phrases with pauses at appropriate linguistic junctures. Work on ERA-SM is integrated with general body relaxation that is carried over into the movements involved in speech. In teaching ERA-SM, Campbell and Gregory take the child through a progression of tasks that begin with one-word responses and end with longer, more complex responses. In going through this hierarchy, they use the following types of activities to elicit speech from the child: choral reading, reading alone, answering questions, describing pictures, and engaging in conversation.

If a child still has residual stutters associated with certain sounds or words, Campbell and Gregory teach the child to modify individual moments of stuttering. To do this, they feign a stutter for the child and ask him to imitate them. They then model a modification of this stutter and ask the child to imitate their modification. This may involve slowing down a repetition or easing the tension on a prolongation. Next, Gregory and Campbell model the child's typical stutter and have the child imitate and experiment with ways to modify it. Eventually, this modification evolves into an easy, relaxed approach with smooth movements.

Campbell and Gregory also believe it is important to deal with an intermediate stutterer's feelings and attitudes about his speech. By being supportive and understanding listeners, they encourage the child to explore areas of concern that he may have about his problem. They also recommend that discussions with the child be concrete and related to specific events. In addition, they may teach a child to use voluntary disfluency if he is overly sensitive about his speech. This involves adding normal disfluencies, such as revisions and insertions, into his speech to help the child realize that some disfluency is a normal part of talking.

In transferring the new speech patterns into the child's environment, Campbell and Gregory teach the child's parents to model ERA-SM in their speech and to reinforce the child's use of it at home. They also work with the child's classroom teacher, so that he or she understands the child's therapy and can be supportive of it. Finally, to help the child maintain improvement, they recommend that the child have monthly rechecks for 12 to 18 months after intensive therapy.

Outcome Measures

Campbell (2003) indicates that about 80% of the children treated with their approach have gained "sufficient confidence to be comfortable about communication and able to speak easily in most situations" (p. 261). About 10% apparently do not succeed in treatment because they are insufficiently motivated to work on their speech at this age, and another 10% make very slow progress and need referral for psychological or educational counseling.

Summary

- In this chapter, a variety of methods of stuttering modification and fluency shaping for intermediate stutterers have been described. All of these approaches teach the child to increase fluency.

■ Some methods focus only on fluent speech; others focus on fluency but also teach the child to manage residual stuttering. Some, but not all, give some attention to attitudes and feelings.

■ My own approach begins with an exploration of stuttering to decrease some of the negative emotions associated with it and then teaches flexible rate, gentle onsets, light contacts, and proprioception to enhance fluency and manage stuttering. The young client then works on reducing his fear and avoidance by being open about stuttering, becoming desensitized to fluency disrupters, and learning to deal with teasing.

■ The other clinicians, whose therapies are described in this chapter, use many of these same techniques. All of them teach fluency-enhancing skills in a hierarchy from words to sentences to conversation in the clinic and then to everyday situations outside the clinic. Most of them foster a change in attitudes about speech and stuttering, not only to provide positive expectations for fluency but also to help clients accept any residual stuttering so that they will deal with it rather than avoid it. Several of these clinicians use relaxation techniques to enhance fluency. Many also prepare the child to deal with teasing. One of these approaches includes teaching communication skills. Thus, the core of these programs is similar, but each clinician adds innovations.

Study Questions

1. What is the "approach" attitude that is recommended for intermediate stutterers to learn? What are some reasons why an "approach" attitude might help a child with intermediate stuttering?

2. Many clinicians, including Ryan, believe that direct work on a child's attitude about speaking is not necessary because operant conditioning can change the child's speaking behaviors, which will automatically change his attitude. Do you agree? Give your rationale.

3. What is a "stuttering-friendly" environment and how could you create one in a child's home and school?

4. Describe what the "exploration" phase of treatment is designed to accomplish and how it meets that goal.

5. Suggest three ways in which you might assess to what extent the goals of the exploration phase of treatment have been met with a particular child.

6. Given what you learned about the nature of stuttering, explain why slowing speech rate (as in "flexible rate") might reduce stuttering.

7. When you are working on a transfer hierarchy and the child seems unable to transfer superfluency to a particular situation, such as giving a book report, what do you do to achieve success on this step?

8. Describe Dell's philosophy of terminating therapy. How do you feel about it?

9. Compare Dell's and Ryan's ways of involving parents in therapy.

10. How do Gregory and Campbell integrate their ERA-SM technique into stuttering modification?

SUGGESTED PROJECTS   ABC

(1) Avoidance reduction is an important componant of the major treatment described in this chapter. Experiment with your own fears and avoidances to see if you can decrease them by using a "seeking out" attitude. For example, if you dislike making phone calls, devote a week to making extra phone calls and seeking out opportunities to make phone calls you usually wouldn't make. After the week is over, assess whether this experience decreased your dislike of making phone calls.

(2) Watch the Stuttering Foundation video *Stuttering: Straight Talk for Teens* and plan how you might use various clips from it to help a child explore his own and others' stuttering.

(3) Draw a "roadmap" with pictures that you could use to help a school-age child at the beginning of therapy learn about what he will be doing over the course of therapy.

(4) Develop new ways, new metaphors, and new activities to help a child learn each of the components of "superfluency."

Suggested Readings

Craig, A., et al. (1996). A controlled clinical trial for stuttering in persons aged 9 to 14 years. *Journal of Speech and Hearing Research,* **39:808-826.**

This article describes three different treatment approaches for intermediate stuttering and assesses the effectiveness of each.

Dell, C. (2000). *Treating the School Age Stutterer: A Guide for Clinicians* **(ed 6). Memphis: Stuttering Foundation of America.**

This bargain-priced booklet contains a wealth of clinical information about stuttering modification with the school-age child, as well as helpful advice on working with parents and teachers.

Guitar, B. and Reville, J. (1997) *Easy Talker: A Fluency Workbook for School Age Childen.* **Austin, TX: Pro-Ed Publishers.**

This is a workbook for elementary school children that tells the story of several children at a camp, working on their stuttering. Along with the story, sequenced concepts and techniques are presented, with workbook activities for children to complete. This book intergrates stuttering modification and fluency shaping.

Manning, W. (1996). *Clinical Decision Making in the Diagnosis and Treatment of Fluency Disorders.* **New York: Delmar Publishers.**

Chapter 5, Treatment of Young Children, contains excellent information on both fluency-shaping and stuttering modification approaches with children between 2 and 12 years old.

Ramig, P., and Dodge, D. (2005). *The Child and Adolescent Stuttering Treatment and Activity Resource Guide.* **Clifton Park, NY: Thomson Delmar Learning.**

Goals of treatment, ideas for IEPs, steps in treatment, activities to teach elements of therapy, tips for involving parents and teachers, and a multitude of handouts (in Spanish and English) are some of the valuable contents of this book. Cluttering evaluation and treatment are also covered.

Van Riper, C. (1973). Treatment of the young confirmed stutterer. In *The Treatment of Stuttering.* **Englewood Cliffs, NJ: Prentice-Hall, pp. 426-451.**

In this chapter, Van Riper provides a comprehensive discussion of a classic stuttering modification approach to the treatment of the intermediate stutterer.

Yaruss, J.S. (Ed) (2003). *Facing the Challenge of Treating Stuttering in the Schools. Part 2: Selecting Goals and Strategies for Success.* **Seminars in Speech and Language, 24, February.**

This journal issue is full of relevant and practical ideas for working with intermediate stuttering in a school setting.

Yaruss, J.S., et al. (2004). *Bullying and Teasing: Helping Children Who Stutter.* **New York: National Stuttering Association.**

The philosophy behind this book is to empower children who stutter to take charge of teasing situations themselves. However, it also provides excellent suggestions for parents, teachers, SLPs, and school administrators.

Zebrowski, P., and Kelly, E. (2002). *Manual of Stuttering Intervention.* **Clifton Park, NY: Singular Publishing Group.**

Chapter 5 of this book (Therapy for the Elementary School-Age Child) describes an approach similar to that described in this text, with many fresh ideas. In addition, a section is devoted to group therapy with this age group.

Chapter 12

Treatment of Advanced Stuttering

Individuals with advanced stuttering are usually older adolescents or adults who have been stuttering for many years. Their patterns, which are well entrenched, consist of blocks, repetitions, and prolongations that are usually accompanied by tension and struggle, as well as escape and avoidance behaviors. Typically, these individuals have developed negative anticipations about speaking situations and listener reactions. Sometimes, their stuttering has been such an important factor in their lives that they have chosen occupations beneath their abilities (Van Riper, for example, worked as a potato digger after he earned his Masters degree in English literature). Adults with advanced stuttering sometimes turn down promotions if more speaking is required than in their present position and will often not participate fully in group discussions, team meetings, and conversations. On the other hand, some seek out therapy in an effort to become more fluent to meet the speaking demands of a higher position available to them.

Because the complex patterns of advanced stuttering involve behaviors, emotions, and cognitions, treatment is most effective if it targets all of these areas. These patterns are so deeply etched into the brain that treatment is best if it is intense, long-lasting, and provides long-term maintenance. My approach to treatment is a brew blended from many sources. I have tried to integrate these procedures so that clients reduce their negative emotions and avoidances and learn to respond differently, with more fluent speech, to old cues that have always triggered stuttering.

An Integrated Approach

Beliefs and Assumptions

The assertions that follow are not facts, but rather my inferences about advanced stuttering and its treatment. The reader should keep in mind that it is filtered through my own experiences as a person who has stuttered since age 3, who received therapy at age 21 from Charles Van Riper, and who has had both successes and failures over the 40 years I have worked as a stuttering therapist.

Nature of Stuttering

As I described in Chapter 5, I believe that the origins of advanced stuttering arise from a physiological predisposition for inefficient neural activation patterns of speech and a vulnerable temperament, interacting with environmental influences, to produce and exacerbate core behaviors of repetitions, prolongations, and blocks. In the early stages, a child responds to these early core behaviors, or disfluencies, with tension and hurry. As the child continues to experience and react to core behaviors, she copes using a variety of escape behaviors, which are reinforced through operant conditioning. During this same period, negative feelings, such as frustration, shame, and fear, become associated with stuttering. These feelings generalize through classical conditioning to more and more words and situations. Finally, the young stutterer begins to avoid feared words and situations, which is perpetuated through intermittant reinforcement. If these underlying processes continue until an individual reaches adolescence or young adulthood, the client will become an advanced stutterer.

Because increased tension, speeding up of speech rate, secondary behaviors, and feelings and attitudes are largely learned, they can be modified. Operant and classical conditioning principles are used to make these changes. However, because predisposing physiological factors contribute to these behaviors and because many years of learning have reorganized the brain in advanced stutterers, *complete* unlearning may not be possible. Thus, it is crucial to help advanced stutterers learn how to cope with residual disruptions in speech if they are going to maintain improvements in fluency.

Speech Behaviors Targeted for Therapy

In this section, I include both *new* behaviors, which should be learned, and *old* behaviors, which must be reduced or eliminated. In most advanced stutterers, well-learned tension and speeding-up responses are cued by anticipated and actual stuttering, which are typically accompanied by a considerable overlay of other learned secondary behaviors. To cope with these learned behaviors and to speak more fluently, advanced stutterers must decrease their fear of stuttering and eliminate their escape and avoidance behaviors. Then, they must learn to respond to anticipated stuttering by speaking slowly and mindfully (but fluently) for several syllables. In the chapter on treatment of intermediate stuttering, I referred to this style of speaking as "superfluency." In this chapter, I call it "controlled fluency." It often works best, however, if clients decide for themselves how to refer to what they do when they use a controlled, mindful form of fluency to replace stuttering.

Another target of therapy are actual, rather than anticipated, moments of stuttering. Individuals with advanced stuttering have deeply learned responses to subtle cues that have been learned through years of stuttering. Thus, some residual stuttering will occur unexpectedly, but it can be diminished if an individual develops a reliable coping response. This response is to loosen muscle tension and slow down speaking rate during stutters so that fluent speech and the feeling of control can be regained soon after. An example that comes to mind is from my own experience as a stutterer. After several years of greatly improved fluency, I tried to shout to a friend who was walking down a hallway, headed away from me, which is usually a tough situation for someone who stutters. When I tried to yell "Paul," I found myself jammed in an old, habitual, tense block without any sound coming out. Once I realized what I was doing, I actually laughed at the return of my old habit, then relaxed my tense posture, almost automatically, and got speech going again, slowly but fluently.

Fluency Goals

The ultimate goal for advanced stutterers is spontaneous "fluency" in all situations or, in other words, normal speech with its normal disfluencies. In my experience, most advanced stutterers do not reach this level of fluency. After treatment, clients may have periods of spontaneous fluency, lasting from a few hours to a month or more, but usually some stuttering returns, especially in stressful situations. At these times, I would like clients to have three options available.

First, when they feel it is important to be fluent, I want them to be able to apply fluency skills successfully, which I will describe in detail later, to achieve controlled fluency. Second, when they feel it is important to be fluent but are unable to achieve controlled fluency,

I want them to be able to apply and feel comfortable using skills to produce easy, mild forms of stuttering. Third, when they feel it is not as important to sound fluent and do not want to put the effort into doing so, I would like them to be comfortable having mild, acceptable stuttering so that they stay relaxed when they stutter, do not avoid speaking, and communicate well. These fluency goals seem realistic to me. However, in the final analysis, it will be the clients who choose which of these options they will use in a particular situation.

Feelings and Attitudes

I believe that advanced stutterers' negative feelings and attitudes often, but not always, need to receive considerable attention in therapy. They also need to eliminate or drastically reduce avoidances. Although this is, technically, part of behavior change, avoidance reduction is intimately tied to fear reduction. Individuals will never reduce their fear of the words and speaking situations that they continue to avoid. Reducing this fear is critical if clients are going to be successful in using either controlled fluency or mild, acceptable stuttering. Otherwise, their fear will create excessive muscular tension and speeding up, and they may be unable to alter their speech production toward fluency under conditions of high fear. I also believe that avoidances and speech fears need to be substantially reduced if clients are going to maintain their improvement over the long run. If they are not significantly diminished, they will become the seeds for relapse, which is prevalent among advanced stutterers.

It is important for clinicians to understand classical conditioning principles when attempting to eliminate clients' avoidance behaviors or to reduce their negative feelings and attitudes. Increased muscle tension, for example, may become classically conditioned when stuttering produces strong negative emotion, which, in turn, triggers an automatic "tension response" (see Chapter 4). Sounds, words, or situations that are associated with this experience eventually become the triggers for increased muscle tension. One strategy for changing classically conditioned responses is *counterconditioning*, which takes place when words and situations that elicit fear (the conditioned stimuli) are experienced over and over again in the presence of positive feelings. For example, when stutterers confront and explore their stuttering in the presence of an accepting and understanding clinician, counterconditioning occurs. The clinician's positive regard and reinforcement of such exploration decrease their clients' fears and negative feelings. Another approach, *deconditioning*, occurs when words and situations that elicit relatively low levels of fear are experienced over and over, in the absence of the feared consequences, until clients' fears are dissipated or extinguished. This is why hierarchies of least-to-most fearful stimuli are helpful for reducing negative emotions. By beginning with clients' least fearful words or situations and gradually working our way up the hierarchy, their fears become systematically reduced. Examples of these strategies are discussed in the section on clinical procedures.

Maintenance Procedures

Effective maintenance depends on clients becoming their own clinicians, which should begin early in therapy. Clients learn to evaluate their own performance in mastering stuttering modification and fluency-shaping techniques and to monitor their speech fears and avoidances. I gradually shift more and more of the responsibility for therapy to clients as they improve, and it is important for them to have a realistic understanding of what they should expect in terms of their long-term fluency. Thus, clients need to understand the concepts of spontaneous fluency, controlled fluency, and acceptable stuttering in setting their own fluency goals. It is also important that they appreciate the relationship between the conscientiousness with which they practice what they have learned in therapy and the attainment of their fluency goals.

Clinical Methods

Like the approach described for intermediate stuttering, my management for advanced stuttering is to begin with stuttering modification activities (specifically exploring the behaviors, cognitions, and emotions) to decrease negative emotion associated with stuttering. Subsequently, I teach fluency skills similar to the superfluency used with the intermediate-level client. Then I help the individual transfer and stabilize those skills with such stuttering modification activities as using a hierarchy of more and more challenging situations, voluntary stuttering, and seeking out feared words and feared situations. The measures I use to assess progress are described in the section titled "Measurement of Progress and Outcome."

Clinical Procedures

Procedures described here for working with advanced stuttering borrow liberally from many clinicians. Three individuals who have had a particularly strong influence on my approach are Gavin Andrews (Andrews and Ingham, 1971), Richard Boehmler (1994), and Charles Van Riper (1973). I am also indebted to numerous colleagues in the field, as well as to my students and clients who have generously shared their ideas.

Key Concepts

1. *Treatment should be tailored to each client's needs.* Although it would be easier if one sequence of treatment fit all clients, stuttering therapy is not so simple. Each person's biological makeup and life experiences differ; therefore, individuals require different therapy ingredients in the overall recipe for their success. Of the procedures presented in this section, *Controlled Fluency* is the heart because all clients will need this. Most clients will also need to follow the procedures at the beginning of treatment that are concerned with mapping the course of treatment and understanding and exploring stuttering. However, mild stutterers who are not uncomfortable with their stuttering and who talk freely and easily with all types of listeners may not need steps 4 and 5 of this section, which deal with reducing fear. Moreover, they may not need the two steps on using voluntary stuttering and feared words and entering feared situations in the section on increasing approach behaviors. The last section, which deals with maintenance, is probably crucial for every client; it is the planning for long-term success.

2. *Successful outcome of treatment requires focused attention to speaking, especially when stuttering is anticipated.* Brain imaging studies of the effects of treatment (e.g, Boberg et al, 1983; Kroll et al, 1997; Neumann et al, 2003; Neumann et al, 2005) suggest

that successfully treated stutterers have increased left-hemisphere activation after treatment compared to before treatment. These researchers interpreted their results as reflecting greater self-monitoring, sequencing, and timing of speech (e.g., DeNil et al, 2003; Neumann et al, 2003). It is probable, given the nature of the treatments used in these studies (fluency-shaping), that the increased left-hemisphere activity was the product of stutterers using skills like those of controlled fluency, which is presented in the treatment approach described in this chapter. These skills include slowed speech rate, easy onset of phonation, light articulatory contact, and proprioception that are used when stuttering is anticipated but practiced in fluent speech.

3. *Successful outcome of treatment depends, in part, on increasing approach behaviors and reducing avoidance.* Evidence from treatment outcome research suggests that successful long-term outcome is associated with positive communication attitudes and low levels of avoidance (e.g., Guitar, 1976; Guitar and Bass, 1978). Work on attitudes, negative emotions, and avoidances takes two forms in an integrated approach to therapy. First, use of controlled fluency, described earlier, will affect attitudes and emotions through repeated experiences of fluency in situations where stuttering previously prevailed. Second, direct work on decreasing fear and avoidance can be effective in reducing stuttering (Van Riper, 1958). Neurophysiologically, the emphasis on approach activities may "kindle" emotional regulation by the left hemisphere, which in turn, may "damp" the avoidance and fear responses regulated by the right hemisphere (Davidson, 1984: Kinsbourne, 1989; Kinsbourne and Bemporad, 1984). Thus, work on controlled fluency and attention to approach behaviors both may be associated with increased left-hemisphere activity.

4. *Adults who stutter may continue to have speech-processing deficits after treatment and may need to continue to compensate for them.* Brain imaging research suggests that, even after successful treatment, adults who stutter are likely to continue to show abnormally low activity in left brain regions that are active for speech processing in non-stutterers (Neumann et al, 2003). Thus, the treatment program described in the following pages includes provisions for dealing with residual stuttering through very long-term work on controlled fluency as well as work on new responses to residual stuttering in a way that is comfortable for both the speaker and listener and thus doesn't interfere with communication.

5. *Measurement of progress and outcome.* I use two principal measures of behavioral change in treatment. As I noted in Chapter 6, "Preliminaries to Assessment," percentage of syllables stuttered (%SS) provides a useful measure of the frequency of stuttering for snapshots of progress during treatment. Frequency of stuttering is particularly handy for assessing audio-recorded samples of speech made outside of the therapy setting. At crucial times in treatment, such as after the Understanding and Exploring Stuttering stage of treatment, after Learning and Generalization of Controlled Fluency, and at the termination of formal treatment and later, I use the SSI-3 to assess overall severity of stuttering.

To assess a client's progress and outcome in terms of her feelings and attitudes about communication, I use the Modified Erickson Scale of Communication Attitudes (S-24), which was also described in Chapter 6. This measure has been adapted for repeated use and has been shown to be predictive of treatment outcomes (Andrews and Cutler, 1974; Andrews and Craig, 1988; Guitar and Bass, 1978). I use this measure before beginning the Maintaining Improvement stage of treatment so that I can assess the extent to which a client has generalized positive feelings and attitudes about communication situations. If a client shows more negative attitudes than the average normal speaker, it is a cue to continue working on approach behaviors and ensure that she has mastered the use of controlled fluency in all situations.

Evidence for the validity and reliability of these measures can be found in Chapter 6.

Beginning Therapy

There are several issues I deal with in the first therapy sessions. The first is to understand what treatment goals the clients has. Frequently, we have discussed this in a preliminary way during the evaluation, but once treatment actually gets underway, it is important to revisit this topic and to clarify for both the client and clinician what they are working toward. During this discussion, I bring up the options of spontaneous fluency, controlled fluency, and acceptable stuttering. The client and I will revisit various situations in her life that are likely to be affected by stuttering, and we explore what level of fluency is important in them. We look for situations in which the client is satisfied with her fluency and discuss what her speech is like at such times.

A second issue is to map out a possible course of treatment. Mindful of what the client's goals are, I provide brief descriptions of the stages of treatment we will go through, matching it to the client's present situation and her desires for improvement. At this point, I don't emphasize the probability that some stuttering may remain after treatment but let the client's hopes be the guide. The general plan I would describe is first for the client to get to know what she does when she stutters, including her behaviors, thoughts, and feelings about her stuttering and her listeners' possible reactions. After that, she would learn to increase overall fluency and deal with anticipated stuttering by employing various controlled fluency skills to reduce tension, slow her speech rate, and monitor her speech. Gradually, working more independently, she would seek out formerly feared words and situations and replace her old avoidance behaviors with a more assertive attitude, more fluency, and a more confident, more relaxed approach to those stutters that remain. Finally, in the later stages of treatment, I would help her work out a plan to use her new fluency in more and more situations and to gradually become her own clinician so that she can diagnose and repair her speech if stuttering creeps back in.

Exploring Stuttering

The aim of this first phase of treatment is to help a client become more objective about her stuttering and to lift the cloud of dread that surrounds stuttering as long as it remains a mystery. Objectivity is fostered through the step-by-step procedures of the client learning about her pattern of stuttering behaviors, as well as through the overall feeling of acceptance she gains from the clinician's support and encouragement. As this process goes on, the client becomes more optimistic about changing her stuttering. She realizes that stuttering consists of behaviors that she can control and feels supported by the clinician's belief in her ability to change.

Understanding Stuttering

The goals of this step are for clients to understand the rationale for exploring their stuttering and to become partners in planning therapy. I begin by giving clients a handout on Understanding Your Stuttering (see gray box) and discussing it with them. As we discuss it, I find out from a client about other domains that she's worked on previously and improved, like skiing, painting, golf, or photography. We discuss how emotions and attitudes can get in the way of new learning and may perpetuate old behaviors. I draw an analogy between the skills that the client has worked on and the tasks before us, which is to learn to increase fluency and modify stuttering. We discuss the idea that if she can learn what she's doing when she stutters, then she may feel more objective and optimistic about her stuttering and be able to change what she's doing and become more fluent. I try to convey the idea in a preliminary way, which will be repeated in many forms, that she has learned to speak in an inefficient way that is influenced by her desire not to stutter. However, despite years of stuttering, she can now learn to replace it with a controlled form of fluency. This process begins by her exploring stuttering and getting to know it and decreasing her understandable tendency to avoid or escape from it. I also discuss the fact that, as with learning other skills, she will need to practice new techniques until they are second nature to her, and even after that.

Understanding Your Stuttering

We want to better understand your stuttering, and we want you to do the same. You may not really know what you do or how you feel when you stutter. Because it's unpleasant, you have probably attempted to hide it from yourself as well as from others. Let's begin to explore your stuttering by discussing the following components of the problem. Once you explore and better understand your stuttering, it will lose its mystery, and you will be less uncomfortable with it.

Core Behaviors

These are the repetitions, prolongations, and blocks (getting completely blocked on a word) that you have; they are the core or heart of the problem. Core behaviors were the first stuttering behaviors you had as a child.

Why do you have these core behaviors? Research suggests that persons who stutter may have "timing" problems related to their control of the speech mechanism. For fluent speech to occur, muscle movements involved in breathing, voice production (voice box), and articulation (tongue, lips, jaw) must all be well coordinated. Evidence suggests that persons who stutter experience a lack of coordination between these muscle groups during speech. Furthermore, research implies that these physical timing problems are so slight that they show up as stuttering only when feelings and emotions are strong enough to cause a breakdown in the coordination of the speech mechanism. We know that our ability to perform any physical skill can be affected by our emotions at the time. When our feelings and emotions are strong, they often may interfere with our performance. This is especially true for the fine coordinations of the speech mechanism in people who stutter. In therapy, we will teach you techniques to assist you in coping more effectively with these core behaviors.

Secondary Behaviors

Secondary behaviors are tricks or crutches you use to avoid stuttering or to help you get a word out. They are behaviors you have learned over the years to help you cope with the core behaviors, and they can be unlearned. There are different types of secondary behaviors. Which of the following do you use?

Avoidance Behaviors

The category of avoidance behaviors covers all the things you might do to keep from stuttering. Word and situation avoidances include substituting words, rephrasing sentences, not entering feared speaking situations, and pretending not to know answers. You might also use "postponements," such as pausing before a difficult word or repeating another word or phrase over and over before trying to say a word on which you expect to stutter. Another avoidance trick some stutterers use is called a "starter." This is when you might say a sound or word quickly just before a difficult word, as in saying "umwould you like to go to a movie?" Hand or body movements might be used in the same way.

Escape Behaviors

These behaviors are things a stutterer does to get out of a word once she is stuttering, such as a head nod, jaw jerk, or eye blink. You may have developed escape behaviors that are so subtle that you don't notice them anymore. Some of them might be called "disguise behaviors" because they are attempts to hide your stuttering as it is happening. These include covering your mouth with your hand or turning your head when you stutter.

Feelings and Attitudes

When you began to stutter as a child, you were probably unaware of your stuttering. Because you have been stuttering for many years, however, you may have experienced many frustrating and embarrassing speaking situations. Consequently, if you're like most stutterers, you have probably acquired some negative feelings and attitudes about your speech. You may feel embarrassed, guilty, fearful, or even angry. Fear is the most common feeling. Stutterers typically fear certain speaking situations and certain sounds or words. What feelings and attitudes do you have regarding your stuttering? As part of your therapy, we will help you reduce these unpleasant feelings and attitudes.

With my help, you will explore and describe the various components of your stuttering problem. Before you can change something, you need to understand what you are changing. And if you can break it down into manageable chunks, you can change it more easily.

Approaching Stuttering

The goal is for clients to make the first steps toward approaching their stuttering, rather than backing away from it. The client needs to learn about the core, escape, and avoidance components of her stuttering and, to some degree, why they occur. The client should also feel that the clinician is genuinely interested in her and in her speech.

The activities associated with this step involve examining moments of stuttering as they occur in the treatment room. I explain to a client that, to begin our work on her stuttering, we will have to work together to understand it and explore what she is doing when she stutters. I warn her that I may interrupt her when she stutters to help us get a sample that we can look closely at together. I have the client read a passage and mark those words on which she stutters for later use. I show genuine interest in her stuttering and make observations about it, such as, "I noticed on that one, it looked like you squeezed your lips together trying to get the word out." I also ask questions like, "Is that how you usually stutter on words that start with B?" As we explore stuttering together, I use my interest and acceptance to begin the process of *desensitization*. During this activity, I teach clients about different components of stuttering, including core, escape, and avoidance behaviors, particularly as they apply to the client's stuttering. This activity goes on at a pace suited to a client's comfort talking about her stuttering. When the client is relatively comfortable examining her stuttering, I may use a mirror to help her explore and confront her stuttering (Fig. 12–1).

It is important to transfer treatment activities to situations outside the clinic, and I use a small audio recorder and go to situations outside the clinic, where the client and I record our speech. Then we go back to the therapy room to listen to it and discuss it calmly and objectively. I then ask the client to take the recorder home and record some

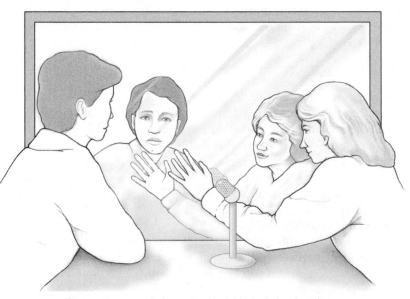

Figure 12–1   *Exploring stuttering with the help of a mirror.*

samples of her stuttering at home or at work and write down her observations about her stuttering when she later listens to it and finally shares it with me.

Analyzing Stuttering

The goals are for the client to (1) become more accurate in analyzing what she does when she stutters and when she avoids stuttering, (2) decrease negative emotions toward her stuttering, and (3) transfer these changes outside the treatment room. The clinician may observe that a client's stuttering is slightly less severe at this point; however, confrontation of stuttering may decrease avoidance behaviors and thereby make stuttering temporarily more severe. The desensitization session in Van Riper's (1975b) videotapes demonstrates this temporary increase in severity of stuttering and the clinician's response to it. Another observable change may be a client's greater willingness to observe and discuss her stuttering. It is advisable to continue this step until a client's negative emotions about stuttering are observably reduced.

I begin by having a client play recordings of her stuttering made outside the therapy room and discuss her descriptions of what she did when she stuttered. If the client has been able to bring in even one stutter from an outside situation, I always reinforce her achievement. Remember that one goal of treatment is to activate "approach" behaviors and lessen avoidance behaviors. If a client has been unable to carry out this task, she and I do the task together and record her stuttering in a situation outside the room or on the telephone.

Before I have her speak in a new situation, I do some pseudo-stuttering to model for an approach orientation toward stuttering and speaking. I show genuine enthusiasm about her ability to enter situations that require speaking and may produce stuttering. Even if the client can only accompany me in these situations, it is a small victory.

As we analyze our recordings, I begin teaching her about the speech mechanism to increase her understanding and objectivity. I also use a drawing or model of the vocal tract that depicts the articulatory, phonatory, and respiratory systems to supplement my descriptions of what we may be doing when I am pseudo-stuttering and she is actually stuttering. For example, we may start by analyzing one of my stutters in which I squeezed my lips together and blocked off air at my larynx. I then imitate it and have her imitate it, as well. Again, I am careful to reinforce her attempts at this to encourage her willingness to approach stuttering. We then analyze her stutters from the recording, thereby creating an attitude of objectivity and interest in her stuttering and washing away some of the "withdrawal" feelings she may have about her stuttering. I try to help a client feel more objective about her stuttering and to understand that it is not something that just takes over her body but something that she does. It's simply a set of behaviors, not a shameful act out of her control. Changes in negative emotion at this point, and every day afterwards, will set the stage for a client being open about her stuttering, which will further reduce negative emotions and decrease tension and speeding up.

During the sessions in which the client and I analyze her stuttering, I look for stutters that are mild, brief, and forward moving and call the client's attention to them. I ask the client to look for them in her samples collected outside and in her stuttering in the therapy room. As we attend to these, I let the client know that these are models of how she can learn to handle her stutters. In fact, she can make them more like fluent speech, so that neither she nor her listeners will hear them as stutters. They will, in fact, become similar to the way persons who don't stutter would handle disruptions in their speech (Boehmler, personal communication, 2004).

The client and I develop transfer activities that continue to strengthen her approach attitudes and behaviors but that are not beyond her present capacity. She continues to record her stuttering in situations outside the clinic and take notes on listener reactions. It is important to ensure that the client is engaged in therapy activities on days when she is not attending treatment, and it helps if she and I keep in telephone or e-mail contact between treatment sessions.

Reducing Fear of Listener Reactions

The goal of this step is for the client to continue to reduce avoidance, self-consciousness, and shame about her stuttering through further "approach" activities, such as being open about her stuttering. The success of these activities can be assessed in terms of reductions in stuttering severity, increases in her speaking in situations that she previously avoided, and reports of greater comfort in talking despite stuttering. This step and the next can be the most difficult part of treatment for many clients, who often require encouragement and support from the clinician. It may help to remind them of where they are in the progression of treatment and to review the rationale for confronting fears associated with their stuttering.

The major activity of this step involves the client talking to others about her stuttering, which I initiate by giving her a handout (see gray box) on being open about her stuttering.

Discussing Stuttering Openly

One way to become more comfortable with your stuttering is to discuss it openly with your family, friends, and acquaintances. When you get to the point of being open about your stuttering, you will lose much of your fear of it and be more relaxed. In most cases, your listeners know you stutter, you know you stutter, but nobody ever says anything about it. It's like an ostrich sticking its head in the sand in the face of danger, pretending it's not there. You would feel much more comfortable about your stuttering if you could talk about it openly. Your listener would also be more comfortable if you were open and at ease with your stuttering. Your listener often takes his cue from you regarding how to respond. If you look uncomfortable, he will probably feel uncomfortable, but if you are open and comfortable with your stuttering, your listener will probably feel at ease.

How can you be more open about your stuttering? Tell family and friends that you are in therapy and explain what you are doing and why you are doing it. After you have talked about it, encourage them to ask you questions about it. Create an opportunity to let them know how you would like them to respond to your stuttering. For example, some of your family and friends may finish words for you when you stutter. Let them know if you would rather for them to wait until you're finished. Or, some of your listeners may look away when you stutter. If this makes you uncomfortable, as it does most people who stutter, let your listeners know that it is helpful if they will maintain eye contact when you stutter.

Another good practice is to make comments about your stuttering. If you feel like it, you can make a funny comment about your stuttering to put yourself and your listeners at ease. For example, if you have to introduce yourself and you think you will stutter on your name, you can say, "Make yourself comfortable, it may take me a few minutes to say my name." Or, just comment casually on a hard block you've had by saying, "Whew, that was a hard one." The more you do this, the less panicked you will feel when you stutter. Another opportunity for being open about your stuttering is when you are faced with making a speech or presentation to a group. Just before you begin speaking, let the audience know that you stutter. They'll find out anyway, but saying it upfront will put everyone, including yourself, much more at ease.

A few advanced stutterers will find these assignments easy, but most will not. I make sure that a client feels she and I are working as a team and that I am supportive and empathetic. I usually help her make lists of the situations in which she will begin to be open about her stuttering and then model an example for her. For example, if commenting on stuttering during a telephone call is on her list, I would call a store, pretend to stutter, and immediately make a comment, such as, "Wow, looks like I'm really stuttering more than usual today." Recently, when working with a young man who was quite sensitive and reluctant to talk openly about his stuttering, I had him videotape me as I interviewed three different people on a busy shopping street. After getting permission to videotape, I asked them a variety of questions about stuttering and found that each gave positive, supportive answers. The young man seemed impressed that the lay public was, after all, not uptight about stuttering. Exercises such as this can help clients test reality and find out that much of their anxiety and disapproval about stuttering is in their mind rather than in those of the listeners. However, I prepare clients for the possibility that there will be a negative listener reaction (although this is rare) by expressing the hope that at least one listener will be impatient or rejecting so that we can see if we can retain our calm under stress.

Usually, by using a hierarchy of situations, stress can be increased slowly. A client and I plan a hierarchy of tasks in which a client is open about her stuttering. We might go, for example, from a casual comment she might make to a store clerk about having a stuttery day all the way up to telling a group of people that she stutters and is working on it. In psychological terms, reductions in negative emotions that are associated with less stressful tasks will generalize to more stressful tasks. Consequently, when a client gets to the more stressful tasks, they will no longer be as difficult.

After the client completes the assignments on her hierarchy, she discusses the outcomes with me. I diligently give her a great deal of praise for confronting her fears and discussing her stuttering openly. At times, I may need to encourage or even push her to move on to the next step; however, I need to be sensitive to the intensity of her feelings so that I don't expect too much too soon. The client needs to feel she is in control of the amount of stress she puts herself under.

The client will probably never completely finish this activity because discussing her stuttering openly will always be an important strategy for her to use, not only during therapy but, possibly, throughout her lifetime. It can help her maintain her improved fluency long after therapy has ended. Thus, I get the client started on her hierarchy, then move on to the next technique, and she will continue to work on discussing her stuttering openly in outside assignments while also working on other techniques or procedures.

Reducing Fear of the Experience of Stuttering

The goal of this step is to reduce the client's fear of stuttering. For years, she has been feeling "trapped" in the stuckness of stutters, helpless and struggling, with little or no reliable way to escape. If she is like most people who stutter, the very act of struggling to escape from stutters increases her muscle tension and consequently the feeling of being stuck. But being able to stop struggling and tolerate her experience of being trapped reduces her tension and perhaps provides more positive sensory feedback to the brain, allowing her to move forward in speech. Progress on this step can be assessed by the client's movement up the hierarchy for this activity. The hierarchy goes from her controlling my pseudo-stuttering with her hand signal, all the way to her holding on to a stutter for several seconds in a conversation with a friend or stranger, while maintaining good eye contact and staying relaxed.

I use the handout in the following gray box to provide clients the rationale for the activities associated with this step.

Freezing or Holding on to the Moment of Stuttering

The experience of being caught in a moment of stuttering (repetition, prolongation, or block) can be frustrating and scary. When your mouth doesn't do what you want it to, you feel out of control. If it goes on for several seconds or your listener is upset or impatient, you may feel devastated. As unpleasant as these core behaviors are, you need to increase your tolerance for them, to learn that you can experience them without panicking. Instead of avoiding them or hurrying to get out of them, you need to learn to experience them and remain calm, so you can change them.

So, how do you learn to remain calm while you're jammed (blocked) in a moment of stuttering? I use a technique called "freezing" or "holding on." By freezing, I mean that when you are stuttering and I signal, you are to hold on to that moment of stuttering until I signal you to come out of it. If you are repeating a syllable, you are to continue repeating it; if you are prolonging a sound, you are to continue prolonging it; and if you are having a block, you are to maintain that phonatory arrest or articulatory posture. By experiencing these core behaviors of repetition, prolongation, and block over and over again while remaining relatively calm or becoming calmer as the freezing continues, you will find your tolerance for them increasing. You will no longer become fearful at the thought of getting stuck on a word, and you will find the core behaviors becoming more relaxed; that is the key to change.

You will begin by signalling me to hold on to a pseudo-stutter for several seconds. Then I will have you hold on to one of your real stutters for only a brief period of time, possibly 1 or 2 seconds. When you get caught in a stutter, I will signal you to hold on to that stutter, and you are to hold on to it and keep it going until I signal you to complete the word slowly. While holding on to a repetition, prolongation, or block, you are to try to stay as calm as possible. Just experience the stutter and be as composed and relaxed as you possibly can. As your tolerance increases, I will gradually increase the length of time you are to hold on to your stutters. Eventually, you will hold on to your stutters until the tension and struggle have dissipated and you can end them easily and slowly. This will involve you signaling yourself and me when you begin a stutter and when you will come out of the stutter. I will also have you watch yourself in a mirror and listen to yourself on a tape recorder as you are holding on to your stutters. Again, just experience your stuttering and try to remain as calm as possible. Remember that after you feel the tension ebb away, finish the word slowly and deliberately.

By experiencing these moments of stuttering over and over again in this manner, you will gradually lose your fear of them. You will find yourself feeling more comfortable when you are talking, and you will be talking more fluently.

After I have made sure that the client understands the rationale and procedures involved in freezing, I explore with her the sequence of activities that we will follow together. Freezing, like the other procedures in this phase of therapy, is implemented most effectively in a hierarchical order. Will she be able to stop in the middle of a block and hold on to it when I signal, or will this be too stressful? Sometimes, I need to put some stutters into my speech and have the client signal me to freeze. How long will she be able to hold on to a core behavior in the beginning? Will it be more unpleasant for her to watch herself in a mirror as she holds on to a block, or will it be more difficult to listen to herself on a tape recorder? After these questions are discussed and a hierarchy is tentatively established, I begin with the easiest task.

Suppose it's decided to begin by having the client hold her stutters for 1 to 2 seconds. This activity would likely go something like this. Whenever she stutters during our conversation, I signal her by raising my finger or touching her arm to freeze or to hold on to whatever she is doing at that moment. I ask her to feel what she's doing that makes the stutter feel stuck. Is she tensing in her throat? Her tongue? Her lips? I tell her to continue her repetitions, prolongations, or blocks for only a second or two, and then I signal her to finish the word slowly and deliberately and then continue speaking. If her tension and struggle have dissipated before my signal, she is to voluntarily continue stuttering until I signal. During these periods, I remain calm, show interest in what she is doing, and praise her ability to hold on to the stutter calmly. If she appears to be frustrated, fearful, or angry, I verbalize these feelings for her and accept them. If she looks away when she is holding her stutters, I encourage her to maintain eye contact with me and strongly reinforce her successes in hanging on to her stutters. When she is successful with this activity, I move on to more stressful steps.

The more stressful steps include gradually increasing the duration with which the client holds on to her core behaviors, as well as having her assume responsibility for signaling when she begins and when she will end a stutter. She should wait until her tension and struggle have dissipated before she ends a stutter. These steps also include having the client listen to herself on recordings and watching herself in a mirror as she holds on to moments of stuttering. Finally, I accompany her into various speaking situations, in which I model holding on to moments of stuttering and have her do it as well. Whenever possible, we audio record these experiences and listen to them together.

For transfer activities, I ask the client to record when she holds on to stutters without my being present. This step will be challenging for most clients and will need much planning and debriefing. In my experience, it helps if we do considerable work together outside the treatment room to help the client become desensitized to working on her stuttering outside the clinic. It will also help if the client can start setting her own goals for assignments, especially those she does on her own.

As we work through holding on to stutters and remaining calm, in the clinic and outside, I continue to be understanding, accepting, and reinforcing of the client's feelings and behaviors, especially when a client is having trouble carrying out assignments on her own. By spending quite a few sessions working on stuttering on phone calls in the clinic and stuttering during conversations with strangers outside, the client will gradually lose much of her strong negative emotion associated with moments of stuttering as she becomes counterconditioned to her stutters.

Reduction of negative emotions often has the effect of reducing the severity of stuttering; this will be reflected in a lower score on the SSI-3, especially in the duration and physical concomitants of stutters. It is advisable to reassess severity with the SSI-3 at this stage, both in the clinic and on recordings of speech outside. If the scores have not decreased and if the client began treatment with a high SSI-3 score as well as evidence of negative communication attitudes on the Modified Erickson scale and high avoidance scores on the Stutterer's Self-Rating of Reactions to Speech Situations, it may be appropriate to continue working on reducing the client's fear before moving on to the next stage of treatment.

Learning and Generalizing Controlled Fluency

Learning Controlled Fluency

The next goal is to have clients learn a controlled type of fluency to replace their stuttering. Some clinicians prefer to delay working on this goal until negative emotions have been reduced further through voluntary stuttering. I find that teaching fluency skills at this point increases motivation and makes the confrontation of stuttering more tolerable for most clients. Progress toward confronting stuttering and reducing negative emotion has been started in the previous work on understanding and exploring stuttering. Further work on reducing negative emotions will be done after controlled fluency is learned.

As a client works on controlled fluency, progress is assessed in the clinic by the clinician's judgment of whether the client can successfully produce speech with each of the components reviewed in the following sections and can use the components together in conversational speech that sounds natural.

The fluency skills learned in this step are the same as those used with intermediate level stuttering, but for the sake of review, I will present them again.

Flexible Rate

Flexible rate is simply slowing down productions of a syllable, most commonly the first and second phonemes of a word (Boehmler, personal communication, 2003). Slowing is thought to be effective in reducing stuttering by allowing more time for language planning and motor execution to occur. This skill is called "flexible rate" rather than "slow rate" to emphasize that only those syllables on which stuttering is expected are slowed, not the surrounding speech. The client learns to vary her rate from syllable to syllable, by slowing one syllable and not another within a word, and from utterance to utterance, depending on her anticipation of stuttering.

Flexible rate is taught by having the clinician first model the production of words in which the first syllable and the transition to the second syllable are said in a way that slows all the sounds equally. Vowels, fricatives, nasals, sibilants, and glides are lengthened, whereas plosives and affricates are produced to sound more like fricatives, without stopping sound or airflow.

Easy Onsets

This refers to an easy or gentle onset of voicing. My perception of my own stuttering is that, if I begin a "feared" sound with a rapid onset of voicing (i.e., a hard glottal attack), I get myself into a "stuck" posture that feels like I can't move it. But if I start my vocal folds vibrating gently at first, I can usually get voicing going without stuttering. For me and probably for many, but not all, people who stutter, vowels in the word-initial position are easier to produce with an easy onset than consonants. Vowels following a word-initial, voiceless consonant, however, are fairly difficult for me. For example, I might prolong the /s/ in "sun" but block on the /u/ unless I consciously employ a gentle onset on the /u/. This also emphasizes another point, that the transitions from a sound or position to those that follow may be the "sticking point" and thus should be a focus of controlled fluency. Teaching easy onsets is like teaching flexible rate. I model the target behavior on lots of different sounds, have the client imitate my model, and reinforce successive approximations.

Light Contacts

Just as hard glottal attacks seem to trigger stuttering, so, too, will hard articulatory contacts. When someone who stutters anticipates difficulty with a sound, she'll often "preset" her articulators in a stuck position before starting the word, or she may even rehearse stuttering behavior (Van Riper, 1936). Producing consonants with light contacts will prevent the stoppage of airflow and/or voicing that seem to trigger stuttering. Light contacts are taught by modeling a style of producing consonants with relaxed articulators and continuous flow of air or voice, depending on the consonant. Plosives and affricates should be slightly distorted so that they sound like fricatives but are still intelligible. For example, when I produce the /b/ in *Barry* using a light contact, I slow my movements into and out of lip "closure" but do not stop airflow or voicing between my lips. Instead, I let my lips vibrate and let the /b/ sound continue for a little longer than normal. For a /p/, my lips barely touch, and air flows out of my loosely closed lips, creating a slight turbulence that sounds a little like an /f/. Teaching clients to use light contacts is accomplished by modeling the target behaviors on a variety of initial consonants in different words and reinforcing clients' successive approximations of these behaviors.

Proprioception

In the present context, proprioception refers to sensory feedback from the mechanoreceptors in muscles of the lips, jaw, and tongue (Abbs, 1996). This feedback may be crucial in controlling speech movements. Its use in stuttering therapy may have originated with Van Riper, who suggested that "...some of the stutterer's difficulties seem to originate in the auditory processing system. [Therefore,] if we can get him to concentrate upon proprioceptive feedback rather than auditory feedback we can bypass these difficulties" (Van Riper, 1973, p. 211). Recent brain imaging studies that were reviewed in Chapter 2 support the contention that the auditory systems of people who stutter may be dysfunctional (e.g., Fox, 2003), but there is also evidence that other sensory systems may not be functioning normally as well (e.g., DeNil and Abbs, 1991). The effectiveness of teaching proprioception may depend on it focusing conscious attention to sensory information from the articulators and perhaps bypassing inefficient automatic sensory monitoring systems, thereby at least temporarily normalizing sensory-motor control.

Proprioceptive awareness can be taught by using masking noise or delayed auditory feedback to interfere with self-hearing during speech. The client should be speaking with very conscious awareness of the movement of the articulators. Sometimes, it helps to have the client speak with her hands over her ears and her eyes closed. Although it is not always easy to judge accurately whether or not a client is using proprioception, I look for slightly exaggerated, slow movements to verify that she is trying to feel the movements of her articulators.

Once a client seems to have acquired the necessary proprioception skill, it can be combined with flexible rate, easy onsets, and light contacts as described in the next section. I refer to this combination as "controlled fluency," which means the same as the term "superfluency," which I used in the chapter on treatment of intermediate stuttering. The clinician should feel free to use whichever term seems appropriate for the client.

Transferring Controlled Fluency into Fluent Speech

The goal of this step is for clients to learn to use controlled fluency in their normally fluent speech to "put money in the bank," as Van Riper used to say. Thus, if a client can use the careful, deliberate style of speech that I call controlled fluency in her normally fluent utterances, she will benefit greatly from the practice. This will improve the chances that, when she anticipates stuttering, she can call upon controlled fluency and it will work for her. She may not always turn a stutter into a fluent utterance, but she may be able to produce the stutter with a feeling of being in control. This requires a well-learned and available behavior (controlled fluency) that can be called upon even under stress. To make the behavior available under stress, the client must practice it over and over until it is second nature to her.

It should be noted that clients don't need to use controlled fluency for an entire sentence every time they practice it. Using controlled fluency on the first word of a sentence or on a word within a sentence can be another way to keep this tool sharp. Some of my clients call these single-word uses of controlled fluency "slideouts." Other clients and my graduate students refer to them as "slides," a term coined by Vivian Sheehan (personal communication, November 1999). Clients should be encouraged to develop their own names for the techniques they find helpful.

Assessing success on this step is a matter of designing a hierarchy of speaking contexts in which controlled fluency can be used to replace normal speech and measuring a client's progress ascending the hierarchy. When I use the term "normally fluent" speech, I am not referring to perfect speech, which is not the goal of treatment, but to speech like that of nonstutterers, which contains its share of normal disfluencies, (e.g., whole-word and phrase repetitions) that the speaker handles easily.

To begin, the client and I design a hierarchy of speaking contexts that progresses from using controlled fluency on single syllables at the beginnings of sentences to using controlled fluency on various syllables in other sentence positions. It is important to remember that this is done only on words on which the client expects to be fluent. We start with conversations between ourselves in the treatment room and progress to outside speaking situations in which the client expects to be fluent. These may include simple telephone conversations in which the client asks what time a store closes, asking questions of store clerks, and stopping unfamiliar people on the street and asking them questions. The client and I then jointly design more transfer activities for a variety of natural situations in her life. At least some of these speaking opportunities should be audio recorded so that we can evaluate the quality of her controlled fluency outside the treatment situation.

Most clients will need considerable practice and feedback to maintain all the components of controlled fluency in real-life situations. To help a client work toward independence, more and more of the analysis of the quality of controlled fluency should be done by the client, with the clinician providing guidance. The client must continue to use controlled fluency in her normal speech, even after she has learned to replace stuttering with controlled fluency, in order to keep this skill at a high level of readiness.

One way to help the client practice controlled fluency on words in her normal speech is to help her set up a quota to meet by noon of every day. She should develop a tallying system, such as using a wrist counter like those used by golfers to tally strokes, or carrying a box of 20 Tic-Tacs and eating one for each word produced with controlled fluency on the first syllable. For my own self-therapy, I prefer to use a golf stroke counter because its noticeable presence on my wrist reminds me to practice controlled fluency on the initial syllables of many sentences throughout the day.

Replacing Stuttering with Controlled Fluency in the Treatment Room

In this step, the goal is for clients to learn to use controlled fluency in response to old stimuli that were followed by stuttering. This means that the client needs to learn to use controlled fluency when she anticipates stuttering and before she finds herself stuck in a block. With lots of practice and success in many situations, she will develop confidence in her ability to speak with controlled fluency instead of stuttering. In time, she will learn to do it in such a way that her controlled fluency becomes more or less indistinguishable from normal fluency for both listeners and the speaker. Progress is assessed by measuring the frequency of stuttering in various situations.

I begin by having a client replace stuttering with controlled fluency during conversation in the treatment room. If she has practiced using controlled fluency in her natural speech, she knows what it feels and sounds like and has started to "groove" it. As a client begins to use controlled fluency to replace stuttering, she may benefit by looking in a mirror as she converses with me, watching for upcoming stutters, and focusing on what she is doing as she starts to respond. Then, as she works to use controlled fluency to replace anticipated stutters, the mirror helps her to monitor her speech in a more focused way. If a client has trouble "downshifting" to controlled fluency before stutters, I have her signal me when she anticipates a stutter and then plan her controlled fluency response. I sometimes use Van Riper's (1973) technique of having a client pantomime her target response before she begins it. Enthusiastic but gradually faded praise is helpful. I also use videotaping and replaying samples of her *successes* to help her learn. Early in this process, I ask the client to evaluate her response, sometimes providing feedback and sometimes not, as I foster the goal of self-evaluation.

As a client is learning controlled fluency, I introduce "cancellations" (Van Riper, 1973) as a way of having her mildly punish herself when she fails to downshift into controlled fluency and stutters instead. Cancellations, which are taught by modeling, involve pausing for several seconds after a stutter (the pause functions as a "time out"), having the speaker mentally prepare to use controlled fluency during the pause, and then using controlled fluency on the word just stuttered and continuing to talk. The opportunity to continue talking is a positive reinforcer for the controlled fluency. I am diligent in rewarding cancellations with verbal praise because they are one of the most powerful tools available for self-therapy. I gradually fade my praise and help the client to develop her own reward system. When used regularly throughout acquisition, transfer, and maintenance stages, cancellations can make controlled fluency a durable replacement for stuttering.

I would like to highlight the point just made because it is important. Cancellations are an operant conditioning procedure. The pause after stutters is a "punishment" that decreases the frequency of stuttering, and the opportunity to continue speaking is a reward that will increase the use of controlled fluency. Cancellations are especially effective because they are self-administered operant procedures that a client eventually uses herself as she takes charge of her own treatment. A good description of cancellations can be found on pages 84 through 90 of the book *Forty Years After Therapy* by George Hellisen, which is listed in the suggested readings for Chapter 1.

Transferring Controlled Fluency to Anticipated Stuttering

When a client seems confident in her responses during conversations with me in the treatment room, she and I design a hierarchy of increasingly difficult contexts to practice in. Typical hierarchies involve (1) inside the clinic with me, (2) outside the clinic with me, (3) everyday speaking situations, and (4) the telephone.

The first hierarchy of inside the clinic with me varies the physical location and social complexity of therapy sessions in the clinic, which means conducting therapy in other locations in the clinic and bringing other people into therapy sessions. The size of the audience can be increased, and people from the client's world, such as family and friends, can also be brought into therapy. The client and I rank such situations from easiest to most difficult, and then she goes through these situations in sequence, using controlled fluency, both in her natural speech and when she expects to stutter, and cancellations if she does stutter. Usually, we work out a point system generating self-rewards to increase her motivation.

Once a client has completed the first hierarchy using controlled fluency, it is time to move on to outside the clinic to hierarchy situations in which I can accompany the client. We jointly select and sequence hierarchy situations and activities for this. Examples of

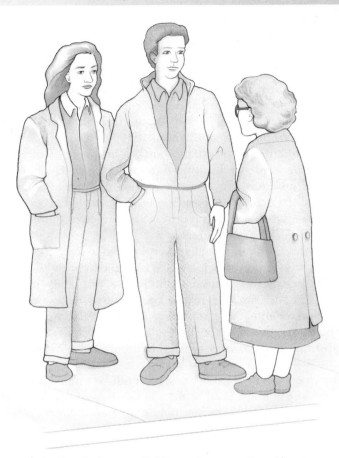

Figure 12–2   *Transferring controlled fluency in conversation with a stranger.*

these situations are asking directions from strangers or obtaining information from store clerks (Fig. 12–2). For this stage of the hierarchy, a survey about stuttering (Does the person know what stuttering is? Do they know anyone who stutters? How do you think you should respond to someone who is stuttering? etc) can be a powerful device to practice replacing anticipated stuttering with controlled fluency. It has the side benefit of discovering what the attitudes about stuttering really are.

For any given situation, the criterion for success is that both the client and clinician agree that the client used these skills as well as she did in the clinic. This means that the controlled fluency she used to replace stutters and in fluent speech feels and sounds as good as it did when she used them in the clinic. Some instances of cancellation are acceptable in achieving success, but most stutters should be replaced by controlled fluency on the first try. This is a subjective evaluation, but realistically, it is the type of evaluation the client will use on her own in the future. It is also important that the client be successful in using controlled fluency in fluent speech and instead of anticipated stuttering in each situation a number of times so that she gains confidence in her ability to use them. After gaining skill and confidence in using controlled fluency in outside situations with the clinician present, it is time for the client to move on to the next, more difficult hierarchy.

The everyday speaking situation hierarchy consists of situations from the client's environment and requires her to complete them on her own. Clients usually rank a dozen or more speaking situations that they encounter in a typical month, from least to most difficult. As a general rule, the client should feel that she has successfully used her transfer skills a number of times in the immediately preceding, easier situation before moving to a more difficult step or situation on the hierarchy. This is important in developing her skills and confidence in using these techniques. During regular therapy sessions, the clinician monitors the client's progress through this hierarchy, praises her when she is successful, encourages her when she is not, and makes suggestions when she has problems. In time, the client will report to the clinician that her speech is becoming much better in her everyday encounters.

I have found that most advanced stutterers need a separate hierarchy for the telephone. The same strategies or principles used in implementing the hierarchies discussed earlier are applied here as well. Thus, telephone calls, with and without the clinician present, are arranged in a hierarchical order. The client practices using controlled fluency in fluent speech and on anticipated stutters or uses cancellations, if needed, during these calls until she meets the criterion for success, and the clinician continues to support and reinforce her during these activities. Soon, the client will report successes in her daily use of the telephone.

By now, the client will be speaking more fluently or with easier stuttering in most situations. Although she is not yet out of the woods, she is well on her way. We now move to the steps that will help clients transfer fluency to even the most challenging situations.

Increasing Approach Behaviors

Using Voluntary Stuttering

Voluntary stuttering can be a very potent procedure for reducing tension and avoidance and, thereby, facilitating the use of controlled fluency to replace stuttering. By using voluntary stuttering, the client is performing an "approach" behavior, which will decrease fear and tension. This makes it more likely that the client will be able to use controlled fluency successfully. Every clinician should be familiar with voluntary stuttering. The handout (gray box), which I give to clients in this stage of therapy, explains the why's and wherefore's of voluntary stuttering.

Using Voluntary Stuttering

One of the most important goals for you to achieve in overcoming your stuttering is to reduce negative feelings associated with it, such as embarrassment, fear, and shame. The more embarrassed you are by your stuttering, the more fearful you are of getting jammed up in a stutter; the more ashamed you are of your stuttering, the more you will try to hide it. The more you try to hide your stuttering, the more tense you will become and the less you will be able to use controlled fluency. This process needs to be reversed.

One way to reduce these feelings is to stutter voluntarily. If you are afraid of something and run away from it, you will always be afraid of it. The way to overcome fear is to confront it and discover that it's not as bad as you thought. By confronting your fear, you will learn that you are tougher than you think. By stuttering on purpose, first in easy situations and later in more difficult situations, you will learn that you can stutter without fear and shame.

You will begin using voluntary stuttering in the clinic, and I will help you start by putting easy repetitions and prolongations in your speech on nonfeared words. Don't be alarmed if you stutter on some of the words on which you use voluntarily stuttering. This is a common experience. Just keep on stuttering voluntarily until you can finish the word comfortably and without struggling. We will continue to practice this until you are able to remain calm while voluntarily stuttering here in the clinic.

The next step will involve you going with me into the real world to do voluntary stuttering together. Again, you will use easy repetitions or prolongations with strangers on nonfeared words. You may be surprised that most people are accepting of stuttering and will wait for you to say what you want to say. A few may frown or try to finish your sentence for you, but these will be trophies to collect, listeners we can discuss together later. While testing reality in this way, you will learn to tolerate your stuttering and any listener's reactions and stay cool.

You will also need to use voluntary stuttering in your own environment to reduce your old fears. Old feelings die slowly! However, if you conscientiously do voluntary stuttering sufficiently often over a long period of time, you will find your old fears decreasing. You will no longer be hiding your stuttering, you will be able to use controlled fluency to replace stuttering, and you will be talking more comfortably and fluently. When you are ready to do voluntary stuttering on your own in your everyday speaking situations, we will work together to help you prepare assignments.

When I first introduce voluntary stuttering to client, many think I must be crazy. After all, they came to therapy to rid themselves of stuttering, not to do more of it. At this point, I explain the rationale behind voluntary stuttering: stuttering is perpetuated by fear of stuttering, and reducing this fear will reduce the stuttering. An analogy often helps. For instance, suppose a person wanted to overcome a fear of dogs. This could not be done by running away from them. Instead, the person would have to begin seeking out contact with dogs with knowledge of how to approach them. The best way to do this would be to have the guidance of someone who was an expert on dogs and was not afraid of them and who would guide the person's contact with dogs in a series of small steps.

For example, the first step might involve only looking at puppies in a pet store; the next step might be talking to a clerk about the puppies. Then, the person might briefly pet a puppy, and then perhaps pick up the puppy and hold it for a short period. This process would need to be repeated over and over again with gradually larger and larger dogs. Eventually, the person would learn how to approach a dog in a friendly way. As the person learned how to approach and make friends with dogs, her fear would gradually decrease.

This same process can be followed with stuttering. With my guidance, the client begins to stutter on purpose and learn that she has nothing to fear. She'll learn that voluntary stuttering frees her from the need to be perfectly fluent and enables her to use controlled fluency because she is less tense and no longer feels a need to "hold back." The success of this process depends a great deal on a clinician who is comfortable with stuttering. Thus, clinicians need to desensitize themselves to stuttering by practicing voluntary stuttering until the experience of stuttering and listeners' reactions to it does not bother them.

After explaining the rationale behind voluntary stuttering, I teach clients how to stutter voluntarily. First, I model brief, easy repetitions or prolongations while remaining calm and relaxed, and I follow this voluntary stuttering with controlled fluency. Then I encourage the client to attempt some voluntary stuttering followed by controlled fluency and enthusiastically reinforce her efforts. If she finds this too difficult, however, I do it with her and have her shadow my voluntary stuttering and controlled fluency. With appropriate modeling and support, most stutterers are able to do some voluntary stuttering within just one session. I continue giving the client lots of praise for her courage in doing something she may find difficult and am careful to point out that what had been so fearful at first no longer seems so scary.

After the client becomes comfortable using voluntary stuttering followed by controlled fluency in the clinic, it is time for her to move out into the world. First, the client and I establish a hierarchy of situations in which she can use voluntary stuttering. The clinician should always go into situations with the client and use voluntary stuttering during the beginning steps of the hierarchy. I ask her to rate my listeners on a scale that reflects a range of qualities. For example, a "1" might be someone who laughs or looks away, and a "10" might be someone who is attentive and listens patiently. The client may want to continue using this rating system when it is her turn to practice voluntarily stuttering as well because it can countercondition old emotions of feeling victimized and helpless.

I voluntarily stutter in such situations as asking directions from strangers or information from store clerks and remain calm as I do it. If all of my listeners are patient and understanding, I ask the client to choose listeners whom she feels might be more difficult. After I've completed several of these, it is the client's turn to stutter voluntarily with strangers. We then continue to take alternate turns, which provides additional counterconditioning as the client and I compare our ratings of listeners and take turns choosing listeners for each other. In time, a stutterer's feelings of assertiveness and exploration usually increase, which diminishes feelings of fear and avoidance.

I am careful not to allow a client to get in "over her head" with listeners who may be too difficult. I also lavish praise on each of the client's attempts, acknowledging how difficult it can be, and try to be sensitive to how much she wants to discuss each event and provide the support needed. After a good workout with store clerks, for example, I may suggest that we take a break for coffee or a soda at a restaurant, where we can practice voluntary stuttering with the waitress and enjoy the counterconditioning effects of drinking and eating while doing something that was previously unpleasant.

The client and I continue working together on voluntary stuttering until she feels comfortable. Then she works her way through the rest of the situations in her hierarchy on her own. She has to continue putting voluntary stuttering into her speech in each situation until her fear subsides before going on to the next situation. I check clients' progress during therapy sessions, commending them when they are successful and supporting, encouraging, and counseling them when they run into problems. Voluntary stuttering is a procedure that clients will continue to use throughout active treatment and maintenance and is not an activity that will soon be discontinued.

Using Feared Words and Entering Feared Situations

Using feared words and entering feared situations are very important "approach" behaviors that will help clients continue their progress in replacing stuttering with controlled fluency. Some clients will have accomplished a great deal in this area during the transfer of controlled fluency to replace stuttering. However, most will benefit from practice in seeking out remaining fears. I use the following handout (see gray box) to begin teaching this step and supplement it with examples and discussion.

Using Feared Words and Entering Feared Situations

An important goal for you to achieve in overcoming your stuttering is to reduce your avoidance of feared words and feared situations. In the past, you have probably changed words that you were sure you would stutter on and have also shied away from people and places that were very difficult for you. The problem in doing this is that avoidance perpetuates stuttering. To make real progress in therapy, you will need to change your avoidance "mind set" to one of approach and begin to seek out words you have stuttered on and situations you have found difficult in the past. These will be opportunities for you to make your controlled fluency stronger and more resistent to stress.

If you have not already developed this habit, you should now begin to approach words and situations that you previously avoided. Even though you may still stutter, the fact that you have an "approach" attitude will keep you from tensing and holding back as much as you usually do, and you will sometimes be surprised to find that you don't stutter as much as you expected.

Starting today, stop substituting easier words for harder ones, stop rephrasing sentences to get around feared words, and stop pretending you don't know the answer to questions when you really do. Instead of using these sorts of tricks, say exactly what you want to say, even if you stutter. If you are afraid you will stutter on a word you are about to say, commit yourself to saying that word, even if you stutter. In time, you will find your old fears decreasing, and with this decrease in word fears, you will find your word and sound avoidances decreasing and your fluency increasing, as well.

From today on, you should try not to avoid talking while in the clinic. In fact, talk as much as you possibly can. If you want to talk about a topic or ask a question, do it. If you think you are going to stutter on a word, go ahead and stutter. In the long run, this is much better than avoiding or postponing. You will learn that you can tolerate your stuttering and will be more comfortable with it and will gradually become more fluent.

Eliminate your avoidance of feared situations by talking in all of those situations that you avoided in the past. For example, introduce yourself to strangers, start using the telephone more than you usually would, and look for opportunities to speak in groups. If you are aware of any fear of a speaking situation, take that as a sign to approach and enter that situation. Your willingness to speak in these situations will make things much easier for you in the long run. You will find your situation fears decreasing and your wanting to avoid these situations also decreasing; a by-product of this decreased fear will be increased fluency.

In addition to not avoiding speaking in the clinic, you should begin today to eliminate the use of word and situation avoidances in the real world. You will need to develop an approach set in your own speaking environment, and I will help you set up a series of outside speaking assignments, from least to most fearful, to help you overcome your use of avoidances. Now and then, old speech fears will be too strong, and you will avoid, but come back the next day and try again. In time, you will find the old fears decreasing and your tolerance for stuttering increasing. You will also be more comfortable with yourself as a speaker and speak more fluently. However, you will need to keep working on this approach attitude for a long time because it is very important that you eliminate your avoidances and keep them eliminated.

After the client has read the handout, I answer any questions she may have. I then encourage her to try not to use any postponements or word avoidances when in therapy from then on. If she does, I have her use a cancellation by redoing the sentence while using controlled fluency on the word(s). When I think she deliberately uses a word that she appeared to want to avoid, I strongly reinforce this approach behavior. I also set up activities in which the client purposefully has to say feared words that we had previously identified and uses controlled fluency when producing these words. These activities may involve her reading word lists and text that is loaded with her feared words or involve her composing sentences loaded with these words. I warmly praise her each time she does not postpone or avoid a feared word, especially when she successfully uses controlled fluency. Sometimes she may be unable to use controlled fluency; however, I am accepting of these occasions and let her know that I understand how hard it can be. This will help her become more comfortable saying these words and will reduce her tendency to want to avoid them.

To help the client eliminate her use of avoidances outside the clinic, I assist her in setting up a hierarchy of word and situation avoidances she commonly uses in daily life. Like all hierarchies, it should be sequenced from least to most difficult for the client. By using this strategy, her fears will be kept to a minimum. A typical step in the hierarchy is the stutterer's deliberate use of certain feared words throughout the day. How often should she use these feared words? They have to be used over and over until she no longer wants to

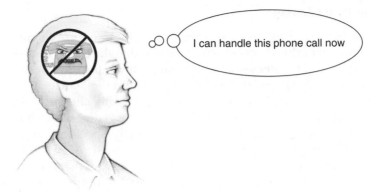

Figure 12–3   *The client reduces fear and avoidance by approaching previously feared situations.*

avoid them. Another step in the hierarchy has the stutterer entering situations that she usually avoids in daily life (Fig. 12–3). As before, she needs to enter these situations until she loses her motivation to avoid them. Many of the latter assignments can be completed as the client goes through her daily routine and will not take any extra time. For instance, she just needs to answer the telephone, whenever it rings, with the feared "hello" said using controlled fluency or introduce herself to a different person each day. Other assignments may have to be created, and she may need to go out of her way to perform them. For example, the client may have to shop for an item whose name contains one of her feared sounds or fabricate reasons for making telephone calls to local businesses.

To help the client get started on an outside hierarchy, it is helpful for me to join her for some of the assignments. Thereafter, she has to complete the assignments by herself but discusses her progress and any problems with me during regular therapy sessions. I make sure that she keeps on track in completing her hierarchy and provide her with the necessary support and sometimes gentle nudging to help her do so. After the client has worked through as many situations as she and I think are sufficient, it is appropriate for her to complete the Modified Erickson Scale of Communication Attitudes. This will give me an indication of whether or not there are still situations that need to be approached and mastered.

Like discussing stuttering openly, eliminating the use of avoidances is a strategy that stutterers will need to use throughout therapy and beyond. So, once a stutterer has begun outside assignments successfully, it is time to move on to steps that will create the foundation for long-term change.

Maintaining Improvement

The goal of this last phase of therapy is to help clients generalize their improvement; that is, transferring their reduced negative feelings, attitudes, avoidances, and increased fluency to all remaining speaking situations and maintaining this improvement following termination of therapy. I introduce the following procedures during this phase: (1) becoming your own clinician and (2) establishing long-term fluency goals.

Becoming Your Own Clinician

If clients with advanced stuttering are going to generalize improvement to all speaking situations and maintain this improvement, I believe that they must assume responsibility for their own therapy. The literature on self-management provides helpful guidance for fostering this transition. The article "Self-Regulation and the Management of Stuttering" (Finn, 2003) is a good example. Finn points out that having clients set their own goals is a key element of success. I would also highlight the importance of teaching clients to formulate their own plans that target specific behaviors for specific changes. An article in *Time* (Ripley, 2005) on surviving disasters suggests that survivors of 9/11 and other catastrophes often had developed a plan of action beforehand, so that they were not affected by the common human response to unexpected stress—freezing. Such plans will help clients become committed and focused in their efforts to improve their fluency.

I use the handout shown in the following grey box to help clients learn how to combat avoidance and continue improving their fluency skills.

Becoming Your Own Clinician

Now that we have covered all the therapy techniques you will need to meet your therapy goals, it is time for you to become your own speech clinician. Although you have improved your fluency and reduced your emotional reactions to stuttering, you will probably still encounter some situations that will give you trouble. Thus, you will need to learn how to handle these situations as well as maintain the fluency you have gained.

Handling the difficult situations that remain will require you to be honest about where you think you may still stutter and what your fears are. Fear doesn't stand still; if you ignore it, it will grow, but if you pursue it, it will die. So you must be vigilant for words and situations that continue to spark fear in you and make you feel as if you won't be able to handle your speech the way you want. For these words and situations, you must be ready to use your techniques to work on these fears, such as controlled fluency in both fluent speech and when you anticipate stuttering, openness about your stuttering, and voluntary stuttering. Up to this point, we have worked together to develop and carry out such plans, but now you will have to take more and more responsibility for them.

Working on feared words and situations is not limited to advances. It also involves maintaining the level of fluency you have now because adult stutterers often relapse or slip back some after they leave therapy. Relapse is not inevitable, but neither is it surprising. After all, you have had years of practice in stuttering. In fact, you are an expert. You have avoided words and situations for a long time, and your negative feelings and attitudes about your speech are well learned. Because stuttering is deeply etched into your brain, you may always have some core behaviors and will need to cope successfully with them. Therefore, you need to become your own speech clinician. You will have to keep applying—on your own and long after you leave therapy—the techniques you have learned in therapy.

So what is involved in being your own clinician? You will need to learn to give yourself assignments to overcome remaining difficult speaking situations and any new ones that crop up. If you still avoid speaking in a certain situation, you will need to design assignments that will eliminate this avoidance. If you are still fearful while talking in some situations, you will need to undertake assignments to reduce this fear. If you are still stuttering a lot in a given situation, you will need to plan assignments that will improve your fluency in this situation. At the beginning of therapy, I helped you create these assignments, but as you improved, more and more of the responsibility was turned over to you. We will continue to do this. With additional practice, you will be able to determine your therapy needs and to develop assignments to meet these needs. When you can do this, you will have become your own speech clinician.

I have found the following approach is effective in meeting this goal. Every day you need to work on reducing any remaining speech fears and eliminating any remaining avoidances. For example, if you still feel fearful while talking in a certain situation, you could give yourself a daily quota of tasks to perform in that situation, including being open about your stuttering and using controlled fluency in your fluent speech and voluntary stuttering. Every day you will also need to work on improving your fluency. If you are still doing a lot of stuttering in a given situation, you could set a daily quota of talking time in that situation during which you will use controlled fluency. These are only examples; the important thing is for you to ask yourself every day which situations are still giving you problems and to give yourself assignments designed to overcome these problems. Now, let's get started in helping you become your own speech clinician.

By this time, a client is probably getting close to completing her everyday speaking situation hierarchy. I point out to her, however, that completing this hierarchy is not enough and that she needs to pursue any other situations that are still giving her trouble. I ask her the following kinds of questions: Is she avoiding talking in any more situations? Is she still unduly afraid while talking in some situations? Is she unable to successfully use controlled fluency in fluent speech and when anticipating stuttering in some situations? Is she hesitant to use voluntary stuttering in some situations? If she answers yes to any of these questions, she needs to target these situations in assignments.

If the client is still avoiding some situations, I remind her of the importance of using feared words and entering feared situations. I may have her re-read the handout and then prepare assignments to overcome her current avoidances. I try not to assume any more responsibility than is necessary. I try to ask helpful questions but want her to figure out on her own what she needs to do. As time goes on, I will gradually have the client assuming more and more responsibility for planning her own assignments.

If the client is still unduly apprehensive about talking in some situations, I remind her of the importance of discussing stuttering openly and of using voluntary stuttering to reduce her negative feelings. I help her create assignments using techniques that will make her feel more comfortable in these situations. Here again, I don't assume any more responsibility than necessary and focus on guiding the client to becoming her own speech clinician.

If she is having difficulties using controlled fluency to replace stuttering in some situations, I explore the nature of her difficulties with her and help her determine what types of assignments she needs to work on to be successful. Maybe she only needs more practice in some less difficult situations before she can reasonably expect to be successful in the more difficult situations. Perhaps she needs to further reduce her speech rate and muscle tension in these difficult situations so that her motor control does not break down as readily. I have found that some clients strive to be as fluent as possible in all situations; however, others are happy with some residual stuttering if it doesn't interfere with their communication. I am accepting of this because I realize that clients must set their own goals. During all of our discussions, I try to keep in mind that my goal is to help the stutterer become independent. So, I gradually become less directive and gradually turn all of the responsibility for her assignments over to her. Throughout this phase of therapy, the client should be working daily on outside assignments and discussing her progress with me during therapy sessions. During this same period, I am more and more of a consultant, helping the client feel that she can go out and fly on her own.

Establishing Long-Term Fluency Goals

Before therapy ends, it is very important for a client to be aware of what she can expect in terms of fluency after termination from therapy. By having realistic goals, she can substantially decrease the possibility of becoming disappointed and frustrated with her speech and not developing feelings that may lead to relapse. To begin this topic, I share with her the handout shown in the following grey box.

Establishing Long-Term Fluency Goals

You are at the point in your therapy when you need to consider your long-term fluency goals. Before you do this, I need to define three of the terms we will be using: "spontaneous fluency," "controlled fluency," and "acceptable stuttering." Spontaneous fluency refers to speech that contains no more than occasional disfluencies, and there is no tension or struggle. This fluency is not maintained by paying attention to or controlling your speech. Therefore, you don't use controlled fluency to be fluent. You just talk and pay attention to your ideas. It is the fluency of normal speakers.

Controlled fluency is another name for normal-sounding fluency that is under your active control. It has the qualities you've practiced: flexible rate, easy onsets, light contacts, and proprioception. It sounds similar to spontaneous fluency except that you must attend to or control your normal-sounding speech to maintain relative fluency. You sound fluent only because you are working on your speech at the time.

Finally, acceptable stuttering refers to speech that contains noticeable but mild stuttering that feels comfortable to you. You are not avoiding words or situations, and you feel okay about yourself as someone who stutters at times. You may have

---

acceptable stuttering when you don't care about working on your speech. Or you may have it when you are trying to use controlled fluency but can't quite get a handle on it. It's healthy to feel okay about the occasional mild stuttering you have in either case.

Now, let's consider long-term fluency goals. A few adults who stutter become spontaneously fluent in all speaking situations on a consistent basis. They become normal speakers. In my experience, however, most adult stutterers do not reach this goal. Instead, they have situations, such as talking to close friends, in which they are spontaneously fluent. In other situations, such as speaking in groups, their stuttering tends to give them trouble. In these troublesome situations, I think it is important for these stutterers—and possibly you—to have the following options.

First, if it *is* important to you to sound fluent in a specific situation, I want you to be able to use your controlled fluency skills. I know this is possible in most situations, especially if you have been putting money in the bank by practicing controlled fluency in your fluent speech. I also know that there will be some situations in which you will not be totally successful. In such situations, I want you to feel comfortable with acceptable stuttering.

Second, if it is *not* important to you to sound fluent in a situation, and you do not want to put the effort into using controlled fluency, I would like you to feel comfortable with acceptable stuttering.

These options, or goals, are both realistic and acceptable. In other words, you don't have to sound perfectly fluent all the time or work on your speech constantly. Indeed, attempting to sound fluent all the time by using controls can become burdensome. Where are you now with regard to these fluency goals? Are you satisfied with your present fluency? Where would you like to be in the future with regard to these goals? We should discuss these issues, and you should begin to make plans based on your answers.

I make sure that the client understands the concepts of spontaneous fluency, controlled fluency, and acceptable stuttering. When I am convinced that she understands what is meant by these terms, I explore with her the types of fluency she currently has in various, everyday speaking situations. If she is unsure, she gives herself assignments to help her find out whether or not she is satisfied with the types of fluency she has in these situations. If she is satisfied, then she has met her goals, and the end of therapy is near. If she is not satisfied, then she needs to continue working along the lines discussed in the previous section on Becoming Your Own Clinician until her goals are met.

I have observed a couple of problems that frequently occur with clients' fluency expectations or goals. First, many clients experience a great deal of spontaneous fluency at this point in therapy. They expect and want this spontaneous fluency to last forever without any effort on their part. It can last, but that will require continued work. A client will need to continue giving herself assignments to keep her negative feelings and attitudes at a minimum and to extinguish her avoidance behaviors. She will also need to continue working on her controlled fluency so that she has confidence in her ability to use it when she chooses. Spontaneous fluency will be a byproduct of these efforts, and

I must help the client understand this. If she doesn't understand, she will be disappointed and possibly panicked when she begins to lose some of her spontaneous fluency, which could lead to relapse.

A second problem frequently involves clients with more severe advanced stuttering. These clients often fail to achieve a great deal of spontaneous fluency. If they are going to talk better, they need to use controlled fluency constantly. Even then, they often achieve only acceptable stuttering, which can be discouraging. It may be too much of a burden for them to constantly monitor and modify their speech. In time, they will become tired and give up doing anything at all, and relapse will soon follow. I need to help these clients accept and become comfortable with their acceptable stuttering. I also need to help them realize that they will need to expend substantial effort to maintain this level of fluency. Clients with severe advanced stuttering may benefit especially from the support provided by a self-help group to help them maintain the motivation needed for continued self-therapy.

Once a client feels she is meeting her fluency goals and has become her own clinician, the frequency of her therapy contacts is systematically reduced. I typically fade contacts to once a week for a month or two, then to once a month for several months, and finally to once a semester for 2 years. This gradual transition provides the client with some continued support. For example, if she is doing well, I reinforce her, and if she is having a few problems, I can help her find solutions. Of course, if she has relapsed completely, she can be re-enrolled in therapy. Ultimately, the day comes to say "goodbye." I commend her for all her efforts and let her know that if she ever needs me again, she should feel free to contact me.

Throughout the fading process, I assess her speech using the SSI-3 for samples gathered in the clinic on videotape and percent syllables stuttered for the samples she brings me from outside situations. The process of us mutually analyzing her fluency and working on areas that need further practice help to keep her focused on using controlled fluency. It also increases the chances that she will become largely spontaneously fluent and her controlled fluency will become more and more automatic.

Other Approaches

Comprehensive Stuttering Program (CSP)

Einer Boberg and Deborah Kully (1985) developed a 3-week treatment program that was initially based on earlier programs that used prolonged speech to induce fluency and then used principles of conditioning to transfer and maintain fluency in clients' every day lives (Ingham and Andrews, 1973; Webster, 1974). Over the last 20 years, Kully and her colleague Marilyn Langevin have refined their approach so that elements of stuttering management, cognitive behavioral therapy, and self-management have become crucial elements of the treatment.

The following description of the program is taken from Kully and Langevin (1999) and Langevin and Kully (in submission). Clients begin by learning very slow, prolonged speech that has the following components: (1) smooth, unrushed breathing patterns with appropriate breath grouping, (2) gentle onset of voicing, (3) continuous airflow and smooth continuous movement of articulators within breath groups, and (4) light contacts of articulators. Once clients learn these skills, they gradually increase their speech rate and monitor their speech naturalness. At the same time, they learn Van Riper's (1973) techniques of cancellation and pullout to deal with stutters that may emerge as clients increase their speech rates. Clients then learn cognitive-behavioral techniques to be comfortable using their techniques in public, to reduce avoidance, and to deal with residual stuttering. They also learn to improve their overall communication skills and attitudes, as well as skills to manage regression and relapse, if they occur.

Once clients have learned these skills and are speaking fluently in the clinic, they begin transfer activities. These are essentially hierarchies, suited to the needs of each client, in which the client uses his newly acquired skills to speak fluently or with managed stuttering in gradually more difficult situations. Clients then consult with their clinicians to design individual maintenance programs to use after they terminate formal therapy. They are encouraged to join support groups and return to the clinic for follow-up treatment if needed.

Outcome data have been reported on both 1-year and 5-year follow-ups. Kully and Langevin (1999) found that in a group of 25 adolescent clients, mean pretreatment %SS was 14.32, and mean score for Erickson Scale of Communication Attitudes (S-24) was 16.81 (mean for nonstutterers reported by Andrews and Cutler, 1974, was 9.4). One year after treatment, mean %SS was found to be 3.89, and mean S-24 scores were reduced to 11.57.

Results of a 5-year follow-up study of 25 clients (mean age = 27 years) revealed the following: (1) mean stuttering frequency, measured as %SS on telephone call, decreased from 15.2 to 4.5; and (2) mean communication attitude score, as measured with S-24, decreased from 17 to 11.5 and 12 of 25 clients were at normal (9.4) or below. In summary, 20 of 25 clients maintained a "clinically meaningful" gain at 5-year follow-up (50% improvement in %SS, and no more than 3% increase in %SS measured immediately after treatment).

Camperdown

Sue O'Brien, Mark Onslow, Angela Cream, and Ann Packman (2003) have developed a treatment program for adults that is based on earlier prolonged speech treatments (e.g. Ingham and Andrews, 1973) but requires less treatment time and gives clients more self-reliance in the establishment, transfer, and maintenance of their controlled fluency.

The Camperdown program has four stages. First are the Individual Teaching Sessions, in which clients learn prolonged speech and practice using a scale of stuttering severity. Unlike traditional methods of teaching prolonged speech via detailed instruction in slow rate, gentle onsets, light contacts, and continuous airflow, the Camperdown approach uses a video of a clinician speaking with prolonged speech at 70 syllables per minute. Clients are coached by the clinician to imitate the model and to continue practice using the model, with the clinician's feedback, until they can produce a 3-minute monologue with fluent prolonged speech. In this stage, clients are taught to use a 9-point scale to rate their stuttering severity, both live and from videotaped samples.

After clients can produce the monologue fluently with prolonged speech, they complete a Group Practice Day, in which they learn to speak at gradually faster rates, fluently and naturally, and to assess their speech on the severity scale as well as a 9-point naturalness scale. Subsequently, they begin Individual Problem-Solving Sessions, consisting of weekly meetings with a clinician, to facilitate generalizing fluent speech to everyday situations. These sessions involve the clinician mentoring clients' planning and carrying out generalization activities, as well as further practice of fluent speech. Clients' speech have to meet two criteria for three consecutive weeks at this stage. Both within-clinic and beyond-clinic conversations must show low levels of stuttering severity (ratings of 1 to 2) and normal levels of speech naturalness (ratings of 1 to 3).

The final stage of the program, Performance-Contingent Maintenance, lasts about a year and involves repeated clinic maintenance visits by clients whose stuttering severity and speech naturalness levels are expected to be equivalent to those required previously. If these severity and naturalness criteria are met, clinic visits are scheduled at fading intervals: 2 weeks, 2 weeks, 4 weeks, 8 weeks, and 24 weeks. If the criteria are not met at any visit, that visit is repeated, and progress is momentarily stalled until it is met.

The authors of the program indicate that this approach is an important advance over previous stuttering treatments because it requires relatively little treatment time (i.e., 20 hours to establish fluency). Because the program doesn't involve extensive teaching and measurement of prolonged speech targets, the authors believe that it can be used by generalist clinicians rather than just stuttering specialists. A more detailed description of the program is available from the treatment manual, which can be downloaded from the Australian Stuttering Research Centre website: www.fhs.usyd.edu.au/asrc//. This can also be reached by googling "Camperdown."

Outcome data on the Camperdown program with 16 subjects who completed four stages indicates that mean %SS of samples recorded in situations beyond the clinic was reduced from 7.9 before treatment to 0.4 one year after maintenance. Self-report measures of severity (on a 1 to 10 scale, with 1 being normal speech) reflected a reduction from 5.4 to 2.8.

Walter Manning

Manning believes that the major handicap of adolescents and adults who stutter is the limitation that stuttering places on their lives academically, socially, and occupationally. Consequently, Manning's therapy procedures, which are tailored to each client, are designed to help clients increase the opportunities and choices in their lives. In his book, *Clinical Decision Making in Fluency Disorders* (2001), and a chapter, "Management of Adult Stuttering" (1999), Manning describes a therapy approach that usually begins with a client identifying what he does *when* he stutters (i.e., core and secondary behaviors) and what he does *because* he stutters (i.e., choices motivated by stuttering, such as avoidance of situations). The client then works to modify his behaviors and choices, learning to feel more comfortable with stuttering in many situations and how to modify stuttering so that it sounds more and more like normal speech.

Manning takes most clients through a sequence of learning experiences that help them gain control of their stuttering. These include desensitization, variation, and modifications (e.g., cancellations, pullouts, and preparatory sets). Manning's aim is to help clients feel in control of the moment of stuttering, to "take charge" of the word being stuttered, and to modify the way they are stuttering on it. After this work on stuttering modification, clients undergo fluency shaping to further enhance the smoothness of their speech.

Manning uses fluency shaping from the beginning of treatment with advanced stutterers who may be unable or unwilling to modify their stuttering. Examples are clients who have psychogenic or neurogenic stuttering or those who are mentally retarded. Manning strongly advocates group therapy as a component of treatment to help clients practice speaking skills and deal with emotional issues, and he urges his stuttering clients to join support groups after therapy to enhance long-term change.

Manning's desired outcome for treatment of adults is not stutter-free speech but a reduction in the handicaps caused by stuttering. That is, he wants clients to feel free to communicate in all situations, and if some stuttering remains, it should be open and smooth, and clients should feel comfortable with it.

Hugo Gregory

Over a 20-year period, Hugo Gregory (1968, 1979, 1986a, 2003) developed and refined a therapy approach that integrated stuttering modification and fluency-shaping therapies. In his most recent discussion of therapy for advanced stutterers, he described four areas of therapeutic activity: (1) getting insight into clients' attitudes (thoughts and feelings), (2) increasing clients' awareness of muscular tension through the use of relaxation exercises, (3) speech analysis and modification, and (4) building new speech skills. Although Gregory viewed these four areas as being interrelated, he believed the first two areas usually precede the last two, which are interwoven.

Gregory believed that it is important for advanced stutterers to change their attitudes about their problem. Thus, he provided stutterers with an accepting and understanding relationship in which stutterers could explore and clarify their feelings and attitudes. These discussions, likewise, help to reduce stutterers' negative feelings about their speech. During this period, Gregory also provided clients with information about stuttering. Toward the end of therapy, as clients' speech improves, Gregory helps them to integrate their new fluency into their daily lives.

Gregory thought that diminishing excessive muscular tension is beneficial for many stutterers, and he uses Jacobson's (1938) progressive relaxation techniques to aid them in doing this. Briefly, this involves having stutterers systematically tense and relax the muscles in one part of the body at a time until the whole body is relaxed. By going through this process over and over, stutterers learn to identify the feelings associated with relaxation and to voluntarily relax their muscles. Gregory reports that many stutterers are able to consciously reduce their bodily tension as they enter a feared speaking situation, including those muscles involved in speaking.

Gregory's third area of therapeutic activity involves analyzing and modifying speech. At this time, Gregory helps stutterers analyze what they do when they stutter by using audio and video recordings. He also helps them to become aware of other aspects of their speech pattern, such as rate, phrasing, and prosody. Following this analysis, he teaches clients to modify their stuttering by relaxing tension, slowing repetitions, and using other similar techniques. A centerpiece of Gregory's treatment is the use of a style of speaking that employs an "easier, more relaxed approach with smooth movements" (ERA-SM) to initiate speech. These relaxed, smooth movements are first practiced in single words, then in phrases, and finally in connected speech, in which phrasing and pausing are also incorporated. When pausing is taught, clients also work on resisting time pressure, so that they give themselves enough time for cognitive, linguistic, and motor planning.

The last area that Gregory worked on in therapy with advanced stutterers is building new speech skills. His goal was to make them good speakers, and he emphasized strengthening normal fluency. Some of the aspects of speech production that are targeted include rate control, loudness, phrasing, and prosody.

Successful Stuttering Management Program (SSMP)

The SSMP was developed by Dorvan Breitenfeldt at Eastern Washington University and is now offered in a residential 3-week treatment program at Eastern Washington University and the University of Utah. There are two phases to the program: the first is reducing fear and avoidance, and the second is learning to manage stuttering and transfer improvements to outside situations. Much of the work in both phases of the program is done outside the clinic.

Phase I begins with stutterers making lists of their covert and overt symptoms, learning to maintain eye contact with listeners when they stutter, and learning to "advertise" their stuttering to listeners. These initial steps are augmented by having clients use a mirror in the clinic to confront their stuttering. Soon afterwards, clients make telephone calls and conduct surveys about stuttering in situations outside the clinic. During this period, clients practice stuttering without using their usual avoidance behaviors, such as starters, postponements, word substitutions, and circumlocutions. The open stuttering pattern that results provides a foundation for the next phase of learning to stutter in an easier way.

Phase II begins with training clients to use light articulatory contacts, prolongation of the first sounds of words, pullouts, and cancellations. These techniques are then combined in "controlled normal speech," which teaches clients to begin words normally, prolong the first sound, and move through the word without stopping. This appears to be similar to Van Riper's "preparatory set." The initial practice in the clinic is followed by practice in many outside situations; at the same time, clients are working on various lifestyle changes, such as organizational ability, appearance, social skills, and physical conditioning. The final step involves planning for long-term success, including learning to become one's own clinician, negative practice, refresher sessions, self-help groups, and networking.

Richard Boehmler

Richard Boehmler's therapy (Boehmler, 1994; Starkweather, 1972) conceives of stuttering as a "speech-flow" disorder that produces a disruption in the processes of speech production involving the synchronized integration of vocal output and language formulation. He categorizes these disruptions into two groups: (1) blocks, which are involuntary disruptions or stoppages of the speech production processes and (2) coping behaviors, which are strategies used to initiate and maintain speech flow. His therapy focuses on minimizing the source of blocks and learning to use the speech flow coping strategies used by normal speakers. Boehmler believes that stuttering individuals need to:

1. use a range of articulatory rates that are compatible with their linguistic and motor abilities,
2. be able to adjust their rate of articulation at the phoneme level in order to effectively synchronize vocal output and language formulation,
3. be able to delay vocal output until language formulation is completed,

4. be able to maintain breath support, even when tense, without using muscles around the larynx, and

5. have confidence in their ability to initiate and maintain speech-flow even when under pressure.

This approach differs from most stuttering modification and fluency-shaping therapies by teaching clients to establish specific skills to be used during all utterances, rather than using unusual or exaggerated styles of speaking only when needed to maintain fluency. The skills that are targeted depend on the specific behavior patterns of the individuals who stutter. Only after the targeted skills are well established during fluent utterances are they used to replace stuttered responses (i.e., ineffective, inefficient coping behaviors) and to minimize the source of blocks.

Pharmacological Approaches

Because the use of drugs in the treatment for stuttering has a long history but has been short on scientific evidence, until recently, this section will be more of a review than a recommendation. Complaints and concerns about the lack of tightly controlled drug studies goes back at least as far as Van Riper (1973), who noted that a valid drug study would involve at least two groups of stutterers: one group would receive the drug, and the other group would receive a placebo that had the same side effects. Another critically important aspect of a good study is "double-blinding"; neither the experimenter nor the participant knows whether he or she was given the drug or the placebo. A third characteristic is that the experimenter should make multiple measures of the drugs' effects on the frequency and severity of stuttering, as well as measures of how the study's stutterers perceived their speech. Van Riper pointed out that the few early studies that used placebos and were double-blind had mixed results, although tranquilizers and sedatives seemed to reduce the severity of stuttering and make subjects feel better about their speech. At that time, there was some hope that an antipsychotic drug called haloperidol, which blocked receptors for the neurotransmitter dopamine, might prove to be effective.

In a later review of pharmacological approaches to stuttering, Brady (1991) reported that improved studies indicated that tranquilizers and sedatives reduced the severity of stuttering compared to placebos, and he also discussed a number of studies on haloperidol. Several authors (Prins, Mandelkorn, and Cerf, 1980; Rosenberger, 1980; Swift, Swift, and Arellano, 1975) who studied haloperidol suggested that its effectiveness might result from diminishing the uptake of dopamine, which could interfere with fluency if it were produced in excess. Although haloperidol seemed to work directly on stuttering symptoms, rather than through overall sedative or tranquilizing mechanisms, major side effects contraindicated its use. Its side effects included drowsiness, sexual dysfunction, excess movement of limbs, and the risk of a permanent, neurologically based movement disorder, tardive dyskinesia. When I worked in Australia, I participated in a haloperidol trial and found that it reduced the tension in my stuttering, allowing blocks to seemingly melt in my mouth, but the side effects were hard to bear. I was always on the verge of falling asleep, but my legs were uncontrollably wiggling.

A recent research review by McGuire et al (2004) updates the evidence that medications that reduce the uptake of dopamine can be effective in reducing stuttering. These authors recently completed a study of olanzapine, a dopamine antagonist, which doesn't have the same side effects as other drugs that reduce dopamine, such as haloperidol or its replacements risperidone and pimozide. In a double-blind study, 5 mg/day of olanzapine was reported to significantly ($P < .05$) reduce stuttering compared with the placebo on each of the following three measures: the SSI-3, the clinician's global impression, and the participant's self-rating of stuttering. The only side effect noted was a tendency for weight gain, but that was minimized via counseling about diet and exercise.

In summary, although case studies appearing in the literature (e.g., Brady and Ali, 2000) frequently report the success of a variety of medications, large-scale double-blind studies most frequently support drugs that block the uptake of dopamine, especially olanzapine. It appears, however, that at this time and for most individuals who stutter, medication for stuttering has not proven any more effective than traditional treatment.

Treatment and Support Groups

My description of treatment groups will largely draw on my own experience as a client in one of Van Riper's stuttering modification treatment groups (see Van Riper, 1958, for a description of his group therapy) and as a clinician in fluency-shaping therapy groups (Guitar, 1976). Manning (2001) provides a good description of group stuttering therapy, in general.

Among the benefits of group therapy is the mutual support that its members experience as they face the challenges of confronting and changing their stuttering. An effective group leader will facilitate extensive interaction among group members so that they encourage each other, share hopes and fears, and provide a safe haven for trying out new behaviors. Many of us in Van Riper's group paired up to do some of our beyond-clinic assignments together. We were able to give each other helpful feedback, both in our group sessions and when we went out together to work on our speech in shopping areas and restaurants. Seeing each other's stuttering made ours more bearable, and vying with each other to bring back "trophies" of successful changes in our speech was healthy competition. The techniques we were taught and the changes we made in our behaviors, feelings, and attitudes were, I suspect, much the same as would have occurred in individual therapy, but the group made the road we had to travel less lonely. Van Riper measured the outcome of his treatment 5 years after the end of therapy, using the following five criteria: (1) the client's speech must be at or below 0.5 on the Iowa Scale of Stuttering Severity (Sherman, 1952), (2) the client must not be avoiding words or situations, (3) stuttering must not be interfering with the client's social or vocational adjustment, (4) the client's word and situation fears must be close to zero, and (5) the client's stuttering must present no concern to himself or others (Van Riper, 1958). The seven members of our group have had our ups and downs, and several of us have had some additional therapy, but most of us would do fairly well, but not perfectly, in terms of Van Riper's criteria.

The fluency-shaping groups I worked with in Australia (Guitar, 1976; Howie and Andrews, 1984) focused first on learning a prolonged speech pattern to replace stuttering and shaping conversational speech to sound essentially normal. Group members then generalized their fluency to their natural environments. In this approach, the group functioned primarily as a setting in which conversational speech could be practiced, with only minor attention to the support that group members provided each other. Treatment in a group promoted an efficient use of the clinician's time as well as opportunities for members to practice using fluent speech in the give-and-take of a conversation among six people. Results of treatment varied widely for individuals (Guitar, 1976), but the overall group mean of percent syllables stuttered went from 14% before treatment to 3.9% a year after treatment, with essentially normal mean speech rates (Howie and Andrews, 1984). Subsequent modifications of the program brought follow-up percentages to even lower levels (1% to 2%SS) (Andrews and Craig, 1982).

Support or self-help groups differ from treatment groups because their main function is to provide an atmosphere in which members can freely share their feelings and develop a sense of connectedness to others who stutter, and they can provide an excellent opportunity for maintenance of improvement made in formal therapy. In my experience, getting together with others who stutter and sharing experiences, especially triumphs and frustrations, motivates continued work on techniques. Our group at the University of Vermont, which has been running for 25 years, is a mix of support and therapy. Participants share their experiences, comment supportively on each others' techniques, give themselves speech assignments, both for that meeting and for the 2 weeks in between meetings, and tell funny stories. There is much therapeutic humor, directed both at stuttering and at difficult listeners.

Ramig (1993) surveyed 62 self-help participants and found that 49 of them believed that their fluency had improved "at least somewhat" as a result of attending meetings regularly. The majority of respondents felt that the group experience improved their feelings about themselves, as well as their comfort in their personal and work environments. Information about the return rate of the survey was not available. Ramig did note that there is a paucity of research on the impact of self-help groups on the lives of people who stutter, and he gave 17 suggestions for designing studies on self-help groups.

Assistive Devices

For hundreds of years, practitioners have offered stutterers an incredible array of devices to help them speak more fluently. These devices have included ivory forks placed under the tongue, auditory feedback-delaying devices inserted in the ear, respiration-monitoring belts snugged around the chest, and masking noise generators triggered by sensors wrapped around the throat. Some have been used alone, and others have been used as an adjunct to therapy. Many have helped stutterers who have not been able to find relief through traditional therapy, but too often, false hopes for a miracle cure have been raised.

Merson (2003) presented a brief overview of devices such as the Edinburgh Masker, the Fluency Master, the Case Futura DAF (delayed auditory feedback), and the SpeechEasy. He reported that he only uses such devices with clients who seem not to be helped by other therapy procedures alone. He noted that he uses these devices only as an adjunct to more traditional stuttering-modification and fluency-shaping therapy techniques. Of the 10 patients who have used the Fluency Master (masking triggered by phonation) for 12 to 24 months, five reported that their stuttering was 100% reduced, two reported a 50% reduction, one stopped using it, and two more could not be contacted. Of the 37 patients who had used the SpeechEasy for 3 to 5 months, 55% reported that its effectiveness was retained, 53% reported less frequent stuttering, 52% reported less tense stuttering, and 28% reported that their speech was more fluent *without* the SpeechEasy. These data are not objective measures of fluency but are the subjective reports of clients who were surveyed and may be unreliable.

Another "soft" source of information about the use of assistive devices is a survey conducted by the Stuttering Foundation (Fraser, 2004; Trautman, 2003). The Foundation contacted 800 adults who had requested information about electronic devices from its website. A little over 100 individuals returned the survey, and of these, only 22 had actually bought a device. Most of those who didn't buy a device cited high costs and the absence of evidence of long-term benefit. Of those who bought devices, 12 bought a SpeechEasy, six bought a Casa Futura DAF, three bought a Fluency Master, and one bought an unspecified device. Initial reports suggested that 14 of the 22 purchasers were happy with their device. A later follow-up survey to learn how they felt after having used their device for a year was able to reach eight of these 14 individuals. Of those eight individuals, three were still happy with their device, three were not happy, and two reported mixed reactions. Some of those who were no longer happy with their device reported that it didn't work when their stutters were those that stop phonation; others reported that their device didn't work well in noisy environments.

Finally, Ramig reported (personal communication, March 8, 2005) that he and his private practice colleagues have evaluated over 60 stuttering patients over a 2-year period, fitting over 40 of them with a SpeechEasy device. Only a few of those patients were able to receive supplemental traditional therapy. He indicates that the device helped one-third of the clients significantly, one-third were helped marginally, and one-third were not helped at all. For some of his clients, it is the only effective treatment they have experienced. Ramig further notes that, for the device to be useful for most clients, the clients must be able to initiate appropriate voicing during their stuttering blocks and they must pay attention to the auditory feedback from the device. He emphasizes that he only dispenses the device for adults, teens, and children over 11 years old, believing that younger children can be helped by other therapeutic approaches. His reluctance to fit very young children stems primarily from the thought that their auditory cortex is not yet fully developed and the fact that the effect of prolonged exposure to delayed auditory feedback and frequency altered pitch is unknown at this time.

Summary

- Advanced stuttering is characterized by repetitions, prolongations, and blocks, accompanied by over-learned patterns of tension, struggle, escape, and avoidance behaviors. Clients will also typically have negative attitudes, feelings, and beliefs about stuttering and about speaking.

- The author believes that because these behaviors are so well learned, treatment must focus on teaching the stutterer new fluency and coping skills as responses to old cues that will still tend to elicit old struggle and avoidance behaviors.

- Treatment begins by increasing motivation to change and decreasing fear and avoidance. Then, new controlled fluency skills are taught in the clinic and generalized to the client's daily life. These skills are practiced on nonfeared words as well as when the client experiences old cues that previously triggered tension, struggle, and avoidance behaviors. For many clients, continued work is needed on increasing approach behaviors and decreasing avoidance behaviors. For all clients, the responsibility for managing their own speech is gradually transferred to them over the course of treatment.

■ A variety of other treatments are available for advanced stuttering, including individual and group approaches, intensive and nonintensive treatment, medication, and assistive devices.

Study Questions

1. Summarize the main differences between *intermediate* and *advanced* stuttering and the treatment approaches used for them.

2. If the aim of therapy is to learn to respond to anticipated stuttering with controlled fluency, why are actual moments of stuttering also targets of treatment?

3. Do you think it is a treatment failure if a client has mild stuttering after treatment? Explain the reasoning behind your answer.

4. Explain the difference between *counterconditioning* and *deconditioning*, using examples from stuttering therapy.

5. If the purpose of treatment is to become more fluent, why do I suggest that the client ought to work on exploring her stuttering?

6. In my approach to treatment, I advocate teaching clients four separate components of "controlled fluency" before they combine them. Clinicians using the Camperdown program prefer to teach clients a variant of controlled fluency using a video model of someone speaking with all the components already combined (speaking with prolonged speech at 70 syllables per minute). What are the advantages and disadvantages of each approach?

7. Why do I advocate learning controlled fluency in fluent speech? How many reasons can you think of?

8. Many clients are reluctant to use voluntary stuttering. What are some reasons you could give them as to why it may be helpful? Are there any clients you would not use it with?

9. Which clients would be most suited for treatment with a pharmacological approach? Which client would be most suited for an assistive device?

10. What do you think are the most valid measures of the benefits of a treatment approach?

SUGGESTED PROJECTS

1 Choose a behavior of yours that you would like to change, and develop a self-therapy plan to explore your present behavior, identify the change you would like to make, and develop a hierarchy to practice the new behavior. Report on your success.

(2) Write out a talk that you could have with a new adult client to described the possible course of treatment (see the section on "Beginning Therapy"). Make your talk both challenging and inspirational.

(3) If you are a nonstutterer, your biggest fear in doing voluntary stuttering is probably that you will be unable to stutter convincingly, and a listener will unmask you. Confront that fear by stuttering to several listeners in a most unconvincing way and see if that decreases your fear.

(4) After you have learned controlled fluency, see if you can use it on just single words ("slideouts") 20 times before noon. In trying to do this, see if you can develop a novel way to remind yourself.

(5) Watch a session of the Van Riper videotapes (for example, the session on desensitization), and see if you can determine what made him so effective as a stuttering therapist.

Suggested Readings and Viewing

Fraser, M. (undated). *Self-Therapy for the Stutterer* **(ed 10). Memphis: Stuttering Foundation.**
This self-help book contains a sequenced program for the adult stutterer to use, either on his own or with the help of a clinician or supportive friend. It describes many of the techniques you have been reading about in this book. In addition, it contains many personal and inspirational messages for the reader. I recommend it not only to individuals who stutter, but also to clinicians so that they may get another perspective on adult stuttering therapy.

Guitar, B., and Guitar, C. (undated). *If You Stutter: Advice for Adults* **(video). Memphis: Stuttering Foundation.**
This video presents a broad spectrum of treatment approaches, and many of them are demonstrated by adults who have benefited from stuttering therapy.

Manning, W. (1999). *Management of Adult Stuttering.* **In R. Curlee (ed),** *Stuttering and Related Disorders of Fluency.* **New York: Thieme Medical Publishers, Inc.**
This is an excellent overview of treatment of advanced stuttering, written by someone who has experienced good treatment himself and has done much self-therapy. Manning's chapter has a strong message that a clinician must learn what is best for each client rather than using a single approach for all.

National Stuttering Association Website: www.westutter.org.
This site contains a wealth of information for adolescents and adults who stutter, including basic information about the nature of stuttering and treatment opportunities. A recent DVD, *Transcending Stuttering,* about the struggle and triumph of many individuals who stutter, is among NSA's recent offerings.

St. Louis, K. (Ed) (1986). *The Atypical Stutterer: Principles and Practices of Rehabilitation.* **New York: Academic Press.**
This book, although somewhat dated now, has information about assessment and treatment of individuals who stutter and who also have one of the following attributes: are exceptionally severe, developmentally delayed, female, or from a minority culture. There are also chapters on psychogenic and neurogenic stuttering, as well as on cluttering.

Stuttering Foundation Website: www.stutteringhelp.org.

Background information on stuttering and its treatment, books, videos, and lists of clinicians who specialize in stuttering are offered on this site.

Stuttering Home Page: www.mnsu.edu/comdis/kuster/stutter.html.

Developed by Judy Kuster at Mankato University, the Stuttering Home Page offers a wide variety of helpful pages and links. On this site, the user can connect to chatrooms and access an annual online conference and its archives, the latest research, and commentary by people who stutter. Links to stuttering sites in other countries are also provided.

Van Riper, C. (undated). *Therapy in Action (video).* **Memphis: Stuttering Foundation.**

This nine-part video shows a master clinician conducting stuttering modification treatment with an adult stutterer. Van Riper takes this young man from the assessment to the final treatment meeting in seven sessions. There are then 1-year and 20-year follow-up interviews. Van Riper introduces each session describing what he has planned for the session and then follows the session with a commentary on what was accomplished.

Chapter 13

Related Disorders of Fluency

Neurogenic Acquired Stuttering

Nature

The term "neurogenic acquired stuttering" denotes stuttering that appears to be caused or exacerbated by neurological disease or damage. It is typically acquired after childhood, and its etiology may be stroke, head trauma, tumor, disease processes such as Parkinson's, or drug toxicity. Additional, although rare, causes are dialysis dementia, seizure disorders, bilateral thalamotomy, and thalamic stimulation (Duffy, 2005). Understanding neurogenic stuttering can help us understand some aspects of typical or "developmental" stuttering. Moreover, neurogenic stuttering in patients may be an early diagnostic sign of a neurological problem. Helm-Estabrooks (1999) describes this eloquently:

Fluent speaking is, perhaps, the most refined motor act performed by humans, requiring complex coordination of many different muscle groups. It can be sensitive, therefore, to even small changes in neurological status, which may be why stuttering occurs in a wide range of neurological disorders, from Parkinson's disease to closed head injury. If this fact is ignored, clinicians may be overlooking an important early indicator of neurological disease. (p. 265)

Some writers prefer to use the term "neurogenic disfluency," because they don't consider neurogenic stuttering to be true stuttering. Such usage may, however, blur the distinction between two different phenomena that may occur with neurological insults. One is an increase in normal types of disfluencies (e.g., whole-word and phrase repetitions, revisions, interjections, and pauses); and the other is a speech disorder presenting stutter-like disfluencies (i.e., part-word repetitions, prolongations, and blocks) sometimes accompanied by tension, struggle, escape, and avoidance behaviors.

Although much of the literature on neurogenic stuttering consists of single-case studies (e.g., Bijleveld, Lebrun, and van Dongen, 1994), there have been several attempts by clinician-researchers to summarize their findings on multiple cases and thereby develop a clearer picture of the disorder. Canter (1971) suggested that neurogenic stuttering comprises three subgroups. One subgroup is dysarthric stuttering, which is seen, for example, in individuals who have Parkinson's disease or have a cerebellar lesion. Dysarthric stuttering is stuttering that appears to emerge from the same lack of muscle control as the primary dysarthic disorder. The second subgroup is apraxic stuttering, in which stuttering may arise from a basic problem in motor planning. Both silent blocks and repetitions occur as the speaker struggles to sequence the appropriate speech movements. The third subgroup is dysnomic stuttering, which sometimes accompanies aphasia. Stuttering symptoms occur as an individual searches for the word he is having trouble retrieving. Canter speculates that there may be a parallel to this type of stuttering in children who have word-retrieval problems and who develop stuttering as a result of their emotional reactions to the word-retrieval difficulty.

Rosenbek (1984) makes the point that neurogenic stuttering should be distinguished from other disfluent behaviors that are associated with neurological problems, such as palalalia (word and phrase repetitions produced with increasing rate and decreasing loudness). Neurogenic stuttering should also be distinguished from repetitions that some patients make as they try to correct their speech motor or linguistic errors. Observations of his own patients led Rosenbek to suggest that stuttering after nervous system damage is characterized primarily by involuntary repetitions of correct sounds and syllables, not those produced in error, that occur at any place in a word (initial, medial, or final). He was distressed by the lack of detail in clinicians' descriptions of patients with this disorder and called for a moratorium on the use of the term "neurogenic stuttering" until more is known about it.

More recently, Helm-Estabrooks (1999) also suggested that the term "neurogenic stuttering" should be replaced; she suggested using "stuttering associated with acquired neurological disorders," which she abbreviates as SAAND. Part of her argument for using this new term is that this diagnostic category should include those adults whose preexisting childhood stuttering either worsened or recurred as a result of an acquired neurological disorder. Her point is that the stuttering in these cases was not initially caused by a neurological disorder. However, "neurogenic" can apply to disorders that are either caused or modified by neurological conditions (Merriam-Webster, 2004), and the term "neurogenic" is commonly used in our field and is a good deal simpler than SAAND. Thus, it is the term I will use in this chapter.

Diagnosis and Evaluation

Helm-Estabrooks (1999) and Ringo and Dietrich (1995) provide a framework for assessing neurogenic stuttering and distinguishing it from other disorders. These authors suggested that the following procedures are important not only for evaluating individual cases, but also for gathering data that may make a contribution to the literature.

1. A complete case history reflecting:
   - onset of stuttering and its association with other neurological or psychological signs
   - the client's level of concern, anxiety, or fear about his stuttering
   - extent to which stuttering interferes with communication
   - changes in stuttering since onset
   - the client's history and family history of speech, language, or learning problems
   - the client's and relatives' handedness
   - neurological and psychological health history

   This information can be gathered initially through a case history and then supplemented during the interview.

2. Direct assessment of speech:
   - Stuttering Severity Instrument-3 should be administered, and speech should be videotaped during conversation and reading samples.
   - Stuttering in speech samples should be analyzed for:

     Proportion of stuttering on function (grammatical) words versus content (substantive) words

     Presence of stuttering on noninitial syllables, such as in the words "exciteme-me-ment," "cowb-b-b-oy," and "canister-er-er"

     Absence of secondary (i.e., escape and avoidance) behaviors, such as eye blinks, head nods, and use of "um" to get a word started

   - Repeating the same short passage reading aloud to determine if stuttering is reduced progressively through six readings. See Chapter 1 for more information and references for this adaptation procedure.
   - Speaking in a variety of fluency-inducing conditions, especially speaking in a rhythm while swinging an arm, speaking while listening to loud masking noise, and speaking slowly under delayed auditory feedback set at 250-msec delay.

3. Other assessment batteries:
   - Helm-Estabrooks (1999) recommended using the Aphasia Diagnostic Profiles (ADP; Helm-Estabrook, 1992) to exclude the possibility that the stuttering actually reflects language formulation problems.
   - Helm-Estabrooks (1999) also recommended that, if other neurological problems might be present that may interfere with treatment, other neuropsychological tests might be important to assess the client's capabilities.

The information gathered from these procedures can be used to improve our understanding of neurogenic stuttering, to differentially diagnose neurogenic stuttering (i.e., distinguishing it from other fluency disorders) in a client, and to help in planning treatment for the client. Beginning with the information gathered in the case history, the data on the client's and relatives' handedness and history of speech, language, or learning problems are primarily used to determine if a client might have a predisposition for stuttering. Left-handedness or ambidexterity, as well as history of speech or language problems in a family, may predispose an individual to stuttering (Geschwind and Galaburda, 1985). If a client began to stutter or if previous stuttering recurred or worsened in association with the occurrence of neurological problems, neurogenic stuttering should be suspected. On the other hand, stuttering that appeared in conjunction with the onset of psychological problems may be of psychogenic origin. Sometimes these etiologies are difficult to sort out and will be discussed further in the section on psychogenic stuttering.

Turning now to direct assessment of speech, the following characteristics have been suggested as *more typical of neurogenic* than developmental stuttering (Canter, 1971; Helm-Estabrooks, 1999; Ringo and Dietrich, 1995; Rosenbek, 1984).

- In neurogenic stuttering, stuttering occurs on *function* words as well as content words. In developmental stuttering, stuttering occurs much more frequently on content words (Bloodstein, 1995).

- In neurogenic stuttering, stuttering is *not restricted to initial* syllables in words, whereas it occurs primarily on initial syllables in developmental stuttering (Bloodstein, 1995).

- In neurogenic stuttering, there are relatively *few* secondary symptoms, and symptoms that do occur are mild. In developmental stuttering, particularly in adults, there are usually escape and avoidance behaviors, which are sometimes severe.

- In neurogenic stuttering, there is *little or no adaptation* with repeated readings of a passage. In developmental stuttering, there is a sudden decrease in frequency of stuttering in the second reading of the passage followed by further decreases that are increasingly smaller and smaller with each successive reading, so that by the fifth reading, there is a 50% reduction, on average (Bloodstein, 1995).

- In neurogenic stuttering, there is *little or no reduction of stuttering* in a variety of fluency-inducing conditions. Most developmental stutterers show noticeable reductions in stuttering under such conditions as speaking in time to a rhythm, speaking under masking noise, or speaking slowly while listening to delayed auditory feedback (Andrews et al, 1982).

- In individuals with neurogenic stuttering, there is relatively little fear and anxiety associated with the act of stuttering or speaking in general, although there may be frustration or annoyance. In developmental stuttering, most adults who stutter have fears and anxiety about stuttering and speaking (Bloodstein, 1995; Van Riper, 1982).

Summarizing the evaluation and diagnostic procedures, I think it is probably impossible to be certain that an individual has neurogenic stuttering rather than disfluencies caused by other impairments. Every effort needs to be made to rule out memory problems, language formulation problems (such as in aphasia), and emotional distress as the source of a client's disfluencies.

Considerations for Treatment

Helm-Estabrooks (1999) suggested several criteria for determining which clients have the potential to benefit from treatment. She noted that some neurogenic stuttering is quite mild and may not result in a handicap that warrants treatment. Other individuals, whose stuttering may be a serious handicap, may have other health problems that are far more serious, such as a progressive or fatal neurological disorder. A third consideration is the extent to which other neurological problems, such as dementia, may interfere with treatment. If a client does have severe and persistent stuttering, is motivated to undergo treatment, and has adequate cognitive and linguistic abilities to benefit from treatment, then several treatment options are available.

Treatment Approaches

Because individuals with neurogenic stuttering do not usually have the cognitive and emotional involvement that characterize developmental stuttering in adults, treatment is often entirely behavioral. An exception is when the neurological etiology of the stuttering is known and can be treated by surgery or drugs.

1. Behavioral Treatments. It has been suggested that neurogenic stuttering can be differentiated from developmental stuttering by the finding that neurogenic stutterers do not become more fluent with rhythmic speech, masking, or speaking slowly. Paradoxically, these very conditions may be therapeutically useful for some patients.

    *   Pacing. This is essentially a technique of speaking one syllable at a time, so that each syllable is spoken separately, without the usual coarticulation across syllables. As a result, speech is produced more slowly and with a regular, staccato rhythm. This treatment was developed by Helm (1979) for patients with palalalia (i.e., rapid repetition of whole words and phrases) but has been used for neurogenic stuttering, as well. To facilitate pacing, especially in those patients who have difficulty slowing their speech, pacing devices can be used. One example is a pacing board (Helm-Estabrooks and Kaplan, 1989); another is a molded form that fits over the patient's finger (Rentschler, Driver, and Callaway, 1984). With either of these devices, the patient moves a finger from place to place, timing each syllable with a finger movement. Helm-Estabrooks (1999) suggested that pacing could begin with a device and progress to simply tapping rhythmically on the thigh to produce fluent speech.

    *   Masking and DAF. Rentschler et al (1984), Marshall and Starch (1984), and Helm-Estabrooks (1999) reported that masking and DAF can be used as therapeutic tools to induce fluency, and in some cases, fluency can then be generalized.

    *   Slow rate and easy onset. Market et al (1990) conducted a survey of clinicians who had worked with acquired stuttering and found that many of them reported success with fluency-shaping tools, such as slow rate and easy onset.

- Stuttering modification. Only a modest percentage of the clinicians surveyed by Market et al (1990) reported that they had used such stuttering modification tools as light contacts, preparatory sets, cancellations, and pull-outs.

- Electromyographic biofeedback for tension reduction. Reports by Helm-Estabrooks (1986) and Rubow, Rosenbek, and Schumaker (1986) suggested that training patients to relax muscles with the help of biofeedback can be effective in reducing neurogenic stuttering.

2. Neurosurgery. Sometimes when a neurological problem requires surgical intervention, the surgery resolves or improves stuttering. Cases reported by Donnan (1979) and Jones (1966) suggested that, for whatever reason, surgery that resolves a neurological problem may also resolve stuttering. The implication is that some disturbance in neurological functioning can result in stuttering, and when the neurosurgery changes this neurological functioning, stuttering can be resolved. This finding is consistent with recent evidence suggesting that brain structure and function may be aberrant in developmental stuttering (e.g., Sommer et al, 2002; Foundas et al, 2001).

3. Drugs. As I described in Chapter 12, a number of drugs, such as haloperidol and olanzapine, have been tried with varying degrees of success in developmental stuttering. These medications have not been tried, however, with neurogenic stuttering. Rather, case studies have reported that drugs for seizure disorders, schizophrenia, depression, anxiety, Parkinson's disease, and asthma can precipitate stuttering in individuals who have not stuttered previously (Baratz and Mesulam, 1981; Duffy, 2005; Elliott and Thomas, 1985; McClean and McClean, 1985; Nurnberg and Greenwald, 1981; Quader, 1977). In most of these cases, stuttering is reduced or eliminated when drug dosage is adjusted or an alternative drug is used.

Summary and Conclusions

Acquired neurogenic stuttering differs from developmental stuttering in a number of ways: neurogenic stuttering usually has a sudden onset in adulthood; stuttering may occur with similar frequency on function and content words; stuttering is less restricted to the initial syllables of words; repeated readings of the same passage have less of an effect on neurogenic stuttering; many fluency-inducing conditions do not reduce stuttering; and often, there is little fear and few secondary behaviors. Effective therapy may include surgery and drug adjustments for the underlying neurological problem, as well as behavioral approaches, such as pacing or slowing speech.

Having highlighted the differences between developmental and neurogenic stuttering in this brief summary, I would also like to consider their similarities by asking this question: What does acquired neurogenic stuttering tell us about developmental stuttering? First, I will assume that both developmental and acquired neurogenic stuttering have a neurological deficit at their core. The evidence regarding acquired neurogenic stuttering suggests that insults to the brain in most regions (except for the occipital lobe and cranial nerves), such as the left hemisphere, right hemisphere, and subcortical areas, can result in at least temporary disfluencies (Duffy, 2005). Thus, it may be that neurological disturbances can affect fluency by interrupting speech and language information flow at many different places in the neural circuitry of these functions. In developmental stuttering, there may be several different inherited or congenital deficits in brain circuitry subserving speech and language, but these differences produce mistimings or discoordinations that have a small range of possible outcomes in disturbances of fluency, such as repetitions, prolongations, and blocks, making it appear as a unitary disorder.

The evidence that acquired neurogenic stuttering is often not accompanied by fear or secondary symptoms suggests that they are independent of the core symptoms, which supports the belief that these aspects of stuttering are reactions that develop as a child experiences more and more negative reactions to his difficulty by listeners and himself. Of course, there are adult developmental stutterers who lack fear and secondary symptoms, hinting at the possibility that there may be a subgroup of developmental stutterers who closely resemble neurogenic stutterers.

Other differences from developmental stuttering are the findings that many neurogenic stutterers stutter as much on medial as on initial consonants, sometimes stutter on final consonants, and are as likely to stutter on function words as on content words. Ringo and Dietrich (1995) pointed out that the profession, as yet, lacks adequate data to be confident of these findings. However, these data hint at the fact that neurogenic stuttering may not be influenced as much by linguistic variables as developmental stuttering. I wonder, therefore, if the linguistic variability of developmental stuttering might be just an artifact of its onset during a critical period of language learning?

In conclusion, professionals working with clients having acquired neurogenic stuttering should be encouraged to develop systematic ways of collecting and sharing data (see Appendix B of Ringo and Dietrich, 1995) so that this infrequently occurring disorder can be better understood. As a consequence, we may better understand stuttering of all kinds.

Psychogenic Acquired Stuttering

Nature

Psychogenic stuttering, like neurogenic stuttering, is a late-onset disorder (late teens and older). Its major identifying feature is that it typically begins after a prolonged period of stress or after a traumatic event. It has sometimes been characterized as a conversion symptom (i.e., a physical or behavioral expression of a psychological conflict) (Lazare, 1981). Unlike malingering or faking, this type of stuttering is not consciously volitional behavior by the client but is involuntary. Several authors (Baumgartner, 1999; Mahr and Leith, 1992; Roth, Aronson, and Davis, 1989) have described the manifestations, diagnosis, and treatment of psychogenic stuttering, and this section borrows a good deal from them.

The stuttering pattern of this disorder resembles developmental stuttering in terms of core behaviors (i.e., repetitions, prolongations, and blocks), but in some cases, secondary behaviors may be unusual and occur independently of attempts to produce stuttered words (Baumgartner, 1999). Psychogenic stuttering may occur alone or together with other signs of psychological or neurological involvement. Strict definitions of psychogenic stuttering exclude cases in which childhood stuttering had been resolved but then reappeared under prolonged or sudden stress. Nonetheless, these cases may respond to treatment as readily as many cases of true psychogenic stuttering.

Diagnosis and Evaluation

Roth et al (1989) pointed out that adult-onset stuttering can have several etiologies that need to be considered: purely neurogenic, purely psychogenic, psychogenic accompanied by psychogenically based neurologic signs, and psychogenic with coexisting (but unrelated) neurologic disease. Thus, one of the first aims of an evaluation is to rule out a neurological etiology, particularly since adult-onset stuttering is sometimes the first sign of a neurologic disorder. A multidisciplinary approach involving neurology, psychiatry, and speech-language pathology may be best, especially if a client has neurological signs, such as headache, dizziness, or numbness of extremities.

The evaluation should include:

1. A complete case history, obtained either exclusively in an interview or followed up with an interview. The case history should obtain information concerning:

   • Onset of stuttering, including circumstances surrounding onset, such as whether it occurred during prolonged or acute stress, and the nature and pattern of the stuttering when it began

   • Changes in stuttering since onset, and whether there have been times of complete fluency

   • Current pattern of stuttering, its situational variability, and its impact on the client's life

   • Whether the individual stuttered previously at any time and, if so, its nature and pattern and the extent of recovery

   • Family history of stuttering and other speech, language, or learning problems

   If the clinician can maintain an interested, accepting attitude, the client is more likely to reveal vital information about the emotions associated with the stuttering. Baumgartner (1999) noted that clients' expression of feelings may be accompanied by increased fluency, which is a sign of psychogenic basis for the stuttering.

2. Baumgartner (1999) suggests giving adult-onset clients a motor speech exam (Duffy, 2005) to rule out such motor speech disorders as apraxia or Parkinson's disease that might underlie stuttering. He also suggests that if clients show signs of language or cognitive problems, these should be further tested.

3. As with neurological stuttering, clients should be asked to speak under traditional fluency-enhancing conditions that were listed in the evaluation procedures for suspected neurogenic stuttering. If a client stutters even more frequently or severely while speaking under these conditions, psychogenic stuttering should be suspected (Baumgartner, 1999).

4. Trial therapy should be carried out, and the clinician should model what is expected of the client and provide praise and support liberally to encourage him. Details are given in Chapter 7, but here is a brief description:

   a. Have the client try to stay in a moment of stuttering. The clinician models this, then instructs the client, and may even need to use a cue to help the client "catch" a moment of stuttering and hold on to it. In this and subsequent steps, the client may stop holding on to a stutter because he has run out of breath or for other reasons. The clinician should accept this and instruct him to get the stutter going again, which at this point, may be voluntary behavior rather than a true stutter.

b. While he's holding on to a stutter, have the client touch places on his face or throat where he appears to be tensing or "holding back" the word that is being stuttered.

c. While he's holding on to a stutter, have the client change the tension, the speeding up, or other elements of the stutter so that the sound becomes prolonged voluntarily.

d. When the client has changed the "holding back" behaviors, the clinician should then coach him to slowly finish the stuttered word, making a slow transition from the stutter into the remainder of the word.

e. After this, the clinician should guide the client to do steps a through d on his own while reading aloud or conversing.

These steps of trial therapy could be replaced by any other treatment the clinician typically uses. The point of trial therapy with psychogenic stuttering is to see if the client becomes dramatically more fluent, which is another sign of psychogenicity.

5. Analysis of stuttering. Samples should be obtained of the client's conversational speech and reading aloud so that baseline measures of stuttering severity can be made with the SSI-3 and the patterns of stuttering can be examined. As mentioned earlier, unusual struggle behaviors, especially if they are independent of moments of stuttering, are signs of possible psychogenicity of stuttering.

Diagnosis of psychogenic stuttering is usually tentative. The clinician must weigh multiple factors, and even then, a conclusive diagnosis might never be reached. The most clear-cut pieces of evidence for this diagnosis are (1) adult onset during psychological stress and (2) the absence of neurological factors associated with the client's stuttering. Three other factors can help support the diagnosis: (3) dramatic improvement with trial therapy, (4) increasing severity when speaking under fluency-inducing conditions, and (5) unusual or bizarre struggle behaviors.

Considerations for Treatment

Individuals who are able to decrease their stuttering in trial therapy and whose psychological adjustment is adequate are often good candidates for stuttering therapy. Even though they may need supportive or uncovering psychotherapy eventually, speech therapy may start immediately. On the other hand, clients who are unable to improve fluency during trial therapy and/or who are dysfunctional because of psychological issues may benefit from receiving psychotherapy concurrently with stuttering therapy. Individuals who resist the idea that their stuttering may have a stress-related basis and who do not improve with trial therapy may not be good candidates for treatment or will need extended treatment.

Treatment Approaches

Several published reports on psychogenic stuttering suggest that speech therapy can be very effective with this group of clients (Baumgartner, 1999; Duffy, 2005; Mahr and Leith, 1992; Roth et al, 1989). Baumgartner emphasized that clients benefit from an understanding that their stuttering is not the result of neurological problems and from the clinician's continuing encouragement about their progress.

It appears that most treatments used with developmental stuttering can be effective with psychogenic stuttering (Roth et al, 1989). In my own experience, a prolonged speech fluency-shaping approach was very beneficial for a young adult who had developed stuttering suddenly when he did not want to pursue a career in classroom teaching but was required to do so because of the financial support he'd received for his education. Roth et al suggested that approaches such as easy onset, light contact, and easy repetitions can be effective. Baumgartner (1999) worked with clients to diminish extra motor behaviors and reduce the physical tension associated with their efforts to speak. Duffy (2005) provided a seven-step procedure in which the clinician helps the client to reduce tension and changes repetitive stutters into more normal-sounding prolongations, while giving support and reassurance for gradual progress. Weiner (1981) employed desensitization combined with vocal control therapy that emphasized adequate respiratory support, gentle onsets, and optimal vocal resonance. Transfer was carried out using a hierarchy of easy-to-difficult situations. Unfortunately, no long-term treatment outcomes for therapy with psychogenic stuttering have been reported.

Summary and Conclusions

In the past 10 years, there has been an increasing acceptance of the idea that disfluencies associated with psychological trauma and stress may actually be a type of stuttering. The main diagnostic markers include: onsets that occur in late adolescence or adulthood; stuttering onset is associated with prolonged or acute stress; unusual struggle behaviors that may not always be associated with moments of stuttering; and, in some individuals, stuttering that increases in fluency-inducing conditions and dramatically improved fluency during trial treatment. Compared with neurogenic stuttering, there are relatively few details concerning the speech characteristics observed in psychogenic stuttering, such as the linguistic loci of stutters, and there is no consensus on the common types of core behaviors associated with this disorder.

There are still many mysteries to be solved about psychogenic stuttering. One is whether the anomalies in brain activity patterns seen in developmental stuttering (Chapter 2) are present in this disorder. Another is whether psychological stress produces mistimings and discoordinations that result in the disorder or whether psychological factors actually result in highly coordinated struggle behaviors that reflect the speaker's efforts to speak despite primitive reflexes holding back speech. It is appropriate to ask, as I did with neurogenic stuttering, what, if anything, does psychogenic stuttering teach us about developmental stuttering. Some electromyographic studies of developmental stuttering have shown co-contraction of speech production muscles in a fashion that impedes speech flow (Freeman and Ushijima, 1975; Guitar et al, 1988). If the same co-contractions are evident in psychogenic stuttering, it may suggest that these muscle activities in developmental stuttering are learned "holding back" responses rather than evidence of discoordination.

Cluttering

Nature

Many years ago, cluttering was described as "...a torrent of half-articulated words, following each other like peas running out of a spout" (Van Riper, 1954). The essence of cluttering, as this quote suggests, is rapid speaking that is difficult to understand. It is often accompanied by disfluencies that differ from those typically heard in stuttering, and instead, cluttering consists of word and phrase repetitions, revisions, and hesitations, all usually without tension. A clutterer's speaking rate is not continuously rapid, however, but instead gives the impression of coming in sudden impulsive bursts that are filled with misarticulations and disfluencies. In contrast to stutterers, clutterers become more fluent, as well as slower and more intelligible, when they make an effort to control their disorder. This rarely happens, unfortunately, because most clutterers are not aware that they are cluttering unless someone brings it to their attention.

Several excellent publications on cluttering have described the disorder as manifesting the speech characteristics I just mentioned, but they have also described the disorder as being characterized by, in many cases, language and neuropsychological problems (Myers and St. Louis, 1986; St. Louis, 1996; St. Louis et al, 2003). The language problems were first recognized by Weiss (1964), who described cluttering as a problem of "central language imbalance" that may reflect a disorganized formulation process. The clutterer seems to be unable to put his thoughts into coherent sentences and link them together in a logical way. Such language behavior is sometimes termed "mazing," which is a metaphor for repeated false starts, hesitations, and revisions that leave listeners puzzled about a speaker's verbal destination. The neuropsychological problems of persons with cluttering may include distractibility, hyperactivity, learning difficulties, and auditory perceptual problems. Cluttering is often accompanied by stuttering.

Cluttering, then, appears to be a disorder whose core signs or symptoms are bursts of rapid speech that are often unintelligible and disfluent. Language and neuropsychological problems may or may not be present. There has been some speculation that the neurological substrata are abnormalities in the basal ganglia (Alm, 2004; Kent, 2002).

Diagnosis and Evaluation

The process of evaluating a client for possible cluttering differs for different ages (school age vs. adult) and will vary, depending on the setting in which the evaluation takes place (e.g., school vs. university or hospital clinic). In many cases, especially with school-age children, a multidisciplinary approach to evaluation is important and may involve the speech-language pathologist, classroom teacher, special educator, psychologist, and audiologist. In the following section, I give some general guidelines that reflect information gleaned from several sources, including Myers and St. Louis (1986), St. Louis (1996), and St. Louis et al (2003).

1. Case History and Interview. The case history can be filled out by a client (or parent) beforehand and used as a guideline for the interview. Among the important areas to be covered in the case history and interview are:

   • The client's, parents', and/or teachers' perceptions of the problem. What aspects of the cluttering "syndrome" are the presenting problem (as seen by whomever is completing the form and participating in the interview)? Because the clutterer himself is often unaware of his own speech, an adult or adolescent may report that his problem is that people say he's sometimes hard to understand. It should be ascertained, however, how cluttering affects him. Does he, for example, have a hard time in school, social situations, or his job because people don't always understand him?

- How long the problem has existed. In some cases, cluttering might have begun in preschool years, but it is usually not until the school years when listeners tell him that he's mumbling or talking too fast or that they simply can't understand him. Nonetheless, it is useful to gather information about the individual's speech and language development—whether it was delayed, advanced, or atypical.

- When and where the problem appears. Cluttering can be variable, so it's important to understand which situations are particularly troublesome. This may depend on the listeners and the demands of the situation. Some children may do well when they are reading or giving one-word answers but may lose intelligibility during narratives. Adults who clutter may be fluent and intelligible when speaking to close friends, but their intelligibility may suffer when speaking in more demanding situations.

- Background on the individual and his family. It is helpful in understanding a client's cluttering to view it in a larger perspective, including whether other members of the client's extended family clutter or have other communication or learning problems, whether the client has other problems, such as stuttering, that interfere with communication, and whether the client has received treatment for his communication problem(s) and its success.

- Reasons for seeking treatment at this time. A major determinant of success in cluttering therapy is the client's motivation. It is important to find out from the case history or interview, whether the client is aware of his cluttering and whether it bothers him enough to undertake the hard work that successful therapy will require.

- Other problems. The case history and interview should determine if the client has any of the other problems that often accompany cluttering, such as receptive or expressive language difficulties, central auditory processing deficits, attention deficit/hyperactivity, reading problems, or learning disabilities.

2. Direct Assessment of Speech. The client's speech should be examined on a variety of tasks in a variety of situations. Cluttering, like stuttering, varies a great deal, so it is easy to gain a false impression from a small sample of speech gathered in the clinic.

- The client should be videotaped while performing a number of speaking tasks, including: (1) a narrative about a topic not related to his speech, such as describing what he did on his last vacation or a favorite movie; (2) reading a passage appropriate for his reading level; and (3) a conversation in which the client talks about something that really interests him. In addition, for clients who report that their cluttering is situational, a sample should be recorded in the relevant environments.

- The speech samples should be analyzed to assess speech rate in syllables per minute (SPM) using the procedures described in Chapter 6. Many individuals who clutter can reduce their overly fast rate when they try, so the narrative and reading samples may show slower rates than conversation samples. If it is the clinician's impression during the evaluation that the client's speech rate was not slower during narrative or reading compared to conversation, she should ask the client to engage in a narrative task and try to speak at a slow, normal rate. The client's ability to slow his speaking rate may be a good prognostic sign because much of cluttering therapy is focused on slowing a client's speaking rate. The sample can be compared to the speech rate norms for different ages that were given in Chapter 7.

Most clutterers don't speak at a consistently fast rate, but instead, they speak at a relatively normal rate with sudden bursts of rapid speech. Assessment, therefore, should include measures of speech rate during these bursts and how frequently they occur. A comparison may be made between the client's articulatory rate (i.e., syllables per second with pauses excluded) during fast bursts of speech and his regular speech. The articulatory rates of typical adults in conversation are six to seven syllables per second (St. Louis et al, 2003).

- Analysis of speech samples should also include separate counts of normal-type disfluencies and stuttering-like disfluencies (see Chapters 5 and 7 for this distinction). The number of syllables that are normally disfluent and the number that are stuttered can be expressed as a proportion of the total number of syllables spoken in the sample. These measures will reflect the proportions of stuttering and cluttering in the client's speech. Some clients have both stuttering and cluttering in their speech, but one usually predominates. It has been suggested that, when stuttering is mixed with cluttering, a client's cluttering may not be noticed until his stuttering is substantially reduced by therapy (Bakker, 2002; St. Louis et al, 2003).

- When I evaluate a client with cluttering, I find it useful to calculate the ratio of the number of syllables spoken that are part of the intended message, if that can be reliably discerned, to the number of syllables spoken that are extraneous to the message. For example, in the utterance, "Well, you see, I think, I think the, the, the sky is well is blue" (15 syllables), we can assume that the speaker meant to convey, "I think the sky is blue" (six syllables). Thus, nine syllables, or 60% of the utterance, are extraneous, which undoubtedly detracts from the speaker's communicative effectiveness. This measure may be helpful also in assessing a client's progress in therapy.

- The intelligibility of a sample should be assessed by having one or more listeners who are unfamiliar with the client gloss (i.e., interpret) each word and each utterance. The percentage of words and utterances that are understood can be calculated, providing pre-therapy measures of a client's intelligibility.

3. Language Assessment. The language skills of clients who clutter are likely to be affected by the disorder. In fact, Weiss (1964) described cluttering as a "Central Language Imbalance," suggesting that language deficits are its core.

Wiig (2002) suggested that many aspects of clutterers' language can be effectively tested using the Clinical Evaluation of Language Fundamentals (CELF-3) (Semel, Wiig, and Secord, 1996). This test assesses "the relationships among semantics, syntax/morphology, and pragmatics and the interrelated domains of receptive and expressive language." Wiig suggested that the test be administered in such a way that a client's responses could be timed because under time pressure, which simulates everyday conversational situations, the clutterer's scores might well be lower.

It may also be helpful to assess a client's pragmatic behaviors in the video-taped conversational sample described earlier. Pragmatic skills that may be lacking include: appropriate turn-taking, supplying complete information to the listener, and repairing communication when it breaks down.

4. Assessment of Cluttering Characteristics. Clients may exhibit a variety of traits that are part of the cluttering syndrome. The clinician may find it helpful to use Daly and Burnett-Stolnack's (1995) checklist and treatment planning analysis to rate a client on a range of speech, language, cognitive, and behavioral characteristics. These ratings help the clinician determine which cluttering characteristics are most salient and are, therefore, most in need of treatment.

5. Assessment of Coexisting Disorders. In the process of gathering information about a client, the clinician may become aware of challenges that affect communication but are not the province of only the speech-language pathologist. These challenges may include auditory processing disorders, attention deficit disorder, hyperactivity, reading difficulties, social adjustment problems, illegible handwriting, and learning disabilities. These challenges may best be assessed with the help of other specialists, such as an audiologist, psychologist, learning specialist, reading specialist, and the classroom teacher.

Considerations for Treatment

Because clients who clutter are usually not aware of their problem and are often surprised when listeners don't understand them, they rarely seek treatment. Indeed, those who do seek treatment are often referred by someone else. Some clutterers, however, can be motivated to work hard in therapy and can make good progress. Two positive prognostic signs are the ability to speak without cluttering if asked to do so and a specific reason for improving, such as keeping a job or receiving a promotion at work. Children who clutter can often be engaged in games and activities that will create motivation for their work in treatment.

Treatment Approaches

The evaluation procedures described earlier should suggest the areas that are particular challenges for each client. Treatment can then focus on these areas of need.

Myers (2002) outlined several cluttering therapy strategies that she and her colleague St. Louis have explored in their work with cluttering over several years. I describe them in the following list, with some minor changes.

1. Increase the client's awareness of his speech rate and his ability to decrease the rate

   • Simulate various speaking rates by having the client move his arm or walk at slow, medium, and fast tempos. Then, teach the client to attend to his sensory feedback while he is doing this so that he learns the feeling of these rates.

   • Alternate between speaking and moving various body parts or walking at various rates, while attending to sensory feedback.

   • Use movements and walking paced by fast and slow music.

   • With children, engage in activities in which they can get speeding tickets or give speeding tickets to the clinician for speaking too fast.

- Teach clients to attend to various verbal and nonverbal cues from a listener that indicates they are speaking too quickly or cannot be understood. For example, listeners may frown or show puzzlement on their face or repeatedly ask the speaker to repeat.

- For readers, put symbols at periods and commas, such as red or yellow lights, to help them slow their speech rate at relevant places in a text.

- Teach phrasing and pausing in conversational speech.

- Use the concept of a speedometer for children and ask them to speak at 75 miles per hour or at 35 miles per hour.

- Teach clients to speak with strong stress patterns by reciting poetry, for example.

2. Improve linguistic skills

- Teach clients to chunk and sequence their thoughts by having them write a story or narrative on cards, sequence them, and then tell the story aloud using the cards.

- Involve clients in skits and plays so that they learn to follow a script and use turn-taking.

- Teach the clients such narrative skills as "adjacency" and "contingency."

- Teach the clients how to use complex sentences with subordinate clauses.

3. Facilitate fluency

- Use delayed auditory feedback to help clients learn to speak in a slower, more fluent manner.

- Use delayed auditory feedback to teach proprioception by having clients speak at a normal rate under maximal delay (i.e., 250 msec) by ignoring auditory feedback.

4. Increase the client's knowledge and awareness of cluttering

- Teach clients about the disorder of cluttering using Daly and Burnett-Stolnack's (1995) checklist to help the client learn which cluttering behaviors he has.

- Have the client transcribe and analyze a recording of his cluttered speech.

- Help the client become aware of his thought processes when he is talking in fast bursts of disorganized speech.

Further suggestions for treatment were presented by St. Louis et al (2003) and include the following.

1. Rather than admonish the client to "slow down," have him match the clinician's speech rate using a computer-based program to display the clinician's and client's utterances. The Visi-Pitch or the Computerized Speech Lab from Kay Elemetrics are examples of programs that can do this.

2. To help clients achieve their potential to use normal speech, have them imagine themselves (i.e., in their mind's eye and ear) speaking effectively and have them use positive self-talk to strengthen their visual and auditory images. It may help also for the client and clinician to record the client's best and worst speech to remind him of the range of his options.

3. When working on intelligibility and organization, begin with short utterances that are spoken clearly, and then gradually increase length and complexity while

ensuring high quality of fluency, articulation, rate, and organization. Video recording and replaying the recordings can help clients establish an auditory-visual image of what they are aiming for.

In his chapter on treatment of cluttering, Daly (1986) provides his own guidelines for many of the treatment strategies described earlier. He believes that video feedback and analysis of audio samples are crucial for increasing a client's self-awareness. He also advocates helping clients learn to use relaxation exercises, mental imagery, and positive self-talk. His chapter has many references that can help clinicians learn more about these activities.

There are very few studies of the treatment outcomes of cluttering therapy, and the ones that do exist consist of only one or two cases. A special edition of the *Journal of Fluency Disorders* (vol. 21, nos. 3-4, September-December 1996) on cluttering has a number of case studies. For example, data on a clutterer-stutterer treated in a 3-week intensive smooth speech program indicated that the client's stuttering and speech rate were reduced to near-normal limits and that the gains appeared to be retained 10 months after treatment.

Summary and Conclusions

Cluttering is a disorder with a probable neurological etiology. It is characterized by an excess of disfluencies, rapid rates of speech that often occur in momentary bursts, and lack of intelligibility, especially in bursts of increased rate. Although there is relatively little research on the nature and treatment of cluttering, there is some consensus that it isn't viewed as a problem until a child has reached school age. Evaluation procedures include (1) obtaining background information to determine, among other things, whether or not the client is aware of the problem and is motivated to undergo therapy; (2) direct assessment of speech on several different tasks to measure (a) frequency and type of disfluencies and (b) speech rate and intelligibility overall and during fast bursts of speech; (3) language testing, particularly pragmatics and other aspects of expressive language; and (4) assessment of other possible concomitant disorders. Treatment should address the interdependent qualities of speech rate, fluency, intelligibility, and expressive language. Although many clinicians report success with motivated clients, there is essentially no outcome data on a particular treatment approach for cluttering.

Because cluttering most often co-occurs with stuttering, the disorders appear to be related in some as-yet undetermined way. Given the strong effect of slow speaking on stuttering and cluttering alike, it is possible that subgroups of stutterers and clutterers have difficulty maintaining a slow enough rate to match their capacity to synchronize the elements of language and speech output. Perhaps each disorder has a particular level at which such dyssynchrony occurs.

Summary

Table 13–1 summarizes the characteristics of neurogenic stuttering, psychogenic stuttering, and cluttering and compares these characteristics with those of typical developmental stuttering.

| Table 13–1 | Comparative Characteristics of Developmental, Neurogenic, and Psychogenic Stuttering and Cluttering |

	Developmental Stuttering	Neurogenic Stuttering	Psychogenic Stuttering	Cluttering
Etiology	Probably neurophysiological (anomalies in left hemisphere) exacerbated by temperament and environment	Stroke, head trauma, tumor, disease process, drug toxicity, dialysis dementia, seizure disorder, bilateral thalamotomy, thalamic stimulation	Prolonged stress, psychological conflict, psychologically traumatic event; emotional arousal or emotional conflict appears to interfere with speech production	Probably neurological, possibly related to dysfunction in basal ganglia
Typical Onset	Usually ages 2-5 years, with some onsets in school years	Usually after childhood, following a neurological event; however, in rare cases, stuttering could be the first sign of a neurological problem	Usually after childhood, following prolonged stress or after a psychologically traumatic event; sometimes occurs in conjunction with apparent neurological problems	May be present in preschool years, but often not diagnosed until problem interferes with school performance
Speech Characteristics	Single-syllable whole-word repetitions, part-word repetitions, prolongations, and blocks; frequency is usually more than 3% syllables stuttered; secondary behaviors (escape and avoidance) common; pattern varies somewhat	Stuttering appears on function as well as content words; stuttering not restricted to word-initial syllables; absence of secondary behaviors; little adaptation in repeated readings; stuttering not markedly reduced in fluency-inducing conditions	Stuttering remains constant or increases while speaking under fluency-inducing conditions; may have unusual struggle behaviors; stuttering may show stereotyped pattern; client may show dramatic improvement with trial therapy	Excess of normal disfluencies, lack of intelligibility, especially during rapid bursts of speech; may slur syllables and leave out others entirely

(Continued)

Table 13–1	Comparative Characteristics of Developmental, Neurogenic, and Psychogenic Stuttering and Cluttering (*Continued*)			
	Developmental Stuttering	**Neurogenic Stuttering**	**Psychogenic Stuttering**	**Cluttering**
Client's Level of Concern	Client typically shows frustration and embarrassment about stuttering, as well as fear of speaking	Client may be annoyed or frustrated, but not fearful or anxious about stuttering	Variable, from indifferent to concerned	Frequently unaware of problem, except when listeners tell him they can't understand what he's said
Other Diagnostic Information	Frequency and severity are often variable from day to day and situation to situation	Need to rule out possibility that disfluencies are from memory or language formulation problems or from emotional distress about neurological problem	Absence of neurological problems that could cause stuttering; client may befit from psychotherapy as well as stuttering therapy if inclined	Often accompanied by stuttering, as well as language, attention, auditory processing, writing, and reading problems, and other learning disabilities
Treatment	School-age children and adults benefit from integration of behavioral, affective, and cognitive focus of stuttering therapy	Pacing, masking, DAF, slow rate, and easy onset	Fluency shaping or tension reduction	Increase awareness of cluttering, particularly fast speech rate; help client self-regulate speech rate and fluency; improve expressive language skills

Study Questions

1. If you had only one activity you could do with a client to differentiate neurogenic from psychogenic stuttering, which activity would you choose and why?

2. After reading about neurogenic stuttering, do you think that Canter's three categories of neurogenic stuttering are adequate? Why or why not?

3. Name four characteristics of stuttering behavior that appear to distinguish neurogenic stuttering from developmental stuttering.

4. What are contraindications (if any) for treatment of neurogenic stuttering?

5. If an adult-onset client had evidence of a neurological disorder, would you rule out psychogenic stuttering? Why or why not?

6. Compare the reported treatment success of psychogenic stuttering and neurogenic stuttering.

7. What are the contraindications (if any) for treatment of psychogenic stuttering?

8. What are the two most salient problems in cluttering?

9. Why might language and learning problems be related to the speech problems of cluttering?

10. What are the contraindications (if any) for treatment of cluttering?

Suggested Readings

Neurogenic Stuttering

Duffy, J. (2005). *Motor Speech Disorders* (ed 2). St. Louis: Elsevier, Mosby.

Chapters 13, 14, 19, and 20 provide excellent coverage of the nature of neurogenic and psychogenic stuttering, as well as their management. Duffy is particularly good at describing etiologies of these disorders and the other conditions with which they may be associated. His sections on management reflect his extensive clinical experience.

Helm-Estabrooks, N. (1999). Stuttering associated with acquired neurological disorders. In R.F. Curlee (Ed), *Stuttering and Related Disorders of Fluency* (ed 2). New York: Thieme Medical Publishers.

This chapter proposes a new term for neurogenic stuttering (the title of the chapter or, as an acronym, SAAND) and describes how to distinguish neurogenic from psychogenic and developmental stuttering. The author describes a wide variety of treatment options gleaned from the recent literature and from her clinical practice. Helm-Estabrooks enriches the chapter with wisdom from her many years of working with SAAND and other neurogenic speech and language disorders. A new edition of this text with an update from Helm-Estabrooks should be available in 2006.

Ringo, C.C., and Dietrich, S. (1995). Neurogenic stuttering: An analysis and critique. *Journal of Medical Speech-Language Pathology*, 3:111–122.

This article is particularly useful in that it critically examines characteristics of neurogenic stuttering that have been proposed by various authors since Canter's (1971) seminal publication about differential diagnosis of neurogenic stuttering. Each of seven characteristics is examined in light of evidence that it is present in neurogenic stuttering in a way that is different from its manifestation in developmental stuttering. Suggestions are made to standardize the data to be collected and reported on individual cases.

Psychogenic Stuttering

Baumgartner, J. (1999). Acquired psychogenic stuttering. In R.F. Curlee (ed), *Stuttering and Related Disorders of Fluency* (ed 2). New York: Thieme Medical Publishers.

This chapter is an excellent starting place for anyone interested in learning about psychogenic stuttering. Baumgartner has been writing about this topic for several years and has first-hand clinical experience with individuals who have psychogenic stuttering, thus making the chapter a solid source for information. A new edition of this text, with an updated chapter by Baumgartner, should be available in 2006.

Roth, C., Aronson, A., and Davis, L. (1989). Clinical studies in psychogenic stuttering of adult onset. *Journal of Speech and Hearing Disorders*, 54:634–646.

This journal article examines the records of 12 patients who were evaluated and treated for psychogenic stuttering. Because the subjects were patients at the Mayo Clinic, they were examined thoroughly for psychological/psychiatric and neurological functioning in a standardized way, providing substantial evidence of the psychogenic nature of the stuttering. A case study is given to illustrate how stuttering can appear as a conversion reaction to emotional conflict. Clinical recommendations are given.

Cluttering

St. Louis, K.O., et al. (2003). Cluttering updated. *The ASHA Leader,* **4–5:20–22.**

This article, which is available online at www.asha.org, provides a clear synopsis of how to identify and evaluate cluttering, as well as specific suggestions for treating the core behaviors. For those who know little about cluttering, this publication is an excellent place to begin.

Myers, F.L., and St. Louis, K.O. (Eds) (1986). *Cluttering: A Clinical Perspective.* **San Diego: Singular Publishing Group, Inc.**

This book, with an interesting forward by Charles Van Riper, is the first text on stuttering since the classic text on cluttering by Deso Weiss (1964). Chapters by the authors and other clinicians working with cluttering provide an overview of the disorder as well as practical suggestions for evaluation and treatment.

St. Louis, K.O. (Ed.) (1996). *Research and Opinion on Cluttering.* **Special Issue of** *Journal of Fluency Disorders,* **21, 1996.**

This special issue of JFD is rich with case studies of evaluations and treatments of individuals who clutter. Therefore, it is one of the few sources with data on treatment outcome, although the heterogeneity of the cases and the manner in which they are studied highlight the fact that research on cluttering is in its infancy. The cases studies are bracketed by overviews of the disorder at the beginning and critical reviews at the end that summarize the case studies and call attention to the poverty of credible data. A chapter by Myers is particularly valuable for its annotated list of publications on stuttering between 1964 and 1996.

References

Abbs, J.H. (1996). Mechanisms of speech motor execution and control. In N. Lass (Ed), *Principles of Experimental Phonetics*. St. Louis: Mosby, pp 93–111.

Adams, M. (1990). The demands and capacities model I: Theoretical elaborations. *Journal of Fluency Disorders*, 15:135–141.

Adams, M., and Hayden, P. (1976). The ability of stutterers and nonstutterers to initiate and terminate phonation during production of an isolated vowel. *Journal of Speech and Hearing Research*, 19:290–296.

Adams, M., and Runyan, C.M. (1981). Stuttering and fluency: Exclusive events or points on a continuum? *Journal of Fluency Disorders*, 6:197–218.

Ahern, G.L., and Schwartz, G.E. (1985). Differential lateralization for positive and negative emotion in the human brain: EEG spectral analysis. *Neuropsychologia*, 23:745–755.

Ainsworth, S., and Fraser, J. (1989). *If Your Child Stutters: A Guide for Parents* (rev ed 3). Memphis: Stuttering Foundation of America.

Alfonso, P.J., Story, R.S., and Watson, B.C. (1987). The organization of supralaryngeal articulation in stutterers' fluent speech production: A second report. *Annual Bulletin Research Institute of Logopedics and Phoniatrics*, 21:117–129.

Allen, G.D., and Hawkins, S. (1980). Phonological rhythm: Definition and development. In G.H. Yeni-Komshian, J.F. Kavanagh, and C.A. Ferguson (Eds), *Child Phonology* (Vol. 1). New York: Academic Press, pp 227–256.

Allen, S. (1988). *Durations of segments in repetitive disfluencies in stuttering and nonstuttering children*. Unpublished manuscript, E.M. Luse Center, University of Vermont, Burlington.

Allman, J.M., Hakeem, A., Erwin, J.M., Nimchinsky, E., and Hof, P. (2001). The anterior cingulate cortex: The evolution of an interface between emotion and cognition. *Annals of the New York Academy of Sciences*, 935:107–117.

Ambrose, N.G., Cox, N.J., and Yairi, E. (1997). The genetic basis of persistence and recovery in stuttering. *Journal of Speech, Language, and Hearing Research*, 40:556–566.

Ambrose, N.G., and Yairi, E. (1995). The role of repetition units in the differential diagnosis of early childhood incipient stuttering. *American Journal of Speech-Language Pathology*, 4:82–88.

Ambrose, N.G., Yairi, E., and Cox, N. (1993). Genetic aspects of early childhood stuttering. *Journal of Speech and Hearing Research*, 36:701–706.

American Speech Language and Hearing Association (1995). Guidelines for practice in stuttering treatment. *ASHA*, 37(Suppl. 14): 26–35.

Anderson, J., Pellowski, M., and Conture, E. (2001, November). *Temperament characteristics of children who stutter*. Paper presented at the Annual Meeting of the American Speech-Language-Hearing Association, New Orleans, LA.

Anderson, J., Pellowski, M., Conture, E., and Kelly, E. (2003). Temperamental characteristics of young children who stutter. *Journal of Speech, Language and Hearing Research*, 46:1221–1233.

Andrews, G. (1982). Stuttering: Overt and covert measurement of the speech of treated subjects. *Journal of Speech and Hearing Disorders*, 47:96–99.

Andrews, G., and Craig, A. (1988). Prediction of outcome after treatment for stuttering. *British Journal of Disorders of Psychiatry*, 153:236–240.

Andrews, G., Craig, A., Feyer, A.-M., Hoddinott, S., Howie, P.M., and Neilson, M.D. (1983). Stuttering: A review of research findings and theories circa 1982. *Journal of Speech and Hearing Disorders*, 48:226–246.

Andrews, G., and Cutler, J. (1974). Stuttering therapy: The relation between changes in symptom level and attitudes. *Journal of Speech and Hearing Disorders,* 39:312–319.

Andrews, G., and Harris, M. (1964). *The Syndrome of Stuttering.* London: Spastics Society Medical Education and Information Unit in association with W. Heinemann Medical Books.

Andrews, G., Howie, P.M., Dozsa, M., and Guitar, B. (1982). Stuttering: Speech pattern characteristics under fluency-inducing conditions. *Journal of Speech and Hearing Research,* 25:208–216.

Andrews, G., and Ingham, R. (1971). Stuttering: Considerations in the evaluation of treatment. *British Journal of Communication Disorders,* 6:129–138.

Andrews, G., Morris-Yates, A., Howie, P., and Martin, N. (1991). Genetic factors in stuttering confirmed. *Archives of General Psychiatry,* 48:1034–1035.

Andrews, G., and Tanner, S. (1982). Stuttering treatment: An attempt to replicate the regulated-breathing method. *Journal of Speech and Hearing Disorders,* 47:138–140.

Arndt, J., and Healey, E.C. (2001). Concomitant disorders in school-age children who stutter. *Language, Speech, and Hearing Services in Schools,* 32:68–78.

Arthur, G. (1952). *Arthur Adaptation of the Leiter International Performance Test.* Los Angeles: Western Psychological Services.

Ayres, J.J.B. (1998). Fear conditioning and avoidance. In W. O'Donohue (Ed), *Learning and Behavior Therapy.* Boston: Allyn and Bacon.

Azrin, N.H., and Nunn, R.G. (1974). A rapid method of eliminating stuttering by a regulated breathing approach. *Behavior Research and Therapy,* 12:279–286.

Baer, D. (1990). The critical issue in treatment efficacy is knowing why treatment was applied. In L.B. Olswand, C.K. Thompson, S.F. Warren, and N.J. Minghetti (Eds), *Treatment Efficacy Research in Communication Disorders.* Rockville, MD: ASHA, pp 31–39.

Baker, D.J. (1967). The amount of information in the Oral Identification of Forms by normal speakers and selected speech-defective groups. In J.F. Bosma (Ed), *Symposium of Oral Sensation and Perception.* Springfield, IL: Thomas, pp 287–293.

Bakker, K. (2002). *Putting cluttering on the map: Looking back/looking ahead.* Paper presented at the Annual Meeting of the American Speech-Language-Hearing Association, Atlanta, GA.

Barasch, C.T., Guitar, B., McCauley, R.J., and Absher, R.G. (2000). Disfluency and time perception. *Journal of Speech, Language and Hearing Research,* 43:1429–1439.

Baratz, R., and Mesulam, M. (1981). Adult-onset stuttering treated with anticonvulsants. *Archives of Neurology,* 38:132–133.

Baumgartner, J.M. (1999). Acquired psychogenic stuttering. In R. Curlee (Ed), *Stuttering and Related Disorders of Fluency* (ed 2). New York: Thieme, pp 269–288.

Beck, J.S. (1995). *Cognitive Therapy: Basics and Beyond.* New York: Guilford Press.

Beitchman, J., Nair, R., Clegg, M., and Patel, P.G. (1986). Prevalence of speech and language in 5–year-old kindergarten children in Ottawa-Carleton region. *Journal of Speech and Hearing Disorders,* 51:98–110.

Berk, L.E. (1991). *Child Development* (ed 2). Boston: Allyn & Bacon.

Bernstein Ratner, N. (1981). Are there constraints on childhood disfluency? *Journal of Fluency Disorders,* 6:341–350.

Bernstein Ratner, N. (1995). Treating the child who stutters with concomitant language and phonological impairment. *Language, Speech, and Hearing in Schools,* 26:180–186.

Bernstein Ratner, N. (1997). Stuttering: A psycholinguistic perspective. In R.F. Curlee, and G.M. Siegel (Eds), *Nature and Treatment of Stuttering: New Directions* (ed 2). Needham Heights, MA: Allyn & Bacon, pp 99–127.

Bernstein Ratner, N., and Sih, C.C. (1987). Effects of gradual increases in sentence length and complexity on children's dysfluency. *Journal of Speech and Hearing Disorders,* 52:278–287.

Bernthal, J. (1994). *Child phonology: Characteristics, Assessment, and Intervention in Special Populations.* New York: Thieme Medical Publishers.

Bernthal, J., and Bankson, N. (1998). *Articulation and Phonological Disorders* (ed 4). Needham Heights, MA: Allyn & Bacon.

Berry, M.F. (1938). Developmental history of stuttering children. *Journal of Pediatrics,* 12:209–217.

Berry, R.C., and Silverman, F.H. (1972). Equality of intervals on the Lewis-Sherman scale of stuttering severity. *Journal of Speech and Hearing Research,* 15:185–188.

Bijleveld, H., Lebrun, Y., and van Dongen, H. (1994). A case of acquired stuttering. *Folia Phoniatrica et Logopedica,* 46:250–253.

Black, J.W. (1951). The effects of delayed sidetone on vocal rate and intensity. *Journal of Speech and Hearing Disorders,* 16:56–60.

Bloch, E.L., and Goodstein, L.D. (1971). Functional speech disorders and personality: A decade of research. *Journal of Speech and Hearing Disorders,* 36:295–314.

Blockcolsky, V.D., Frazer, J.M., and Frazer, D.H. (1987). *40,000 Selected Words: Organized by Letter, Sound, and Syllable.* Tucson, AZ: Communication Skill Builders.

Blood, G. (1985). Laterality differences in child stutterers: Heterogeneity, severity levels, and statistical treatment. *Journal of Speech and Hearing Disorders,* 50:66–72.

Blood, G., Blood, I., Tellis, G., and Gabel, R. (2001). Communication apprehension and self-perceived communication competence in adolescents who stutter. *Journal of Fluency Disorders,* 26:161–178.

Bloodstein, O. (1944). Studies in the psychology of stuttering: XIX. The relationship between oral reading rate and severity of stuttering. *Journal of Speech Disorders,* 9:161–173.

Bloodstein, O. (1948). *Conditions under which stuttering is reduced or absent.* Unpublished doctoral dissertation, University of Iowa, Iowa City, IA.

Bloodstein, O. (1950). Hypothetical conditions under which stuttering is reduced or absent. *Journal of Speech and Hearing Disorders,* 15:142–153.

Bloodstein, O. (1958). Stuttering as an anticipatory struggle reaction. In J. Eisenson (Ed), *Stuttering: A Symposium.* New York: Harper & Row.

Bloodstein, O. (1960a). The development of stuttering: I. Changes in nine basic features. *Journal of Speech and Hearing Disorders,* 25:219–237.

Bloodstein, O. (1960b). The development of stuttering: II. Developmental phases. *Journal of Speech and Hearing Disorders,* 25:366–376.

Bloodstein, O. (1961). The development of stuttering: III. Theoretical and clinical implications. *Journal of Speech and Hearing Disorders,* 26:67–82.

Bloodstein, O. (1974). The rules of early stuttering. *Journal of Speech and Hearing Disorders,* 39:379–394.

Bloodstein, O. (1975). Stuttering as tension and fragmentation. In J. Eisenson (Ed), *Stuttering: A Second Symposium.* New York: Harper & Row.

Bloodstein, O. (1987). *A Handbook on Stuttering* (ed 4). Chicago: National Easter Seal Society.

Bloodstein, O. (1993). *Stuttering: The Search for a Cause and a Cure.* Boston: Allyn & Bacon.

Bloodstein, O. (1995). *A Handbook on Stuttering* (ed 5). San Diego: Singular.

Bloodstein, O. (1997). Stuttering as an anticipatory struggle reaction. In R.F. Curlee and G.M. Siegel (Eds), *The Nature and Treatment of Stuttering: New Directions* (ed 2). Boston: Allyn & Bacon, pp 169–181.

Bloodstein, O. (2001). Incipient and developed stuttering as two distinct disorders: Resolving a dilemma. *Journal of Fluency Disorders,* 26:67–73.

Bloodstein, O. (2002). Early stuttering as a type of language difficulty. *Journal of Fluency Disorders,* 27:163–167.

Bloodstein, O., and Gantwerk, B.F. (1967). Grammatical function in relation to stuttering in young children. *Journal of Speech and Hearing Research,* 10:786–789.

Bluemel, C.S. (1932). Primary and secondary stuttering. *Quarterly Journal of Speech,* 18:187–200.

Boberg, E., Yeudall, L., Schopflocher, D., and Bo-Lassen, P. (1983). The effect of an intensive behavioral program on the distribution of EEG alpha power in stutterers during the processing of verbal and visuospatial information. *Journal of Fluency Disorders,* 8:245–263.

Bobrick, B. (1995). *Knotted Tongues: Stuttering in History and the Quest for a Cure.* New York: Simon & Schuster.

Boehme, G. (1968). Stammering and cerebral lesions in early childhood: Examinations of 802 children and adults with cerebral lesions. *Folia Phoniatrica,* 20:239–249.

Boehmler, R.M. (1994). *The treatment of stuttering as a speech-flow disorder.* Unpublished manuscript.

Boone, D., and McFarlane, S. (1988). *The Voice and Voice Therapy* (ed 4). Englewood Cliffs, NJ: Prentice-Hall.

Borden, G.J. (1983). Initiation versus execution time during manual and oral counting by stutterers. *Journal of Speech and Hearing Research,* 26:389–396.

Boscolo, B., Ratner, N.B., and Rescorla, L. (2002). Fluency of school-aged children with a history of Specific Expressive Language Impairment. *American Journal of Speech-Language Pathology,* 11:41–49.

Bothe, A. (2004). *Evidence-Based Treatment of Stuttering: Empirical Bases and Clinical Applications.* Mahwah, NJ: Erlbaum.

Brady, J.P., and Ali, Z. (2000). Alprazolam, citalopram, and clomipramine for stuttering. *Journal of Clinical Psychopharmacology,* 20:287.

Brady, J.P., and Berson, J. (1975). Stuttering, dichotic listening, and cerebral dominance. *Archives of General Psychiatry,* 32:1449–1452.

Branigan, G. (1979). Some reasons why successive single word utterances are not. *Journal of Child Language,* 6:411–421.

Braun, A., Varga, M., Stager, S., Schulz, G., Selbie, S., Maisog, J.M., et al. (1997). Altered patterns of cerebral activity during speech and language production in developmental stuttering: An H2(15)O positron emission tomography study. *Brain,* 120:761–784.

Braun, A.R., Varga, M., Stager, S., Schulz, G., Selbie, S., Maisog, J.M., et al. (1997). A typical lateralization of hemispheral activity in developmental stuttering: An H2 (15) 0 positron emission tomography study. In W. Hulstijn, H.F.M. Peters, and P.H.H.M. van Lieshout (Eds), *Speech Production: Motor Control, Brain Research and Fluency Disorders.* Amsterdam: Elsevier, pp 279–292.

Brayton, E.R., and Conture, E.G. (1978). Effects of noise and rhythmic stimulation on the speech of stutterers. *Journal of Speech and Hearing Research,* 21:285–294.

Brosch, S., Haege, A., Kalehne, P., and Johannsen, S. (1999). Stuttering children and the probability of remission: The role of cerebral dominance and speech production. *International Journal of Pediatric Otorhinolaryngology,* 47:71–76.

Brown, S.F. (1937). The influence of grammatical function on the incidence of stuttering. *Journal of Speech Disorders,* 2:207–215.

Brown, S.F. (1938a). A further study of stuttering in relation to various speech sounds. *Quarterly Journal of Speech,* 24:390–397.

Brown, S.F. (1938b). Stuttering with relation to word accent and word position. *Journal of Abnormal Social Psychology,* 33:112–120.

Brown, S.F. (1938c). The theoretical importance of certain factors influencing the incidence of stuttering. *Journal of Speech Disorders,* 3:223–230.

Brown, S.F. (1943). An analysis of certain data concerning loci of "stutterings" from the viewpoint of general semantics. *Papers from the Second American Congress of General Semantics,* 2:194–199.

Brown, S.F. (1945). The loci of stutterings in the speech sequence. *Journal of Speech Disorders,* 10:181–192.

Brown, S.F., and Moren, A. (1942). The frequency of stuttering in relation to word length during oral reading. *Journal of Speech Disorders,* 7:153–159.

Brundage, S., and Bernstein Ratner, N. (1989). The measurement of stuttering frequency in children's speech. *Journal of Fluency Disorders,* 14:351–358.

Brutten, G.J., and Dunham, S. (1989). The Communication Attitude Test: A normative study of grade school children. *Journal of Fluency Disorders,* 14:371–377.

Brutten, G.J., and Shoemaker, D.J. (1967). *The Modification of Stuttering.* Englewood Cliffs, NJ: Prentice-Hall.

Calkins, S.D. (1994). Origins and outcomes of individual differences in emotion regulation. In N.A. Fox, and J. Campos (Eds), *The Development of Emotional Regulation: Biological and Behavioral Considerations.* Chicago: Society for Research in Child Development.

Calkins, S.D., and Fox, N.A. (1994). Individual differences in the biological aspects of temperament. In J.E. Bates, and T.D. Wachs (Eds), *Temperament: Individual Differences at the Interface of Biology and Behavior.* Washington, D.C.: American Psychological Association, pp 199–217.

Callen, D.E., Kent, R.D., Guenther, F.H., and Vorperian, H.K. (2000). An auditory-feedback based neural network model of speech production that is robust to developmental changes in the size and shape of the articulatory system. *Journal of Speech, Language and Hearing Research,* 43:721–736.

Canter, G. (1971). Observations on neurogenic stuttering: A contribution to differential diagnosis. *British Journal of Communication Disorders,* 6:139–143.

Caplan, D. (1987). *Neurolinguistics and Linguistic Aphasiology.* Cambridge, UK: Cambridge University Press.

Carlisle, J. (1985). *Tangled Tongue: Living with a Stutter.* Toronto: University of Toronto Press.

Caruso, A.J., Abbs, J.H., and Gracco, V. (1988). Kinematic analysis of multiple movement coordination during speech in stutterers. *Brain,* 111:439–455.

Caruso, A.J., Chodzko-Zajko, W., Bidinger, D., and Sommers, R. (1994). Adults who stutter: Responses to cognitive stress. *Journal of Speech and Hearing Research,* 37:746–754.

Caruso, A.J., Chodzko-Zajko, W., and McClowry, M. (1995). Emotional arousal and stuttering: The impact of cognitive stress. In C.W. Starkweather, and H.F.M. Peters (Eds), *Stuttering: Proceedings of the First World Congress on Fluency Disorders.* Nijmegen, The Netherlands: International Fluency Association.

Chase, C.H. (1996). Neurobiology of learning disabilities. *Seminars in Speech, Language and Hearing,* 17:173–181.

Chmela, K.A., and Reardon, N.A. (2001). *The School-Aged Child Who Stutters: Working Effectively with Attitudes and Emotions: A Workbook.* Memphis: Stuttering Foundation of America.

Chuang, C.K., Fromm, D.S., Ewanowski, S.J., and Abbs, J.H. (1980, November). *Nonspeech articulatory sensorimotor control differences between stutterers and nonstutterers.* Paper presented at the Annual Meeting of the American Speech and Hearing Association, Detroit, MI.

Clarke-Stewart, A., and Friedman, S. (1987). *Child Development: Infancy Through Adolescence*. New York: John Wiley & Sons.

Cohen, M.S., and Hanson, M.L. (1975). Intersensory processing efficiency of fluent speakers and stutterers. *British Journal of Disorders of Communication*, 10:111–122.

Colburn, N., and Mysak, E.D. (1982a). Developmental disfluency and emerging grammar. I. Disfluency characteristics in early syntactic utterances. *Journal of Speech and Hearing Research*, 25:414–420.

Colburn, N., and Mysak, E.D. (1982b). Developmental disfluency and emerging grammar. II. Co-occurrence of disfluency with specified semantic-syntactic structures. *Journal of Speech and Hearing Research*, 25: 421–427.

Colcord, R.D., and Adams, M.R. (1979). Voicing duration and vocal SPL changes associated with stuttering reduction during singing. *Journal of Speech and Hearing Research*, 22:468–479.

Coleman, T.J. (2000). *Clinical Management of Communication Disorders in Culturally Diverse Children*. Boston: Allyn & Bacon.

Colton, R., and Casper, J. (1996). *Understanding Voice Problems: A Physiological Perspective for Diagnosis and Therapy*. Baltimore: Williams & Williams.

Conrad, C. (1996). Fluency in multicultural populations. In L. Cole, and V.R. Deal (Eds), *Communication Disorders in Multicultural Populations*. Rockville, MD: American Speech-Language-Hearing Association.

Conture, E. (2002). *Stuttering and Your Child: Questions and Answers* (ed 3). Memphis: Stuttering Foundation of America.

Conture, E.G. (1982). *Stuttering*. Englewood Cliffs, NJ: Prentice-Hall.

Conture, E.G. (1990). *Stuttering* (ed 2). Englewood Cliffs, NJ: Prentice-Hall.

Conture, E.G. (1991). Young stutterers' speech production. In H.F.M. Peters, W. Hulstijn, and C.W. Starkweather (Eds), *Speech Motor Control and Stuttering*. Amsterdam: Excerpta Medica, pp 365–384.

Conture, E.G. (2001). *Stuttering: Its Nature, Diagnosis, and Treatment*. Boston: Allyn & Bacon.

Conture, E.G., and Fraser, J. (1989). *Stuttering and Your Child: Questions and Answers*. Memphis: Stuttering Foundation of America.

Conture, E.G., Louko, L., and Edwards, M.L. (1993). Simultaneously treating stuttering and disordered phonology in children. *American Journal of Speech-Language Pathology*, 2:72–81.

Conture, E.G., McCall, G.N., and Brewer, D.W. (1977). Laryngeal behavior during stuttering. *Journal of Speech and Hearing Research*, 20:661–668.

Conture, E., and Melnick, K. (1999). Parent-child group approach to stuttering in preschool and school-age children. In M. Onslow, and A. Packman (Eds), *Early Stuttering: A Handbook of Intervention Strategies*. San Diego: Singular, pp 17–51.

Cooper, E.B., and Cooper, C.S. (1993). Fluency disorders. In D.E. Battle (Ed), *Communication Disorders in Multicultural Organizations*. Boston: Andover Medical Publishers, pp 189–211.

Cox, N., and Yairi, E. (2000, November). *Genetics of stuttering: Insights and recent advances*. Paper presented at the Annual Meeting of the American Speech-Language-Hearing Association, Washington, D.C.

Craig, A., and Andrews, G. (1985). The prediction and prevention of relapse in stuttering. *Behavior Modification*, 9:427–442.

Craig, A., Franklin, J., and Andrews, G. (1984). A scale to measure locus of control of behavior. *British Journal of Medical Psychology*, 57:173–180.

Cross, D.E., and Cooke, P. (1979). Vocal and manual reaction times of adult stutterers and nonstutterers. (Abstract). *ASHA*, 21:693.

Cross, D.E., and Luper, H.L. (1979). Voice reaction time of stuttering and nonstuttering children and adults. *Journal of Fluency Disorders*, 4:58–77.

Cross, D.E., and Luper, H.L. (1983). Relation between finger reaction time and voice reaction time in stuttering and nonstuttering children and adults. *Journal of Speech and Hearing Research*, 26:356–361.

Cross, D.E., Sweet, J., and Bates, D. (1985). *Mental imagery and stuttering: Electroencephalographic and physiological characteristics*. Paper presented at the Annual Meeting of the American Speech and Hearing Association, Washington, D.C.

Crystal, D. (1987). Towards a "bucket" theory of language disability: Taking account of interaction between linguistic levels. *Clinical Linguistics and Phonetics*, 1:7–22.

Culatta, R., and Goldberg, S. (1995). *Stuttering Therapy: An Integrated Approach to Theory and Practice*. Boston: Allyn & Bacon.

Cullinan, W.L., and Springer, M.T. (1980). Voice initiation times in stuttering and nonstuttering children. *Journal of Speech and Hearing Research*, 23:344–360.

Curlee, R. (1993). Identification and management of beginning stuttering. In R. Curlee (Ed), *Stuttering and Related Disorders of Fluency*. New York: Thieme Medical Publishers.

Curlee, R. (1999). Identification and case selection guidelines for early childhood stuttering. In R. Curlee (Ed), *Stuttering and Related Disorders of Fluency* (ed 2). New York: Thieme Medical Publishers.

Curlee, R. (2004). Stuttering. In R.D. Kent (Ed), *The MIT Encyclopedia of Communication Disorders*. Cambridge, MA: MIT Press, pp 220–223.

Curlee, R., and Siegel, G. (1997). *Nature and Treatment of Stuttering: New Directions* (ed 2). Boston: Allyn & Bacon.

Curry, F., and Gregory, H. (1969). The performance of stutterers on dichotic listening tasks thought to reflect cerebral dominance. *Journal of Speech and Hearing Research*, 12:73–82.

Dalton, P., and Hardcastle, W.J. (1977). *Disorders of Fluency*. New York: Elsevier.

Daly, D.A. (1986). The clutterer. In K. St. Louis (Ed), *The Atypical Stutterer*. New York: Academic Press.

Daly, D.A. (1993). Cluttering: Another fluency syndrome. In R. Curlee (Ed), *Stuttering and Related Disorders of Fluency*. New York: Thieme Medical Publishers, pp 151–175.

Daly, D.A., and Burnett-Stolnack, M.L. (1995). Identification of and treatment planning for stuttering clients: Two practical tools. *The Clinical Connection*, 8:15.

Darley, F.L. (1955). The relationship of parental attitudes and adjustments to the development of stuttering. In W. Johnson, and R.R. Leutenegger (Eds), *Stuttering in Children and Adults*. Minneapolis: University of Minnesota Press.

Darley, F.L., and Spriestersbach, D. (1978). *Diagnostic Methods in Speech Pathology* (ed 2). New York: Harper & Row.

Davenport, R.W. (1977). *Dichotic ear preferences of stuttering adults*. Unpublished doctoral dissertation, Iowa State University, Ames, IA.

Davidson, R.J. (1984). Affect, cognition, and hemispheric specialization. In C.E. Izard, J. Kagan, and R. Zajonc (Eds), *Emotion, Cognition and Behavior*. New York: Cambridge University Press.

Davidson, R.J. (1995). Cerebral asymmetry, emotion, and affective style. In R.J. Davidson, and K. Hugdahl (Eds), *Brain Asymmetry*. Cambridge, MA: MIT Press, pp 361–387.

Davis, D.M. (1940). The relation of repetitions in the speech of young children to certain measures of language maturity and situational factors: Parts II & III. *Journal of Speech Disorders*, 5:235–246.

DeJoy, D.A., and Gregory, H.H. (1973). The relationship of children's disfluencies to the syntax, length, and vocabulary of their sentences. (Abstract). *ASHA*, 15:472.

DeJoy, D.A., and Gregory, H.H. (1985). The relationship between age and frequency of disfluency in preschool children. *Journal of Fluency Disorders*, 10:107–122.

De Nil, L.F. (1995, November). *Linguistic and motor approaches to stuttering: Exploring unification*. Paper presented at the Annual Meeting of the American Speech-Language-Hearing Association, Orlando, FL.

De Nil, L.F. (2004). Recent developments in brain imaging research in stuttering. In B. Maassen, L.R. Kent, H.F.M. Peters, P.H.H.M. van Lieshout, and W. Hulstijn (Eds), *Speech Motor Control in Normal and Disordered Speech*. Oxford: Oxford University Press, pp 113–137.

De Nil, L.F., and Abbs, J.H. (1991). Kinaesthetic activity of stutterers and non-stutterers for oral and non-oral movement. *Brain*, 114:2145–2158.

De Nil, L.F., and Bosshardt, H.G. (2001). Studying stuttering from a neurological and cognitive information processing perspective. In H.G. Bosshardt, J.S. Yaruss, and H.F.M. Peters (Eds), *Stuttering Research: Research, Therapy and Self-Help: Proceedings of the 3rd World Congress on Fluency Disorders*. Nijmegen, The Netherlands: Nijmegen University Press, pp 53–58.

De Nil, L.F., and Brutten, G.J. (1991). Speech-associated attitudes of stuttering and normally fluent children. *Journal of Speech and Hearing Research*, 34:60–66.

De Nil, L.F., Kroll, R.M., and Houle, S. (2001). Functional neuroimaging of cerebellar activation during single word reading and verb generation in stuttering and nonstuttering adults. *Neuroscience Letters*, 302:77–80.

De Nil, L.F., Kroll, R.M., Houle, S., Ludlow, C.L., Braun, A., Ingham, R., et al. (1995, November). *Advances in stuttering research using positron emission tomography brain imaging*. Paper presented at the Annual Meeting of the American Speech-Language-Hearing Association, Orlando, FL.

De Nil, L.F., Kroll, R.M., Kapur, S., and Houle, S. (2000). A positron emission tomography study of silent and oral single word reading in stuttering and nonstuttering adults. *Journal of Speech, Language, and Hearing Research*, 43:1038–1053.

De Nil, L.F., Kroll, R.M., Lafaille, S.J., and Houle, S. (2003). A positron emission tomography study of short- and long-term treatment effects on functional brain activation in adults who stutter. *Journal of Fluency Disorders*, 28:357–380.

Devinsky, O., Morrell, M.J., and Vogt, B.A. (1995). Contributions of anterior cingulate cortex to behaviour. *Brain,* 118:279–306.

Dietrich, S. (1995). Middle latency auditory responses in males who stutter. *Journal of Speech and Hearing Research,* 38:5–17.

Donnan, G.A. (1979). Stuttering as a manifestation of stroke. *Medical Journal of Australia,* 1:44–45.

Dorman, M., and Porter, R. (1975). Hemispheric lateralization for speech perceptions in stutterers. *Cortex,* 11:181–185.

Douglass, L.C. (1943). A study of bilaterally recorded electroencephalograms of adult stutterers. *Journal of Experimental Psychology,* 32:247–265.

Drayna, D. (1997). Genetic linkage studies of stuttering: Ready for prime time? *Journal of Fluency Disorders,* 22:237–241.

Duffy, J. (2005). *Motor Speech Disorders* (ed 2). St. Louis: Elsevier, Mosby.

Edelman, G. (1992). *Bright Air, Brilliant Fire: On the Matter of Mind.* New York: Basic Books.

Elliott, R.L., and Thomas, B.J. (1985). A case report of alprazolam-induced stuttering. *Journal of Clinical Psychopharmacology,* 5:159–160.

Embrechts, M., and Ebben, H. (2000). A comparison between the interactions of stuttering and nonstuttering children and their parents. In K.L. Baker, L. Rustin, and F. Cook (Eds), *Proceedings of the Fifth Oxford Dysfluency Conference, 7th-10th July, 1999.* Oxford: Kevin Baker, pp 125–133.

Faver, A., and Mazlish, E. (1999). *How to Talk So Kids Will Listen and How to Listen So Kids Will Talk.* New York: Harper Resource.

Felsenfeld, S. (1997). Epidemiology and genetics of stuttering. In R. Curlee, and G. Siegel (Eds), *The Nature and Treatment of Stuttering: New Directions* (ed 2). Boston: Allyn & Bacon, pp 3–23.

Felsenfeld, S., Kirk, K.M., Zhu, G., Statham, D.J., Neale, M.C., and Martin, N.G. (2000). A study of the genetic and environmental etiology of stuttering in a selected twin sample. *Behavior Genetics,* 30:359–366.

Fibiger, S. (1971). Stuttering explained as a physiological tremor. *Quarterly Progress and Status Report: Speech Transmission Laboratory,* 2–3.

Fibiger, S. (1972). Further discussion on stuttering explained as a physiological tremor. *Quarterly Progress and Status Report: Speech Transmission Laboratory.*

Finn, P. (2003). Self-regulation and the management of stuttering. *Seminars in Speech and Language,* 24:27–32.

Flugel, F. (1979). Erhebungen von Personlichkeitsmerk-malen an Muttern stotternder Kinder und Jugendicher. *DSH Abstracts,* 19:226.

Fosnot, S.M. (1995). Clinical forum. *Language, Speech, and Hearing Services in Schools,* 26:115–200.

Fosnot, S.M., and Woodford, L.L. (1992). *The Fluency Development System for Young Children.* Buffalo: United Educational Services.

Foundas, A.L., Bollich, A.M., Corey, D.M., Hurley, M., and Heilman, K.M. (2001). Anomalous anatomy of speech-language areas in adults with persistent developmental stuttering. *Neurology,* 57:207–215.

Foundas, A.L., Bollich, A.M., Feldman, J., Corey, D.M., Hurley, M., Lemen, L.C., Heilman, K.M. (2004). Aberrant auditory processing and a typical planum temporale in developmental stuttering. *Neurology,* 63:1640–1646.

Fowlie, G.M., and Cooper, E.B. (1978). Traits attributed to stuttering and nonstuttering children by their mothers. *Journal of Fluency Disorders,* 3:233–246.

Fox, N., and Davidson, R. (1984). Hemispheric substrates of affect: Developmental model. In N. Fox, and R. Davidson (Eds), *The Psychobiology of Affective Development.* Hillsdale, NJ: Lawrence Erlbaum Associates.

Fox, P., Ingham, R.J., Ingham, J.C., Zamarripa, F., Xiong, J.-H., and Lancaster, J.L. (2000). Brain correlates of stuttering and syllable production: A PET performance-correlation analysis. *Brain,* 123:1985–2004.

Fox, P.T. (2003). Brain imaging in stuttering: Where next? *Journal of Fluency Disorders,* 28:265–272.

Fox, P.T., Ingham, R., Ingham, J.C., Hirsch, T.B., Downs, J.H., Martin, C., et al. (1996). A PET study of the neural systems of stuttering. *Nature,* 382:158–162.

Fraisse, P. (1963). *The Psychology of Time.* New York: Harper & Row.

Franken, M.C.J., Kielstra-van der Schalk, C.J., and Boelens, H.H. (in press). Experimental treatment of early stuttering: A preliminary study. *Journal of Fluency Disorders.*

Fraser, J. (2004). Results of survey on electronic devices. *Stuttering Foundation Newsletter* (Winter) 3:7.

Fraser, J., and Perkins, W.H. (1987). *Do You Stutter: A Guide for Teens.* Memphis: Speech Foundation of America.

Frattali, C.M. (1998). *Measuring Outcomes in Speech-Language Pathology.* New York: Thieme.

Freeman, F.J., and Ushijima, T. (1975). Laryngeal activity accompanying the moment of stuttering: A preliminary report of EMG investigations. *Journal of Fluency Disorders,* 1:36–45.

Freeman, F.J., and Ushijima, T. (1978). Laryngeal muscle activity during stuttering. *Journal of Speech and Hearing Research,* 21:538–562.

Gaines, N.D., Runyan, C.M., and Meyers, S.C. (1991). A comparison of young stutterers' fluent versus stuttered utterances on measures of length and complexity. *Journal of Speech and Hearing Research,* 34:37–42.

Garber, S., and Martin, R. (1977). Effects of noise and vocal intensity on stuttering. *Journal of Speech and Hearing Research,* 20:233–240.

Garfinkel, H.A. (1995). Why did Moses stammer? And was Moses left-handed? *Journal of the Royal Society of Medicine,* 88:256–257.

Geschwind, N., and Galaburda, A.M. (1985). Cerebral lateralization: Biological mechanisms, associations, and pathology: I. A hypothesis and a program for research. *Archives of Neurology,* 42:429-459.

Gibson, E. (1972). Reading for some purpose. In J.F. Kavanaugh, and I. Mattingly (Eds), *Language by Ear and by Eye.* Cambridge, MA: MIT Press.

Gildston, P. (1967). Stutterers' self-acceptance and perceived parental acceptance. *Journal of Abnormal Psychology,* 72:59–64.

Goldberg, G. (1985). Supplementary motor area structure and function: Review and hypothesis. *Behavioral and Brain Sciences,* 8:567–616.

Goldman-Eisler, F. (1968). *Psycholinguistics: Experiments in Spontaneous Speech.* New York: Academic Press.

Goldstein, B. (2000). *Cultural and Linguistic Diversity Resource Guide for Speech-Language Pathologists.* San Diego: Singular Publishing Group.

Goodstein, L.D. (1956). MMPI profiles of stutterers' parents: A follow-up study. *Journal of Speech and Hearing Disorders,* 21:430–435.

Goodstein, L.D., and Dahlstrom, W.G. (1956). MMPI difference between parents of stuttering children and nonstuttering children. *Journal of Consulting Psychology,* 20:365–370.

Gordon, P.A., Luper, H.L., and Peterson, H.A. (1986). The effects of syntactic complexity on the occurrence of disfluencies in 5 year old stutterers. *Journal of Fluency Disorders,* 11:151–164.

Gottwald, S., and Starkweather, C.W. (1984, November). *Stuttering prevention: Rationale and method.* Paper presented at the Annual Meeting of the American Speech and Hearing Association, San Francisco, CA.

Gottwald, S., and Starkweather, C.W. (1985, November). *The prognosis of stuttering.* Paper presented at the Annual Meeting of the American Speech and Hearing Association, Washington, D.C.

Gottwald, S., and Starkweather, C.W. (1999). Stuttering prevention and early intervention: A multiprocess approach. In M. Onslow, and A. Packman (Eds), *Handbook of Early Stuttering Intervention.* San Diego: Singular, pp 53–82.

Gray, J.A. (1987). *The Psychology of Fear and Stress* (ed 2). Cambridge: Cambridge University Press.

Greenspan, S.I. (1993). Making time for your child. *Parents,* August: 111–114.

Gregory, H.H. (1968). Application of learning theory concepts in the management of stuttering. In H.H. Gregory (Ed), *Learning Theory and Stuttering Therapy.* Evanston, IL: Northwestern University Press.

Gregory, H.H. (1979). Controversial issues: Statement and review of the literature. In H.H. Gregory (Ed), *Controversies About Stuttering Therapy.* Baltimore: University Park Press.

Gregory, H.H. (1986). *Stuttering: Differential Evaluation and Therapy.* Austin, TX: Pro-Ed.

Gregory, H.H. (2003). *Stuttering Therapy: Rationale and Procedures.* Boston: Allyn & Bacon.

Gregory, H.H., and Campbell, J.H. (1988). Stuttering in the school-age child. In D.E. Yoder, and R.D. Kent (Eds), *Decision Making in Speech-Language Pathology.* Toronto: B.C. Decker.

Gregory, H.H., Campbell, J.H., and Hill, D. (2003). Differential evaluation of stuttering problems. In H.H. Gregory (Ed), *Stuttering Therapy: Rationale and Procedures.* Boston: Allyn & Bacon, pp 78–141.

Gregory, H.H., and Hill, D. (1980). Stuttering therapy for children. *Seminars in Speech, Language and Hearing,* 1:351–363.

Guitar, B. (1976). Pretreatment factors associated with the outcome of stuttering therapy. *Journal of Speech and Hearing Research,* 19:590–600.

Guitar, B. (1978). Between parent and (stuttering) child. *WMU Journal of Speech, Language and Hearing,* 14:3–5.

Guitar, B. (1984). Indirect treatment of childhood stuttering. In J.M. Costello (Ed), *Speech Disorders in Children: Recent Advances.* San Diego: College-Hill Press, pp 291–311.

Guitar, B. (1997). Therapy for children's stuttering and emotions. In R.F. Curlee, and G.M. Siegel (Eds), *Nature and Treatment of Stuttering: New Directions* (ed 2). Boston: Allyn & Bacon, pp 280–291.

Guitar, B. (1998). *Stuttering: An Integrated Approach to Its Nature and Treatment* (ed 2). Philadelphia: Lippincott Williams & Wilkins.

Guitar, B. (2000). Emotion, temperament and stuttering: Some possible relationships. In K.L. Baker, L. Rustin, and F. Cook (Eds), *Proceedings of the Fifth Oxford Dysfluency Conference, 7th–10th July, 1999*. Berkshire, UK: K. L. Baker, pp 1–6.

Guitar, B. (2003). Acoustic startle responses and temperament in individuals who stutter. *Journal of Speech, Language and Hearing Research,* 46:233–240.

Guitar, B. (2004). Burn your textbooks! Evidence-based practice in stuttering treatment. In A. Packman, A. Meltzer, and H.F.M. Peters (Eds), *Theory, Research and Therapy in Fluency Disorders: Proceedings of the Fourth World Congress in Fluency Disorders*. Nijmegen, The Netherlands: Nijmegan University Press, pp 21–27.

Guitar, B., and Bass, C. (1978). Stuttering therapy: The relation between attitude change and long-term outcome. *Journal of Speech and Hearing Disorders,* 43:392–400.

Guitar, B., and Conture, E. (1996). *Do you stutter: Straight talk for teens* [Videotape]. Memphis: Stuttering Foundation of America.

Guitar, B., and Grims, S. (1977, November). *Developing a scale to assess communication attitudes in children who stutter.* Paper presented at the Annual Meeting of the American Speech-Language-Hearing Association, Atlanta, GA.

Guitar, B., and Guitar, C. (2003). *Stuttering: Straight talk for teens* [Videotape]. Memphis: Stuttering Foundation.

Guitar, B., Guitar, C., and Fraser, J. (2000). *Stuttering and the preschool child: Help for families* [Videotape]. Memphis: Stuttering Foundation of America.

Guitar, B., Guitar, C., Neilson, P.D., O'Dwyer, N.J., and Andrews, G. (1988). Onset sequencing of selected lip muscles in stutterers and nonstutterers. *Journal of Speech and Hearing Research,* 31:28–35.

Guitar, B., Kopff-Schaefer, H., Donahue-Kilburg, G., and Bond, L. (1992). Parent verbal interaction and speech rate. *Journal of Speech and Hearing Research,* 35:742–754.

Guitar, B., and Peters, T.J. (1980). *Stuttering: An Integration of Contemporary Therapies*. Memphis: Speech Foundation of America.

Habib, M., Daquin, G., Milandre, L., Royere, M.L., Rey, M., Lanteri, A., et al. (1995). Mutism and auditory agnosia due to bilateral insular damage—Role of the insula in human communication. *Neuropsychologia,* 33:327–339.

Hadders-Algra, M., and Forssberg, H. (2002). Development of motor function in health and disease. In H. Lagercrantz, M.L. Hanson, P. Evrard, and C. H. Rodeck (Eds), *The Newborn Brain: Neuroscience and Clinical Applications*. Cambridge: Cambridge University Press.

Hall, J.W., and Jerger, J. (1978). Central auditory function in stutterers. *Journal of Speech and Hearing Research,* 21:324–337.

Hall, N.E., Yamashita, T.S., and Aram, D.M. (1993). Relationship between language and fluency in children with developmental language disorders. *Journal of Speech and Hearing Research,* 36:568–579.

Hannley, M., and Dorman, M.F. (1982). Some observations on auditory function and stuttering. *Journal of Fluency Disorders,* 7:93–108.

Hanson, P.E., and Rodeck, C.H. (Eds) (2002). *The Newborn Brain: Neuroscience and Clinical Applications*. Cambridge, MA: Cambridge University Press.

Harris, V., Onslow, M., Packman, A., Harrison, E., and Menzies, R. (2002). An experimental investigation of the impact of the Lidcombe Program on early stuttering. *Journal of Fluency Disorders,* 27:203–214.

Haynes, W.O., and Hood, S.B. (1978). Disfluency changes in children as a function of the systematic modification of linguistic complexity. *Journal of Communication Disorders,* 11:79–83.

Heinze, B., and Johnson, K. (1985). *Easy Does It: Fluency Activities for Young Children*. East Moline, IL: LinguiSystems.

Helliesen, G.G. (2002). *Forty Years After Therapy: One Man's Story*. Newport News, VA: Apollo Press.

Helm, N.A. (1979). Management of palilalia with a pacing board. *Journal of Speech and Hearing Disorders,* 44:350–353.

Helm-Estabrooks, N. (1986). Diagnosis and management of neurogenic stuttering in adults. In K. St. Louis (Ed), *The Atypical Stutterer*. New York: Academic Press.

Helm-Estabrooks, N. (1992). *Aphasia Diagnostic Profiles*. Chicago: Applied Symbolix.

Helm-Estabrooks, N. (1999). Stuttering associated with acquired neurological disorders. In R. Curlee (Ed), *Stuttering and Related Disorders of Fluency* (ed 2). New York: Thieme, pp 255–268.

Helm-Estabrooks, N., and Kaplan, E. (1989). *Boston Stimulus Boards*. Chicago: Applied Symbolix.

Hickok, G. (2001). Functional anatomy of speech perception and speech production: Psycholinguistic implications. *Journal of Psycholinguistic Research,* 30:225–235.

Hill, H. (1954). An experimental study of disorganization of speech and manual responses in normal subjects. *Journal of Speech and Hearing Disorders,* 19:295–305.

Hillman, R.E., and Gilbert, H.R. (1977). Voice onset time for voiceless stop consonants in the fluent reading of stutterers and nonstutterers. *Journal of the Acoustical Society of America,* 61:610–611.

Hiscock, M., and Kinsbourne, M. (1977). Selective listening asymmetry in preschool children. *Developmental Psychology,* 13:217–224.

Hiscock, M., and Kinsbourne, M. (1980). Asymmetry of verbal-manual time sharing in children: A follow-up study. *Neuropsychologia,* 18:151–162.

Hodge, G., Rescorla, L., and Ratner, N.B. (1999, November). *Fluency in toddlers with SLI: A preliminary investigation.* Paper presented at the Annual Meeting of the American Speech-Language-Hearing Association, San Francisco, CA.

Hodson, B.W. (1986). *The Assessment of Phonological Processes–Revised.* Austin, TX: Pro-Ed.

Hoffman, P., Schuckers, G., and Daniloff, R. (1989). *Children's Phonetic Disorders: Theory and Treatment.* Boston: College-Hill Press.

Hood, L. (1987, November). *Middle latency responses in stutterers.* Paper presented at the Annual Meeting of the American Speech-Language-Hearing Association, New Orleans, LA.

Horovitz, L.J., Johnson, S.B., Pearlman, R.C., Schaffer, E.J., and Hedin, A.K. (1978). Stapedial reflex and anxiety in fluent and disfluent speakers. *Journal of Speech and Hearing Research,* 21:762–767.

Howell, P., El-Yaniv, N., and Powell, D.J. (1987). Factors affecting fluency in stutterers when speaking under altered auditory feedback. In H.F.M. Peters, and W. Hulstijn (Eds), *Speech Motor Dynamics in Stuttering.* New York: Springer, pp 361–369.

Howie, P.M. (1981). Concordance for stuttering in monozygotic and dizygotic twin pairs. *Journal of Speech and Hearing Research,* 24:317–321.

Howie, P.M., and Andrews, G. (1984). Treatment of adult stutterers: Managing fluency. In R. Curlee and W. Perkins (Eds), *Nature and Treatment of Stuttering: New Directions.* San Diego: College-Hill Press, pp 425–445.

Hubbard, C.P., and Yairi, E. (1988). Clustering of disfluencies in the speech of stuttering and nonstuttering preschool children. *Journal of Speech and Hearing Research,* 31:228–233.

Ingham, J. (1999). Behavioral treatment of young children who stutter. In R. Curlee (Ed), *Stuttering and Related Disorders of Fluency.* New York: Thieme, pp 80–109.

Ingham, R.J. (1979). Comment on "Stuttering therapy: The relation between attitude change and long-term outcome." *Journal of Speech and Hearing Disorders,* 44:397–400.

Ingham, R.J. (2001). Brain imaging studies of developmental stuttering. *Journal of Communication Disorders,* 34:493–516.

Ingham, R.J. (2003). Brain imaging and stuttering: Some reflection on current and future developments. *Journal of Fluency Disorders,* 28:411–420.

Ingham, R.J., and Andrews, G. (1973). Details of a token economy stuttering therapy programme for adults. *Australian Journal of Human Communication Disorders,* 1:13–20.

Ingham, R.J., Cordes, A., and Finn, P. (1993). Time-interval measurement of stuttering: Systematic replication of Ingham, Cordes & Gow (1993). *Journal of Speech and Hearing Research,* 36:1168–1176.

Ingham, R.J., Cordes, A., and Gow, M. (1993). Time-interval measurement of stuttering: Modifying interjudge agreement. *Journal of Speech and Hearing Research,* 36:503–515.

Ingham, R.J., Fox, P.T., Ingham, J.C., Zamarripa, F., Martin, C., Jerabek, P., et al. (1996). Functional-lesion investigation of developmental stuttering with positron emission tomography. *Journal of Speech and Hearing Research,* 39:1208–1227.

Ingham, R.J., Gow, M., and Costello, J. M. (1985). Stuttering and speech naturalness: Some additional data. *Journal of Speech and Hearing Disorders,* 50:217–219.

Ingham, R.J., Ingham, J.C., Finn, P., and Fox, P.T. (2003). Towards a functional neural systems model of developmental stuttering. *Journal of Fluency Disorders,* 28:297–318.

Ito, T. (1986). Speech dysfluency and the acquisition of syntax in children 2–6 years old. (Abstract). *Folia Phoniatrica,* 38:310.

Jacobson, E. (1938). *Progressive Relaxation.* Chicago: University of Chicago Press.

Jaffe, J., and Anderson, S.W. (1979). Prescript to Chapter 1: Communication rhythms and the evolution of language. In A.W. Siegman, and S. Feldman (Eds), *Of Speech and Time: Temporal Speech Patterns in Interpersonal Contexts.* Hillsdale, NJ: Lawrence Erlbaum Associates.

Jensen, P.J., Sheehan, J.G., Williams, W.M., and LaPointe, L.L. (1975). Oral-sensory-perceptual integrity of stutterers. *Folia Phoniatrica,* 27:106–115.

Jezer, M. (1997). *Stuttering: A Life Bound Up in Words*. New York: Basic Books.

Johnson, K., and Heinze, B. (1994). *The Fluency Companion: Strategies for Stuttering*. East Moline, IL: LinguiSystems.

Johnson, W. (1955). A study of the onset and development of stuttering. In W. Johnson, and R.R. Leutenegger (Eds), *Stuttering in Children and Adults*. Minneapolis: University of Minnesota Press.

Johnson, W., et al. (1942). A study of the onset and development of stuttering. *Journal of Speech Disorders*, 7:251–257.

Johnson, W., and associates (1959). *The Onset of Stuttering*. Minneapolis: University of Minnesota Press.

Johnson, W., and Brown, S.F. (1935). Stuttering in relation to various speech sounds. *Quarterly Journal of Speech*, 21:481–496.

Johnson, W., Darley, F., and Spriestersbach, D. (1952). *Diagnostic Manual in Speech Correction: A Professional Training Workbook*. New York: Harper & Brothers.

Johnson, W., and Inness, M. (1939). Studies in the psychology of stuttering: XIII. A statistical analysis of the adaptation and consistency effects in relation to stuttering. *Journal of Speech Disorders*, 4:79–86.

Johnson, W., and Knott, J.R. (1937). Studies in the psychology of stuttering: I. The distribution of moments of stuttering in successive readings of the same material. *Journal of Speech Disorders*, 2:17–19.

Johnson, W., and Leutenegger, R.R. (1955). *Stuttering in Children and Adults*. Minneapolis: University of Minnesota Press.

Johnson, W., and Rosen, L. (1937). Studies in the psychology of stuttering: VII. Effects of certain changes in speech pattern upon frequency of stuttering. *Journal of Speech Disorders*, 2:105–109.

Johnson, W., and Solomon, A. (1937). Studies in the psychology of stuttering: IV. A quantitative study of expectation of stuttering as a process involving a low degree of consciousness. *Journal of Speech Disorders*, 2:95–97.

Jones, J.E., and Niven, P. (1993). *Voices and Silences*. New York: Charles Scribner's Sons.

Jones, R.K. (1966). Observations on stammering after localized cerebral injury. *Journal of Neurology, Neurosurgery and Psychiatry*, 29:192–195.

Jurgens, U. (2002). Neural pathways underlying vocal control. *Neuroscience and Biobehavioral Reviews*, 26:235–258.

Kagan, J. (1981). *The Second Year: The Emergence of Self-Awareness*. Cambridge, MA: Harvard University Press.

Kagan, J. (1994a). The realistic view of biology and behavior. *The Chronicle of Higher Education*, October 5:A64.

Kagan, J. (1994b). *Galen's Prophecy: Temperament in Human Nature*. New York: Basic Books.

Kagan, J., Reznick, J.S., and Snidman, N. (1987). The physiology and psychology of behavioral inhibition in children. *Child Development*, 58:1459–1473.

Kagan, J., and Snidman, N. (1991). Temperamental factors in human development. *American Psychologist*, 46:856–862.

Kasprisin-Burrelli, A., Egolf, D.B., and Shames, G.H. (1972). A comparison of parental verbal behavior with stuttering and nonstuttering children. *Journal of Communication Disorders*, 5:335–346.

Kelly, E. (1994). Speech rates and turn-taking behaviors of children who stutter and their fathers. *Journal of Speech and Hearing Research*, 37:1284–1267.

Kelly, E., and Conture, E. (1992). Speaking rates, response time latencies, and interrupting behaviors of young stutterers, nonstutterers, and their mothers. *Journal of Speech and Hearing Research*, 35:1256–1267.

Kelly, E., Smith, A., and Goffman, L. (1995). Orofacial muscle activity of children who stutter. *Journal of Speech and Hearing Research*, 38:1025–1036.

Kent, L.R., and Williams, D.E. (1963). Alleged former stutterers in grade two. (Abstract). *ASHA*, 5:772.

Kent, R.D. (1981). Sensorimotor aspects of speech development. In R.D. Alberts, and M.R. Peterson (Eds), *The Development of Perception: Psycho-Biological Perspectives*. New York: Academic Press.

Kent, R.D. (1984). Stuttering as a temporal programming disorder. In R.F. Curlee, and W.H. Perkins (Eds), *Nature and Treatment of Stuttering: New Directions*. San Diego: College-Hill Press, pp 283–301.

Kent, R.D. (1985). Developing and disordered speech: Strategies for organization. *ASHA Reports*, 15:29–37.

Kent, R.D. (1997). *The Speech Sciences*. San Diego, CA: Singular Publishing Company.

Kent, R.D., and Perkins, W. (1984). *Oral-verbal fluency: Aspects of verbal formulation, speech motor control and underlying neural systems*. Unpublished manuscript.

Kent, R.D., and Vorperian, H.K. (1995). Anatomic development of the craniofacial-oral-laryngeal systems: A review. *Journal of Medical Speech-Language Pathology*, 3:145–190.

Kenyon, E.L. (1942). The etiology of stammering: Fundamentally a wrong psychophysiologic habit in control of the vocal cords for the production of an individual speech sound. *Journal of Speech Disorders*, 7:97–104.

Kidd, K.K. (1977). A genetic perspective on stuttering. *Journal of Fluency Disorders*, 2:259–269.

Kidd, K.K. (1984). Stuttering as a genetic disorder. In R.F. Curlee, and W.H. Perkins (Eds), *Nature and Treatment of Stuttering: New Directions*. San Diego: College-Hill Press, pp 149–169.

Kidd, K.K., Kidd, J.R., and Records, M.A. (1978). The possible causes of the sex ratio in stuttering and its implications. *Journal of Fluency Disorders,* 3:13–23.

Kidd, K.K., Reich, T., and Kessler, S. (1973). A genetic analysis of stuttering suggesting a single major locus. *Genetics,* 74:(2, Part 2)s137.

Kimura, D. (1961). Cerebral dominance and the perception of verbal stimuli. *Canadian Journal of Psychology,* 15:166–177.

Kinsbourne, M. (1989). A model of adaptive behavior related to cerebral participation in emotional control. In G. Gianotti, and C. Caltagirone (Eds), *Emotions and the Dual Brain.* New York: Springer-Verlag.

Kinsbourne, M., and Bemporad, E. (1984). Lateralization of emotion: A model and the evidence. In N.A. Fox, and R.J. Davidson (Eds), *The Psychology of Affective Development.* Hillsdale, NJ: Lawrence Erlbaum Associates.

Kinsbourne, M., and Hicks, R. (1978). Functional cerebral space: A model for overflow, transfer and interference effects in human performance: A tutorial review. In M. Kinsbourne (Ed), *Asymmetrical Function of the Brain.* Cambridge, UK: Cambridge University Press, pp 345–362.

Kleinow, J., and Smith, A. (2000). Influences of length and syntactic complexity on the speech motor stability of the fluent speech of adults who stutter. *Journal of Speech, Language, and Hearing Research,* 43:548–559.

Kline, M.L., and Starkweather, C.W. (1979). Receptive and expressive language performance in young stutterers. (Abstract). *ASHA,* 21:797.

Kloth, S., Janssen, P., Kraaimaat, F., and Brutten, G. (1995). Speech-motor and linguistic skills of young stutterers prior to onset. *Journal of Fluency Disorders,* 20:157–170.

Kloth, S.A.M., Kraaimaat, F.W., Janssen, P., and Brutten, G.J. (1999). Persistence and remission of incipient stuttering among high-risk children. *Journal of Fluency Disorders,* 24:253–265.

Knott, J.R., Johnson, W., and Webster, M.J. (1937). Studies in the psychology of stuttering: II. A quantitative evaluation of expectation of stuttering in relation to the occurrence of stuttering. *Journal of Speech Disorders,* 2:20–22.

Kolk, H., and Postma, A. (1997). Stuttering as a covert repair phenomenon. In R.F. Curlee, and G.M. Siegel (Eds), *Nature and Treatment of Stuttering: New Directions* (ed 2). Boston: Allyn & Bacon, pp 182–203.

Kramer, M., Green, D., and Guitar, B. (1987). A comparison of stutterers and nonstutterers on masking level differences and synthetic sentence identification tasks. *Journal of Communication Disorders,* 20:379–390.

Kroll, R.M., De Nil, L.F., Kapur, S., and Houle, S. (1997). A positron emission tomography investigation of post-treatment brain activation in stutterers. In W. Hulstijn, H.F.M. Peters, and P.H.H.M. van Lieshout (Eds), *Speech Production: Motor Control, Brain Research and Fluency Disorders.* Amsterdam: Elsevier, pp 307–319.

Kully, D., and Langevin, M. (1999). Intensive treatment for stuttering adolescents. In R. Curlee (Ed), *Stuttering and Related Disorders of Fluency* (ed 2). New York: Thieme Medical Publishers, 139–159.

Lai, C.S., Fisher, S.E., Hurst, J.A., Vargha-Khadem, F., and Monaco, A.P. (2001). A forkhead-domain gene is mutated in a severe speech and language disorder. *Nature,* 413:519–523.

Langlois, A., Hanrahan, L.L., and Inouye, L.L. (1986). A comparison of interactions between stuttering children, nonstuttering children, and their mothers. *Journal of Fluency Disorders,* 11:263–273.

Langlois, A., and Long, S.H. (1988). A model for teaching parents to facilitate fluent speech. *Journal of Fluency Disorders,* 13:163–172.

LaSalle, L. (1999, November). *Temperament in preschoolers who stutter: A preliminary investigation.* Paper presented at the Annual Meeting of the American Speech-Language-Hearing Association, San Francisco, CA.

LaSalle, L.R., and Conture, E. (1995). Disfluency clusters of children who stutter: Relation of stutterings to self-repairs. *Journal of Speech and Hearing Research,* 38:965–977.

Lauter, J.L. (1995). Visions of speech and language: Noninvasive imaging techniques and their applications to the study of human communication. In H. Winitz (Ed), *Current Approaches to the Study of Language Development and Disorders.* Timonium, MD: York Press, pp 277–390.

Lauter, J.L. (1997). Noninvasive brain imaging in speech motor control and stuttering: Choices and challenges. In W. Hulstijn, H.F.M. Peters, and P.H.H.M. van Lieshout (Eds), *Speech Production: Motor Control, Brain Research, and Fluency Disorders.* Amsterdam: Elsevier, pp 233–258.

Lazare, A. (1981). Current concepts in psychiatry: Conversion symptoms. *New England Journal of Medicine,* 305:745.

LeDoux, J.E. (1996). *The Emotional Brain: The Mysterious Underpinnings of Emotional Life.* New York: Simon & Schuster.

LeDoux, J.E. (2002). *Synaptic Self: How Our Brains Become Who We Are.* New York: Viking.

Lee, B.S. (1951). Artificial stutter. *Journal of Speech and Hearing Disorders,* 16:53–55.

Lefton, L.A. (1997). *Psychology* (ed 6). Boston: Allyn & Bacon.

Lewis, M. (2000). Self-conscious emotions: Embarrassment, pride, shame and guilt. In M. Lewis, and J.M. Haviland-Jones (Eds), *Handbook of Emotions* (ed 2). New York: Guilford Press.

Lidz, T. (1968). *The Person: His Development Throughout the Life Cycle.* New York: Basic Books.

Liebetrau, R., and Daly, D. (1981). Auditory processing and perceptual abilities of "organic" and "functional" stutterers. *Journal of Fluency Disorders,* 6:219–231.

Lincoln, M., and Onslow, M. (1997). Long-term outcome of an early intervention for stuttering. *American Journal of Speech-Language Pathology,* 6:51–58.

Lindsay, J.S. (1989). Relationship of developmental disfluency and episodes of stuttering to the emergence of cognitive stages in children. *Journal of Fluency Disorders,* 14:271–284.

Logan, K., and Conture, E. (1995). Length, grammatical complexity, and rate differences in stuttered and fluent conversational utterances of children who stutter. *Journal of Fluency Disorders,* 20:35–61.

Luchsinger, R. (1944). Biological studies on monozygotic and dizgotic twins relative to size and form of the larynx. *Archiv Julius Klaus-Stiftung fur Verergungsforchung,* 19:3–4.

Ludlow, C.L., and Loucks, T. (2003). Stuttering: A dynamic motor control disorder. *Journal of Fluency Disorders,* 28:273–295.

Luper, H.L., and Mulder, R.L. (1964). *Stuttering: Therapy for Children.* Englewood Cliffs, NJ: Prentice-Hall.

Luterman, D.M. (2001). *Counseling Persons With Communications Disorders and Their Families* (ed 4). Austin, TX: ProEd.

Maassen, B., Kent, R.D., Peters, H.F.M., van Lieshout, P.H.H.M., and Hulstijn, W. (Eds) (2004). *Speech Motor Control in Normal and Disordered Speech.* Oxford: Oxford University Press.

MacFarland, D.H., and Moore, W. (1982, November). *Alpha hemispheric asymmetries during an electromyographic biofeedback procedure for stuttering.* Paper presented at the Annual Meeting of the American Speech-Language-Hearing Association, Toronto, Canada.

MacNeilage, P. (1987). The evolution of hemispheric specialization for manual function and language. In S.P. Wise (Ed.), *Higher Brain Functions.* New York: John Wiley and Sons, pp 285–309.

Maguire, G., Yu, B.P., Franklin, D.L., and Riley, G.D. (2004). Alleviating stuttering with pharmacological interventions. *Expert Opinion in Pharmacotherapy,* 5:1565–1571.

Mahr, G., and Leith, W. (1992). Psychogenic stuttering of adult onset. *Journal of Speech and Hearing Research,* 35:283–286.

Manning, W.H. (1999). Management of adult stuttering. In R. Curlee (Ed.), *Stuttering and Related Disorders of Fluency* (ed 2). New York: Thieme, pp 160–180.

Manning, W.H. (2001). *Clinical Decision Making in Fluency Disorders* (ed 2). San Diego: Singular.

Mansson, H. (2000). Childhood stuttering: Incidence and development. *Journal of Fluency Disorders,* 25:47–57.

Market, K.E., Montague, J.C., Buffalo, M.D., and Drummond, S.A. (1990). Acquired stuttering: Descriptive data and treatment outcomes. *Journal of Fluency Disorders,* 15:21–33.

Marshall, R.C., and Starch, S.A. (1984). Behavioral treatment of acquired stuttering. *Australian Journal of Communication Disorders,* 12:87–92.

Martin, R., Haroldson, S.K., and Triden, K.A. (1984). Stuttering and speech naturalness. *Journal of Speech and Hearing Disorders,* 49:53–58.

Maske-Cash, W., and Curlee, R. (1995). Effect of utterance length and meaningfulness on the speech initiation times of children who stutter and children who do not stutter. *Journal of Speech and Hearing Research,* 38:18–25.

Max, L., Guenther, F.H., Gracco, V.L., Ghosh, S.S., and Wallace, M.E. (2004). Unstable or insufficiently activated internal models and feedback-biased motor-control as sources of dysfluency: A theoretical model of stuttering. *Contemporary Issues in Communication Science and Disorders,* 31:105–122.

McCauley, R.J. (1996). Familiar strangers: Criterion-referenced measures in communication disorders. *Language, Speech, and Hearing Services in Schools,* 27:122–131.

McClean, M.D. (1990). Neuromotor aspects of stuttering: Levels of impairment and disability. In J. Cooper (Ed), *Research Needs in Stuttering: Roadblocks and Future Directions (ASHA Reports, 18).* Rockville, MD: American Speech-Language-Hearing Association, pp 64–71.

McClean, M.D., Kroll, R.M., and Loftus, N.S. (1990). Kinematic analysis of lip closure in stutterers' fluent speech. *Journal of Speech and Hearing Research,* 33:755–760.

McClean, M.D., and McClean, A. (1985). Case report of stuttering acquired in association with phenytoin use for post-head-injury seizures. *Journal of Fluency Disorders,* 10:241–255.

McDearmon, J.R. (1968). Primary stuttering at the onset of stuttering: A reexamination of data. *Journal of Speech and Hearing Research,* 11:631–637.

McDevitt, S.C., and Carey, W.B. (1978). The measurement of temperament in 3–7 year old children. *Journal of Child Psychology and Psychiatry and Allied Disciplines,* 19:245–253.

McDevitt, S.C., and Carey, W.B. (1995). *Behavioral Style Questionnaire.* West Chester, PA: TemperaMetrics.

McFarlane, S.C., and Prins, D. (1978). Neural response time of stutterers and nonstutterers in selected oral motor tasks. *Journal of Speech and Hearing Research,* 21:768–778.

McLoughlin, J., and Lewis, R. (1990). *Assessing Special Students* (ed 3). Columbus, OH: Charles E. Merrill.

Meyers, S.C., and Freeman, F.J. (1985a). Interruptions as a variable in stuttering and disfluency. *Journal of Speech and Hearing Research,* 28:428–425.

Meyers, S.C., and Freeman, F.J. (1985b). Mother and child speech rate as a variable in stuttering and disfluency. *Journal of Speech and Hearing Research,* 28:436–444.

Miles, S., and Ratner, N.B. (2001). Parental language input to children at stuttering onset. *Journal of Speech Language and Hearing Research,* 44:1116–1130.

Milisen, R. (1938). Frequency of stuttering with anticipation of stuttering controlled. *Journal of Speech Disorders,* 3:207–214.

Miller, S. (1993). *Multiple measures of anxiety and psychophysiologic arousal in stutterers and nonstutterers during non-speech and speech tasks of increasing complexity.* Unpublished doctoral dissertation, University of Texas at Dallas, Dallas, TX.

Mineka, S. (1985). Animal models of anxiety-based disorders: Their usefulness and limitations. In A.H. Tuma, and J. Mase (Eds), *Anxiety and the Anxiety Disorders.* Hillsdale, NJ: Lawrence Erlbaum Associates.

Minifie, F.D., and Cooker, H.S. (1964). A disfluency index. *Journal of Speech and Hearing Disorders,* 29:189–192.

Molt, L.F. (1997). *Event-related cortical potentials and language processing in stutterers.* Paper presented at the 2nd World Congress on Fluency Disorders, San Francisco, CA.

Molt, L.F., and Guilford, A.M. (1979). Auditory processing and anxiety in stutterers. *Journal of Fluency Disorders,* 4:255–267.

Moncur, J.P. (1952). Parental domination in stuttering. *Journal of Speech and Hearing Disorders,* 17:155–165.

Moore-Brown, B.J., and Montgomery, J.K. (2001). *Making a Difference for America's Children: Speech-Language Pathologists in Public Schools.* Eau Claire, WI: Thinking Publications.

Moore, W.H., Jr., and Haynes, W.O. (1980). Alpha hemispheric asymmetry and stuttering: Some support for a segmentation dysfunction hypothesis. *Journal of Speech and Hearing Research,* 23:229–247.

Morgenstern, J.J. (1956). Socio-economic factors in stuttering. *Journal of Speech and Hearing Disorders,* 21:25–33.

Murphy, B. (1999). The school-age child who stutters: Dealing effectively with guilt and shame. On *Practical Ideas for the School Clinician Series* [videotape]. Memphis: Stuttering Foundation of America.

Murray, F.P. (2001). *A Stutterer's Story* (ed 2). Memphis: Stuttering Foundation of America.

Murray, H.L., and Reed, C.G. (1977). Language abilities of preschool stuttering children. *Journal of Fluency Disorders,* 2:171–176.

Myers, F.L. (1978). Relationship between eight physiological variables and severity of stuttering. *Journal of Fluency Disorders,* 3:181–191.

Myers, F.L. (2002). *Putting cluttering on the map: Looking back/looking ahead.* Paper presented at the Annual Meeting of the American Speech Language and Hearing Association, Atlanta, GA.

Myers, F.L., and St. Louis, K. (1986). *Cluttering: A Clinical Perspective.* San Diego: Singular.

Navon, D. (1984). Resources—A theoretical stone soup. *Psychological Review,* 91:216–234.

Neilson, M.D. (1980). *Stuttering and the control of speech: A systems analysis approach.* Unpublished doctoral dissertation, University of New South Wales, Kensington, Australia.

Neilson, M.D., Howie, P.M., and Andrews, G. (1987, August). *Does foetal testosterone play a role in the aetiology of stuttering?* Paper presented at the Fifth International Australasian Winter Conference on Brain Research, Queenstown, New Zealand.

Neilson, M.D., and Neilson, P.D. (1987). Speech motor control and stuttering: A computational model of adaptive sensory-motor processing. *Speech Communication,* 6:325–333.

Neilson, M.D., and Neilson, P.D. (1988). *Sensory-motor integration capacity of stutterers and nonstutterers.* Paper presented at the Second Australian International Conference on Speech Science and Technology, Sydney, Australia.

Neilson, P.D., Neilson, M.D., and O'Dwyer, N.J. (1992). Adaptive model theory: Application to disorders of motor control. In J.J. Summers (Ed), *Approaches to the Study of Motor Control and Learning.* Amsterdam: Elsevier Science Publishers.

Neilson, P.D., Quinn, P.T., and Neilson, M.D. (1976). Auditory tracking measures of hemispheric asymmetry in normals and stutterers. *Australian Journal of Human Communication*, 4:121–126.

Nelson, L. (1985). Language formulation related to dysfluency and stuttering. In *Stuttering Therapy: Prevention and Intervention with Children*. Memphis: Stuttering Foundation of America.

Netsell, R. (1981). The acquisition of speech motor control: A perspective with direction for research. In R. Stark (Ed), *Language Behavior in Infancy and Early Childhood*. New York: Elsevier-North Holland.

Neumann, K., Euler, H.A., Wolff von Gudenberg, A., Giraud, A.-L., Lanfermann, H., Gall, V., et al. (2003). The nature and treatment of stuttering as revealed by fMRI: A within- and between-group comparison. *Journal of Fluency Disorders*, 28:381–410.

Neumann, K., Preibisch, C., Euler, H.A., Wolff von Gudenberg, A., Lanfermann, H., Gall, V., and Giraud, A.L. (2005). Cortical plasticity associated with stuttering therapy. *Journal of Fluency Disorders*, 30:23–29.

Nippold, M.A. (1990). Concomitant speech and language disorders in stuttering children: A critique of the literature. *Journal of Speech and Hearing Disorders*, 55:51–60.

Nippold, M.A., and Rudzinski, M. (1995). Parents' speech and children's stuttering: A critique of the literature. *Journal of Speech and Hearing Research*, 38:978–989.

Nittrouer, S., Studdert-Kennedy, M., and McGowan, R.S. (1989). The emergence of phonetic segments: Evidence from the spectral structure of fricative-vowel syllables spoken by children and adults. *Journal of Speech and Hearing Research*, 32:120–132.

Nudelman, H.B., Herbrich, K.E., Hess, K.R., Hoyt, B.D., and Rosenfield, D.B. (1992). A model of the phonation response time of stutterers and fluent speakers to frequency-modulated tones. *Journal of the Acoustical Society of America*, 92(4, Part 1):1882–1888.

Nudelman, H.B., Herbrich, K.E., Hoyt, B.D., and Rosenfield, D.B. (1987). Dynamic characteristics of vocal frequency tracking in stutterers and nonstutterers. In H.F.M. Peters, and W. Hulstijn (Eds), *Speech Motor Dynamics in Stuttering*. Wien: Springer-Verlag.

Nudelman, H.B., Herbrich, K.E., Hoyt, B.D., and Rosenfield, D.B. (1989). A neuro-science model of stuttering. *Journal of Fluency Disorders*, 14:399–427.

Numminen, J., Salmelin, R., and Hari, R. (1999). Subject's own speech reduces reactivity of the human auditory cortex. *Neuroscience Letters*, 265:119–122.

Nurnberg, H. G., and Greenwald, B. (1981). Stuttering: An unusual side effect of phenothiasines. *American Journal of Psychiatry, 138*, 386–387.

O'Brian, S., Onslow, M., Cream, A., and Packman, A. (2003). The Camperdown Program: Outcomes of a new prolonged-speech treatment model. *Journal of Speech Language and Hearing Research*, 46:933–946.

O'Brian, S., Packman, A., and Onslow, M. (2004). Self-rating of stuttering severity as a clinical tool. *American Journal of Speech-Language Pathology*, 13:219–226.

Okasha, A., Bishry, Z., Kamel, M., and Hassan, A.H. (1974). Psychosocial study of stammering in Egyptian children. *British Journal of Psychiatry*, 124:531–533.

Onslow, M., Andrews, C., and Costa, L. (1990). Parental severity scaling of early stuttered speech: Four case studies. *Australian Journal of Human Communication*, 18:47–61.

Onslow, M., Andrews, C., and Lincoln, M. (1994). A control/experimental trial of an operant treatment for early stuttering. *Journal of Speech and Hearing Research*, 37:1244–1259.

Onslow, M., Costa, L., and Rue, S. (1990). Direct early intervention with stuttering: Some preliminary data. *Journal of Speech and Hearing Disorders*, 55:405–416.

Onslow, M., Harrison, E., Jones, M., and Packman, A. (2002). Beyond-clinic speech measures during the Lidcombe Program of early stuttering intervention. *Acquiring Knowledge in Speech, Language, and Hearing*, 4:82–85.

Onslow, M., Packman, A., and Harrison, E. (2003). *The Lidcombe Program of Early Stuttering Intervention: A Clinician's Guide*. Austin, TX: Pro-Ed.

Oyler, M.E. (1992, November). *Self perception and sensitivity in stuttering adults*. Paper presented at the Annual Meeting of the American Speech-Language-Hearing Association, San Antonio, TX.

Oyler, M.E., and Ramig, P.R. (1995, December). *Vulnerability in stuttering children*. Paper presented at the Annual Meeting of the American Speech-Language-Hearing Association, Orlando, FL.

Paden, E.P. (2005). Development of phonological ability: For clinicians by clinicians. In E. Yairi, and N.G. Ambrose (Eds), *Early Childhood Stuttering*. Austin, TX: Pro-Ed, pp 197–234.

Paden, E.P., Yairi, E., and Ambrose, N.G. (1999). Early childhood stuttering II: Initial status of phonological abilities. *Journal of Speech, Language and Hearing Research*, 42:1113–1124.

Paul, R. (1995). *Language Disorders From Infancy Through Adolescence: Assessment and Intervention.* St. Louis: Mosby-Year Book.

Paulesu, E., Frith, C.D., and Frackowiak, R.S.J. (1993). The neural correlates of the verbal component of working memory. *Nature,* 362:342–345.

Paulesu, E., Frith, U., Snowling, M., Gallagher, A., Morton, J., Frackowiak, R.S.J., et al. (1996). Is developmental dyslexia a disconnection syndrome? Evidence from PET scanning. *Brain,* 119:143–157.

Pearl, S.Z., and Bernthal, J.E. (1980). The effect of grammatical complexity upon disfluency behavior of non-stuttering preschool children. *Journal of Fluency Disorders,* 5:55–68.

Peters, H.F.M., and Hulstijn, W. (1984). Stuttering and anxiety: The difference between stutterers and non-stutterers in verbal apprehension and physiologic arousal during the anticipation of speech and non-speech tasks. *Journal of Fluency Disorders,* 9:67–84.

Peters, T.J. (1968). Oral language skills of children who stutter. (Abstract). *Speech Monographs,* 35:325.

Peters, T.J., and Guitar, B. (1991). *Stuttering: An Integrated Approach to Its Nature and Treatment.* Baltimore: Williams & Wilkins.

Piertranton, A. (2003, June). *Evidence based practice.* Paper presented at the Special Interest Division 4 Leadership Conference (ASHA), St. Louis, MO.

Pindzola, R., Jenkins, M., and Lokken, K. (1989). Speaking rates of young children. *Language, Speech, and Hearing Services in Schools,* 20:133–138.

Pinsky, S., and McAdams, D. (1980). Electroencephalographic and dichotic indices of cerebral intensity of stutterers. *Brain and Language,* 11:374–397.

Platt, J., and Basili, A. (1973). Jaw tremor during stuttering block: An electromyographic study. *Journal of Communication Disorders,* 6:102–109.

Ponsford, R.E., Brown, W.S., Marsh, J.T., and Travis, L.E. (1975). Proceedings: Evoked potential correlates of cerebral dominance for speech perception in stutterers and non-stutterers. *Electroencephalography and Clinical Neurophysiology,* 39:434.

Pool, K.D., Devous, M.D., Freeman, F.J., Watson, B.C., and Finitzo, T. (1991). Regional cerebral blood flow in developmental stutterers. *Archives of Neurology,* 48:509–512.

Preus, A. (1981). *Identifying Subgroups of Stutterers.* Oslo: Universitetsforlaget.

Prins, D. (1991). Theories of stuttering as event and disorder: Implications for speech production processes. In H.F.M. Peters, W. Hulstijn, and C.W. Starkweather (Eds), *Speech Motor Control and Stuttering.* Amsterdam: Elsevier Science Publishers.

Prins, D. (1999). Describing the consequences of disorders: Comment on Yaruss (1998). *Journal of Speech, Language and Hearing Research,* 42:1395–1397.

Proceedings of the NIDCD Workshop on Treatment Efficacy Research in Stuttering. (1993). *Journal of Fluency Disorders,* 18:121–361.

Quader, S.E. (1977). Dysarthria: An unusual side effect of trycyclic antidepressants. *British Medical Journal,* 9:97.

Quinn, P. (1972). Stuttering, cerebral dominance, and the dichotic word test. *Medical Journal of Australia,* 2:639–642.

Rahman, P. (1956). *The self-concept and ideal self-concept of stutterers as compared to nonstutterers.* Unpublished masters thesis, Brooklyn College, Brooklyn, NY.

Ramig, P.R. (1993). The impact of self-help groups on persons who stutter: A call for research. *Journal of Fluency Disorders,* 18:351–361.

Ramig, P.R., and Dodge, D.M. (2005). *Child and Adolescent Stuttering Treatment and Activity Resource Guide.* Clifton Park, NJ: Thomson Delmar Learning.

Rentschler, G.I., Driver, L.E., and Callaway, E.A. (1984). The onset of stuttering following drug overdose. *Journal of Fluency Disorders,* 9:265–284.

Reville, J. (1988). *The Many Voices of Paws.* Princeton Junction, NJ: The Speech Bin.

Riley, G. (1972). A stuttering severity instrument for children and adults. *Journal of Speech and Hearing Disorders,* 37:314–322.

Riley, G. (1994). *Stuttering Severity Instrument for Children and Adults* (ed 3). Austin, TX: Pro-Ed.

Riley, G.D., and Riley, J. (1984). A component model for treating stuttering in children. In M. Peins (Ed), *Contemporary Approaches in Stuttering Therapy.* Boston: Little, Brown.

Ringo, C.C., and Dietrich, S. (1995). Neurogenic stuttering: An analysis and critique. *Journal of Medical Speech-Language Pathology,* 3:111–122.

Ripley, A. (2005, May 2). How to get out alive: From hurricanes to 9/11: What the science of evacuation reveals about how humans behave in the worst of times. *Time,* 165:58–62.

Roessler, R., and Bolton, B. (1978). *Psychosocial Adjustment to Disability*. Baltimore: University Park Press.

Rogers, C.R. (1957). The necessary and sufficient conditions of therapeutic personality change. *Journal of Consulting Psychology,* 21:95–103.

Rogers, C.R. (1961). *On Becoming a Person*. Boston: Houghton Mifflin.

Rommel, D., Hage, P., Kalehne, P., and Johannsen, H. (2000). Development, maintenance, and recovery of childhood stuttering: Prospective longitudinal data 3 years after first contact. In K.L. Baker, L. Rustin, and F. Cook (Eds), *Proceedings of the Fifth Oxford Disfluency Conference, 7th–10th July, 1999*. Berkshire, UK: Kevin L. Baker, pp 168–182.

Rosenbek, J.C. (1984). Stuttering secondary to nervous system damage. In R.F. Curlee, and W.H. Perkins (Eds), *Nature and Treatment of Stuttering: New Directions*. San Diego: College-Hill Press, pp 31–48.

Rosenfield, D., and Goodglass, H. (1980). Dichotic testing of cerebral dominance in stutterers. *Brain and Language,* 11:170–180.

Roth, C., Aronson, A., and Davis, L. (1989). Clinical studies in psychogenic stuttering of adult onset. *Journal of Speech and Hearing Disorders,* 54:634–646.

Rubow, R.T., Rosenbek, J.C., and Schumaker, J.G. (1986). Stress management in the treatment of neurogenic stuttering. *Biofeedback and Self Regulation,* 11:77–78.

Rustin, L. (1991). *Parents, Families, and the Stuttering Child*. London: Whurr.

Ryan, B.P. (1984). Treatment of stuttering in school children. In W.H. Perkins (Ed), *Stuttering Disorders*. New York: Thieme -Stratton.

Ryan, B.P. (1992). Articulation, language, rate, and fluency characteristics of stuttering and nonstuttering preschool children. *Journal of Speech and Hearing Research,* 35:333–342.

Ryan, B.P. (2000). *Programmed Therapy for Stuttering in Children and Adults* (ed 2). Springfield, IL: C. C. Thomas.

Ryan, B.P., and Ryan, B.V. (1995). Programmed stuttering treatment for children: Comparison of two establishment programs through transfer, maintenance, and follow-up. *Journal of Speech and Hearing Research,* 38:61–75.

Sackett, D., Straus, S., Richardson, W., Rosenberg, W., and Haynes, R. (2000). *Evidence-Based Medicine: How to Practice and Teach EBM*. New York: Churchill Livingstone.

Salmelin, R., Schnitzler, A., Schmitz, F., and Freund, H.-J. (2000). Single word reading in developmental stutterers and fluent speakers. *Brain,* 123:1184–1202.

Salmelin, R., Schnitzler, A., Schmitz, F., Jancke, L., Witte, O.W., and Freund, H.-J. (1998). Functional organization of the auditory cortex is different in stutterers and fluent speakers. *NeuroReport,* 9:2225–2229.

Schiavetti, N., and Metz, D.E. (1997). Stuttering and the measurement of speech naturalness. In R.F. Curlee, and G.M. Siegel (Ed.), *Nature and Treatment of Stuttering: New Directions* (ed 2). Boston: Allyn & Bacon, pp 398–412.

Schwartz, M.F. (1974). The core of the stuttering block. *Journal of Speech and Hearing Disorders,* 39:169–177.

Sedaris, D. (2000). *Me Talk Pretty One Day*. Boston: Little, Brown & Co.

Seeman, M. (1937). The significance of twin pathology for the investigation of speech disorders. *Archive gesamte Phonetik 1, Part II,* 88–92.

Seider, R.A., Gladstien, K.L., and Kidd, K.K. (1982). Language-onset and concomitant speech and language problems in subgroups of stutterers and their siblings. *Journal of Speech and Hearing Research,* 25:482–486.

Semel, E., Wiig, E., and Secord, W.A. (1996). *Clinical Evaluation of Language Fundamentals–3*. San Antonio: Psychological Corporation.

Shapiro, A.I. (1980). An electromyographic analysis of the fluent and dysfluent utterances of several types of stutterers. *Journal of Fluency Disorders,* 5:203–231.

Shapiro, A.I., and DeCicco, B.A. (1982). The relationship between normal dysfluency and stuttering: An old question revisited. *Journal of Fluency Disorders,* 7:109–121.

Shapiro, D.A. (1999). *Stuttering Intervention: A Collaborative Journey to Fluency Freedom*. Austin, TX: Pro-Ed.

Shaywitz, B.A., Shaywitz, S.E., Pugh, K.R., Constable, R.T., Skudlarski, P., Fulbright, R.K., et al. (1995). Sex differences in the functional organization of the brain for language. *Nature,* 373:607–609.

Sheehan, J.G. (1970). *Stuttering: Research and Therapy*. New York: Harper & Row.

Sheehan, J.G. (1974). Stuttering behavior: A phonetic analysis. *Journal of Communication Disorders,* 7:193–212.

Sheehan, J.G. (1975). Conflict theory and avoidance-reduction therapy. In J. Eisenson (Ed), *Stuttering: A Second Symposium*. New York: Harper & Row.

Sherman, D. (1952). Clinical and experimental use of the Iowa scale of severity of stuttering. *Journal of Speech and Hearing Disorders,* 17:316–320.

Shields, D. (1989). *Dead Languages.* New York: Knopf.

Shugart, Y.Y., Mundorff, J., Kilshaw, J., Doheny, K., Doan, B., Wanyee, J., et al. (2004). Results of a genome-wide linkage scan for stuttering. *American Journal of Medical Genetics,* 124A:133–135.

Silverman, E.-M. (1974). Word position and grammatical function in relation to preschoolers' speech disfluency. *Perceptual and Motor Skills,* 39:267–272.

Silverman, F.H. (1988). The "monster" study. *Journal of Fluency Disorders,* 13:225–231.

Skinner, E., and McKeehan, A. (1996). *Preventing stuttering in the preschool child: A video program for parents* [Videotape]. San Antonio, TX: Communication Skill Builders.

Slorach, N., and Noer, B. (1973). Dichotic listening in stuttering and dyslexic children. *Cortex,* 9:295–300.

Smith, A. (1989). Neural drive to muscles in stuttering. *Journal of Speech and Hearing Research,* 32:252–264.

Smith, A., and Luschei, E.S. (1983). Assessment of oral-motor reflexes in stutterers and normal speakers: Preliminary observations. *Journal of Speech and Hearing Research,* 26:322–328.

Smith, A., McCauley, R.J., and Guitar, B. (2000). Development of the Teacher Assessment of Student Communicative Competence (TASCC) in grades 1 through 5. *Communication Disorders Quarterly,* 22:3–11.

Snidman, N., and Kagan, J. (1994). The contribution of infant temperamental differences to the acoustic startle response. (Supplement, Abstract). *Psychophysiology,* 31:S92.

Sommer, M., Koch, M.A., Paulus, W., Weiller, C., and Buchel, C. (2002). Disconnection of speech-relevant brain areas in persistent developmental stuttering. *Lancet,* 360:380–383.

Sommers, R., Brady, W.A., and Moore, W.H., Jr. (1975). Dichotic ear preferences of stuttering children and adults. *Perceptual and Motor Skills,* 41:931–938.

St. Louis, K. (1991). The stuttering/articulation disorders connection. In H.F.M. Peters, W. Hulstijn, and C.W. Starkweather (Eds), *Speech Motor Control and Stuttering.* Amsterdam: Excerpta Medica.

St. Louis, K. (1996). Research and opinion on cluttering. [Special issue]. *Journal of Fluency Disorders,* 21.

St. Louis, K. (2001). *Living with Stuttering: Stories, Basics, Resources, and Hope.* Morgantown, WV: Populore Publishing Company.

St. Louis, K., Raphael, L.J., Myers, F.L., and Bakker, K. (2003). Cluttering updated. *ASHA Leader,* 4–5:20–22.

St. Louis, K.O., and Myers, F.L. (1997). Management of cluttering and related fluency disorders. In R.F. Curlee, and G.M. Siegel (Eds), *The Nature and Treatment of Stuttering: New Directions* (ed 2). Boston: Allyn & Bacon, pp 313–332.

St. Onge, K. (1963). The stuttering syndrome. *Journal of Speech and Hearing Research,* 6:195–197.

Stager, S., Jeffries, K.J., and Braun, A.R. (2003). Common features of fluency-evoking conditions studied in stuttering subjects and controls: An H2–15–0 PET study. *Journal of Fluency Disorders,* 28:319–336.

Starkweather, C.W. (1972). *Stuttering: An Account of Intensive Demonstration Therapy.* Memphis: Speech Foundation of America.

Starkweather, C.W. (1980). A multiprocess behavioral approach to stuttering therapy. *Seminars in Speech, Language and Hearing,* 1:327–337.

Starkweather, C.W. (1983). *Speech and Language: Principles and Processes of Behavior Change.* Englewood Cliffs, NJ: Prentice-Hall.

Starkweather, C.W. (1985). The development of fluency in normal children. In *Stuttering Therapy: Prevention and Intervention with Children.* Memphis: Speech Foundation of America.

Starkweather, C.W. (1987). *Fluency and Stuttering.* Englewood Cliffs, NJ: Prentice-Hall.

Starkweather, C.W. (1991). Stuttering: The motor-language interface. In H.F.M. Peters, W. Hulstijn, and C.W. Starkweather (Eds), *Speech Motor Control and Fluency.* Amsterdam: Excerpta Medica.

Starkweather, C.W., and Gottwald, S. (1990). The demands and capacities model II: Clinical application. *Journal of Fluency Disorders,* 15:143–157.

Starkweather, C.W., Gottwald, S.R., and Halfond, M.H. (1990). *Stuttering Prevention: A Clinical Method.* Englewood Cliffs, NJ: Prentice-Hall.

Starkweather, C.W., Hirschman, P., and Tannenbaum, R.S. (1976). Latency of vocalization onset: Stutterers versus nonstutterers. *Journal of Speech and Hearing Research,* 19:481–492.

Starkweather, C.W., and Myers, M. (1979). Duration of subsegments within the intervocalic interval in stutterers and nonstutterers. *Journal of Fluency Disorders,* 4:205–214.

Stephanson-Opsal, D., and Bernstein Ratner, N. (1988). Maternal speech rate modification and childhood stuttering. *Journal of Fluency Disorders,* 13:49–56.

Sternberger, J.P. (1982). The nature of segments in the lexicon: Evidence from speech errors. *Lingua,* 56: 235–259.

Stocker, B., and Goldfarb, R. (1995). *The Stocker Probe for Fluency and Language.* Vero Beach, FL: The Speech Bin.

Stocker, B., and Usprich, C. (1976). Stuttering in young children and level of demand. *Journal of Childhood Communication Disorders,* 1:116–131.

Stromsta, C. (1957). A methodology related to the determination of the phase angle of bone-conducted speech sound energy in stutterers and nonstutterers. (Abstract). *Speech Monographs* 24:147–148.

Stromsta, C. (1972). Interaural phase disparity of stutterers and nonstutterers. *Journal of Speech and Hearing Research,* 15:771–780.

Stromsta, C. (1986). *Elements of Stuttering.* Oshtemo, MI: Atsmorts Publishing.

Strong, J.C. (1977). *Dichotic speech perception: A comparison between stutterers and nonstutterers ages five to nine.* Unpublished doctoral dissertation, Pennsylvania State University, University Park, PA.

Studdert-Kennedy, M. (1987). The phoneme as a perceptuomotor structure. In A. Allport, D. McKay, D. Prinz, and E. Scheerer (Eds), *Language Perception and Production.* London: Academic Press.

Sussman, H., and MacNeilage, P. (1975). Hemispheric specialization for speech production and perception in stutterers. *Neuropsychologia,* 13:19–26.

Taylor, O. (1986). *Treatment of Communication Disorders in Culturally and Linguistically Diverse Populations.* San Diego: College-Hill Press.

Taylor, O. (1994). *Communication and Communication Disorders in a Multicultural Society.* San Diego: Singular Publishing Group.

Taylor, R.M., and Morrison, L.P. (1996). *Taylor-Johnson Temperament Analysis Manual.* Thousand Oaks, CA: Psychological Publications, Inc.

Thomas, A., and Chess, S. (1977). *Temperament and Development.* New York: Brunner/Mazel, Inc.

Throneburg, R., and Yairi, E. (1994). Temporal dynamics of repetitions during the early stage of childhood stuttering: An acoustic study. *Journal of Speech and Hearing Research,* 37:1067–1075.

Till, J.A., Reich, A., Dickey, S., and Sieber, J. (1983). Phonatory and manual reaction times of stuttering and nonstuttering children. *Journal of Speech and Hearing Research,* 26:171–180.

Toscher, M.M., and Rupp, R.R. (1978). A study of the central auditory processes in stutterers using the Synthetic Sentence Identification (SSI) test battery. *Journal of Speech and Hearing Research,* 21:779–792.

Trautman, L.S. (2003). SFA conducts survey on satisfaction with electronic devices. *Stuttering Foundation Newsletter,* (Fall) 6.

Trautman, L.S., and Guitar, C. (2002). *Stuttering: Straight talk for teachers* [Videotape]. Memphis: Stuttering Foundation.

Trautman, L.S., and Guitar, C. (2004). *Stuttering: For kids, by kids* [Videotape]. Memphis: Stuttering Foundation.

Travis, L. (1931). *Speech Pathology.* New York: Appleton-Century.

Travis, L.E., and Knott, J.R. (1937). Bilaterally recorded brain potentials from normal speakers and stutterers. *Journal of Speech Disorders,* 2:239–241.

Tudor, M. (1939). *An experimental study of the effect of evaluative labeling on speech fluency.* Unpublished master's thesis, University of Iowa, Iowa City, IA.

Turnbaugh, K.R., and Guitar, B.E. (1981). Short-term intensive stuttering treatment in a public school setting. *Language, Speech, and Hearing Services in Schools,* 12:107–114.

Turnbaugh, K.R., Guitar, B.E., and Hoffman, P.R. (1979). Speech clinicians' attribution of personality traits as a function of stuttering severity. *Journal of Speech and Hearing Research,* 22:37–45.

Van Borsel, J., Maes, E., and Foulon, S. (2001). Stuttering and bilingualism: A review. *Journal of Fluency Disorders,* 26:179–205.

Van Riper, C. (1936). Study of the thoracic breathing of stutterers during expectancy and occurrence of stuttering spasm. *Journal of Speech Disorders,* 1:61–72.

Van Riper, C. (1954). *Speech Correction: Principles and Methods* (ed 3). Englewood Cliffs, NJ: Prentice-Hall.

Van Riper, C. (1958). Experiments in stuttering therapy. In J. Eisenson (Ed), *Stuttering: A Symposium.* New York: Harper & Row, pp 273–290.

Van Riper, C. (1971). *The Nature of Stuttering.* Englewood Cliffs, NJ: Prentice-Hall.

Van Riper, C. (1973). *The Treatment of Stuttering.* Englewood Cliffs, NJ: Prentice-Hall.

Van Riper, C. (1975a). The stutterer's clinician. In J. Eisenson (Ed), *Stuttering: A Second Symposium.* New York: Harper & Row.

Van Riper, C. (1975b). Therapy in action. On *3 videotapes.* Memphis: Stuttering Foundation of America.

Van Riper, C. (1982). *The Nature of Stuttering* (ed 2). Englewood Cliffs, NJ: Prentice Hall.

Van Riper, C. (1990). Final thoughts about stuttering. *Journal of Fluency Disorders,* 15:317–318.

Van Riper, C., and Hull, C.J. (1955). The quantative measurement of the effect of certain situations on stuttering. In W. Johnson, and R.R. Leutenegger (Eds), *Stuttering in Children and Adults.* Minneapolis: University of Minnesota Press.

Vanryckeghem, M., and Brutten, G. (1993). The Communication Attitude Test: A test-retest reliability investigation. *Journal of Fluency Disorders,* 17:177–190.

Vanryckeghem, M., and Brutten, G. (2002). *KittyCAT: A measure of stuttering and nonstuttering preschoolers' attitudes.* Paper presented at the Annual Meeting of the American Speech-Language-Hearing Association, Atlanta, GA.

Vrana, S.R., Spence, E.L., and Lang, P.J. (1988). The startle probe: A new measure of emotion? *Journal of Abnormal Psychology,* 97:487–491.

Wakaba, Y. (1998). *Research on temperament of stuttering children with early onset.* Paper presented at the 2nd World Conference on Fluency Disorders, San Francisco, CA.

Wall, M.J. (1980). A comparison of syntax in young stutterers and nonstutterers. *Journal of Fluency Disorders,* 5:345–352.

Wall, M.J., and Myers, F.L. (1984). *Clinical Management of Childhood Stuttering.* Baltimore: University Park Press.

Wall, M.J., and Myers, F.L. (1995). *Clinical Management of Childhood Stuttering* (ed 2). Austin, TX: Pro-Ed.

Wallen, V. (1960). A Q-technique study of the self-concepts of adolescent stutterers and nonstutterers. (Abstract). *Speech Monographs* 27:257–258.

Watkins, R.V. (2005). Language abilities of young children who stutter. In E. Yairi, and N.G. Ambrose (Eds), *Early Childhood Stuttering: For clinicians by Clinicians.* Austin, TX: Pro-Ed, pp 235–251.

Watkins, R.V., Yairi, E., and Ambrose, N.G. (1999). Early childhood stuttering III: Initial status of expressive language abilities. *Journal of Speech, Language and Hearing Research,* 42:1125–1135.

Watson, B.C., and Alfonso, P.J. (1987). Physiological bases of acoustic LRT in nonstutterers, mild stutterers, and severe stutterers. *Journal of Speech and Hearing Research,* 30:434–447.

Watson, J.B., and Kayser, H. (1994). Assessment of bilingual/bicultural children and adults who stutter. *Seminars in Speech, Language and Hearing,* 15:149–163.

Weber, C.M., and Smith, A. (1990). Autonomic correlates of stuttering and speech assessed in a range of experimental tasks. *Journal of Speech and Hearing Research,* 33:690–706.

Webster, R.L. (1974). A behavioral analysis of stuttering: Treatment and theory. In K.S. Calhoun, H.E. Adams, and K.M. Mitchell (Eds), *Innovative Treatment Methods in Psychopathology.* New York: John Wiley & Sons.

Webster, W.G. (1993a). Evidence in bimanual finger tapping of an attentional component to stuttering. *Behavioural Brain Research,* 37:93–100.

Webster, W.G. (1993b). Hurried hands and tangled tongues: Implications of current research for the management of stuttering. In E. Boberg (Ed), *Neuropsychology of Stuttering.* Edmonton, Alberta, Canada: University of Alberta Press, pp 73–111.

Webster, W.G. (1997). Principles of human brain organization related to lateralization of language and speech motor functions in normal speakers and stutterers. In W. Hulstijn, H.F.M. Peters, and P.H.H.M. van Lieshout (Eds), *Speech Production: Motor Control, Brain Research and Fluency Disorders.* Amsterdam: Elsevier, pp 119–139.

Weiller, C., Isensee, C., Rijntjes, M., Huber, W., Muller, S., Bier, D., et al. (1995). Recovery from Wernicke's aphasia: A positron emission tomographic study. *Annals of Neurology,* 37:723–732.

Weiner, A.E. (1981). A case of adult onset of stuttering. *Journal of Fluency Disorders,* 6:181–186.

Weiss, A.L., and Zebrowski, P. (1992). Disfluencies in the conversations of young children who stutter: Some answers about questions. *Journal of Speech and Hearing Research,* 35:1230–1238.

Weiss, C., Gordon, M., and Lillywhite, H. (1987). *Clinical Management of Articulatory and Phonologic Disorders* (ed 2). Baltimore: Williams & Wilkins.

Weiss, D.A. (1964). *Cluttering.* Englewood Cliffs, NJ: Prentice-Hall.

Welch, J., and Byrne, J.A. (2001). *Jack: Straight from the Gut.* New York: Warner Books.

West, R. (1931). The phenomenology of stuttering. In R. West (Ed), *A Symposium on Stuttering.* Madison, WI: College Typing Company.

Westby, C.E. (1979). Language performance of stuttering and nonstuttering children. *Journal of Communication Disorders,* 12:133–145.

Wexler, K.B., and Mysack, E.D. (1982). Disfluency characteristics of 2-, 4- and 6-year old males. *Journal of Fluency Disorders,* 7:37–46.

Wiig, E. (2002). *Putting cluttering on the map: Looking back/looking ahead.* Paper presented at the Annual Meeting of the American Speech Language and Hearing Association, Atlanta, GA.

Wijnen, F. (1990). The development of sentence planning. *Journal of Child Language,* 17:651–675.

Wilkenfeld, J.R., and Curlee, R.F. (1997). The relative effects of questions and comments on children's stuttering. *American Journal of Speech-Language Pathology,* 6:79–89.

Williams, D., Darley, F., and Spriestersbach, D. (1978). Appraisal of rate and fluency. In F. Darley, and D. Spriestersbach (Eds), *Diagnostic Methods in Speech Pathology* (ed 2). New York: Harper & Row, pp 256–283.

Williams, D.E. (1978). The problem of stuttering. In F. Darley, and D. Spriestersbach (Eds), *Diagnostic Methods in Speech Pathology.* New York: Harper & Row, pp 284–321.

Williams, D.E., Melrose, B.M., and Woods, C.L. (1969). The relationship between stuttering and academic achievement in children. *Journal of Communication Disorders,* 2:87–98.

Williams, D.E., Silverman, F.H., and Kools, J.A. (1968). Disfluency behavior of elementary-school stutterers and nonstutterers: The adaptation effect. *Journal of Speech and Hearing Research,* 11:622–630.

Wingate, M.E. (1964). Recovery from stuttering. *Journal of Speech and Hearing Disorders,* 29:312–321.

Wingate, M.E. (1983). Speaking unassisted: Comments on a paper by Andrews et al. *Journal of Speech and Hearing Disorders,* 48:255–263.

Wingate, M.E. (1988). *The Structure of Stuttering: A Psycholinguistic Approach.* New York: Springer-Verlag.

Winnicott, D.W. (1971). *Playing and Reality.* New York: Routledge.

Wood, F., Stump, D., McKeehan, A., Sheldon, S., and Proctor, J. (1980). Patterns of regional cerebral blood flow during attempted reading aloud by stutterers both on and off haloperidol medication: Evidence for inadequate left frontal activation during stuttering. *Brain and Language,* 9:141–144.

Woods, C.L., and Williams, D.E. (1976). Traits attributed to stuttering and normally fluent males. *Journal of Speech and Hearing Research,* 19:267–278.

Woolf, G. (1967). The assessment of stuttering as struggle, avoidance, and expectancy. *British Journal of Disorders of Communication,* 2:158–171.

Wu, J., Maguire, G., Riley, G., Fallon, J., LaCasse, L., Chin, S., et al. (1995). A positron emission tomography [18F]deoxyglucose study of developmental stuttering. *NeuroReport,* 6:501–505.

Wynne, M.K., and Boehmler, R.M. (1982). Central auditory function in fluent and disfluent normal speakers. *Journal of Speech and Hearing Research,* 25:54–57.

Yairi, E. (1981). Disfluencies of normally speaking two-year old children. *Journal of Speech and Hearing Research,* 24:490–495.

Yairi, E. (1982). Longitudinal studies of disfluencies in two-year old children. *Journal of Speech and Hearing Research,* 25:155–160.

Yairi, E. (1983). The onset of stuttering in two- and three-year old children: A preliminary report. *Journal of Speech and Hearing Disorders,* 48:171–178.

Yairi, E. (1997a). Early stuttering. In R.F. Curlee, and G.M. Siegel (Eds), *Nature and Treatment of Stuttering: New Directions* (ed 2). Boston: Allyn & Bacon.

Yairi, E. (1997b). Home environment and parent-child interaction in childhood stuttering. In R.F. Curlee, and G.M. Siegel (Eds), *Nature and Treatment of Stuttering: New Directions* (ed 2). Boston: Allyn & Bacon, pp 24–48.

Yairi, E., and Ambrose, N.G. (1992a). A longitudinal study of stuttering in children: A preliminary report. *Journal of Speech and Hearing Research,* 35:755–760.

Yairi, E., and Ambrose, N.G. (1992b). Onset of stuttering in preschool children: Selected factors. *Journal of Speech and Hearing Research,* 35:782–788.

Yairi, E., and Ambrose, N.G. (1996). *Disfluent speech in early childhood stuttering.* Unpublished manuscript, University of Illinois, IL.

Yairi, E., and Ambrose, N.G. (1999). Early childhood stuttering I: Persistency and recovery rates. *Journal of Speech, Language and Hearing Research,* 42:1097–1112.

Yairi, E., and Ambrose, N.G. (2005). *Early Childhood Stuttering: For Clinicians by Clinicians.* Austin, TX: Pro-Ed.

Yairi, E., Ambrose, N.G., and Cox, N.J. (1996). Genetics of stuttering: A critical review. *Journal of Speech and Hearing Research,* 39:771–784.

Yairi, E., Ambrose, N.G., Paden, E., and Throneburg, R. (1996). Predictive factors of persistence and recovery: Pathways of childhood stuttering. *Journal of Communication Disorders,* 29:51–77.

Yairi, E., and Lewis, B. (1984). Disfluencies at the onset of stuttering. *Journal of Speech and Hearing Research,* 27:154–159.

Yaruss, J.S. (1998). Describing the consequences of disorders: Stuttering and the international classification of impairments, disabilities, and handicaps. *Journal of Speech, Language, and Hearing Research,* 41:249–257.

Yaruss, J.S. (1999). Utterance length, syntactic complexity, and childhood stuttering. *Journal of Speech, Language and Hearing Research,* 42:329–344.

Yaruss, J.S., and Conture, E.G. (1995). Mother and child speaking rates and utterance lengths in adjacent fluent utterances: Preliminary observations. *Journal of Fluency Disorders*, 20:257–278.

Yaruss, J.S., Murphy, B., Quesal, R.W., and Reardon, N.A. (2004). *Bullying and Teasing–Helping Children Who Stutter: A Manual for Speech-Language Pathologists, Teachers, Administrators, and Children Who Stutter.* New York: National Stuttering Association.

Yaruss, J.S., Newman, R.M., and Flora, T. (1999). Language and disfluency in nonstuttering children's conversational speech. *Journal of Fluency Disorders*, 24:185–207.

Young, M.A. (1961). Predicting ratings of severity of stuttering. *Journal of Speech and Hearing Disorders, Monograph Supplement*, 7:31–54.

Young, M.A. (1981). A reanalysis of "Stuttering therapy: The relation between attitude change and long-term outcome." *Journal of Speech and Hearing Disorders*, 46:221–222.

Young, M.A. (1984). Identification of stuttering and stutterers. In R.F. Curlee, and W.H. Perkins (Eds), *The Nature and Treatment of Stuttering: New Directions.* San Diego: College-Hill, pp 13–30.

Zebrowski, P. (1991). Duration of the speech disfluencies of beginning stutterers. *Journal of Speech and Hearing Research*, 34:483–491.

Zebrowski, P. (1995). Temporal aspects of the conversations between children who stutter and their parents. *Topics in Language Disorders*, 15:1–17.

Zebrowski, P., Guitar, B., and Guitar, C. (2002). Counseling: Listening to and talking with parents of children who stutter [videotape]. Memphis: Stuttering Foundation.

Zebrowski, P.M., and Kelly, E. (2002). *Manual of Stuttering Intervention.* Clifton Park, NY: Singular.

Zenner, A.A., Ritterman, S.I., Bowen, S.K., and Gronhovd, K.D. (1978). Measurement and comparison of anxiety levels of parents of stuttering, articulatory defective, and normal-speaking children. *Journal of Fluency Disorders*, 3:273–283.

Zimmerman, G.N. (1980). Articulatory dynamics of fluent utterances of stutterers and nonstutterers. *Journal of Speech and Hearing Research*, 23:95–107.

Zimmerman, G.N., and Knott, J.R. (1974). Slow potentials of the brain related to speech processing in normal speakers and stutterers. *Electroencephalography & Clinical Neurophysiology*, 37:599–607.

Zimmerman, I., Steiner, V., and Pond, R. (1979). *Preschool Language Scale.* San Antonio, TX: Psychological Corp.

Names Index

Note: Page numbers followed by f indicate figures; those followed by t indicate tables.

Subject Index

Note: Page numbers followed by f indicate figures; those followed by t indicate tables.